Lecture Notes in Computer Science   9350

Commenced Publication in 1973
Founding and Former Series Editors:
Gerhard Goos, Juris Hartmanis, and Jan van Leeuwen

More information about this series at http://www.springer.com/series/7412

Nassir Navab · Joachim Hornegger
William M. Wells · Alejandro F. Frangi (Eds.)

Medical Image Computing and Computer-Assisted Intervention – MICCAI 2015

18th International Conference
Munich, Germany, October 5–9, 2015
Proceedings, Part II

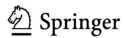 Springer

Editors

Nassir Navab
Technische Universität München
Garching
Germany

Joachim Hornegger
Friedrich-Alexander-Universität
    Erlangen-Nürnberg
Erlangen
Germany

William M. Wells
Brigham and Women's Hospital
Harvard Medical School
Boston
USA

Alejandro F. Frangi
University of Sheffield
Sheffield
UK

ISSN 0302-9743   ISSN 1611-3349   (electronic)
Lecture Notes in Computer Science
ISBN 978-3-319-24570-6   ISBN 978-3-319-24571-3   (eBook)
DOI 10.1007/978-3-319-24571-3

Library of Congress Control Number: 2015949456

LNCS Sublibrary: SL6 – Image Processing, Computer Vision, Pattern Recognition, and Graphics

Springer Cham Heidelberg New York Dordrecht London

Printed on acid-free paper

Springer International Publishing AG Switzerland is part of Springer Science+Business Media
(www.springer.com)

Preface

In 2015, the 18th International Conference on Medical Image Computing and Computer-Assisted Intervention (MICCAI 2015) was held in Munich, Germany. It was organized by the Technical University Munich (TUM) and the Friedrich Alexander University Erlangen-Nuremberg (FAU). The meeting took place in the Philharmonic Hall "Gasteig" during October 6-8, one week after the world-famous Oktoberfest. Satellite events associated with MICCAI 2015 took place on October 5 and October 9 in the Holiday Inn Hotel Munich City Centre and Klinikum rechts der Isar. MICCAI 2015 and its satellite events attracted word-leading scientists, engineers, and clinicians, who presented high-standard papers, aiming at uniting the fields of medical image processing, medical image formation, and medical robotics.

This year the triple anonymous review process was organized in several phases. In total, 810 valid submissions were received. The review process was handled by one primary and two secondary Program Committee members for each paper. It was initiated by the primary Program Committee member, who assigned a minimum of three expert reviewers. Based on these initial reviews, 79 papers were directly accepted and 248 papers were rejected. The remaining papers went to the rebuttal phase, in which the authors had the chance to respond to the concerns raised by reviewers. The reviews and associated rebuttals were subsequently discussed in the next phase among the reviewers leading to the acceptance of another 85 papers and the rejection of 118 papers. Subsequently, secondary Program Committee members issued a recommendation for each paper by weighing both the reviewers' recommendations and the authors' rebuttals. This resulted in "accept" for 67 papers and in "reject" for 120 papers. The remaining 92 papers were discussed at a Program Committee meeting in Garching, Germany, in May 2015, where 36 out of 75 Program Committee members were present. During two days, the 92 papers were examined by experts in the respective fields resulting in another 32 papers being accepted. In total 263 papers of the 810 submitted papers were accepted which corresponds to an acceptance rate of 32.5%.

The frequency of primary and secondary keywords is almost identical in the submitted, the rejected, and the accepted paper pools. The top five keywords of all submissions were machine learning (8.3%), segmentation (7.1%), MRI (6.6%), and CAD (4.9%).

The correlation between the initial keyword counts by category and the accepted papers was 0.98. The correlation with the keyword distribution of the rejected papers was 0.99. The distributions of the intermediate accept and reject phases was also above 0.9 in all cases, i.e., there was a strong relationship between the submitted paper categories and the finally accepted categories. The keyword frequency was essentially not influenced by the review decisions. As a conclusion, we believe the review process was fair and the distribution of topics reflects no favor of any particular topic of the conference.

This year we offered all authors the opportunity of presenting their work in a five-minute talk. These talks were organized in 11 parallel sessions setting the stage for further scientific discussions during the poster sessions of the main single-track conference. Since we consider all of the accepted papers as excellent, the selection of long oral presentations representing different fields in a single track was extremely challenging. Therefore, we decided to organize the papers in these proceedings in a different way than in the conference program. In contrast to the conference program, the proceedings do not differentiate between poster and oral presentations. The proceedings are only organized by conference topics. Only for the sake of the conference program did we decide on oral and poster presentations. In order to help us in the selection process, we asked the authors to submit five-minute short presentations. Based on the five-minute presentations and the recommendations of the reviewers and Program Committee members, we selected 36 papers for oral presentation. We hope these papers to be to some extent representative of the community covering the entire MICCAI spectrum. The difference in raw review score between the poster and oral presentations was not statistically significant ($p > 0.1$). In addition to the oral presentation selection process, all oral presenters were asked to submit their presentations two months prior to the conference for review by the Program Committee who checked the presentations thoroughly and made suggestions for improvement.

Another feature in the conference program is the industry panel that features leading members of the medical software and device companies who gave their opinions and presented their future research directions and their strategies for translating scientific observations and results of the MICCAI community into medical products.

We thank Aslı Okur, who did an excellent job in the preparation of the conference. She took part in every detail of the organization for more than one year. We would also like to thank Andreas Maier, who supported Joachim Hornegger in his editorial tasks following his election as president of the Friedrich Alexander University Erlangen-Nuremberg (FAU) in early 2015. Furthermore, we thank the local Organizing Committee for arranging the wonderful venue and the MICCAI Student Board for organizing the additional student events ranging from a tour to the BMW factory to trips to the world-famous castles of Neuschwanstein and Linderhof. The workshop, challenge, and tutorial chairs did an excellent job in enriching this year's program. In addition, we thank the MICCAI society for provision of support and insightful comments as well as the Program Committee for their support during the review process. Last but not least, we thank our sponsors for the financial support that made the conference possible.

We look forward to seeing you in Istanbul, Turkey in 2016!

October 2015

Nassir Navab
Joachim Hornegger
William M. Wells
Alejandro F. Frangi

Organization

General Chair

Nassir Navab   Technische Universität München, Germany

General Co-chair

Joachim Hornegger   Friedrich-Alexander-Universität
                                    Erlangen-Nürnberg, Germany

Program Chairs

Nassir Navab   Technische Universität München, Germany
Joachim Hornegger   Friedrich-Alexander-Universität
                                    Erlangen-Nürnberg, Germany
William M. Wells   Harvard Medical School, USA
Alejandro F. Frangi   University of Sheffield, Sheffield, UK

Local Organization Chairs

Ralf Stauder   Technische Universität München, Germany
Aslı Okur   Technische Universität München, Germany
Philipp Matthies   Technische Universität München, Germany
Tobias Zobel   Friedrich-Alexander-Universität
                                    Erlangen-Nürnberg, Germany

Publication Chair

Andreas Maier   Friedrich-Alexander-Universität
                                    Erlangen-Nürnberg, Germany

Sponsorship and Publicity Chairs

Stefanie Demirci   Technische Universität München, Germany
Su-Lin Lee   Imperial College London, UK

Workshop Chairs

Purang Abolmaesumi   University of British Columbia, Canada
Wolfgang Wein   ImFusion, Germany
Bertrand Thirion   Inria, France
Nicolas Padoy   Université de Strasbourg, France

Challenge Chairs

Björn Menze   Technische Universität München, Germany
Lena Maier-Hein   German Cancer Research Center, Germany
Bram van Ginneken   Radboud University, The Netherlands
Valeria De Luca   ETH Zurich, Switzerland

Tutorial Chairs

Tom Vercauteren   University College London, UK
Tobias Heimann   Siemens Corporate Technology, USA
Sonia Pujol   Harvard Medical School, USA
Carlos Alberola   University of Valladolid, Spain

MICCAI Society Board of Directors

Stephen Aylward   Kitware, Inc., NY, USA
Simon Duchesne   Université Laval, Quebéc, Canada
Gabor Fichtinger (Secretary)   Queen's University, Kingston, ON, Canada
Alejandro F. Frangi   University of Sheffield, Sheffield, UK
Polina Golland   MIT, Cambridge, MA, USA
Pierre Jannin   INSERM/INRIA, Rennes, France
Leo Joskowicz   The Hebrew University of Jerusalem
Wiro Niessen
   (Executive Director)   Erasmus MC - University Medical Centre,
                                         Rotterdam, The Netherlands
Nassir Navab   Technische Universität, München, Germany
Alison Noble (President)   University of Oxford, Oxford, UK
Sebastien Ourselin (Treasurer)   University College, London, UK
Xavier Pennec   INRIA, Sophia Antipolis, France
Josien Pluim   Eindhoven University of Technology,
                                         The Netherlands
Dinggang Shen   UNC, Chapel Hill, NC, USA
Li Shen   Indiana University, IN, USA

MICCAI Society Consultants to the Board

Alan Colchester   University of Kent, Canterbury, UK
Terry Peters   University of Western Ontario, London, ON,
                Canada
Richard Robb   Mayo Clinic College of Medicine, MN, USA

MICCAI Society Staff

Society Secretariat   Janette Wallace, Canada
Recording Secretary   Jackie Williams, Canada
Fellows Nomination
   Coordinator   Terry Peters, Canada

Program Committee

Acar, Burak
Barbu, Adrian
Ben Ayed, Ismail
Castellani, Umberto
Cattin, Philippe C.
Chung, Albert C.S.
Cootes, Tim
de Bruijne, Marleen
Delingette, Hervé
Fahrig, Rebecca
Falcão, Alexandre
Fichtinger, Gabor
Gerig, Guido
Gholipour, Ali
Glocker, Ben
Greenspan, Hayit
Hager, Gregory D.
Hamarneh, Ghassan
Handels, Heinz
Harders, Matthias
Heinrich, Mattias Paul
Huang, Junzhou
Ionasec, Razvan
Isgum, Ivana
Jannin, Pierre
Joshi, Sarang
Joskowicz, Leo

Kamen, Ali
Kobashi, Syoji
Langs, Georg
Li, Shuo
Linguraru, Marius George
Liu, Huafeng
Lu, Le
Madabhushi, Anant
Maier-Hein, Lena
Martel, Anne
Masamune, Ken
Moradi, Mehdi
Nielsen, Mads
Nielsen, Poul
Niethammer, Marc
Ourselin, Sebastien
Padoy, Nicolas
Papademetris, Xenios
Paragios, Nikos
Pernus, Franjo
Pohl, Kilian
Preim, Bernhard
Prince, Jerry
Radeva, Petia
Rohde, Gustavo
Sabuncu, Mert Rory
Sakuma, Ichiro

Salcudean, Tim
Salvado, Olivier
Sato, Yoshinobu
Schnabel, Julia A.
Shen, Li
Stoyanov, Danail
Studholme, Colin
Syeda-Mahmood, Tanveer
Taylor, Zeike
Unal, Gozde
Van Leemput, Koen

Wassermann, Demian
Weese, Jürgen
Wein, Wolfgang
Wu, Xiaodong
Yang, Guang Zhong
Yap, Pew-Thian
Yin, Zhaozheng
Yuan, Jing
Zheng, Guoyan
Zheng, Yefeng

Additional Reviewers

Abolmaesumi, Purang
Achterberg, Hakim
Acosta-Tamayo, Oscar
Aerts, Hugo
Afacan, Onur
Afsari, Bijan
Aganj, Iman
Ahad, Md. Atiqur Rahman
Ahmidi, Narges
Aichert, André
Akbari, Hamed
Akhondi-Asl, Alireza
Aksoy, Murat
Alam, Saadia
Alberola-López, Carlos
Aljabar, Paul
Allan, Maximilian
Allassonnieres, Stephanie
Antani, Sameer
Antony, Bhavna
Arbel, Tal
Auvray, Vincent
Awate, Suyash
Azzabou, Noura
Bagci, Ulas
Bai, Wenjia
Baka, Nora
Balocco, Simone
Bao, Siqi
Barmpoutis, Angelos

Bartoli, Adrien
Batmanghelich, Kayhan
Baust, Maximilian
Baxter, John
Bazin, Pierre-Louis
Berger, Marie-Odile
Bernal, Jorge
Bernard, Olivier
Bernardis, Elena
Bhatia, Kanwal
Bieth, Marie
Bilgic, Berkin
Birkfellner, Wolfgang
Blaschko, Matthew
Bloch, Isabelle
Boctor, Emad
Bogunovic, Hrvoje
Bouarfa, Loubna
Bouix, Sylvain
Bourgeat, Pierrick
Brady, Michael
Brost, Alexander
Buerger, Christian
Burgert, Oliver
Burschka, Darius
Caan, Matthan
Cahill, Nathan
Cai, Weidong
Carass, Aaron
Cardenes, Ruben

Cardoso, Manuel Jorge
Carmichael, Owen
Caruyer, Emmanuel
Cathier, Pascal
Cerrolaza, Juan
Cetin, Mustafa
Cetingul, Hasan Ertan
Chakravarty, M. Mallar
Chamberland, Maxime
Chapman, Brian E.
Chatelain, Pierre
Chen, Geng
Chen, Shuhang
Chen, Ting
Cheng, Jian
Cheng, Jun
Cheplygina, Veronika
Chicherova, Natalia
Chowdhury, Ananda
Christensen, Gary
Chui, Chee Kong
Cinar Akakin, Hatice
Cinquin, Philippe
Ciompi, Francesco
Clarkson, Matthew
Clarysse, Patrick
Cobzas, Dana
Colliot, Olivier
Commowick, Olivier
Compas, Colin
Corso, Jason
Criminisi, Antonio
Crum, William
Cuingnet, Remi
Daducci, Alessandro
Daga, Pankaj
Dalca, Adrian
Darkner, Sune
Davatzikos, Christos
Dawant, Benoit
Dehghan, Ehsan
Deligianni, Fani
Demirci, Stefanie
Depeursinge, Adrien
Dequidt, Jeremie

Descoteaux, Maxime
Deslauriers-Gauthier, Samuel
DiBella, Edward
Dijkstra, Jouke
Ding, Kai
Ding, Xiaowei
Dojat, Michel
Dong, Xiao
Dowling, Jason
Dowson, Nicholas
Du, Jia
Duchateau, Nicolas
Duchesne, Simon
Duncan, James S.
Dzyubachyk, Oleh
Eavani, Harini
Ebrahimi, Mehran
Ehrhardt, Jan
Eklund, Anders
El-Baz, Ayman
El-Zehiry, Noha
Ellis, Randy
Elson, Daniel
Erdt, Marius
Ernst, Floris
Eslami, Abouzar
Fallavollita, Pascal
Fang, Ruogu
Fenster, Aaron
Feragen, Aasa
Fick, Rutger
Figl, Michael
Fischer, Peter
Fishbaugh, James
Fletcher, P. Thomas
Florack, Luc
Fonov, Vladimir
Forestier, Germain
Fradkin, Maxim
Franz, Alfred
Freiman, Moti
Freysinger, Wolfgang
Fripp, Jurgen
Frisch, Benjamin
Fritscher, Karl

Fundana, Ketut
Gamarnik, Viktor
Gao, Fei
Gao, Mingchen
Gao, Yaozong
Gao, Yue
Gaonkar, Bilwaj
Garvin, Mona
Gaser, Christian
Gass, Tobias
Gatta, Carlo
Georgescu, Bogdan
Gerber, Samuel
Ghesu, Florin-Cristian
Giannarou, Stamatia
Gibaud, Bernard
Gibson, Eli
Gilles, Benjamin
Ginsburg, Shoshana
Girard, Gabriel
Giusti, Alessandro
Goh, Alvina
Goksel, Orcun
Goldberger, Jacob
Golland, Polina
Gooya, Ali
Grady, Leo
Gray, Katherine
Grbic, Sasa
Grisan, Enrico
Grova, Christophe
Gubern-Mérida, Albert
Guevara, Pamela
Guler, Riza Alp
Guo, Peifang B.
Gur, Yaniv
Gutman, Boris
Gómez, Pedro
Hacihaliloglu, Ilker
Haidegger, Tamas
Hajnal, Joseph
Hamamci, Andac
Hammers, Alexander
Han, Dongfeng
Hargreaves, Brian

Hastreiter, Peter
Hatt, Chuck
Hawkes, David
Hayasaka, Satoru
Haynor, David
He, Huiguang
He, Tiancheng
Heckel, Frank
Heckemann, Rolf
Heimann, Tobias
Heng, Pheng Ann
Hennersperger, Christoph
Holden, Matthew
Hong, Byung-Woo
Honnorat, Nicolas
Hoogendoorn, Corné
Hossain, Belayat
Hossain, Shahera
Howe, Robert
Hu, Yipeng
Huang, Heng
Huang, Xiaojie
Huang, Xiaolei
Hutter, Jana
Ibragimov, Bulat
Iglesias, Juan Eugenio
Igual, Laura
Iordachita, Iulian
Irving, Benjamin
Jackowski, Marcel
Jacob, Mathews
Jain, Ameet
Janoos, Firdaus
Janowczyk, Andrew
Jerman, Tim
Ji, Shuiwang
Ji, Songbai
Jiang, Hao
Jiang, Wenchao
Jiang, Xi
Jiao, Fangxiang
Jin, Yan
Jolly, Marie-Pierre
Jomier, Julien
Joshi, Anand

Joshi, Shantanu
Jung, Claudio
K.B., Jayanthi
Kabus, Sven
Kadoury, Samuel
Kahl, Fredrik
Kainmueller, Dagmar
Kainz, Bernhard
Kakadiaris, Ioannis
Kandemir, Melih
Kapoor, Ankur
Kapur, Tina
Katouzian, Amin
Kelm, Michael
Kerrien, Erwan
Kersten-Oertel, Marta
Khan, Ali
Khurd, Parmeshwar
Kiaii, Bob
Kikinis, Ron
Kim, Boklye
Kim, Edward
Kim, Minjeong
Kim, Sungmin
King, Andrew
Klein, Stefan
Klinder, Tobias
Kluckner, Stefan
Kobayahsi, Etsuko
Konukoglu, Ender
Kumar, Puneet
Kunz, Manuela
Köhler, Thomas
Ladikos, Alexander
Landman, Bennett
Lang, Andrew
Lapeer, Rudy
Larrabide, Ignacio
Lasser, Tobias
Lauze, Francois
Lay, Nathan
Le Reste, Pierre-Jean
Lee, Han Sang
Lee, Kangjoo
Lee, Su-Lin

Lefkimmiatis, Stamatis
Lefèvre, Julien
Lekadir, Karim
Lelieveldt, Boudewijn
Lenglet, Christophe
Lepore, Natasha
Lesage, David
Li, Gang
Li, Jiang
Li, Quanzheng
Li, Xiang
Li, Yang
Li, Yeqing
Liang, Liang
Liao, Hongen
Lin, Henry
Lindeman, Robert
Lindner, Claudia
Linte, Cristian
Litjens, Geert
Liu, Feng
Liu, Jiamin
Liu, Jian Fei
Liu, Jundong
Liu, Mingxia
Liu, Sidong
Liu, Tianming
Liu, Ting
Liu, Yinxiao
Lombaert, Herve
Lorenz, Cristian
Lorenzi, Marco
Lou, Xinghua
Lu, Yao
Luo, Xiongbiao
Lv, Jinglei
Lüthi, Marcel
Maass, Nicole
Madooei, Ali
Mahapatra, Dwarikanath
Maier, Andreas
Maier-Hein (né Fritzsche),
   Klaus Hermann
Majumdar, Angshul
Malandain, Gregoire

Mansi, Tommaso
Mansoor, Awais
Mao, Hongda
Mao, Yunxiang
Marchesseau, Stephanie
Margeta, Jan
Marini Silva, Rafael
Mariottini, Gian Luca
Marsden, Alison
Marsland, Stephen
Martin-Fernandez, Marcos
Martí, Robert
Masutani, Yoshitaka
Mateus, Diana
McClelland, Jamie
McIntosh, Chris
Medrano-Gracia, Pau
Meier, Raphael
Mendizabal-Ruiz, E. Gerardo
Menegaz, Gloria
Menze, Bjoern
Meyer, Chuck
Miga, Michael
Mihalef, Viorel
Miller, James
Miller, Karol
Misaki, Masaya
Modat, Marc
Moghari, Mehdi
Mohamed, Ashraf
Mohareri, Omid
Moore, John
Morales, Hernán G.
Moreno, Rodrigo
Mori, Kensaku
Morimoto, Masakazu
Murphy, Keelin
Müller, Henning
Nabavi, Arya
Nakajima, Yoshikazu
Nakamura, Ryoichi
Napel, Sandy
Nappi, Janne
Nasiriavanaki, Mohammadreza
Nenning, Karl-Heinz

Neumann, Dominik
Neumuth, Thomas
Ng, Bernard
Nguyen Van, Hien
Nicolau, stephane
Ning, Lipeng
Noble, Alison
Noble, Jack
Noblet, Vincent
O'Donnell, Lauren
O'Donnell, Thomas
Oda, Masahiro
Oeltze-Jafra, Steffen
Oh, Junghwan
Oktay, Ayse Betul
Okur, Aslı
Oliver, Arnau
Olivetti, Emanuele
Onofrey, John
Onogi, Shinya
Orihuela-Espina, Felipe
Otake, Yoshito
Ou, Yangming
Ozarslan, Evren
Pace, Danielle
Papa, Joao
Parsopoulos, Konstantinos
Paul, Perrine
Paulsen, Rasmus
Peng, Tingying
Pennec, Xavier
Peruzzo, Denis
Peter, Loic
Peterlik, Igor
Petersen, Jens
Petitjean, Caroline
Peyrat, Jean-Marc
Pham, Dzung
Piella, Gemma
Pitiot, Alain
Pizzolato, Marco
Plenge, Esben
Pluim, Josien
Poline, Jean-Baptiste
Prasad, Gautam

Prastawa, Marcel
Pratt, Philip
Preiswerk, Frank
Preusser, Tobias
Prevost, Raphael
Prieto, Claudia
Punithakumar, Kumaradevan
Putzer, David
Qian, Xiaoning
Qiu, Wu
Quellec, Gwenole
Rafii-Tari, Hedyeh
Rajchl, Martin
Rajpoot, Nasir
Raniga, Parnesh
Rapaka, Saikiran
Rathi, Yogesh
Rathke, Fabian
Rauber, Paulo
Reinertsen, Ingerid
Reinhardt, Joseph
Reiter, Austin
Rekik, Islem
Reyes, Mauricio
Richa, Rogério
Rieke, Nicola
Riess, Christian
Riklin Raviv, Tammy
Risser, Laurent
Rit, Simon
Rivaz, Hassan
Robinson, Emma
Roche, Alexis
Rohling, Robert
Rohr, Karl
Ropinski, Timo
Roth, Holger
Rousseau, François
Rousson, Mikael
Roy, Snehashis
Rueckert, Daniel
Rueda Olarte, Andrea
Ruijters, Daniel
Samaras, Dimitris
Sarry, Laurent

Sato, Joao
Schaap, Michiel
Scheinost, Dustin
Scherrer, Benoit
Schirmer, Markus D.
Schmidt, Frank
Schmidt-Richberg, Alexander
Schneider, Caitlin
Schneider, Matthias
Schultz, Thomas
Schumann, Steffen
Schwartz, Ernst
Sechopoulos, Ioannis
Seiler, Christof
Seitel, Alexander
Sermesant, Maxime
Seshamani, Sharmishtaa
Shahzad, Rahil
Shamir, Reuben R.
Sharma, Puneet
Shen, Xilin
Shi, Feng
Shi, Kuangyu
Shi, Wenzhe
Shi, Yinghuan
Shi, Yonggang
Shin, Hoo-Chang
Simpson, Amber
Singh, Vikas
Sinkus, Ralph
Slabaugh, Greg
Smeets, Dirk
Sona, Diego
Song, Yang
Sotiras, Aristeidis
Speidel, Michael
Speidel, Stefanie
Špiclin, Žiga
Staib, Lawrence
Stamm, Aymeric
Staring, Marius
Stauder, Ralf
Stayman, J. Webster
Steinman, David
Stewart, James

Styles, Iain
Styner, Martin
Su, Hang
Suinesiaputra, Avan
Suk, Heung-Il
Summers, Ronald
Sun, Shanhui
Szekely, Gabor
Sznitman, Raphael
Takeda, Takahiro
Talbot, Hugues
Tam, Roger
Tamura, Manabu
Tang, Lisa
Tao, Lingling
Tasdizen, Tolga
Taylor, Russell
Thirion, Bertrand
Thung, Kim-Han
Tiwari, Pallavi
Toews, Matthew
Toh, Kim-Chuan
Tokuda, Junichi
Tong, Yubing
Tornai, Gábor János
Tosun, Duygu
Totz, Johannes
Tournier, J-Donald
Toussaint, Nicolas
Traub, Joerg
Troccaz, Jocelyne
Tustison, Nicholas
Twinanda, Andru Putra
Twining, Carole
Ukwatta, Eranga
Umadevi Venkataraju, Kannan
Unay, Devrim
Urschler, Martin
Uzunbas, Mustafa
Vaillant, Régis
Vallin Spina, Thiago
Vallotton, Pascal
Van assen, Hans
Van Ginneken, Bram
Van Tulder, Gijs

Van Walsum, Theo
Vandini, Alessandro
Vannier, Michael
Varoquaux, Gael
Vegas-Sánchez-Ferrero, Gonzalo
Venkataraman, Archana
Vercauteren, Tom
Veta, Mtiko
Vignon-Clementel, Irene
Villard, Pierre-Frederic
Visentini-Scarzanella, Marco
Viswanath, Satish
Vitanovski, Dime
Voigt, Ingmar
Von Berg, Jens
Voros, Sandrine
Vrtovec, Tomaz
Wachinger, Christian
Waechter-Stehle, Irina
Wahle, Andreas
Wang, Ancong
Wang, Chaohui
Wang, Haibo
Wang, Hongzhi
Wang, Junchen
Wang, Li
Wang, Liansheng
Wang, Lichao
Wang, Linwei
Wang, Qian
Wang, Qiu
Wang, Song
Wang, Yalin
Wang, Yuanquan
Wee, Chong-Yaw
Wei, Liu
Wels, Michael
Werner, Rene
Wesarg, Stefan
Westin, Carl-Fredrik
Whitaker, Ross
Whitney, Jon
Wiles, Andrew
Wörz, Stefan
Wu, Guorong

Wu, Haiyong
Wu, Yu-Chien
Xie, Yuchen
Xing, Fuyong
Xu, Yanwu
Xu, Ziyue
Xue, Zhong
Yagi, Naomi
Yamazaki, Takaharu
Yan, Pingkun
Yang, Lin
Yang, Ying
Yao, Jianhua
Yaqub, Mohammad
Ye, Dong Hye
Yeo, B.T. Thomas
Ynnermann, Anders
Young, Alistair
Yushkevich, Paul
Zacharaki, Evangelia
Zacur, Ernesto
Zelmann, Rina
Zeng, Wei
Zhan, Liang

Zhan, Yiqiang
Zhang, Daoqiang
Zhang, Hui
Zhang, Ling
Zhang, Miaomiao
Zhang, Pei
Zhang, Shaoting
Zhang, Tianhao
Zhang, Tuo
Zhang, Yong
Zhao, Bo
Zhao, Wei
Zhijun, Zhang
Zhou, jinghao
Zhou, Luping
Zhou, S. Kevin
Zhou, Yan
Zhu, Dajiang
Zhu, Hongtu
Zhu, Yuemin
Zhuang, ling
Zhuang, Xiahai
Zuluaga, Maria A.

Contents – Part II

Computer Aided Diagnosis II: Automation

Registration: Method and Advanced Applications

Modeling and Simulation for Diagnosis and Interventional Planning

Reconstruction, Image Formation, Advanced Acquisition - Computational Imaging

Computer Aided Diagnosis II:
Automation

Computer-Aided Detection and Quantification of Intracranial Aneurysms

Tim Jerman, Franjo Pernuš, Boštjan Likar, and Žiga Špiclin

Faculty of Electrical Engineering, Laboratory of Imaging Technologies,
University of Ljubljana, Tržaška 25, 1000 Ljubljana, Slovenia
{tim.jerman,ziga.spiclin,bostjan.likar,franjo.pernus}@fe.uni-lj.si

Abstract. Early detection, assessment and treatment of intracranial aneurysms is important to prevent rupture, which may cause death. We propose a framework for detection and quantification of morphology of the aneurysms. A novel detector using decision forests, which employ responses of blobness and vesselness filters encoded in rotation invariant and scale normalized frequency components of spherical harmonics representation is proposed. Aneurysm location is used to seed growcut segmentation, followed by improved neck extraction based on intravascular ray-casting and robust closed-curve fit to the segmentation. Aneurysm segmentation and neck curve are used to compute three morphologic metrics: neck width, dome height and aspect ratio. The proposed framework was evaluated on ten cerebral 3D-DSA images containing saccular aneurysms. Sensitivity of aneurysm detection was 100% at 0.4 false positives per image. Compared to measurements of two expert raters, the values of metrics obtained by the proposed framework were accurate and, thus, suitable for assessing the risk of rupture.

Keywords: intracranial aneurysm, rupture, detection, multiscale enhancement, random forests, segmentation, neck extraction, morphology.

1 Introduction

The prevalence of intracranial aneurysms is between 2%-5% of the world population and, although aneurysm rupture is a rather rare event, the majority of patients that experience the rupture die of subarachnoid hemorrhage [3]. To prevent such fatal events, aneurysms should be detected, assessed and treated as early as possible. After an aneurysm is detected, the risk of rupture is assessed through quantitative studies of its morphology and hemodynamics so as to prioritize the treatment of patients. Quantifying the morphology of aneurysms can be performed manually using a 3D angiographic image like 3D digital subtraction angiography (3D-DSA). However, tasks like manual detection, segmentation, isolation and measurement of the aneurysm in a complex 3D vascular tree, usually based on observing 2D cross-sections of the 3D image, are tedious and time consuming to perform for a clinician. To assist the clinician, but also to improve the accuracy, reliability and reproducibility of the outcome [1], there is a need for computer-aided detection and quantification of the aneurysms.

© Springer International Publishing Switzerland 2015
N. Navab et al. (Eds.): MICCAI 2015, Part II, LNCS 9350, pp. 3–10, 2015.
DOI: 10.1007/978-3-319-24571-3_1

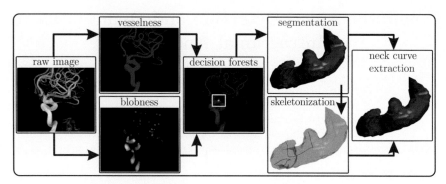

Fig. 1. Image analysis framework for aneurysm detection, segmentation and neck extraction based on a 3D angiogram.

Although several methods for detecting intracranial aneurysms [6,4], segmenting vascular structures [7] and extracting the aneurysm's neck curve [1], were proposed in the past, to the best of our knowledge, these methods still need to be further improved before being incorporated into a computer-aided detection and quantification framework. Of the aneurysm detection, segmentation, and quantification tasks, detection seems to be the most difficult. The specific hemodynamics of each aneurysm causes large variations of image intensity between different aneurysms, which, besides variations in aneurysm size and shape, adversely impact the performance of detection methods [6,4]. The intensity, size and shape variations typically result in lower sensitivity and specificity of computer-aided detection of aneurysms.

To aid the detection and quantification of intracranial aneurysms, we propose an image analysis framework that involves: a) enhancement of the 3D cerebral angiogram, b) novel detection of aneurysms based on random forests and rotation invariant and scale normalized visual features, c) a growcut segmentation of the aneurysm and attached vasculature, followed by d) neck curve extraction based on intravascular ray-casting to find points on the neck and a robust RANSAC-type closed-curve fitting. The proposed framework was evaluated on ten cerebral 3D-DSA images containing aneurysms, which were quantified by three morphologic metrics: neck width, dome height and aspect ratio. The achieved sensitivity of aneurysm detection was 100% at 0.4 false positives per image, while, compared to aneurysm measurements of two expert raters, the automatic measurements were accurate and thus suitable for assessing the risk of aneurysm rupture.

2   Methods

Main steps of the image analysis framework for the detection and morphologic quantification of cerebral aneurysms are illustrated in Fig. 1. The following subsections detail the aneurysm detection, segmentation and neck curve extraction. Based on aneurysm segmentation and neck curve, the morphologic metrics like neck width, dome height and aspect ratio of the aneurysm can be quantified.

2.1   Aneurysm Detection

Computer-aided detection of aneurysms in angiographic images should exhibit high sensitivity, but at the same time, reduce the number of false detections to a minimum. Since aneurysms are blob-like structures a simple approach to their detection is to employ blob enhancement on the images, e.g. multiscale filters based on analysis of Hessian eigenvalues [8]. Although the response of a blob enhancement filter is high at aneurysms and thus promising for computer-aided detection of aneurysms, the response may also be high at bifurcations and vessel bents, which, on a certain scale, resemble a blob-like structure. Hence, a blob enhancement filter will likely indicate many false positives (FPs). To better discriminate between the aneurysm regions, i.e. true positives (TPs), and other structures, and to further reduce FPs, we use random decision forests (RDFs) [2] trained on visual features obtained from the responses of enhancement filters.

Visual Features. For each location $\mathbf{x}_i \in \mathbb{R}^3$ in a 3D angiographic image $I(\mathbf{x})$ an ensemble of rotation invariant and scale normalized features that describe the local neighborhood of $\mathbf{x}_i$ are computed. First, the aneurysms and vessels of various sizes are enhanced by a multiscale Hessian-based filtering of $I(\mathbf{x})$ using blobness and vesselness [8] filters, with normalized responses denoted by $\mathcal{B}(\mathbf{x})$ and $\mathcal{V}(\mathbf{x})$, respectively. These two responses are locally resampled about $\mathbf{x}_i$ over concentric spheres (Fig. 2.b,c) parameterized by (θ, ϕ) and radii $r_k, k = 1, \ldots, K$ and then projected onto spherical harmonics basis $Y_l^m(\theta, \phi)$ [5] to represent, e.g., the blobness response over a sphere as:

$$\hat{\mathcal{B}}(\theta, \phi | \mathbf{x}_i, r_k) = \sum_{l=0}^{L} \sum_{m=-l}^{m=l} a_{lm} Y_l^m(\theta, \phi), \tag{1}$$

where L is the maximal bandwidth of spherical basis functions m, and coefficients a_{lm} are computed from $\mathcal{B}(\theta, \phi | \mathbf{x}_i, r_k)$. Analoguously, we get $\hat{\mathcal{V}}(\theta, \phi | \mathbf{x}_i, r_k)$. A rotation invariant representation (Fig. 2.d) is obtained by computing the L_2-norm of spherical functions with respect to frequency l as [5]:

$$\hat{\mathcal{B}}_l^{i,k} = \left\| \sum_{m=-l}^{m=l} a_{lm} Y_l^m(\theta, \phi) \right\|, \tag{2}$$

where a simpler notation was used to indicate the dependence on $\mathbf{x}_i$ and r_k. Analoguously, we get $\hat{\mathcal{V}}_l^{i,k}$. To normalize the scale we first compute the rotation invariant features for K concentric spheres with $r_K = R$, where R is some fixed radius larger than the structures of interest, and estimate the cutoff radius r_C:

$$r_C \leftrightarrow C = \sup\{ k = 1, \ldots, K : \hat{\mathcal{B}}_0^{i,k} / \overline{\mathcal{B}}^{i,k} \geq 0.75 \}, \tag{3}$$

where $\overline{\mathcal{B}}^{i,k} = [\sum_{l=0}^{L} \hat{\mathcal{B}}_l^{i,k}]^{1/2}$. Scale and rotation invariant features are then computed for K concentric spheres with the outer sphere of radius $r_K = 2 \cdot r_C$. Finally, the ensemble of visual features for point $\mathbf{x}_i$ is obtained as:

$$\phi(\mathbf{x}_i) = \{\hat{\mathcal{B}}_0^{i,k}, \ldots, \hat{\mathcal{B}}_L^{i,k}, \hat{\mathcal{V}}_0^{i,k}, \ldots, \hat{\mathcal{V}}_L^{i,k} : k = 1, \ldots, K\}. \tag{4}$$

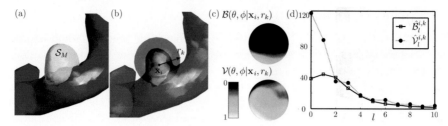

Fig. 2. (a) Reference segmentation $\mathcal{S}_M$ (yellow) of an aneurysm. (b) Blobness $\mathcal{B}(\mathbf{x}_i)$ and vesselness $\mathcal{V}(\mathbf{x}_i)$ sampled on a sphere with radius r_k around $\mathbf{x}_i$ are (c) projected onto a spherical harmonics basis, from which (d) rotation invariant features $\hat{\mathcal{B}}_l^{i,k}$ and $\hat{\mathcal{V}}_l^{i,k}$ are computed and used in a RDF based detector.

RDF Based Detector. RDF is trained on N angiographic images $I_n(\mathbf{x}); n = 1, \ldots, N$, in which the aneurysms were manually segmented by a neuroradiologist (Fig. 2). RDF requires visual features of two sets of points, one of TPs ($\mathcal{S}_{TP}$) and one of FPs ($\mathcal{S}_{FP}$). The set $\mathcal{S}_{TP}$ contains points with a high blobness response $\mathcal{B}(\mathbf{x}) > \tau_{\mathcal{B}}$ that lie within the manual segmentation $\mathcal{S}_M$ (Fig. 2.a), i.e. $\mathcal{S}_{TP} = \{\mathbf{x} : \mathbf{x} \in \mathcal{S}_M \wedge \mathcal{B}(\mathbf{x}) > \tau_{\mathcal{B}}\}$. Threshold $\tau_{\mathcal{B}}$ is manually determined. The set of FPs is obtained as $\mathcal{S}_{FP} = \{\mathbf{x} : \mathbf{x} \notin \mathcal{S}_{TP} \wedge \mathcal{B}(\mathbf{x}) > \tau_{\mathcal{B}}\}$. Since $\mathcal{B}(\mathbf{x})$ usually indicates many FPs, the cardinality of the two point sets may be unbalanced, i.e. $|\mathcal{S}_{TP}| \ll |\mathcal{S}_{FP}|$, thus points in $\mathcal{S}_{TP}$ are multiplied such that $|\mathcal{S}_{TP}| \approx |\mathcal{S}_{FP}|$.

Visual features are computed using (4) as $\{\phi(\mathbf{x}) : \mathbf{x} \in \mathcal{S}_{TP} \vee \mathbf{x} \in \mathcal{S}_{FP}\}$, while for each $\phi(\mathbf{x}_j)$ a class indicator variable $c(\mathbf{x}_j) \in \{\text{TP}, \text{FP}\}$ is set accordingly. The features are used to train a RDF of T independent trees Ψ_t; $t = 1, \ldots, T$ of depth D, in which information gain is maximized to determine optimal node splits [2]. The number of points in the training sets $\mathcal{S}_{TP}$, $\mathcal{S}_{FP}$ that reach a certain leaf is used to compute the posterior probabilities $p_t(c|\phi(\mathbf{x}))$ at each leaf in t-th tree.

Aneurysm detection on a test image $I(\mathbf{x})$ proceeds by extracting a set of candidate points $\mathcal{S}_{CP} = \{\mathbf{x} : \mathcal{B}(\mathbf{x}) > \tau_{\mathcal{B}}\}$. For each $\mathbf{x}_j \in \mathcal{S}_{CP}, j = 1, \ldots, |\mathcal{S}_{CP}|$ we compute the ensemble of visual features $\phi(\mathbf{x}_j)$ and then evaluate and average the posterior probabilities over all trees as:

$$p(c = \text{TP}|\phi(\mathbf{x}_j)) = \mathcal{L}(\mathbf{x}_j) = \frac{1}{T} \sum_{t=1}^{T} p_t(c = \text{TP}|\phi(\mathbf{x}_j)), \qquad (5)$$

where $\mathcal{L}(\mathbf{x}_j)$ is the aneurysm likelihood map. For a fixed threshold $0 < \tau_A < 1$, the set of points within aneurysms is detected as $\mathcal{S}_A = \{\mathbf{x} : \mathcal{L}(\mathbf{x}) > \tau_A\}$.

2.2   Aneurysm Segmentation and Neck Extraction

Based on a local segmentation of the aneurysm, intravascular ray-casting from the center of aneurysm to the vessel wall is used to find points on the aneurysm neck as the points with a high gradient in ray distance map. These points are fitted with a closed-curve to obtain the neck curve and isolate the aneurysm's dome, which is used to quantify the aneurysm.

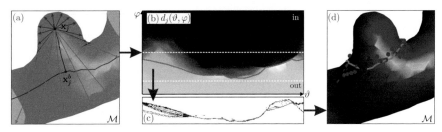

Fig. 3. (a) Intravascular ray-casting from the centerlines to segmentation surface $\mathcal{M}$ yields (b) distance maps $d_j(\vartheta, \varphi)$. (c) The edges in (b) are tentative points on the neck, which are used in a RANSAC-type fitting of closed-curve to obtain the final neck curve.

Segmentation of each aneurysm and neighboring vessels is performed by grow-cut [9], which requires seed points within the vascular structures and on background. First, the center $\mathbf{x}^c$ of each aneurysm is set as the center of the corresponding connected component in $\mathcal{S}_A$. Each $\mathbf{x}_j^c \in \mathcal{S}_A$ is merged to corresponding connected component in $\{\mathbf{x} : \mathcal{B}(\mathbf{x}) > \tau_\mathcal{B}\}$ to obtain a volume of interest (VOI) $\mathcal{S}_{j,VOI}$, set twice the size of bounding box of the connected component. Seeds within the vascular structures $\mathcal{S}_{j,+}$ are the 6-connected neighboors of $\mathbf{x}_j^c$, while seeds $\mathcal{S}_{j,-}$ on background are points within the VOI with low blobness and low vesselness response, i.e. $\{\mathbf{x} : ero(\mathcal{V}(\mathbf{x})) < \tau_\mathcal{V} \wedge \mathcal{B}(\mathbf{x}) < \tau_\mathcal{B}) \wedge \mathbf{x} \in \mathcal{S}_{j,VOI}\}$, where ero denotes binary erosion. Using the segmentation of vascular structure we extract its centerlines [7] and choose the aneurysm's centerline $\mathcal{S}_l$ as the centerline closest to $\mathbf{x}_j^c$ and then find a bifurcation point $\mathbf{x}_j^b$ connecting the aneurysm's centerline to the feeding vessel.

Extraction of aneurysm's neck curve is based on casting rays from $\mathbf{x}_j^c$ [10] in directions defined by $\vartheta \in [-\pi, \pi], \varphi \in [0, \pi]$ towards the surface mesh $\mathcal{M}$ of the segmented vascular structures, measuring the ray distance to intersection and thresholding a corresponding distance map $d(\vartheta, \varphi)$. The idea is that between rays intersecting the neck (Fig. 3.a red) and those passing through the neck aperture (Fig. 3.a green), the distance increases noticeably. While the original method [10] is not robust to initial source point and thus requires user interaction, we perform ray casting from several points $\mathbf{x}_j \in \mathcal{S}_l$ with respect to $\mathbf{x}_j^b$ and then map the corresponding $d_j(\vartheta, \varphi)$ into a common coordinate frame (Fig. 3.b). A tentative neck curve is computed for each $d_j(\vartheta, \varphi)$ by initial Otsu thresholding and level set based segmentation determining the edge between the vessel and the aneurysm. All edges are mapped into common distance map and a 1D median filter is applied along φ (Fig. 3.c). The obtained points are projected onto $\mathcal{M}$, yielding possible neck curve points $\mathcal{C}$ (Fig. 3.d). The points in $\mathcal{C}$ are binned according to ϑ, with the bin size $\Delta\vartheta$. Using a RANSAC-type method, in which multiple subsets of points $\mathbf{x} \in \mathcal{C}' \subset \mathcal{C}$ are randomly selected by drawing at least one point from each bin, and then connected by shortest path across $\mathcal{M}$, the final neck curve is determined by subset $\mathcal{C}'$ that yields the shortest neck curve (Fig. 3.d).

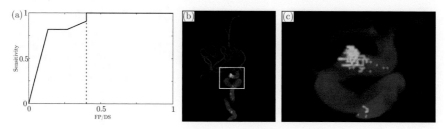

Fig. 4. (a) Free-response ROC curve of the RDF-based aneurysm detector showing sensitivity versus false positives per dataset (FP/DS) and (b,c) a maximum intensity projection of 3D-DSA with superimposed aneurysm likelihood map $\mathcal{L}(\mathbf{x}_j)$.

3   Experiments and Results

The proposed framework for the detection, segmentation, and neck curve extraction of cerebral aneurysms was trained on cerebral 3D-DSAs of $N = 15$ patients containing at least one intracranial saccular aneurysm. Another ten 3D-DSA images containing 15 intracranial saccular aneurysms were used for evaluation of the aneurysm detection, segmentation and neck curve extraction methods.

The RDFs were constructed with $T = 10$ trees of depth $D = 10$. For training and testing the RDFs we used points $\mathbf{x}$ with blobness $\mathcal{B}(\mathbf{x})$ above $\tau_{\mathcal{B}} = 0.15$. The visual features for RDFs were computed on $K = 10$ spheres with radii r_k increasing in equidistant steps. The maximum radius was $R = 10$, while the spherical harmonics bandwidth was set to $L = 15$. These parameters were determined by maximizing the overall detection performance on the test images.

The neck curve extraction was evaluated on 15 aneurysms from the test dataset. For evaluation, the neck curve was manually delineated by two experts on the surface of segmented aneurysm. Intravascular ray-casting was performed from 10 skeleton points $\mathbf{x}_j \in \mathcal{S}_l$ to obtain distance maps $d_j(\vartheta, \varphi)$.

Sampling of the tentative neck points used bin size of $\Delta\vartheta = 30°$. To quantitatively compare the neck curves extracted manually and automatically, we computed three morphologic metrics of the aneurysms: average neck width (NW), dome height (DH), and aspect ratio: AR = DH/NW. AR has been studied widely and has consistently been found to correlate with risk of aneurysm rupture [3].

Results. For each of the 10 test images, the aneurysm likelihood map $\mathcal{L}(\mathbf{x})$ was computed and thresholded with τ_A to obtain points $\mathcal{S}_A$ on aneurysms, whereas connected components smaller than 15 voxels were eliminated. The sensitivity and the amount of false positives per dataset (FP/DS) were determined at various threshold values $0 < \tau_A < 1$ so as to obtain the free-response receiver operating characteristic (FROC) curve shown in Fig. 4.a. The proposed detection method achieved a 100% sensitivity at 0.4 FP/DS. A maximum intensity projection (MIP) of a test image is shown in Fig. 4.b, in which the yellow component represents the superimposed aneurysm likelihood map with values above $\tau_A = 0.5$. The aneurysm location is clearly visible as a cluster of points (Fig. 4.c).

Fig. 5 shows Bland-Altman diagrams with the bias and standard deviation (SD) of error of NW, DH and AR measures between the two expert raters and

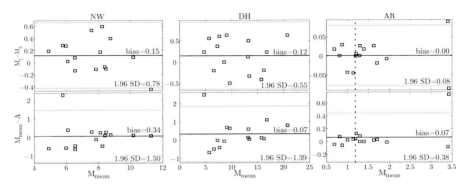

Fig. 5. Bland-Altman diagrams of quantitative aneurysm measures: average neck width (NW), dome height (DH) and aspect ratio (AR=H/NW), computed from two expert (M) and one automatic (A) neck curve delineations. Aneurysms with AR>1.18 (vertical dashed line) have a high risk of rupture [3].

between averaged values of the two raters and values obtained by the proposed neck extraction method. The agreement between the two raters was high as the bias and the SD were low, while in the comparison between the raters and the proposed method bias was low, but SD was slightly higher. The SD was higher because of one small aneurysm that had a low curvature on the neck, thus, the neck curves of both the expert raters and the automatic method differed substantially. Ignoring this outlier reduced the bias and SD of AR to 0.02 and 0.11, which is similar to the values obtained between the raters.

4   Discussion

To assist the clinician, we proposed a framework for computer-aided detection and morphologic quantification of cerebral aneurysms that involves a novel detection approach, local aneurysm segmentation, and improved neck curve extraction of intracranial aneurysms. The segmentation and neck curve are used for aneurysm isolation and quantification of its morphology, which is important for assessing the risk of rupture and planning the treatment.

The proposed aneurysm detection is based on random decision forests, which employ novel visual features based on responses of blob and vessel enhancement filters [8], Locations with high blobness are considered in feature extraction that proceeds by sampling the two response maps over concentric spheres, which are encoded by rotation invariant and scale normalized spherical harmonics. Thereby, characteristic aneurysm shape is encoded, while the variability, non-informative for the detection, is minimized. On ten 3D-DSAs containing 15 aneurysms, the proposed method achieved a 100% sensitivity at 0.4 FP/DS.

Although the results of other methods were obtained on other datasets, and are thus not directly comparable, their performance is slightly worse with 95% at 2.6 FP/DS [4] and 100% at 0.66 FP/DS [6]. Moreover, Lauric et al. [6] require a highly accurate segmentation of the entire vasculature, which is difficult to obtain because of intensity variations of the 3D-DSA [7]. Herein the proposed framework executes a VOI-based aneurysm segmentation [9] after the detection.

To robustly isolate and quantify the aneurysm, we improved neck curve extraction by repeated intravascular ray-casting [10] to sample neck edge points, to which a closed-curve was fit by a RANSAC-type approach. Validation was performed by observing the bias and standard deviation of three morphologic measures of the aneurysms, i.e. NW, DH, AR, with respect to manual delineations of two expert raters (Fig. 5). Except for one small aneurysm, in which the extracted neck curve substantially differed from manual delineations, the computed measures were consistent over all aneurysms.

Aspect ratio (AR) is widely used as a measure of risk rupture [1], thus the methods for its assessment need to be accurate and reproducible. For aneurysms with AR>1.18 (dashed vertical line in Fig. 5) the risk of rupture is considered high, thus an immediate treatment is required [3]. Compared to four methods analyzed on a different database of aneurysms in [1] that had a mean relative error of 9.1, 7.5, 6.9, and 6.8% of AR versus a manual reference, the proposed method had the lowest mean relative error of 5.2%. Hence, the obtained low mean relative error renders the proposed method highly suited for assessing the risk of aneurysm rupture. Evaluation of the proposed framework shows encouraging results on 3D-DSA images. Since aneurysm detection and isolation rely on highly sensitive blob and vessel enhancement filters the approach also seems promising for other angiographic modalities like CTA and MRA.

References

1. Cardenes, R., Larrabide, I., et al.: Performance assessment of isolation methods for geometrical cerebral aneurysm analysis. Med. Biol. Eng. Comput. 51(3) (2012)
2. Criminisi, A., Shotton, J. (eds.): Decision Forests for Computer Vision and Medical Image Analysis. Springer, London (2013)
3. Dhar, S., Tremmel, M., Mocco, J., et al.: Morphology Parameters for Intracranial Aneurysm Rupture Risk Assessment. Neurosurgery 63(2), 185–197 (2008)
4. Hentschke, C.M., Beuing, O., Paukisch, H., et al.: A system to detect cerebral aneurysms in multimodality angiographic data sets. Med. Phys. 41(9), 091904 (2014)
5. Kazhdan, M., Funkhouser, T., Rusinkiewicz, S.: Rotation invariant spherical harmonic representation of 3D shape descriptors. In: Proc. Symp. on Geom. Proc. (2003)
6. Lauric, A., Miller, E., Frisken, S., et al.: Automated detection of intracranial aneurysms based on parent vessel 3D analysis. Med. Image. Anal. 14(2), 149–159 (2010)
7. Lesage, D., Angelini, E.D., et al.: A review of 3D vessel lumen segmentation techniques: Models, features and extraction schemes. Med. Image Anal. 13(6) (2009)
8. Sato, Y., Westin, C.-F., et al.: Tissue classification based on 3D local intensity structures for volume rendering. IEEE T. Vis. Comput. Gr. 6(2), 160–180 (2000)
9. Vezhnevets, V., Konushin, V.: Growcut - interactive multi-label n-d image segmentation by cellular automata. In: Proc. GraphiCon (2005)
10. van der Weide, R., Zuiderveld, K., Mali, W.P.T.M., et al.: CTA-based angle selection for diagnostic and interventional angiography of saccular intracranial aneurysms. IEEE Trans. Med. Imag. 17(5), 831–841 (1998)

Discriminative Feature Selection for Multiple Ocular Diseases Classification by Sparse Induced Graph Regularized Group Lasso

Xiangyu Chen[1], Yanwu Xu[1], Shuicheng Yan[2], Tat-Seng Chua[2],
Damon Wing Kee Wong[1], Tien Yin Wong[2], and Jiang Liu[1]

[1] Institute for Infocomm Research, Agency for Science,
Technology and Research, Singapore
[2] National University of Singapore, Singapore

Abstract. Glaucoma, Pathological Myopia (PM), and Age-related Macular Degeneration (AMD) are three leading ocular diseases worldwide. Visual features extracted from retinal fundus images have been increasingly used for detecting these three diseases. In this paper, we present a discriminative feature selection model based on multi-task learning, which imposes the exclusive group lasso regularization for competitive sparse feature selection and the graph Laplacian regularization to embed the correlations among multiple diseases. Moreover, this multi-task linear discriminative model is able to simultaneously select sparse features and detect multiple ocular diseases. Extensive experiments are conducted to validate the proposed framework on the *SiMES* dataset. From the Area Under Curve (AUC) results in multiple ocular diseases classification, our method is shown to outperform the state-of-the-art algorithms.

1 Introduction

Many of the leading causes of vision impairment and blindness worldwide are irreversible and cannot be cured [1]. Glaucoma, Pathological Myopia (PM), and Age-related Macular Degeneration (AMD) are three leading ocular diseases worldwide. Early detection of these ocular diseases utilizing effective visual features is highly needed [2][11].

With the advancement of retinal fundus imaging, several computer-aided diagnosis (CAD) methods and systems have been developed to automatically detect these three leading ocular diseases from retinal fundus images [6][4]. However, current work mainly focus on detecting Glaucoma, PM, and AMD individually. Classifying these three leading diseases simultaneously is still an open research direction. There are some correlations among these three leading ocular diseases. In recent decades, the problem of low vision and blindness in elderly people became a major and socially significant issue. The number of patients having age-related macular degeneration (AMD) in association with glaucoma is growing all over the world [8], which attaches great medical and social value to this multiple diseases diagnosis problem. Moreover, in a recent study, myopic eyes are less likely to have AMD and diabetic retinopathy (DR) but more likely to have nuclear cataracts and glaucoma [9].

© Springer International Publishing Switzerland 2015
N. Navab et al. (Eds.): MICCAI 2015, Part II, LNCS 9350, pp. 11–19, 2015.
DOI: 10.1007/978-3-319-24571-3_2

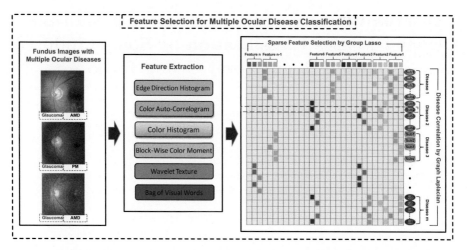

Fig. 1. System overview of our proposed discriminative feature selection scheme for multiple ocular diseases classification. Here "Sub1" stands for a sub-type disease of a leading ocular disease. As indicated within red dashed borders in the right of the figure, a sparse feature will be learned for each disease. For better viewing, please see the color pdf file.

In this paper, we adopt a Multi-task Learning (MTL) based method for discriminatively selecting sparse features, harmoniously integrating the correlation information of multiple diseases, and investigating the problem of learning to simultaneously diagnose them for a given fundus image. Different from previous algorithms that detect ocular disease independently, the proposed method formulates the correlation information of different diseases by a graph Laplacian regularizer and models the sparse feature selection by an exclusive group lasso regularizer. It then utilizes a multi-task linear model to learn a linear mapping from features to diseases. Since a patient may have two or three ocular diseases at the same time, multiple ocular diseases detection is well suited for real-world diagnosis scenarios.

2   Discriminative Feature Selection by Graph Regularized Group Lasso

2.1   Graph Regularized Group Lasso Multi-task Learning

For a multiple ocular disease dataset $\{x_i, l_i\}_{i=1}^{N}$, $x_i \in R^d$ is the feature vector of the i-th fundus image and $l_i = \{l_i^k\}_{k=1}^{K}$ is the associated disease label. For simplicity and clarity, we set $K = 2$ and denote the Cartesian product of $\mathcal{L}^1$ and $\mathcal{L}^2$ as $\mathcal{L} = \mathcal{L}^1 \times \mathcal{L}^2$, as done in [10]. In addition, $y_i \in R^{|\mathcal{L}|}$ is the zero-one disease label vector ($|\mathcal{L}| = |\mathcal{L}^1| \times |\mathcal{L}^2|$) indicating whether x_i is jointly labeled as $l^1 \in \mathcal{L}^1$ and $l^2 \in \mathcal{L}^2$. For the case of multiple ocular diseases, $|\mathcal{L}^1|$ is equal to the number of types of ocular diseases and $|\mathcal{L}^2|$ stands for the number of sub-types of each disease. For example, since AMD is classified into dry AMD (non-exudative

AMD) and wet AMD (exudative AMD), $|\mathcal{L}^2|$ is equal to 2. Given the training feature-label set $\{x_i, y_i\}_{i=1}^N$, the disease label of a test image can be predicted via learning a linear model $y = Mx$. Our employed learning model is based on the following basic MTL formulation [5]:

$$\Theta(M) = \frac{1}{2} \sum_{j=1}^{|\mathcal{L}|} \|Y_j - M_j X\|^2, \tag{1}$$

where $Y_j \in \mathbb{R}^n$ and $M_j \in \mathbb{R}^d$ are the j-th row of Y and M, respectively. $X = [x_1, ..., x_n] \in \mathbb{R}^{d \times n}$ is the feature matrix with each column representing a training image feature, $Y = [y_1, ..., y_n] \in \mathbb{R}^{|\mathcal{L}| \times n}$ is the label matrix with each column as a training image label vector, and $M \in \mathbb{R}^{|\mathcal{L}| \times d}$ is the parameter to be estimated. We are to learn $|\mathcal{L}|$ different linear regression models (tasks) $Y_j = M_j X$, $j = 1, ..., |\mathcal{L}|$. In this naive formulation, the tasks are learned independently of each other.

In order to learn the discriminative features for multiple diseases detection, we consider the relationships across tasks by imposing two regularizers (*Exclusive Group Lasso Regularizer* and *Graph Laplacian Regularizer*) to the objective $\Theta(M)$ in (1) as in [10]. Before we start to utilize the improved objective $\Theta(M)$, let us introduce some notation for group lasso and graph Laplacian. Let $\mathcal{G}^1$ of size $|\mathcal{L}^1|$ be a group of label index sets in $\mathcal{L}$ constructed as follows: each element $g \in \mathcal{G}^1$ is an index set of combinational labels $(l^1, l^2) \in \mathcal{L}$ which share a common $l^1 \in \mathcal{L}^1$. And $\mathcal{G}^2$ of size $|\mathcal{L}^2|$ is constructed with label set $\mathcal{L}^2$. Given a similarity matrix $S \in \mathbb{R}^{|\mathcal{L}| \times |\mathcal{L}|}$ that stores the pairwise similarity scores between concepts, the larger S_{jk} is, the more similar two concepts j and k are, and vice versa. Hence, the objective $\Theta(M)$ in (1) can be written as:

$$\Theta(M) = \frac{1}{2} \sum_{j=1}^{|\mathcal{L}|} \|Y_j - M_j X\|^2 + \mu \sum_{i=1}^{d} \left(\|M_{\mathcal{G}^1}^i\|_{2,1}^2 + \|M_{\mathcal{G}^2}^i\|_{2,1}^2 \right)$$

$$+ \eta \sum_{j,k=1}^{|\mathcal{L}|} S_{jk} \| M_j - M_k \|^2, \tag{2}$$

where $\sum_{i=1}^{d} \left(\|M_{\mathcal{G}^1}^i\|_{2,1}^2 + \|M_{\mathcal{G}^2}^i\|_{2,1}^2 \right)$ is the *Exclusive Group Lasso Regularizer* (denoted as $\Gamma(M)$) and $\sum_{j,k=1}^{|\mathcal{L}|} S_{jk} \| M_j - M_k \|^2$ is the *Graph Laplacian Regularizer*. $\|M_{\mathcal{G}^k}^i\|_{2,1}^2 = \left(\sum_{g \in \mathcal{G}^k} \|M_g^i\|_2 \right)^2$, $k = 1, 2$, and $M^i \in \mathbb{R}^{|\mathcal{L}|}$ is the i-th column of M, and $M_g^i \in \mathbb{R}^{|\mathcal{L}|}$ is the restriction of vector M^i on the subset g by setting $M_j^i = 0$ for $j \neq g$.

According to [13], $\|M_{\mathcal{G}^k}^i\|_{2,1}^2$ is sparseness inducing and it encourages exclusive selection of features at the level of group $g \in \mathcal{G}^k$. Hence, for each feature i, it tends to assign larger weights to some important groups while assigning small or even zero weights to the other groups. Different from the *Exclusive Group Lasso Regularizer* that describes the negative correlation among tasks, the *Graph Laplacian*

Regularizer models the positive correlation among tasks by transferring the weight information among multiple ocular diseases.

2.2   Solution

The objective $\Theta(M)$ in (2) is convex but non-smooth since all the three components are convex whereas the *Exclusive Group Lasso Regularizer* $\Gamma(M)$ is non-smooth. The non-smooth structure of $\Gamma(M)$ makes the optimization of problem $\min_M \{\Theta(M)\}$ a non-trivial task. The subgradient method as used in [13] is applicable but it typically ignores the structure of the problem and suffers from a slow rate of convergence. As indicated in [14], the optimization can be achieved by approximating the original non-smooth objective by a smooth function, and then solving the latter by utilizing some off-the-shelf fast algorithms. Here, we introduce a Nesterov-like smoothing optimization method [3] to achieve this purpose. Once the optimal parameter M^* is obtained, the multiple diseases labels of a test fundus image with feature x are learned by $y = M^*x$. The whole algorithm of the proposed feature selection and multiple diseases detection is described in Algorithm 1.

For any vector $z \in \mathbb{R}^n$, its ℓ_2-norm $\|z\|_2$ has a max-structure representation $\|z\|_2 = \max_{\|v\|_2 \le 1}\langle z, v \rangle$. Based on this simple property and the smoothing approximation techniques originally from [3], function $\Gamma(M)$ can be approximated by the following smooth function:

$$\Gamma_\delta(M) = \frac{1}{2}\sum_{i=1}^{d}\left(z_{\mathcal{G}^1,\delta}^2(M^i) + z_{\mathcal{G}^2,\delta}^2(M^i)\right), \tag{3}$$

where $z_{\mathcal{G}^k,\delta}(M^i) := \max_{\|V_{\mathcal{G}^k}^{i,k}\|_{2,\infty} \le 1}\langle M^i, V^{i,k} \rangle - \frac{\delta}{2}\|V^{i,k}\|_2^2$, and δ is a parameter to control the approximation accuracy. We use the following Theorem [10] to show that $\Gamma_\delta(M)$ is differentiable and its gradient can be easily calculated.

Algorithm 1. Discriminative Feature Selection for Multiple Ocular Diseases Detection

---

Input: Feature matrix of training data $X \in \mathbb{R}^{d \times n}$, diseases label matrix $Y \in \mathbb{R}^{|\mathcal{L}| \times d}$, groups $\mathcal{G}^1$ and $\mathcal{G}^2$, parameters μ, η, δ.
Output: Learned feature selection matrix $M^t \in \mathbb{R}^{|\mathcal{L}| \times d}$
Initialization: Initialize M_0, V_0 and let $\alpha_0 \leftarrow 1$, $t \leftarrow 0$.
repeat
    $U_t = (1 - \alpha_t)M_t + \alpha_t V_t$,
    Calculate $\nabla\Gamma_\delta(U_t)$ based on (4), (5), and obtain L_δ according to (6).
    $V_{t+1} = V_t - \frac{1}{\alpha_t L_\delta}\left(-(Y - MX)X^T + \mu\nabla\Gamma_\delta(U_t) + \eta L_\delta M\right)$,
    $M_{t+1} = (1 - \alpha_t)M_t + \alpha_t V_{t+1}$,
    $\alpha_{t+1} = \frac{2}{t+1}$, $t \leftarrow t + 1$.
until Convergence

Table 1. The Baseline Algorithms.

Name	Methods
KNN	k-Nearest Neighbors
SVM	Support Vector Machine
LNP	Linear Neighborhood Propagation [10]
MTL	Naive Multi-task Learning in (1)
SPM	State-of-the-art algorithm for PM Detection [4]
SAMD	State-of-the-art algorithm for AMD Detection [15]
SGL	State-of-the-art algorithm for Glaucoma Detection [2]
GRML	State-of-the-art algorithm for Multiple Ocular Diseases Detection [7]

Theorem 1. *Function $\Gamma_\delta(M)$ is well defined, convex and continuously differentiable with gradient*

$$\nabla \Gamma_\delta(M) = \left[\nabla \Gamma_\delta(M^1), ..., \nabla \Gamma_\delta(M^d) \right], \tag{4}$$

where for $i = 1, ..., d$,

$$\nabla \Gamma_\delta(M^i) = q_{\mathcal{G}^1,\delta}(M^i)V^{i,1}(M^i) + q_{\mathcal{G}^2,\delta}(M^i)V^{i,2}(M^i). \tag{5}$$

Moreover, $\nabla \Gamma_\delta(M)$ is Lipschitz continuous with the constant

$$L_\delta = \left(\frac{2\sqrt{2}R}{\delta} + |\mathcal{L}^1|^2 + |\mathcal{L}^2|^2 \right) d. \tag{6}$$

3   Experiments

3.1   Dataset and Evaluation Criteria

We conduct the experiments on the SiMES dataset [12], in which the detection of Glaucoma, AMD, and PM have been made by clinicians. We choose a subset of SiMES for experiments, which contains 2,258 subjects. In this subset dataset, there are 100 with glaucoma, 122 with AMD, and 58 with PM. For each disease, the distribution of the subjects who contracted the disease in the selected dataset is representative of the disease prevalence in the population. We extract three different types of visual features (popular global and local features as adopted in [7]) for conducting experiments, and study the performance of the proposed approach with a total of four settings: 1) global features; 2) grid-based features; 3) bag of words; 4) global features + grid-based features + bag of words. The notation + indicates a combination of four types of features in the corresponding setting. We utilize the area under the curve (AUC) of the receiver operation characteristic curve (ROC) to evaluate the performance of classification.

3.2   Experiment Analysis

In order to evaluate the performance of our proposed algorithm, we provide a quantitative study on SiMES, with an emphasis on the comparison with eight state-of-the-art related methods as listed in Table 1. Below are the parameters and the adopted values for each method:

- For the SVM algorithm, we adopt the RBF kernel. For its two parameters γ and C, we set $\gamma = 0.6$ and $C = 1$ in the experiments after fine tuning.
- For KNN, there is only one parameter k for tuning, which stands for the number of nearest neighbors and is set to 150.
- For SGL, SPM, SAMD and GRML, we use the same settings as in their papers.
- For our proposed approach, we set $|\mathcal{L}^1| = 3$ and $|\mathcal{L}^2| = 1$ because the selected dataset lacks ground truth labels of the sub-types of each ocular disease for each fundus image. For the control parameters, we set $\mu = 0.5$, $\eta = 0.2$,

The AUCs of the baseline methods for detecting the three leading ocular diseases on the SiMES dataset are illustrated in Table 2. The combined visual features (global features + grid-based features + bag of words) are utilized for

Table 2. The AUCs of different algorithms for simultaneously detecting Glaucoma, PM and AMD on the SiMES dataset. The combined visual features (global features + grid-based features + bag of words) are utilized by the eight baseline methods. The AUC results marked in boldface are significantly better than the others.

Methods	KNN	SVM	LNP	MTL	SGL	SPM	SAMD	GRML	Our Proposed
Glaucoma	74.2 %	76.7 %	78.8%	80.0%	81.0%	-	-	82.5%	**85.3%**
PM	86.5 %	89.1 %	90.1%	90.6%	-	91.0%	-	92.3%	**94.4%**
AMD	72.9 %	75.0%	76.6%	77.0%	-	-	77.8%	79.3%	**81.8%**

Table 3. The AUCs of different algorithms under four settings of features on the SiMES dataset for Glaucoma diagnosis. The AUC results marked in boldface are significantly better than the others.

Methods	KNN	SVM	LNP	MTL	GRML	Our Proposed
Global Features	71.2 %	73.5 %	75.2%	77.5%	78.7%	79.6%
Grid based Features	69.1 %	71.2 %	73.0%	75.4%	76.7%	78.0%
Bag of Words	68.4 %	70.9%	72.6%	73.9%	75.0%	76.6%
Combined Features	**74.2 %**	**76.7%**	**78.8 %**	**80.0%**	**82.5%**	**85.3%**

Table 4. The AUCs of different algorithms under three settings of features on the SiMES dataset for AMD diagnosis. The AUC results marked in boldface are significantly better than the others.

Methods	KNN	SVM	LNP	MTL	GRML	Our Proposed
Global Features	70.2 %	72.5%	73.9 %	75.0%	76.4%	76.9%
Grid based Features	69.3 %	71.8 %	72.5%	73.8%	75.1%	75.8%
Bag of Words	68.1 %	70.3%	71.6%	72.1%	73.5%	74.9%
Combined Features	**72.9 %**	**75.0%**	**76.6 %**	**77.0%**	**79.3%**	**81.8%**

Table 5. The AUCs of different algorithms under three settings of features on the SiMES dataset for PM diagnosis. The AUC results marked in boldface are significantly better than the others.

Methods	KNN	SVM	LNP	MTL	GRML	Our Proposed
Global Features	81.5 %	84.1%	85.6 %	86.4%	87.3%	89.1%
Grid based Features	79.3 %	82.3 %	83.7%	84.2%	85.2%	87.3%
Bag of Words	83.8 %	86.5%	87.9%	88.4%	89.5%	91.6%
Combined Features	**86.5 %**	**89.1%**	**90.1 %**	**90.6%**	**92.3%**	**94.4%**

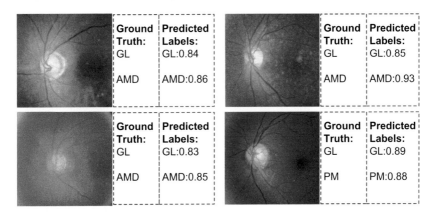

Fig. 2. Sample diagnosis results from our proposed algorithm.

all methods in this experiment. Our proposed algorithm performs the feature selection on the combined visual features, which outperforms the other baseline algorithms significantly. For example, our proposed method has an improvement of 11.2% over SVM, 15.0% over KNN, and 8.2% over LNP for detecting Glaucoma. For PM, our proposed method has an improvement of 5.9% over SVM, 9.1% over KNN, and 4.2% over LNP. For AMD, Ours has an improvement of 9.1% over SVM, 12.2% over KNN, and 6.8% over LNP. Compared with the state-of-the-art algorithms of individual disease detection, the proposed method outperforms SGL, SPM, and SAMD by achieving an AUC of 85.3%, 94.4%, 81.8%, respectively. The improvement stems from the fact that our proposed algorithm encodes the exclusive group lasso regularization for competitive sparse feature selection, and the graph Laplacian regularization to impose the correlations among multiple ocular diseases. GRML considers inter-label constraints but does not model the exact correlations of diseases in the objective formulation. Moreover, GRML is based on genetic features and is not able to select discriminative features for each disease.

The comparison results for detection performance under the four feature settings are listed in Table 3, 4, 5. Since the state-of-the-art detection algorithms (SGL, SPM, SAMD) of individual ocular diseases are based on their own special visual features and retinal structures, the AUC results are not given in these tables. From Table 3, we are able to observe that, for glaucoma detection, our proposed algorithm outperforms the five baseline algorithms based on the combined features. The AUC of the receiver operating characteristic curve in glaucoma detection is 85.3%. Similar results are shown in Table 4 and 5 for AMD and PM detection respectively. Figure 2 gives four sample results by our proposed algorithm. Each fundus image is presented with the ground truth diagnosed by clinicians and the predicted labels with probabilities by our algorithm. GL stands for Glaucoma. Though the second row has low image quality, our method still detects the glaucoma, PM, and AMD, indicating its robustness and stability.

4   Conclusion

In this paper, we develop a discriminative feature selection scheme for multiple ocular diseases classification. We formulate this challenging problem as a multi-task discriminative analysis model, where individual tasks are defined by learning the linear discriminative model for each disease. We considered all the tasks in a joint manner by utilizing two types of regularization on parameters, namely the graph Laplacian regularization and exclusive group lasso regularization. A Nesterov-type smoothing approximation method is adopted for model optimization. In the future, we will attach a few sub-categories to each category of the three leading ocular diseases to expand our classification range.

References

1. Quigley, H.A., Broman, A.T.: The number of people with glaucoma worldwide in 2010 and 2020. Br. J. Ophthalmol. 90(3), 262–267 (2006)
2. Xu, Y., Lin, S., Wong, D.W.K., Liu, J., Xu, D.: Efficient reconstruction-based optic cup localization for glaucoma screening. In: Mori, K., Sakuma, I., Sato, Y., Barillot, C., Navab, N. (eds.) MICCAI 2013, Part III. LNCS, vol. 8151, pp. 445–452. Springer, Heidelberg (2013)
3. Nesterov, Y.: Smooth minimization of non-smooth functions. Mathematical Programming 103(1), 127–152 (2005)
4. Xu, Y., Liu, J., Zhang, Z., Tan, N.M., Wong, D.W.K., Saw, S.M., Wong, T.Y.: Learn to recognize pathological myopia in fundus images using bag-of-feature and sparse learning approach. In: International Symposium on Biomedical Imaging (2013)
5. Yuan, X., Yan, S.: Visual classification with multi-task joint sparse representation. In: Computer Vision and Pattern Recognition (CVPR) (2010)
6. Bressler, N.M., Bressler, S.B., Fine, S.L.: Age-related macular degeneration. Survey of Ophthalmology 32(6), 375–413 (1988)
7. Chen, X., Xu, Y., Duan, L., Zhang, Z., Wong, D.W.K., Liu, J.: Multiple ocular diseases detection by graph regularized multi-label learning. In: Proceedings of the Ophthalmic Medical Image Analysis First International Workshop (OMIA) Held in Conjunction with MICCAI (2014)

8. Avetisov, S.E., Erichev, V.P., Budzinskaia, M.V., Karpilova, M.A., Gurova, I.V., Shchegoleva, I.V., Chikun, E.A.: Age-related macular degeneration and glaucoma: intraocular pressure monitoring after intravitreal injections. Vestn. Oftalmol. 128(6), 3–5 (2012)
9. Pan, C.W., Cheung, C.Y., Aung, T., Cheung, C.M., Zheng, Y.F., Wu, R.Y., Mitchell, P., Lavanya, R., Baskaran, M., Wang, J.J., Wong, T.Y., Saw, S.M.: Differential associations of myopia with major age-related eye diseases: the Singapore Indian Eye Study. Ophthalmol. 20(2), 284–291 (2013)
10. Chen, X., Yuan, X., Yan, S., Tang, J., Rui, Y., Chua, T.-S.: Towards multi-semantic image annotation with graph regularized exclusive group lasso. In: ACM Multimedia (2011)
11. Xu, Y., Duan, L., Lin, S., Chen, X., Wong, D.W.K., Wong, T.Y., Liu, J.: Optic cup segmentation for glaucoma detection using low-rank superpixel representation. In: Golland, P., Hata, N., Barillot, C., Hornegger, J., Howe, R. (eds.) MICCAI 2014, Part I. LNCS, vol. 8673, pp. 788–795. Springer, Heidelberg (2014)
12. Foong, A.W.P., Saw, S.M., Loo, J.L., Shen, S., Loon, S.C., Rosman, M., Aung, T., Tan, D.T.H., Tai, E.S., Wong, T.Y.: Rationale and methodology for a population-based study of eye diseases in Malay people: The Singapore Malay eye study (SiMES). Ophthalmic Epidemiology 14(1), 25–35 (2007)
13. Zhou, Y., Jin, R., Hoi, S.C.: Exclusive lasso for multi-task feature selection. In: International Conference on Artificial Intelligence and Statistics (AISTATS) (2010)
14. Chen, X., Yuan, X., Chen, Q., Yan, S., Chua, T.-S.: Multi-label visual classification with label exclusive context. In: International Conference on Computer Vision (ICCV) (2011)
15. Wong, D.W.K., Liu, J., Cheng, X., Zhang, J., Yin, F., Bhargava, M., Cheung, C.M.G., Wong, T.Y.: THALIA - An automatic hierarchical analysis system to detect drusen lesion images for amd assessment. In: ISBI, pp. 884–887 (2013)

Detection of Glands and Villi by Collaboration of Domain Knowledge and Deep Learning*

Jiazhuo Wang[1], John D. MacKenzie[2],
Rageshree Ramachandran[3], and Danny Z. Chen[1]

[1] Department of Computer Science & Engineering, University of Notre Dame, USA
[2] Department of Radiology & Biomedical Imaging, UCSF, USA
[3] Department of Pathology, UCSF, USA

Abstract. Architecture distortions of glands and villi are indication of chronic inflammation. However, the "duality" nature of these two structures causes lots of ambiguity for their detection in H&E histology tissue images, especially when multiple instances are clustered together. Based on the observation that once such an object is detected for certain, the ambiguity in the neighborhood of the detected object can be reduced considerably, we propose to combine deep learning and domain knowledge in a unified framework, to simultaneously detect (the closely related) glands and villi in H&E histology tissue images. Our method iterates between exploring domain knowledge and performing deep learning classification, and the two components benefit from each other. (1) By exploring domain knowledge, the generated object proposals (to be fed to deep learning) form a more complete coverage of the true objects and the segmentation of object proposals can be more accurate, thus improving deep learning's performance on classification. (2) Deep learning can help verify the class of each object proposal, and provide feedback to repeatedly "refresh" and enhance domain knowledge so that more reliable object proposals can be generated later on. Experiments on clinical data validate our ideas and show that our method improves the state-of-the-art for gland detection in H&E histology tissue images (to our best knowledge, we are not aware of any method for villi detection).

1   Introduction

Architecture distortions of glands and villi are strong signs of chronic inflammation [9]. Also, a quantitative measurement of the degree of such distortions may help determine the severity of the chronic inflammation. A crucial step towards these goals is the ability to detect accurately these two biological structures.

As shown in Fig. 1(a)-(b), both glands and villi are actually composed of the same structure: epithelium. A gland encloses lumen and is surrounded by extracellular material, while a villus encloses extracellular material but is surrounded

---

* This research was supported in part by NSF Grant CCF-1217906, a grant of the National Academies Keck Futures Initiative (NAKFI), and NIH grant K08-AR061412-02 Molecular Imaging for Detection and Treatment Monitoring of Arthritis.

N. Navab et al. (Eds.): MICCAI 2015, Part II, LNCS 9350, pp. 20–27, 2015.
DOI: 10.1007/978-3-319-24571-3_3

by lumen. In H&E histology tissue images, the detection challenges of glands and villi are mainly due to such "duality" of the two structures (especially when multiple instances are clustered together), as well as the complex tissue background (containing different biological structures, e.g., different types of cells, connective tissue, etc), and the variable appearances of glands and villi due to morphology, staining, and scale.

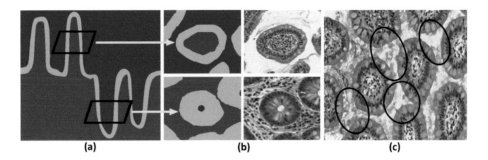

Fig. 1. (a) A 3-D illustration of the dual glands and villi: Villi (top) are evagination of epithelium (green) into lumen (blue), and glands (bottom) are invagination of epithelium into extracellular material (red); (b) histology tissue images are 2-D slices of the 3-D structures; (c) some areas (black circles) that may cause false positives of glands.

Some methods [4,8,10] were proposed for glands detection in H&E histology tissue images, which used a similar framework: (1) Find lumen regions; (2) for each lumen region, perform a region-growing like process to find the epithelium enclosing the lumen which is considered as the boundary of a gland. Applying such a method in the presence of villi clusters could generate many false positives for glands, because a lumen region among different villi may be found in the first step, and then the epithelium regions bounding these villi may be taken incorrectly as the boundaries of a gland enclosing the lumen (see Fig. 1(c)). Also, due to certain slicing angles for the images, the lumen regions inside some glands may not be very obvious; thus, this methodology may tend to produce false negatives for such glands. A recent glands detection method [2] was proposed for H-DAB images, and it also did not consider the influence of the dual villi. To our best knowledge, we are not aware of any previous work on detecting villi.

In this paper, we propose to combine domain knowledge and deep learning to simultaneously detect glands and villi (since they are closely related) in H&E histology tissue images. Our method is based on the observation that once we detect an object (of some class, i.e., glands or villi) for certain, we can propagate this information to the neighborhood of the detected object, so that the detection ambiguity nearby is reduced. The main steps of our method are as follows.

(1) We extract (pseudo-)probability maps (PPMs) for possible candidates of the target objects, by using domain knowledge on the appearances of glands and villi. (2) Using PPMs, we generate object proposals and feed them to deep

convolutional neural networks (CNN) [6], to verify whether each object is really of the class claimed by PPMs (reflecting domain knowledge). (3) If the object proposals pass the verification, then we update PPMs (essentially, propagating the information that we have detected some objects for certain), so that new object proposals can be generated using the updated domain knowledge. We repeat the last two steps until no more object can be detected for certain.

Our work shows that the close collaboration between domain knowledge and deep learning allows multiple instances of glands and villi to be detected effectively. Experimental results (summarized in Table 1) on clinical data validate our ideas and show that we improve the state-of-the-art for glands detection.

2   Methodology

2.1   Extraction of (Pseudo-)Probability Maps

Each histology tissue slide may contain multiple instances of glands and villi, possibly in different scales. Thus, the first step of our method aims to initially extract (pseudo-)probability maps (PPMs) that contain information of both the locations and scales for all objects of the two target classes (glands and villi). We will generate object proposals based on the PPMs in the next step. Our main idea for this step is to conduct a generalized Hough transform voting process.

This idea is based on two considerations after exploring domain knowledge of the appearances of glands and villi. (I) Each epithelium region suggests that a target object is nearby, but its class (i.e., gland or villus), location, and scale are not yet clear, at least from the perspective of this single epithelium region. (II) A more clear and complete picture of all objects could be obtained after each epithelium region votes (based on its own view). This is because, collectively, true positives of objects are more likely to receive more votes from such epithelium regions. Our idea and steps are discussed in more detail below.

(1) We first obtain a superpixel segmentation [1] (Fig. 2(b)) of the image. We then classify each superpixel as epithelium, lumen, or extracellular material (since they are all related to the appearances of glands and villi), using Random Forest and hand-crafted features (e.g., colors, texture based on Gabor filters).

(2) Since each epithelium superpixel suggests that a target object is nearby, it would vote for some points in a 4-D object voting space (voting process is illustrated below), where each dimension corresponds to a factor of each single object, i.e., its class (glands or villi), x and y coordinates in the image, and scale (we empirically use 8 scales corresponding to roughly $S=\{0.011, 0.014, 0.025, 0.05, 0.067, 0.111, 0.167, 0.25\}$ times LS, the length of the shorter side of the image).

(2.a) We first find the lumen (LM) and extracellular material (EM) within a distance of $d = S(i) \times LS$ from this epithelium superpixel (ES), if any. (2.b) For each class and each scale, we map the ES to some locations, based on the following observation for choosing the mapping/voting direction (which narrows down the voting space to be covered): If the ES is part of a gland, then the gland is likely to lie on the same side as LM, but on the opposite side from EM (found in (2.a) near this ES); if it is actually part of a villus, then due to the "duality"

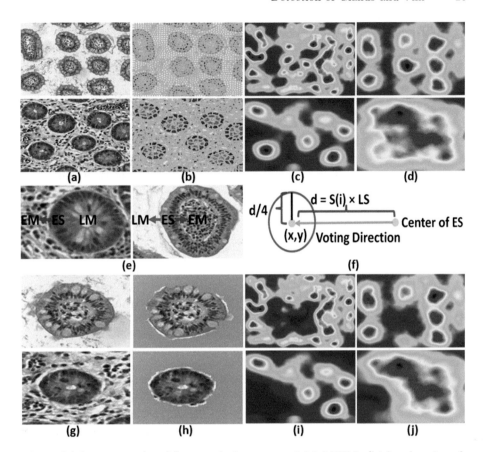

Fig. 2. (a) Image samples; (b) superpixel segments; initial PPMs (high values in red; low values in blue) for respectively glands (c) and villi (d) at a single scale; (e) blue and red arrows are voting directions for glands and villi, respectively; (f) the voted points in a circle (blue) by an ES at a single scale for one class; (g) image patches containing detected objects (the presented villus (top) is around the center of the top image in (a), and the presented gland (bottom) is at the bottom left of the bottom image in (a)); (h) image patches with background masked out; updated PPMs for respectively glands (i) and villi (j) at a single scale, after the information of the objects in (g) detected is propagated to the neighborhood (note the changes of the (pseudo-)probability values around the detected objects).

of glands and villi, the villus is likely to lie on the same side as EM, but on the opposite side from LM (see Fig. 2(e)). More specifically, the ES would vote for the points in a circle (of a radius $d/4$) centered at the (x, y) coordinates, which are of a distance d away from the center of the ES, towards the chosen directions accordingly, for respectively glands and villi, and the 8 scales (see Fig. 2(f)).

(3) We view the corresponding 3-D hyper-plane w.r.t. to the class dimension in the built 4-D voting space as the initial PPMs of each class, containing the location and scale information for the candidate objects (see Fig. 2(c)-(d)).

2.2   Object Proposals Generation and Class Verification

Overview. This step aims to make sure that detected objects are indeed true positive objects, so that in the next step, we would not propagate wrong information to their neighborhoods for resolving ambiguity. We first apply graph search [5] (which uses high level priors) to conduct segmentation for object proposals (generated based on PPMs), and then feed two small image patches containing the same object proposal (with or without the background masked out) to respectively **two** convolutional neural networks (CNN) with the same architecture, to verify whether the class of that object proposal is the one claimed by PPMs.

The observation that object proposals generated using domain knowledge can help CNN is critical. (1) If being blind to domain knowledge (e.g., in [3,11,6]), many true objects might be missed by the generated object proposals. Thus, during training, CNN cannot well model the target objects; during testing, false negatives can be produced. (2) Although the segmented form of object proposals at the pixel level can help improve CNN's performance on object classification [6], segmentation in [6] is done in a bottom-up fashion, using only low level image cues. Based on which class of the PPMs (reflecting domain knowledge) that an object proposal is generated from, we can obtain more accurate segmentation in a top-down fashion, by utilizing class-specific high level semantic priors.

CNN Training. For every class, we find, in the corresponding **initial** PPM, each local maximum point above a certain threshold as one object proposal, and perform graph search based segmentation for it. If the segmented foreground region R_{Seg} and a manually marked ground truth object region R_{GT} of that class satisfy $\frac{|R_{Seg} \cap R_{GT}|}{|R_{Seg}|} > 0.6$ and $\frac{|R_{Seg} \cap R_{GT}|}{|R_{GT}|} > 0.6$, then we take the object proposal as a positive training example of that class; otherwise, a negative one. Note the relatively high overlap threshold 0.6 is to make trained CNN be conservative so that false positives are less likely to pass CNN verification during testing.

We crop a small image patch containing the object proposal, warp it to 256×256 pixels, and use in training one CNN. We further mask out the background region in it by the mean values of all training image patches (see Fig. 2(g)-(h)), and use it in training the other CNN. Our two CNNs have the same architecture and are trained using the same learning algorithm as [7]; we also apply data augmentation and drop out to reduce overfitting as [7].

Note CNN once trained using **initial** PPMs, will be used in all rest iterations.

CNN Testing. During CNN testing, we also perform graph search based segmentation for each object proposal (generated using the **current** PPMs, as described in detail below), and feed the two image patches (with or without background masked out) to respectively the two CNNs. We use the average probabilities output by the two CNNs to predict the class. Once an object proposal is verified by CNNs as a true positive for either glands or villi (i.e., the prediction result is not a non-object), we will propagate this information to the neighborhood regions by updating the PPMs (to be described in Section 2.3). We stop the algorithm if CNN cannot verify any true object.

Since during the testing, the PPMs change dynamically as more and more object proposals pass the verification by CNNs, and object proposals are generated based on the new versions of PPMs after update, we need to determine what would be an appropriate order to generate and process object proposals. One possible order is of a greedy and one-by-one fashion: Each time, we find a point with the **largest** (pseudo-)probability value in current PPMs, verify the corresponding object proposal by CNNs, and update PPMs if necessary.

Another possible way is of a batch fashion: Each time, we generate a batch of object proposals, verify all of them by CNNs, and update PPMs if necessary. Of course, object proposals generated within the same batch should not be closely related to one another (otherwise, we may have conflicting information to propagate subsequently). We formulate the problem of finding a non-conflicting batch as computing a *maximal weighted independent set* (MWIS) in a vertex weighted graph G, constructed as follows: Each vertex of G is for a local maximal point above a certain threshold in the PPM of either class; connect two vertices by an edge if the (x, y) coordinates of one vertex in the image are within 2 times the scale of those of the other vertex; the weight of each vertex is the (pseudo-)probability value of the corresponding point. (Hence, we may view MWIS as being partially greedy.)

Graph Search. We apply graph search [5] to segment each object proposal. We utilize various category-specific high level semantic priors to construct the needed input for graph search, as follows. We use the scale information of each object proposal to set the lengths of the re-sampling rays and the geometric smoothness constraint. We simply apply distance transform to the border pixels between detected epithelium and extracellular material (resp., lumen) to set up on-boundary cost of glands (resp., villi). We simply set in-region cost for glands (resp., villi) to be low for pixels inside epithelium or lumen (resp., extracellular material), and high for pixels inside extracellular material (resp., lumen). Note better segmentation may be obtained with more sophisticated cost functions.

2.3   Information Propagation

This step aims to propagate the information that an object, Obj, is detected, so that the detection ambiguity in its neighborhood is reduced. This is why we generate object proposals dynamically (to take advantage of the reduced ambiguity) instead of all in one-shot as in [3,11,6]. Our idea is to update PPMs (see Fig. 2(i)-(j)) which are used to generate new object proposals. Specifically, for the segmented foreground region of Obj, R_{Obj}, we find each epithelium superpixel (ES) such that its region R_{ES} satisfies $\frac{|R_{ES} \cap R_{Obj}|}{|R_{ES}|} > 0.8$ and $\frac{|R_{ES} \cap R_{Obj}|}{|R_{Obj}|} > 0.8$. Since these ESs are quite unlikely to be part of other target objects, we remove their votes for all points that they have voted for in the 4-D voting space, thus resulting in new PPMs, with the information of Obj's detection being incorporated and propagated.

3 Experiments and Discussions

We collected clinical H&E histology tissue slides (scanned at 40X magnification) from patients suspected of having inflammatory bowl disease (the study was performed under an IRB and in compliance with the privacy provisions of HIPPA of 1996). We manually marked 1376 glands and 313 villi and their boundaries as ground truth. We used 2-fold cross validation (CNN training for each fold takes a week on a single CPU) to evaluate the performance using three metrics, $precision = \frac{TP}{TP+FP}$, $recall = \frac{TP}{TP+FN}$, and $Fscore = \frac{2 \times precision \times recall}{precision + recall}$. A detected object is counted as TP if its segmented foreground region R_{Seg} and a ground truth region R_{GT} (not corresponding to any other detected object) satisfy $\frac{|R_{Seg} \cap R_{GT}|}{|R_{Seg}|} > 0.6$ and $\frac{|R_{Seg} \cap R_{GT}|}{|R_{GT}|} > 0.6$; otherwise, it is counted as FP. If a ground truth region corresponds to no detected object, it is counted as FN.

Table 1. Quantitative performance of different methods.

	Precision		Recall		F score	
	Glands	Villi	Glands	Villi	Glands	Villi
DK-Only	0.79	0.73	0.75	0.86	0.77	0.79
CNN-Only	0.82	0.71	0.69	0.81	0.75	0.76
DK-CNN-Greedy	0.95	0.94	0.80	0.85	0.87	0.89
DK-CNN-MWIS	0.96	0.95	0.78	0.79	0.86	0.86
Glands-Detect [10]	0.42	-	0.54	-	0.47	-

To validate the key ideas we proposed, we construct several versions of our method (DK-Only, CNN-Only, DK-CNN-Greedy, and DK-CNN-MWIS), by either simply taking away or replacing by alternatives some important components of our method, as follows. DK-Only depends only on exploring domain knowledge (i.e., we take away the CNN verification) to detect objects. In CNN-Only, all object proposals and their segmentation are generated in one-shot, in a bottom-up fashion, and being blind to domain knowledge as in [6]; instead of dynamically and in a top-down fashion by exploring domain knowledge. We use the greedy fashion to address the object proposals during testing in these two versions. DK-CNN-Greedy uses both domain knowledge and CNN, and is based on the greedy fashion. DK-CNN-MWIS also uses both domain knowledge and CNN, but is based on the maximal weighted independent set approach.

Table 1 shows the quantitative performance of these four versions and the state-of-the-art glands detection method [10] (referred to as Glands-Detect). One can see the following points. (1) The two complete versions DK-CNN-Greedy and DK-CNN-MWIS perform much better than DK-Only, indicating that CNN is suitable for the verification task on object detection, which reduces the amount of incorrect information propagated to the neighborhoods to resolve ambiguity. (2) These two complete versions also outperform CNN-Only, indicating that it is better to dynamically generate object proposals and their segmentation, based on the gradually "refreshed" domain knowledge, than generating them all at once and being blind to suggestions of domain knowledge. (3) Combining the above two points, it shows that the close collaboration between domain knowledge and deep learning can effectively detect multiple instances of glands and villi. (4) DK-CNN-Greedy and DK-CNN-MWIS perform similarly well. This means that generating object proposals in a greedy or batch fashion (partially greedy) is not quite critical, as long as domain knowledge and the power of deep learning are fully explored. (5) Glands-Detect does not use an appropriate verification scheme to address the situation when villi, with a dual structure (causing lots of ambiguity), are also present in the images; it requires lumen regions inside glands to be obvious, and thus does not perform well on our images. (6) All four versions of our method have a higher precision than recall, this is because we use relatively high overlap thresholds. We plan to do complete ROC analysis by varying overlap thresholds.

References

1. Achanta, R., Shaji, A., Smith, K., Lucchi, A., Fua, P., Susstrunk, S.: Slic superpixels compared to state-of-the-art superpixel methods. IEEE Trans. Pattern Anal. Mach. Intell. 34(11), 2274–2282 (2012)
2. Fu, H., Qiu, G., Shu, J., Ilyas, M.: A novel polar space random field model for the detection of glandular structures. IEEE Trans. Med. Imaging 33, 764–776 (2014)
3. Girshick, R.B., Donahue, J., Darrell, T., Malik, J.: Rich feature hierarchies for accurate object detection and semantic segmentation. In: CVPR, pp. 580–587 (2013)
4. Gunduz-Demir, C., Kandemir, M., Tosun, A.B., Sokmensuer, C.: Automatic segmentation of colon glands using object-graph. Medical Image Analysis 14(1) (2010)
5. Haeker, M., Wu, X., Abràmoff, M.D., Kardon, R., Sonka, M.: Incorporation of regional information in optimal 3-D graph search with application for intraretinal layer segmentation of optical coherence tomography images. In: Karssemeijer, N., Lelieveldt, B. (eds.) IPMI 2007. LNCS, vol. 4584, pp. 607–618. Springer, Heidelberg (2007)
6. Hariharan, B., Arbeláez, P., Girshick, R., Malik, J.: Simultaneous detection and segmentation. In: Fleet, D., Pajdla, T., Schiele, B., Tuytelaars, T. (eds.) ECCV 2014, Part VII. LNCS, vol. 8695, pp. 297–312. Springer, Heidelberg (2014)
7. Krizhevsky, A., Sutskever, I., Hinton, G.E.: ImageNet classification with deep convolutional neural networks. In: NIPS, pp. 1106–1114 (2012)
8. Naik, S., Doyle, S., Feldman, M., Tomaszewski, J., Madabhushi, A.: Gland segmentation and computerized gleason grading of prostate histology by integrating low-, high-level and domain specific information. In: MIAAB (2007)
9. Naini, B.V., Cortina, G.: A histopathologic scoring system as a tool for standardized reporting of chronic (ileo) colitis and independent risk assessment for inflammatory bowel disease. Human Pathology 43, 2187–2196 (2012)
10. Nguyen, K., Sarkar, A., Jain, A.K.: Structure and context in prostatic gland segmentation and classification. In: Ayache, N., Delingette, H., Golland, P., Mori, K. (eds.) MICCAI 2012, Part I. LNCS, vol. 7510, pp. 115–123. Springer, Heidelberg (2012)
11. Sermanet, P., Eigen, D., Zhang, X., Mathieu, M., Fergus, R., LeCun, Y.: Overfeat: Integrated recognition, localization and detection using convolutional networks. In: ICLR (2014)

Minimum S-Excess Graph for Segmenting and Tracking Multiple Borders with HMM*

Ehab Essa, Xianghua Xie**, and Jonathan-Lee Jones

Department of Computer Science, Swansea University, UK
x.xie@swan.ac.uk

Abstract. We present a novel HMM based approach to simultaneous segmentation of vessel walls in Lymphatic confocal images. The vessel borders are parameterized using RBFs to minimize the number of tracking points. The proposed method tracks the hidden states that indicate border locations for both the inner and outer walls. The observation for both borders is obtained using edge-based features from steerable filters. Two separate Gaussian probability distributions for the vessel borders and background are used to infer the emission probability, and the transmission probability is learned using a Baum-Welch algorithm. We transform the segmentation problem into a minimization of an s-excess graph cost, with each node in the graph corresponding to a hidden state and the weight for each node being defined by its emission probability. We define the inter-relations between neighboring nodes based on the transmission probability. We present both qualitative and quantitative analysis in comparison to the popular Viterbi algorithm.

1 Introduction

Tracking object contour is usually carried out for complex and nonrigid shapes where a contour provides more accurate representation than a bounding box. In this paper, we propose a hidden Markov model (HMM) based approach to track lymphatic anatomical borders over the cross-sectional images in order to achieve coherent segmentations in 3D. HMM is a stochastic model in which the Markov property is assumed to be satisfied in a finite set of states and these states are hidden. Many applications have demonstrated the advantages of HMM in dealing with time-varying series, such as [3,4,14]. In [11], the authors used HMM to detect abnormal local wall motion in stress echocardiography. In [5], HMM is used in conjunction with a particle filter to track hand motion. The particle filter is used to estimate the hand region that is most likely to appear. HMM estimates the hand shape using the Viterbi algorithm where the hidden state is a set of quantized pre-learned exemplars. However, the number of exemplars can grow exponentially depending on the complexity of the object. In [2], the authors

---

* The project is funded by NISCHR MIAV-BRU. E. Essa was funded by Swansea University as a PhD student and NISCHR as a postdoc, and he is also affiliated with Mansoura University, Egypt.
** Corresponding author.

N. Navab et al. (Eds.): MICCAI 2015, Part II, LNCS 9350, pp. 28–35, 2015.
DOI: 10.1007/978-3-319-24571-3_4

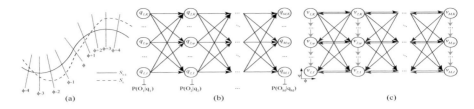

Fig. 1. (a) an illustration of segmenting border S_t based on S_{t-1}. The border is divided into M points with RBF interpolation and at each point a normal line is drawn with length K. (b) conventional HMM construction. (c) proposed HMM construction.

used the Kalman filter with pseudo 2-dimensional HMM to perform tracking. The Viterbi algorithm is used to find the best sequence of states to perform object and background classification. However, this system becomes increasingly more complex and time-consuming with the increase of object size. In [3,4], the authors incorporated region and edge features in HMM. The contour is sampled as a set of discrete points, and the features are extracted along the normal direction at each contour point. An ellipse is fitted to the contour and the unscented Kalman filter is used for tracking. Sargin *et al.* [14] extended the work to deal with variable length open contours and investigated using arc emission instead of traditional state emission in defining the observational probabilities for the HMM. Notably, Viterbi algorithm is commonly used to find the best sequence of hidden states. However, the search process can be hampered by occlusions in the image where the emission probability is not reliable and transition probability does not guarantee smooth transition of the border. Moreover, the Viterbi algorithm cannot handle the case when starting and ending points are the same. Nor does it work well to simultaneously search multiple borders.

In this paper, we propose a multi-border segmentation and tracking method based on HMM, and we demonstrate the technique through simultaneously delineating the inner and outer borders in lymphatic vessel images that are corrupted by noise, intensity inhomogeneity and occlusions. A new optimization method is proposed to find the optimal sequence of the hidden states based on the minimization of an s-excess graph. Instead of using the traditional Viterbi algorithm, we transform the problem into finding the minimum-cost closet set graph that corresponds to the desired border and can be efficiently solved in polynomial time. The emission probability is defined based on two probability distributions of the vessel border and background respectively that are derived directly from edge-based features. The training of the transition probability is achieved by using the Baum-Welch algorithm.

2 Proposed Method

2.1 Border Parameterization

The border of interest can be either an open curve/surface or a closed contour/surface. For the purpose of efficient graph optimization, we unravel the images so that the border of interest appears to be an open contour in 2D or an open surface in 3D. The first columns and the last columns of the image data are connected so that the continuity of the original data is unaffected. In effect, the images are transformed from Cartesian coordinates to polar coordinates. This is particularly suitable for vessel segmentation. We thus treat the segmentation of the two vessel walls in 3D as tracking two non-overlapping and non-crossing contours in the longitudinal direction. Compared to the optimal surface method [9], which also adopts image unravelling, our approach has very limited computational overhead when dealing with 3D data in that only adjacent cross sections are needed to construct the graph for segmentation. We further simplify the border of interest in 2D cross sections through radial basis function (RBF) based parameterization, since it is unnecessary to track each every point along the boarder. As illustrated in Fig. 1(a), the border of interest is approximated by RBFs where the hidden states of the HMM are considered as the potential RBF centers. The border is evenly sampled into M points and at each point a line segment is drawn perpendicular to the tangent line of the border and each line segment has K points. The RBF centers are indexed by $\phi \in \{1, \ldots, M\}$ and points on perpendicular line segments are indexed by $\psi \in \{1, \ldots, K\}$. The initial RBF centers for the current cross section or frame are defined using the result from the previous frame, see Fig. 1(a).

2.2   HMM Formulation

The segmentation of both vessel walls in 3D is then transformed into tracking of two sets of RBF centers in longitudinal direction. For the proposed HMM, we denote all possible sequences of hidden states as $Q = \{q\}$, where $q = \{q_1, \ldots, q_\phi, \ldots, q_M\}$ is one possible state sequence and q_ϕ is the state on the normal at ϕ. These sequences correspond to possible RBF center locations. The HMM observations $O = \{O_1, \ldots, O_\phi, \ldots, O_M\}$ are extracted from the normal lines. HMM is specified by three probability measures $\lambda = (A, B, \pi)$, where A, B and π are the probabilities for the transition, emission and initial states. The transition between states q at two normals ϕ and $\phi + 1$ are governed by a set of probabilities, i.e. transition probabilities $P(q_\phi | q_{\phi+1})$, and any state can only be observed by an output event according to associated probability distribution, i.e. emission probabilities $P(O_\phi | q_\phi)$. The output event is the image features extracted from each state at the normal line.

Image observations are modeled by two probability density functions: one for the vessel wall and the other for the background. Let $O_\phi = \{o_{\phi,1}, \ldots, o_{\phi,\psi}, \ldots, o_{\phi,K}\}$ be a set of features along the normal ϕ and $o_{\phi,\psi}$ a feature extracted from point ψ on the line. $P(o_{\phi,\psi} | F)$ and $P(o_{\phi,\psi} | B)$ represent the probabilities of that feature belonging to the border of interest and the background respectively. The state-emission probability is defined as: $P(O_\phi | q_\phi) \propto P(o_{\phi,\psi} | F) \prod_{\psi \neq q_\phi} P(o_{\phi,\psi} | B)$. The likelihood of the observed variables O_ϕ from a state q_ϕ is computed by measuring the likelihood of each feature $o_{\phi,\psi}$ at index ψ on the line ϕ belonging to the contour and all the rest of features on that line belonging to the background. From a set of training data with a manually labeled borders of interest, we use first order derivatives of Gaussian filters [6] in six different orientations to highlight the edge features along the border, and extract features that correspond to the border and the background, in order to learn the mean and variance of two Gaussian distributions $P(F)$ and $P(B)$.

For the transition probability, we use the Baum-Welch (Forward-Backward) algorithm [13] to learn both the transition and initial probabilities. The process is iterative and each iteration increases the likelihood of the data $P(O|\hat{\lambda}) \geq P(O|\lambda)$ until convergence. Note the emission probability is already computed as described before and there is no need for it to be re-estimated. The initial probability is only needed in case of Viterbi algorithm is used.

2.3   Minimum S-Excess Graph Optimization

Minimization of closure graph and s-excess problems have been applied in image segmentation, e.g. [9,15]. In [9], the authors formulated the problem as a minimization of a closed graph to find the optimal surfaces on d-dimensional multi-column graphs ($d \geq 3$). However, only weighted graph nodes is used in the segmentation by assuming the surface is changing within a global constant constraint which is difficult to define and may lead to abrupt changes of the surface due to its sensitivity to nodal weights. Recently, its graph construction has been extended to handle volumetric data without image unravelling. For example, in [12], Petersen *et al.* proposed to use graph columns defined from non-intersecting, non-parallel flow lines obtained from an initial segmentation. In [15], prior information is incorporated by encoding the prior shapes as a set of convex functions defined between every pair of adjacent columns. Our work is similar to Song *et al.* [15] in that aspect. However, we formulate the problem as tracking borders in consecutive frames, i.e. defining the pair-wise cost based on the transition probability learned from the training data and treating it as a stochastic process, whilst the optimal surface method searches the border as a surface in volumetric image, which is much more computationally expensive. Moreover, the proposed method can tackle more complex shapes, such as open, closed, and variable length contours.

The minimum s-excess problem [8] is a relaxation of minimum closure set problem. A closed set is a subset of graph where all successors of any nodes in the set are also taken in the set. The successors of nodes may not be contained in the set but with their cost equal to the edge costs heading to such successors. Given a directed graph $G(V, E)$, each node $v \in V$ is assigned to a certain weight $w(v)$ and each edge $e \in E$ have a positive cost. The task is to obtain a subset of graph nodes $S \subset V$ where the total nodal cost and the cost of separating the set from the rest of the graph $S' = V - S$ are minimized: $\mathcal{E} = \sum_{v \in S} w(v) + \sum_{\substack{(u,v) \in E \\ u \in S, v \in S'}} c(u, v)$.

For each border of interest $\mathcal{S}$, a graph G_s is constructed in $M \times K$. Each node in the graph corresponds to one hidden state and each normal line is referred to as a column chain. We have three type of graph arcs: intra-chain, inter-chain and inter-border arcs as shown in Fig. 1(c). For intra-chain, along each chain

32   E. Essa, X. Xie and J.-L. Jones

$C(\phi, \psi)$, every node $v(\phi, \psi)$ ($\phi \in \{1, \ldots, M\}$, $\psi \in \{1, \ldots, K\}$, and here $\psi > 1$) has a directed arc to the node $v(\phi, \psi-1)$ with $+\infty$ weight assigned to the edge to ensure that the desired border intersects with each chain once and once only. In the case of inter-chain, for every pair of adjacent chains $C(\phi_1, \psi_1)$ and $C(\phi_2, \psi_2)$, a set of directed arcs are established to link node $v(\phi_1, \psi_1)$ to nodes $v(\phi_2, \psi_2')$ in $C(\phi_2, \psi_2)$, where $1 \leq \psi_2' \leq \psi_1$. Similarly, directed arcs are used to link node $v(\phi_2, \psi_2)$ to node $v(\phi_1, \psi_1')$ in the $C(\phi_1, \psi_1)$ where $1 \leq \psi_1' \leq \psi_2$. Since each hidden state is represented by a node in the graph, the cost of arcs between a pair of adjacent chains is defined by the HMM transition matrix $A(q_{\phi_1, \psi_1}, q_{\phi_2, \psi_2})$. The last row of each graph is connected to each other to form the base of the closed graph. Since the images are unravelled into the polar coordinates, the first and last chains are also connected in the same manner as the inter-chain arcs to ensure connectivity. Inter-border arcs are defined to impose the non-overlapping constraint between two vessel borders, i.e. $\underline{\Delta} \leq S_1 - S_2 \leq \bar{\Delta}$. Let $C_1(\phi, \psi)$ and $C_2(\phi, \psi)$ denote two corresponding chains from G_1 and G_2, $\hat{\psi}$ be the spatial coordinate equivalent to ψ in the graph domain, and $X \times Y$ denote the spatial domain size. For any node $v_1(\phi, \hat{\psi})$ in $C_1(\phi, \psi)$, a direct arc is established between $v_1(\phi, \hat{\psi})$ and $v_2(\phi, \hat{\psi} - \bar{\Delta})$ where $\hat{\psi} \geq \bar{\Delta}$ and $v_2 \in C_2(\phi, \psi)$. Also, nodes $v_2(\phi, \hat{\psi})$ in $C_2(\phi, \psi)$ are connected to $v_1(\phi, \hat{\psi} + \underline{\Delta})$ where $\hat{\psi} < Y - \underline{\Delta}$ and $v_1 \in C_1(\phi, \psi)$. The cost of these arcs is assigned as $+\infty$ such that the minimum and maximin distances are imposed as hard constraints.

Fig. 1(b,c) shows the comparison between the conventional HMM and the proposed HMM construction. The intra-chain arcs and the arcs in the last row are necessary in order to compute the closed set graph. The transition between states is defined as a set of inter-chain arcs from left-to-right and right-to-left to ensure that the cost of cut is proportional to the distance of border location between two neighboring chains.

The emission probability for every node is converted to graph cost according to $W(\phi, \psi) = -log(P(o_{\phi, \psi} | q_{\phi, \psi}))$ and it is inversely proportional to the likelihood that the border of interest passes through the node (ϕ, ψ). The weight for each node $w(\phi, \psi)$ on the directed graph is defined as $w(\phi, \psi) = W(\phi, \psi) - W(\phi, \psi-1)$, except for the bottom chain, i.e. $w(\phi, 1) = W(\phi, 1)$. Hochbaum [7] showed that the minimum s-excess problem is equivalent to solving the minimum $s - t$ cut [1] defined on a proper graph. Hence, the s-t cut algorithm is used to find the minimum closed set in polynomial time. The cost of the cut is the total edge cost in separating the graph into source and sink sets.

Table 1. Inner border quantitative results (mean value and standard deviation).

	AMD	HD	AO	Sens.	Spec.
Optimal Surface [9]	7.1 ± 3.5	50.6 ± 22.1	90.1 ± 5.6	91.2 ± 5.6	99.3 ± 0.6
Using Viterbi Alg.	35.4 ± 18.5	82.2 ± 17.7	53.1 ± 20.9	53.2 ± 21.0	$\mathbf{99.9 \pm 0.1}$
Single border s-excess	4.9 ± 3.2	15.6 ± 10.0	93.0 ± 4.9	93.6 ± 4.9	99.6 ± 0.6
Double border s-excess	$\mathbf{3.1 \pm 1.9}$	$\mathbf{9.8 \pm 4.3}$	$\mathbf{95.5 \pm 3.2}$	$\mathbf{96.9 \pm 3.1}$	99.2 ± 0.8

Table 2. Outer border quantitative results (mean value and standard deviation).

	AMD	HD	AO	Sens.	Spec.
Optimal Surface [9]	7.0 ± 5.9	54.9 ± 26.1	91.7 ± 7.3	92.7 ± 7.5	99.2 ± 0.5
Using Viterbi Alg.	3.2 ± 1.2	13.6 ± 5.6	96.4 ± 1.3	97.6 ± 1.3	98.9 ± 1.3
Single border s-excess	2.4 ± 0.8	8.1 ± 3.7	97.2 ± 1.2	97.8 ± 1.3	$\mathbf{99.5 \pm 0.5}$
Double border s-excess	$\mathbf{2.0 \pm 0.8}$	$\mathbf{7.4 \pm 3.1}$	$\mathbf{97.6 \pm 1.0}$	$\mathbf{98.7 \pm 1.1}$	99.1 ± 0.6

3 Application and Results

The proposed method is applied to segmenting lymphatic vessel images that are obtained using confocal microscopy. Confocal microscopy is a method that allows for the visualization and imaging of 3D volume objects that are thicker than the focal plane of a conventional microscope. For the purpose of our evaluation, a total of 48 segments were obtained from in vitro confocal microscopy images and 16 of those were randomly selected for training the HMM. Anisotropic vessel diffusion [10] was applied to enhance image features and to improve vessel connectivity, as well as to reduce the amount of image noise that is typical in this type of images. Each 3D segment is measured at $512 \times 512 \times 512$ voxels. The evaluation was carried out on every frame where manual labeling was performed. Five different evaluation metrics were used, i.e. absolute mean difference (AMD), Hausdorff distance (HD) in pixel, sensitivity (Sens. %), specificity (Spec. %), and Area Overlap (AO %). The inner region is considered as positive for Sens. and Spec. measurements. The normal line segments were measured at a length of 101 pixels, and 42 RBF centers in polar coordinates were used, i.e. one RBF centre every 30 pixels. The minimum and maximum distance between two borders, $\underline{\Delta}$ and $\bar{\Delta}$, are fixed to 5 and 25 respectively.

Tables 1 and 2 present the quantitative results of segmenting both the inner and outer vessel walls, respectively. Some typical segmentation results are shown in Fig. 2. The proposed s-excess optimization clearly outperformed the Viterbi algorithm in tracking both borders. The Viterbi based method was easily distracted by lymphatic valves attached to the inner wall and produced high distance error and low sensitivity. It also requires a much larger amount of data to train the transition and prior probabilities. The proposed method was also compared against the optimal surface segmentation [9]. The results of the optimal surface method were found sensitive to the distance parameters between columns. The proposed method has full connection of arcs between chains and produced better and more consistent results. The result of simultaneous segmentation of both borders was found better than segmenting the borders separately. Particularly for inner border segmentation (shown in Table 1), the inter-border constraint significantly improved its performance against distraction from lymphatic valves. The proposed s-excess optimization also achieved much smoother border transition, particularly when there was an occlusion or missing feature (see Fig. 2). Fig. 3 shows 3D visualization of some segmentation results.

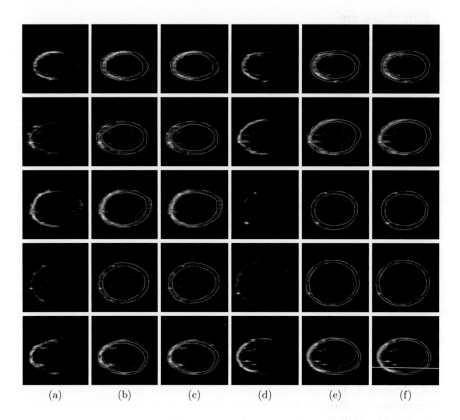

(a)   (b)   (c)   (d)   (e)   (f)

Fig. 2. Comparison between ground-truth (green) and segmentation results (red: inner, blue: outer). (a,d) original image (b,e) proposed single border method. (c,f) proposed double border method.

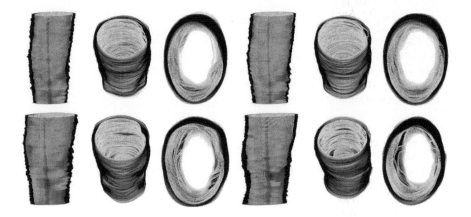

Fig. 3. Visualization of the results in 3D by the proposed method (inner wall: yellow, outer wall: red).

4   Conclusions

We presented an HMM based method for simultaneously segmenting the inner and outer lymphatic vessel borders in confocal images. The method searches for the border along a set of normal lines based on the segmentation of the previous frame. Boundary based features were extracted to infer the emission probability. We show that the optimal sequence of the hidden states corresponds to RBFs of the border can be effectively obtained by solving a minimum s-excess problem. Qualitative and quantitative results on lymphatic images showed the superior performance of the proposed method.

Acknowledgement. The authors like thank D. Zawieja for the data.

References

1. Boykov, Y., Kolmogorov, V.: An experimental comparison of min-cut/max-flow algorithms for energy minimization in vision. IEEE PAMI 26(9), 1124–1137 (2004)
2. Breit, H., Rigoll, G.: Improved person tracking using a combined pseudo-2D-HMM and kalman filter approach with automatic background state adaptation. In: ICIP (2001)
3. Chen, Y., Rui, Y., Huang, T.S.: JPDAF based HMM for real-time contour tracking. In: CVPR (2001)
4. Chen, Y., Rui, Y., Huang, T.S.: Multicue HMM-UKF for real-time contour tracking. IEEE PAMI 28(9), 1525–1529 (2006)
5. Fei, H., Reid, I.D.: Joint bayes filter: A hybrid tracker for non-rigid hand motion recognition. In: Pajdla, T., Matas, J(G.) (eds.) ECCV 2004. LNCS, vol. 3023, pp. 497–508. Springer, Heidelberg (2004)
6. Freeman, W.T., Adelson, E.H.: The design and use of steerable filters. IEEE PAMI 13(9), 891–906 (1991)
7. Hochbaum, D.: An efficient algorithm for image segmentation, markov random fields and related problems. J. ACM 48(4), 686–701 (2001)
8. Hochbaum, D.: Anniversary article: Selection, provisioning, shared fixed costs, maximum closure, and implications on algorithmic methods today. Manage. Sci. 50(6), 709–723 (2004)
9. Li, K., Wu, K., Chen, D.Z., Sonka, M.: Optimal surface segmentation in volumetric images-a graph-theoretic approach. IEEE PAMI 28(1), 119–134 (2006)
10. Manniesing, R., Viergever, M., Niessen, W.: Vessel enhancing diffusion: A scale space representation of vessel structures. MIA 10(6), 815 (2006)
11. Mansor, S., Noble, J.A.: Local wall motion classification of stress echocardiography using a hidden markov model approach. In: ISBI (2008)
12. Petersen, J., et al.: Optimal surface segmentation using flow lines to quantify airway abnormalities in chronic obstructive pulmonary disease. MIA 18, 531–541 (2014)
13. Rabiner, L.: A tutorial on hidden markov models and selected applications in speech recognition. Proceedings of the IEEE 77(2), 257–286 (1989)
14. Sargin, M.E., Altinok, A., Manjunath, B.S., Rose, K.: Variable length open contour tracking using a deformable trellis. IEEE TIP 20(4), 1023–1035 (2011)
15. Song, Q., et al.: Optimal multiple surface segmentation with shape and context priors. IEEE TMI 32(2), 376–386 (2013)

Automatic Artery-Vein Separation from Thoracic CT Images Using Integer Programming

Christian Payer[1,2,*], Michael Pienn[2], Zoltán Bálint[2],
Andrea Olschewski[2], Horst Olschewski[3], and Martin Urschler[4,1]

[1] Institute for Computer Graphics and Vision,
BioTechMed, Graz University of Technology, Austria
[2] Ludwig Boltzmann Institute for Lung Vascular Research, Graz, Austria
[3] Department of Pulmonology, Medical University of Graz, Austria
[4] Ludwig Boltzmann Institute for Clinical Forensic Imaging, Graz, Austria

Abstract. Automated computer-aided analysis of lung vessels has shown to yield promising results for non-invasive diagnosis of lung diseases. In order to detect vascular changes affecting arteries and veins differently, an algorithm capable of identifying these two compartments is needed. We propose a fully automatic algorithm that separates arteries and veins in thoracic computed tomography (CT) images based on two integer programs. The first extracts multiple subtrees inside a graph of vessel paths. The second labels each tree as either artery or vein by maximizing both, the contact surface in their Voronoi diagram, and a measure based on closeness to accompanying bronchi. We evaluate the performance of our automatic algorithm on 10 manual segmentations of arterial and venous trees from patients with and without pulmonary vascular disease, achieving an average voxel based overlap of 94.1% (range: 85.0% – 98.7%), outperforming a recent state-of-the-art interactive method.

1 Introduction

The automatic extraction of vascular tree structures is highly relevant in medical image analysis. Especially the investigation of the pulmonary vascular tree, the complex lung vessel network responsible for oxygen uptake and carbon dioxide release, is of great interest in clinical practice. Applications include detection of early stage pulmonary nodules [1], pulmonary embolism [2], or pulmonary hypertension [3]. The recent trend towards quantitative pulmonary computer-aided diagnosis (CAD) was enabled by the rapid progress in medical imaging technologies, with state-of-the-art computed tomography (CT) scanners allowing depiction of anatomical structures in the lung at a sub-millimeter level at low radiation doses. This remarkable resolution can help in CAD of diseases like chronic obstructive pulmonary disease [4] or pulmonary hypertension [5]. However, the higher amount of data leads to an increased demand for fully automatic

* We thank Peter Kullnig for radiological support, Vasile Fóris for medical support and data analysis and Martin Wurm for his help in the manual artery-vein separations.

© Springer International Publishing Switzerland 2015
N. Navab et al. (Eds.): MICCAI 2015, Part II, LNCS 9350, pp. 36–43, 2015.
DOI: 10.1007/978-3-319-24571-3_5

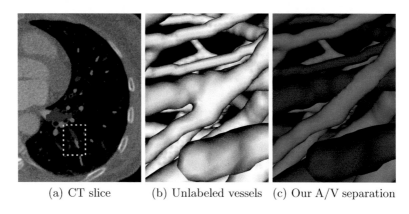

(a) CT slice   (b) Unlabeled vessels   (c) Our A/V separation

Fig. 1. Thoracic CT case where arteries (blue) and veins (red) are close to each other.

extraction and computer-aided quantitative analysis of pulmonary structures, including the automated separation of arterial and venous trees (see Fig. 1). This can improve the diagnosis of lung diseases affecting both trees differently.

Automatic artery-vein (A/V) separation is a very complex problem, due to the similar intensity values of both vessel trees in CT. Further, the pulmonary arterial and venous trees are intertwined and the vessels are in close proximity, making their distinction even harder. Most of the few existing A/V separation algorithms start with vessel segmentation, often using tubularity filters combined with region growing or fast marching methods based on seed points [6]. The work of [7] proposes to solely detect pulmonary arteries by using the anatomical constraint that arteries usually run along the bronchi, whereas the method of [8] involves global structural information by constructing a minimum-spanning-tree from weights derived from local vessel geometry measures and a cutting step for A/V separation. However, using this method, an interactive refinement is often necessary to finalize the separation. In [9] A/V separation utilizes the close proximity of arteries and veins. By morphological operations with differently sized kernels, equal intensity structures are split and locally separated regions are traced. [10] extended this method with a GUI enabling efficient refinement. Another promising method is [11], who formulate an automatic voxel labeling problem based on root detection for both trees. However, it requires a training step and, due to locally restricted image features, it still has problems near the hilum of the lung, i.e. where arteries and veins are in close proximity.

In this work we present a novel, automatic A/V separation algorithm for thoracic CT images, which requires no manual correction and takes the global structural information about vascular trees as well as local features like vessel orientation and bronchus proximity into account. Based on a vessel segmentation step we formulate both the extraction of subtrees and the labeling of arteries and veins as integer programs. We evaluate our method on a database of 10 thoracic CT images with manually segmented A/V trees as a reference and demonstrate the benefits of our method compared to the state-of-the-art method in [8].

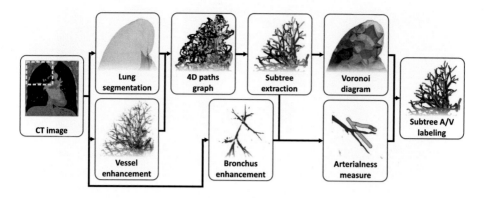

Fig. 2. Overview of our proposed A/V separation algorithm.

2   Method

Our proposed algorithm for A/V separation from contrast-enhanced thoracic CT images is shown in Fig. 2. After a lung segmentation from [5], subsequent processing is performed for both lungs independently. A multi-scale vessel enhancement filter [12] produces a vessel orientation estimate as well as a 4D tubularity image for the three spatial coordinates and the radius. Next, we calculate a graph $G = (V, E)$ of regularly spaced local maxima V of the vessel enhanced image, which are connected by edges E in a local neighborhood similar to [13]. For every edge, a path between its two endpoints is extracted, which minimizes the geodesic distance, penalizing small tubularity values along the path [12]. To drastically prune these edges, a filtering step is performed removing all paths that fully contain any other path. The resulting graph still contains many spurious edges, but also the real arterial and venous vessel paths. These are subsequently organized in subtrees and separated using two integer programs.

2.1   Subtree Extraction

In order to identify anatomically meaningful vascular trees and prepare the input for A/V separation, we contribute a novel method to extract a set of connected subtrees from the overcomplete maxima graph G, using an optimization procedure based on an integer program. Different from [13], we do not need explicitly declared root nodes, but include their search into the optimization. Formally, we find multiple tree-like structures in G, defined by edge tuples $\langle e_{ij}, t_{ij} \rangle$, where binary variable $t_{ij} = 1$ indicates that the path from node i to node j is active, i.e. contained in one of the resulting subtrees. The quadratic objective function is a sum of weights $w_{ijk} \in \mathbb{R}$ of adjacent oriented edge pairs described by t_{ij} and t_{jk} to model the tree structure, and a term controlling the creation of subtrees formalized by a binary variable $r_{ij} \in \{0, 1\}$ indicating if e_{ij} is a root of a subtree:

$$\underset{t,r}{\arg\min} \sum_{e_{ij},\ e_{jk}\in E} w_{ijk}\, t_{ij}\, t_{jk} \ + \ \sigma \sum_{e_{ij}\in E} r_{ij}$$

$$\text{s.t.}\quad \begin{aligned} &\sum_{e_{hi}\in E} t_{hi} + r_{ij} \geq t_{ij}, \quad &&\sum_{e_{hi}\in E} t_{hi} + r_{ij} \leq 1, \\ &t_{ij} \geq r_{ij}, \quad &&t_{ij} + t_{ji} \leq 1, \end{aligned} \quad \forall e_{ij}\in E \tag{1}$$

The linear constraints in (1) enforce tree-like structures by ensuring that an active edge $t_{ij} = 1$ has exactly one predecessor $t_{hi} = 1$ in the set e_{hi} of all preceding edges, or is a root node $r_{ij} = 1$. The fourth constraint guarantees that a directed edge and its opposite are not active simultaneously. With $\sigma \in \mathbb{R}_0^+$ the number of created subtrees is globally controlled, where in contrast to [13] we allow growing of numerous subtrees throughout the whole local maxima graph, and select the best root nodes of anatomically meaningful subtrees implicitly. The key component of the integer program is the weight w_{ijk} of adjacent oriented edge pairs. It consists of three parts, the first one derived from the costs of traveling along the path from node i to k via j according to the tubularity measure, the second one penalizing paths with strong orientation changes computed by the mean of the dot products of directions along a path, and the final part penalizing radius increases from start node i to end node k. While all other components are positive, a global parameter $\delta \in \mathbb{R}^-$ is further added to w_{ijk} to allow for negative weights, otherwise the trivial solution, i.e. no extracted paths and subtrees, would always minimize the objective function (1).

After minimizing the objective function, the integer program results in a list of individual connected subtrees, which is post-processed to locate the anatomical branching points instead of local tubularity maxima.

2.2   Subtree A/V Labeling

Next, each individual subtree is labeled as either artery or vein using two anatomical properties. First, we exploit that arteries and veins are roughly uniformly distributed in the lung. The second property uses the fact, that bronchi run parallel and in close proximity to arteries, as previously proposed in [7]. The main contribution of our work lies in a novel optimization model calculating the final A/V labeling by an integer program, that assigns to every individual subtree t_i either $a_i = 1$ (artery) or $v_i = 1$ (vein). This is achieved by maximizing

$$\underset{a,v}{\arg\max} \sum_{t_i,\ t_j\in T} a_i\, v_j\, w_{ij}^{border} + \lambda \sum_{t_i\in T} a_i\, w_i^{artery} \tag{2}$$

$$\text{s.t.}\quad a_i + v_i = 1, \quad \forall t_i\in T,$$

where the first term counts the number of voxels $w_{ij}^{border} \in \mathbb{R}_0^+$ on the contact surface between artery and vein regions modeled by a generalized Voronoi diagram. For each voxel inside the lung segmentation this Voronoi diagram determines the nearest subtree. By maximizing the sum of all w_{ij}^{border} of neighboring artery and vein regions, a uniform distribution of arteries and veins throughout the whole lung is ensured. The second term of (2) uses a measure of arterialness $w_i^{artery} \in \mathbb{R}_0^+$ for every tree t_i to incorporate a distinction between arteries and veins. Our arterialness measure is inspired by [7], but instead of searching for bronchus points in the input CT image, we employ the multi-scale tubularity filter from [12] for locating dark on bright bronchus structures. At each voxel along the segments of a subtree, we locally search for similarly oriented bronchial structures giving high tubularity response in a plane orthogonal to the vessel direction. After fitting a line through all bronchus candidate locations of a vessel segment, we compute an arterialness measure from their distance and deviation in direction. This gives higher values for arteries running closer and in parallel to bronchi, while veins, typically more distant and deviating stronger from the bronchus direction, will receive lower values. The arterialness value w_i^{artery} of a tree t_i is the sum of all arterialness values of its vessel segments. Finally, the constraint from (2) ensures, that not both labels are active at the same time for the same tree t_i. A factor λ weights the sums. The result of solving this integer program is the final labeling of arteries and veins for all subtrees.

3   Experimental Setup and Results

Experimental Setup: To validate our algorithm, we used 10 datasets from patients (6 female/4 male) with and without lung vascular disease who underwent thoracic contrast-enhanced, dual-energy CT examinations. The CT scans were acquired either with a Siemens Somatom Definition Flash (D30f reconstruction kernel) or with a Siemens Somatom Force (Qr40d reconstruction kernel) CT scanner. The size of the isotropic 0.6mm CT volumes was $512 \times 512 \times 463$ pixels.

Manual reference segmentations of all 10 patients, that include pulmonary artery and left atrium, as well as A/V trees down to a vessel diameter of 2mm, were created requiring 5–8 h per dataset. These data served as basis for validating our algorithm together with a re-implementation of [8], which is similar to our proposed method, as it extracts and labels subtrees. The interactive step of [8], i.e. the final A/V labeling of subtrees, was done manually by looking for connections to the heart for every subtree. Similarly, we additionally performed user-defined labeling of the extracted subtrees of our algorithm, to evaluate the A/V labeling part. As the compared segmentations may differ substantially in the included vessel voxels, we compared only those voxels which are present in the segmentation and the manual reference.

Table 1. Overlap ratio in % of automatic, Park et al. [8] and user-defined (UD) labeling methods with manual reference segmentations for the 10 datasets.

Patient #	1	2	3	4	5	6	7	8	9	10	μ
Automatic	**95.0**	93.3	**98.4**	87.3	**97.4**	85.0	**95.0**	**98.7**	**98.5**	92.4	**94.1**
Park et al. [8]	90.2	**93.9**	91.2	**90.4**	91.9	**88.0**	90.6	94.7	95.3	**93.3**	91.9
UD labeling	99.1	99.4	98.6	98.5	97.9	97.6	99.2	99.8	98.6	99.1	98.8

Table 2. Comparison of user-defined subtree labeling and fully automatic segmentation for the 10 datasets. The amount of mislabeled vessel voxels (Mislabeled) and the amount of detected structures, which are not vessels (Non-vessel) is provided in %.

Patient #	1	2	3	4	5	6	7	8	9	10	μ
Mislabeled	3.9	6.1	0.2	11.6	1.8	10.4	4.6	1.4	0.6	7.9	4.9
Non-vessel	5.1	0.2	1.4	2.2	4.7	3.0	0.1	0.3	0.4	0.0	1.7

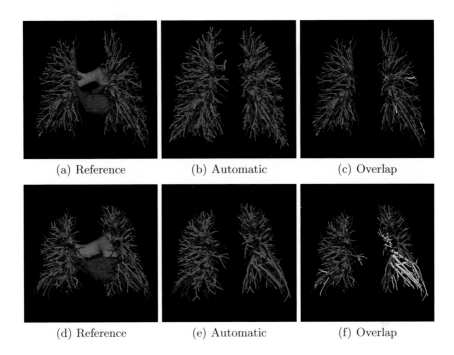

(a) Reference   (b) Automatic   (c) Overlap

(d) Reference   (e) Automatic   (f) Overlap

Fig. 3. Visualization of reference segmentation (left), automatic segmentations (center) and their overlap (right). Only voxels, that are set in both segmentations, are visualized in the overlap image. Red: vein, blue: arteries, yellow: disagreement between segmentations. Top row: 98.4% agreement (#3), bottom row: 85% agreement (#6).

The development and testing platform for our C++ algorithm consisted of a Windows 7 Intel Core i5-4670 @ 3.40 GHz with 16 GB RAM. For multi-scale vessel enhancement and 4D path extraction, the publicly available code from [12] was used. Gurobi Optimizer[1] was applied to solve integer programs. The parameters $\sigma = 0.2$ and $\delta = -0.2$ were determined empirically within a few try-outs providing satisfactory results for the subtree extraction. The parameter $\lambda = 6.0$ was determined by grid search, as the A/V labeling is not time consuming.

---

[1] Gurobi Optimizer Version 6.0 with academic license from http://www.gurobi.com/

Results: The automatic algorithm generated an average of 1210 individual vessel segments, composed of 619 arteries and 591 veins, with diameters ranging from 2 to 10mm. The average voxel-based overlap of correct labels for all 10 datasets between automatic and manual reference segmentation was 94.1%. The re-implementation of [8] achieved 91.9%, whereas the user-defined subtree labeling based on the output of our subtree extraction achieved an overlap of 98.8%. The individual values are listed in Table 1, with two datasets visualized in Fig. 3.

Furthermore, in order to evaluate the subtree A/V labeling in more detail, we validated our automatic segmentation against the user-defined labeling (Table 2). The average ratio of voxels, where arteries and veins were switched (mislabeled) was 4.9%. As additional voxels cannot be added by the manual labeling, the number of mistakenly detected vessels can be quantified as well. The average ratio of misclassified structures (non-vessel), i.e., the ratio of voxels that are not in the manually labeled result, but present in the automatic one, was 1.7%.

The average time needed for generating a single, fully automatic A/V segmentation with our unoptimized method was 5 hours, while [8] required 0.5 hours of computation time with additional 2 hours of interaction time.

4   Discussion and Conclusion

Our proposed novel algorithm for separating arteries and veins in thoracic CT images achieves a higher average correct overlap compared to the method of [8], although the latter method includes explicit manual correction, while our approach is fully automated. We assume that our integer program is better modeling the anatomical constraints involved in A/V separation compared to the minimum-spanning-tree of [8] by exploiting the uniform distribution of arteries and veins throughout the lungs as well as proximity and similar orientation of arteries and bronchi. Our extracted vascular subtrees are very well separated, which can be observed in Fig. 3 or by comparing the user-defined labeling with the manual reference in Table 2. Furthermore, our main contribution, the automatic A/V labeling step, removes the need for manual post-processing.

We observed that mislabeled subtrees often are neighbors in the generalized Voronoi diagram, due to the maximization of their contact surfaces. This may lead to switched labels of all subtrees within a lung lobe. Therefore, restricting the uniform distribution of arteries and veins to lung lobes instead of whole lungs could further improve performance and robustness. Because of the lack of a standardized dataset and openly available A/V separation algorithms, our algorithm was only compared to the most recently published work in [8]. The evaluation of our algorithm on a larger dataset is ongoing. As our algorithm is not optimized in its current state, we expect that improvements in runtime are still possible. Another interesting idea could be to combine subtree extraction and labeling into one integer program, like in [14]. We conclude, that our novel method provides an opportunity to become an integral part of computer aided diagnosis of lung diseases.

References

1. Murphy, K., van Ginneken, B., Schilham, A.M.R., de Hoop, B.J., Gietema, H.A., Prokop, M.: A large-scale evaluation of automatic pulmonary nodule detection in chest CT using local image features and k-nearest-neighbour classification. Med. Image Anal. 13(5), 757–770 (2009)
2. Masutani, Y., MacMahon, H., Doi, K.: Computerized detection of pulmonary embolism in spiral CT angiography based on volumetric image analysis. IEEE Trans. Med. Imaging 21(12), 1517–1523 (2002)
3. Linguraru, M.G., Pura, J.A., Van Uitert, R.L., Mukherjee, N., Summers, R.M., Minniti, C., Gladwin, M.T., Kato, G., Machado, R.F., Wood, B.J.: Segmentation and quantification of pulmonary artery for noninvasive CT assessment of sickle cell secondary pulmonary hypertension. Med. Phys. 37(4), 1522–1532 (2010)
4. Estépar, R.S.J., Kinney, G.L., Black-Shinn, J.L., Bowler, R.P., Kindlmann, G.L., Ross, J.C., Kikinis, R., Han, M.K., Come, C.E., Diaz, A.A., Cho, M.H., Hersh, C.P., Schroeder, J.D., Reilly, J.J., Lynch, D.A., Crapo, J.D., Wells, J.M., Dransfield, M.T., Hokanson, J.E., Washko, G.R.: Computed tomographic measures of pulmonary vascular morphology in smokers and their clinical implications. Am. J. Respir. Crit. Care Med. 188(2), 231–239 (2013)
5. Helmberger, M., Pienn, M., Urschler, M., Kullnig, P., Stollberger, R., Kovacs, G., Olschewski, A., Olschewski, H., Bálint, Z.: Quantification of tortuosity and fractal dimension of the lung vessels in pulmonary hypertension patients. PLoS One 9(1), e87515 (2014)
6. van Rikxoort, E.M., van Ginneken, B.: Automated segmentation of pulmonary structures in thoracic computed tomography scans: a review. Phys. Med. Biol. 58, R187–R220 (2013)
7. Bülow, T., Wiemker, R., Blaffert, T., Lorenz, C., Renisch, S.: Automatic extraction of the pulmonary artery tree from multi-slice CT data. In: Proc. SPIE 5746, Med. Imaging Physiol. Funct. Struct. from Med. Images, pp. 730–740 (2005)
8. Park, S., Lee, S.M., Kim, N., Seo, J.B., Shin, H.: Automatic reconstruction of the arterial and venous trees on volumetric chest CT. Med. Phys. 40(7), 071906 (2013)
9. Saha, P.K., Gao, Z., Alford, S.K., Sonka, M., Hoffman, E.A.: Topomorphologic separation of fused isointensity objects via multiscale opening: Separating arteries and veins in 3-D pulmonary CT. IEEE Trans. Med. Imaging 29(3), 840–851 (2010)
10. Gao, Z., Grout, R.W., Holtze, C., Hoffman, E.A., Saha, P.K.: A new paradigm of interactive artery/vein separation in noncontrast pulmonary CT imaging using multiscale topomorphologic opening. IEEE Trans. Biomed. Eng. 59(11), 3016–3027 (2012)
11. Kitamura, Y., Li, Y., Ito, W., Ishikawa, H.: Adaptive higher-order submodular potentials for pulmonary artery-vein segmentation. In: Proc. Fifth Int. Work. Pulm. Image Anal., pp. 53–61 (2013)
12. Benmansour, F., Türetken, E., Fua, P.: Tubular Geodesics using Oriented Flux: An ITK Implementation. The Insight Journal (2013)
13. Türetken, E., Benmansour, F., Andres, B., Pfister, H., Fua, P.: Reconstructing loopy curvilinear structures using integer programming. In: IEEE Conf. Comput. Vis. Pattern Recognit., pp. 1822–1829 (2013)
14. Robben, D., Türetken, E., Sunaert, S., Thijs, V., Wilms, G., Fua, P., Maes, F., Suetens, P.: Simultaneous segmentation and anatomical labeling of the cerebral vasculature. In: Golland, P., Hata, N., Barillot, C., Hornegger, J., Howe, R. (eds.) MICCAI 2014, Part I. LNCS, vol. 8673, pp. 307–314. Springer, Heidelberg (2014)

Automatic Dual-View Mass Detection in Full-Field Digital Mammograms

Guy Amit, Sharbell Hashoul, Pavel Kisilev, Boaz Ophir,
Eugene Walach, and Aviad Zlotnick

IBM Research - Haifa, Israel

Abstract. Mammography is the first-line modality for screening and diagnosis of breast cancer. Following the common practice of radiologists to examine two mammography views, we propose a fully automated dual-view analysis framework for breast mass detection in mammograms. The framework combines unsupervised segmentation and random-forest classification to detect and rank candidate masses in cranial-caudal (CC) and mediolateral-oblique (MLO) views. Subsequently, it estimates correspondences between pairs of candidates in the two views. The performance of the method was evaluated using a publicly available full-field digital mammography database (INbreast). Dual-view analysis provided area under the ROC curve of 0.94, with detection sensitivity of 87% at specificity of 90%, which significantly improved single-view performance (72% sensitivity at 90% specificity, 78% specificity at 87% sensitivity, P<0.05). One-to-one mapping of candidate masses from two views facilitated correct estimation of the breast quadrant in 77% of the cases. The proposed method may assist radiologists to efficiently identify and classify breast masses.

Keywords: Digital Mammography, Automatic Mass Detection, Dual-View, Machine Learning.

1   Introduction

Mammography is the most common imaging modality for breast cancer screening, with over 38 million tests performed annually in the US. The majority of certified breast imaging facilities in the US already use full-field digital mammography (FFDM) [1]. When interpreting a mammogram, radiologists typically examine images obtained from two anatomical projections: the cranial-caudal (CC) view and the mediolateral-oblique (MLO) view. A breast mass is a lesion seen in both views. However, since the two projected images are acquired by applying different compression on the non-rigid breast tissue, deriving the dual-view correspondence between potential masses is a non-trivial task.

Computer-aided detection of breast masses in mammography has been studied extensively. Earlier work focused on single-view analysis using either supervised, model-based methods or unsupervised techniques, including region-based segmentation, boundary detection, and pixel clustering (see [2] for a thorough review). Previous

© Springer International Publishing Switzerland 2015
N. Navab et al. (Eds.): MICCAI 2015, Part II, LNCS 9350, pp. 44–52, 2015.
DOI: 10.1007/978-3-319-24571-3_6

work on multi-view mass detection in mammograms introduced various correspondence features including distance to the nipple, region- and histogram correlations, and texture gradients [3, 4]. These features were used either to restrict the search region in the second view [5, 6] or to jointly classify pairs of masses, using machine learning techniques such as linear discriminant analysis [3, 7], artificial neural networks [4] or Bayesian networks [8]. The mammograms used in the abovementioned work were either proprietary image datasets, used for a particular research, or publicly available datasets such as DDSM and MIAS, which consist of digitized film images. As FFDM becomes the standard clinical technology, automated analysis methods should be adapted [9] and evaluated on FFDM benchmarks. INbreast (courtesy of Breast Research Group, INESC Porto, Portugal) is a new publicly-available full-field digital mammography database, which includes detailed annotations of masses [10].

The current work introduces a new fully automated dual-view analysis framework for breast mass detection in FFDM images. Our work entails three major contributions: (1) A hybrid unsupervised-supervised approach for segmentation and ranking of candidate masses in single-view images; (2) A learning-based method for estimating the correspondence between candidate masses in two views; (3) An evaluation of the proposed automatic detection methods on the INbreast database.

2   Methods

2.1   Single View Detection

The single view mass detection pipeline [11] consists of image preprocessing, detection of candidate seeds, generation of candidate contours, feature extraction, and candidate ranking (Fig 1a).

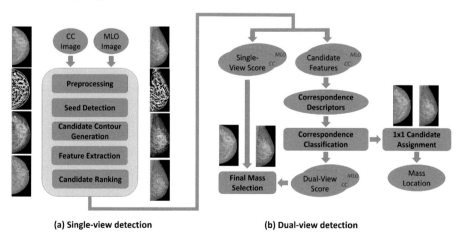

Fig. 1. Single-view analysis framework (a) detects and ranks mass candidates separately in CC and MLO images. The dual-view correspondence between pairs of candidates is estimated and a combined dual-view score is used to select true masses and reject false-positives (b). Dual-view candidate assignment is also used to estimate mass location.

Images were first preprocessed by separating the breast from the background and identifying the pectoral muscles and the nipple. Seed detection was based on applying semantic thresholding [12], followed by a distance transform. Semantic thresholding classifies image pixels as locally dark or locally bright, and finds a global binarization threshold that balances the number of locally dark pixels that are brighter than the threshold and locally bright pixels that are darker than the threshold. The image is partitioned into 20x20 tiles and a threshold is computed for each tile. The resulting 20x20 threshold matrix is smoothed by a Gaussian filter, interpolated to the image dimensions and used as a per-pixel threshold for binarization (Fig. 2b). A distance transform is then applied to the binary image (Fig 2c) and large connected components are selected as candidate seeds, using experimentally-set thresholds (Fig. 2d). The selected seeds are sorted by the maximal value of the distance transform in the connected component. This value is used as an initial unsupervised detection score, denoted S_i^0. To account for large lesions, the process is repeated with a coarser image portioning (5x5 tiles), and the largest connected component is added to the selected seeds.

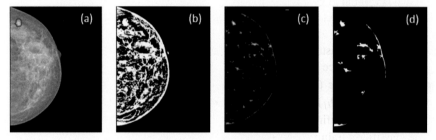

Fig. 2. Seed detection. A mammogram (a) is processed by semantic thresholding to produce a binary image (b). A distance transform is applied (c), and large connected components are selected (d). The contour annotation in (a) indicates a ground-truth mass.

The contours of mass candidates were generated by finding an optimal path in a polar representation of the image around the seeds, similar to [13] and [14]. The maximal value of the seed's distance transform was used as an initial estimate for the radius of the polar image.

For each ground-truth and candidate mass contour, we extract a multitude of features, including: (1) Shape features: area, aspect ratio, curvature along the boundaries, orientation, and eccentricity of a fitted ellipse; (2) Intensity features: intensity statistics, normalized intensity histograms inside and outside the contour; (3) Texture features: local entropy of gray-level values, calculated at different scales [15].

Mass ranking was done with a random forest (RF) classifier [16] using a leave-one-patient-out cross validation scheme. For each patient, a model was trained using a balanced set of true- and false-detected mass contours from all other patients. True-detection observations were the ground-truth contours, m_{gt}, as well as detected candidate masses m_i with large ground-truth overlap $dice(m_i, m_{gt}) \geq \delta$, where $dice(A, B) = 2|A \cap B|/(|A| + |B|)$ and $\delta = 0.5$. False-detection observations were candidate masses without any ground-truth overlap $(dice(m_i, m_{gt}) = 0)$. For each test candidate contour, a class label $l(m_i) \in \{0,1\}$ was predicted, classifying the candidate as a true or false mass. The candidate's *single-view score* $S_i^1 \in [-1,1]$ was defined by $S_i^1 = \mathcal{P}(l(m_i) = 1) - \mathcal{P}(l(m_i) = 0)$, where $\mathcal{P}(l(m_i) = \mathcal{L})$ is calculated as the fraction of trees in the random-forest model that voted for class label $\mathcal{L}$.

2.2   Dual View Detection

The analysis framework for detecting corresponding mass candidates in two views is illustrated in Figure 1b. Given a pair of CC and MLO mammograms $I = (I^{CC}, I^{MLO})$, each having a set of candidate masses $M^{CC} = \{m_1^{CC}, \dots, m_N^{CC}\}$, $M^{MLO} = \{m_1^{MLO}, \dots, m_N^{MLO}\}$, the analysis aims to find a relation from M^{CC} to M^{MLO} that contains all the corresponding candidate pairs from the two views. A *correspondence descriptor* D_{ij} is a dual-view feature vector encoding the matching between single-view features of m_i^{CC} and m_j^{MLO}. D_{ij} consists of the following features: (1) Location features: ratio of the distances between the centroid of the candidate mass and the nipple, ratio of the distances between the centroid of the candidate mass and a line tangential to the nipple and parallel to the pectoral muscle; (2) Shape features: ratios between single-view shape features, including area, perimeter, eccentricity, ellipse axis-length, solidity; (3) Image features: contrast difference, differences of intensity statistics, histogram distance (Earth Mover's Distance) and histogram flow [17].

The correspondence between candidate masses m_i^{CC} and m_j^{MLO} is assessed by a *correspondence score* $C_{ij} \in [-1,1]$. To estimate C_{ij}, a classifier is trained and used to predict a label $l(D_{ij}) \in \{0,1\}$ for each correspondence descriptor D_{ij}. The *correspondence score* is defined by: $C_{ij} = \mathcal{P}(l(D_{ij}) = 1) - \mathcal{P}(l(D_{ij}) = 0)$.

The classifier's training data is composed of correspondence descriptors of matching ('*positive*') and non-matching ('*negative*') pairs of masses. For an image pair I, D_{gt}^I is the correspondence descriptor of the ground-truth mass contours $(m_{gt}^{CC}, m_{gt}^{MLO})$. The set of positive observations in our training set consists of ground-truth descriptors, as well as the pairs of candidate contours with sufficiently-large overlap with the ground-truth:

$$Observ_+^I = \{D_{gt}^I\} \cup \{D_{ij}^I \mid dice(m_i^{CC}, m_{gt}^{CC}) \geq \delta, dice(m_j^{MLO}, m_{gt}^{MLO}) \geq \delta\}$$

Likewise, the set of negative observations consists of correspondence descriptors of candidate pairs, where the contour in one view overlaps with the ground-truth, while the contour in the other view is a false detection, which does not overlap with the ground-truth:

$$Observ_-^I = \{D_{ij}^I \mid dice(m_i^{CC}, m_{gt}^{CC}) \geq \delta, dice(m_j^{MLO}, m_{gt}^{MLO}) = 0\}$$
$$\cup \{D_{ij}^I \mid dice(m_i^{CC}, m_{gt}^{CC}) = 0, dice(m_j^{MLO}, m_{gt}^{MLO}) \geq \delta\}$$

Similar to mass classification, the correspondence descriptors of each image pair were classified by a random-forest classifier using leave-one-patient-out cross validation.

The likelihood of a test candidate having a corresponding mass candidate in the other view was estimated by a *dual-view score* $S_i^2 = \max_j\{C_{ij}\}$.

To estimate the spatial location of the candidate masses, a one-to-one correspondence between pairs of candidates was derived by solving the linear assignment problem, minimizing $\sum_i \sum_j (1 - C_{ij}) x_{ij}$, where $x_{ij} = \begin{cases} 1, & \text{if } m_i^{CC} \text{ is assigned to } m_j^{MLO} \\ 0, & \text{otherwise} \end{cases}$

2.3   Evaluation Experiments

Our analysis included 90 images from 43 patients. All selected images had a single annotated mass. In order to simplify the interpretation of the results, images with multiple mass annotations or cases with missing annotation in one of the views were excluded (18 images). For each image, unsupervised seed detection was applied, and candidate mass contours were generated from the 30 first seeds, ordered by the detection score, S_i^0. A seed that resided within the ground-truth contour was considered a true detection. The candidate contours were then ranked by computing the single-view score S_i^1, using leave-one-patient-out cross validation. The quality of the candidate contours was assessed by their Dice-index overlap with the ground-truth contours. The single-view detection performance was measured by the area under the receiver operating characteristic curve (AUROC) and the detection sensitivity at a false-positive rate (FPR) of 10%. Dual-view analysis was carried out using the first 10 mass candidates from each view. For each pair of CC-MLO images, the analysis consisted of classification of correspondence descriptors, calculation of dual-view scores S_i^2 and breast quadrant estimation, following one-to-one candidate assignment. The AUROC of the combined dual-view score $S_i^1 + S_i^2$ was compared to the single-view score, and the differences in detection sensitivity and specificity were assessed using McNemar's chi-square test.

3   Results

Sorting the detected seeds by the unsupervised score S_i^0, a true detection was found within the first 30 seeds, 10 seeds and 1 seed in 96%, 79% and 37% of the images, respectively. The average Dice-index overlap between the best automatically detected candidate mass contour and the ground-truth mass contour was 0.8±0.2. This overlap was > 0.5 in 96% of the images. Candidate mass classification with S_i^0 achieved an AUROC of 0.71, with sensitivity of 36% at specificity of 90% (Fig 3).

Following learning-based candidate ranking, the 10 highest-ranked candidates included a true detection (Dice > 0.5) in 89% of the images. In 70% of the images the first-ranked candidate was a true detection, which corresponds to an average FPR of 0.3 per image. With 2.2 false-positives per image, the detection sensitivity was 83%. The AUROC of candidate classification by the single-view score S_i^1 was 0.92 (Fig. 3), with detection sensitivity of 72% at a specificity of 90%.

Classification of the correspondence descriptors into true- and false pairwise matches provided an AUROC of 0.96, with optimal sensitivity and specificity of 89%

and 96%, respectively. Following the one-to-one candidate assignment, correct pairs of true CC-MLO mass candidates were found in 67% of the pairs, and the correct breast quadrant was estimated in 77% of the cases.

The combined dual-view score $S_i^1 + S_i^2$ improved the candidate classification compared to the single-view score (Fig 3), with AUROC of 0.94 and detection sensitivity of 87% vs. 72%, at specificity of 90% (P<0.05). At the same detection sensitivity of 87%, the specificity of the single-view score was lower at 78% (P<0.05).

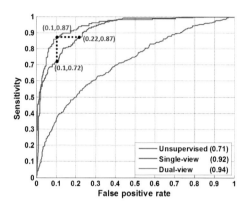
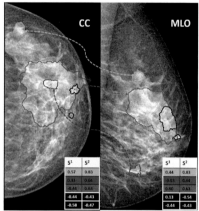

Fig. 3. ROC curves and AUROC of unsupervised- single-view- and combined dual-view detection scores. The marked points indicate the differences in sensitivity and specificity between single- and dual-view analyses.

Fig. 4. CC-MLO candidate correspondence example. S^1 and S^2 are the single- and dual-view scores for each candidate. A combined score is used to reject unpaired candidates (black) and select the best pair (green).

Figure 4 shows a typical example of dual-view correspondence between detected candidates. In this example, three pairs of candidates were linked with high dual-view scores, while two additional candidates in each view were rejected as false detections. The combination of S_i^1 and S_i^2 scores enabled correct selection of the true mass candidate (green) in both views, although its MLO single-view score was not the maximal.

4   Discussion

Oliver et al. [2] evaluated seven different single-view detection algorithms, using two mammography databases. The reported AUROC ranged from 0.56 to 0.79. None of the evaluated algorithms provided an overall best performance, and there was a trend of decreased performance when using FFDM images, compared to digitized mammograms. Wei et al. [18] analyzed a proprietary FFDM dataset and reported sensitivity of 70% at a FPR of 0.72 per image, using morphological and gray-level texture features and a combination of rule-based and linear discriminant analysis (LDA) classifiers. Paquerault et al. [7] reported single-view sensitivity of 62%, with 1 false-positive per image, while their two-view detection scheme increased the sensitivity to 73%. Van Engeland et al. [3] used LDA to classify correct and incorrect pairs of suspicious mass regions. Using features such as difference of mass-nipple distances, contrast difference and histogram correlation, a correct pairing of true positive regions was found in 82% of the cases. Yuan et al. [4] applied a Bayesian artificial neural network to estimate the probability of correspondence between lesions from different views, reporting AUROC of 0.87. Velicova et al. [8] proposed a fixed Bayesian network framework for modeling multi-view dependences, which increased the AUROC by 0.01 to 0.05. Recently, Kozegar et al. [19] assessed their mass detection method using INbreast mammograms. Their proposed ensemble of classifiers achieved sensitivity of 87% at FPR of 3.67 per image. At a lower FPR of 0.5 per image, the sensitivity decreased to 32%. Our single-view analysis framework, based on a similar approach achieved 87% sensitivity at a lower FPR of 3.13 per image, and maintained a fair detection sensitivity of 70% at a low FPR of 0.3 per image. Fusing the dual-view correspondence score with the single-view ranking score boosted the detection performance, reducing either the false-negative or the false-positive rate by more than half, compared to the single-view performance (Fig. 3). The pairwise correspondence classification was highly accurate, with AUROC of 0.96. These results strengthen the potential of the automated dual-view analysis. Our proposed approach also provided an estimation of the three-dimensional spatial location of the mass, based on deriving one-to-one correspondence between candidate masses. As breast quadrants have different likelihoods for incidence of cancer, accurate estimation of the quadrant may be useful for further semantic classification of the detected masses into benign or malignant lesions.

While training a random forest classifier, the relative importance of each feature can be measured by randomly perturbing every variable and computing the average difference in accuracy. In our experiments, the most prominent features for two-view correspondence classification were the ratios of mass-nipple distances, mass areas, ellipse axis lengths, normalized distances to the center of the image, and earth mover's distance between the local histograms. The proposed analysis framework is highly scalable in terms of the feature set used for single- and dual-view detection, enabling experimentation with new informative features, as well as with feature selection strategies.

The use of INbreast FFDM database to assess the framework's performance takes advantage of the detailed ground-truth mass annotations, which allows the definition of fine shape correspondences between annotated contours. Moreover, the major benefit of using INbreast lies in its availability to the research community, allowing the use of standard benchmarking of mammogram analysis algorithms. A current limitation of this dataset is its relatively-small number of mass-containing images. This limitation was addressed by evaluating the classifiers using leave-one-out cross validation. However, further validation of the method on additional datasets is needed. Another limitation of this work is the restriction of analysis to mammograms with a single annotated mass. A natural extension would be to evaluate the method on multiple-mass images, as well as images with different numbers of masses in each view.

The proposed dual-view analysis framework could assist radiologists in decreasing their workload, by automatically indicating suspicious regions that require attention. Such fusion of human knowledge and computer algorithms bears a true promise for future cognitive systems in diagnostic radiology.

References

1. Mammography Quality Standards Act's National Statistics.
   http://www.fda.gov/Radiation-EmittingProducts/
   MammographyQualityStandardsActandProgram/
2. Oliver, A., Freixenet, J., Martí, J., Pérez, E., Pont, J., Denton, E.R.E., Zwiggelaar, R.: A review of automatic mass detection and segmentation in mammographic images. Med. Image Anal. 14, 87–110 (2010)
3. Van Engeland, S., Timp, S., Karssemeijer, N.: Finding corresponding regions of interest in mediolateral oblique and craniocaudal mammographic views. Med. Phys. 33, 3203–3212 (2006)
4. Yuan, Y., Giger, M.L., Li, H., Sennett, C.: Correlative feature analysis on FFDM. Med. Phys. 35, 5490–5500 (2008)
5. Zheng, B., Leader, J.K., Abrams, G.S., Lu, A.H., Wallace, L.P., Maitz, G.S., Gur, D.: Multiview-based computer-aided detection scheme for breast masses. Med. Phys. 33, 3135–3143 (2006)
6. Wiemker, R., Kutra, D., Heese, H., Buelow, T.: Identification of corresponding lesions in multiple mammographic views using star-shaped iso-contours. In: Aylward, S., Hadjiiski, L.M. (eds.) SPIE Medical Imaging, p. 90351A. International Society for Optics and Photonics (2014)
7. Paquerault, S., Petrick, N., Chan, H.-P., Sahiner, B., Helvie, M.A.: Improvement of computerized mass detection on mammograms: fusion of two-view information. Med. Phys. 29, 238–247 (2002)
8. Velikova, M., Samulski, M., Lucas, P.J.F., Karssemeijer, N.: Improved mammographic CAD performance using multi-view information: a Bayesian network framework. Phys. Med. Biol. 54, 1131–1147 (2009)
9. Li, H., Giger, M.L., Yuan, Y., Chen, W., Horsch, K., Lan, L., Jamieson, A.R., Sennett, C.A., Jansen, S.A.: Evaluation of computer-aided diagnosis on a large clinical full-field digital mammographic dataset. Acad. Radiol. 15, 1437–1445 (2008)
10. Moreira, I.C., Amaral, I., Domingues, I., Cardoso, A., Cardoso, M.J., Cardoso, J.S.: INbreast: Toward a Full-field Digital Mammographic Database. Acad. Radiol. 19, 236–248 (2012)
11. Zlotnick, A., Ophir, B., Kisilev, P.: Hybrid Unsupervised-Supervised Lesion Detection in Mammograms. SPIE Medical Imaging (2015)
12. Zlotnick, A., Lozinskii, E.: Semantic thresholding. Pattern Recognit. Lett. 5, 321–328 (1987)
13. Timp, S., Karssemeijer, N.: A new 2D segmentation method based on dynamic programming applied to computer aided detection in mammography. Med. Phys. 31, 958–971 (2004)
14. Rojas Domínguez, A., Nandi, A.K.: Improved dynamic-programming-based algorithms for segmentation of masses in mammograms. Med. Phys. 34, 4256–4269 (2007)
15. Gonzalez, R.C., Woods, R.E.: Digital Image Processing, 3rd edn (2006)

16. Breiman, L.: Random Forests. Mach. Learn. 45, 5–32 (2001)
17. Kisilev, P., Freedman, D., Wallach, E., Tzadok, A., Naveh, Y.: DFlow and DField: New features for capturing object and image relationships. In: 21st International Conference on Pattern Recognition (ICPR), pp. 3590–3593. IEEE (2012)
18. Wei, J., Sahiner, B., Hadjiiski, L.M., Chan, H.-P., Petrick, N., Helvie, M.A., Roubidoux, M.A., Ge, J., Zhou, C.: Computer-aided detection of breast masses on full field digital mammograms. Med. Phys. 32, 2827–2838 (2005)
19. Kozegar, E., Soryani, M., Minaei, B., Domingues, I.: Assessment of a novel mass detection algorithm in mammograms. J. Cancer Res. Ther. 9, 592–600 (2013)

Leveraging Mid-Level Semantic Boundary Cues for Automated Lymph Node Detection*

Ari Seff, Le Lu, Adrian Barbu, Holger Roth, Hoo-Chang Shin, and Ronald M. Summers

Imaging Biomarkers and Computer-Aided Diagnosis Laboratory, Radiology and Imaging Sciences, National Institutes of Health Clinical Center, Bethesda, MD 20892-1182, USA

Abstract. Histograms of oriented gradients (HOG) are widely employed image descriptors in modern computer-aided diagnosis systems. Built upon a set of local, robust statistics of low-level image gradients, HOG features are usually computed on raw intensity images. In this paper, we explore a learned image transformation scheme for producing higher-level inputs to HOG. Leveraging semantic object boundary cues, our methods compute data-driven image feature maps via a supervised boundary detector. Compared with the raw image map, boundary cues offer mid-level, more object-specific visual responses that can be suited for subsequent HOG encoding. We validate integrations of several image transformation maps with an application of computer-aided detection of lymph nodes on thoracoabdominal CT images. Our experiments demonstrate that semantic boundary cues based HOG descriptors complement and enrich the raw intensity alone. We observe an overall system with substantially improved results ($\sim 78\%$ versus 60% recall at 3 FP/volume for two target regions). The proposed system also moderately outperforms the state-of-the-art deep convolutional neural network (CNN) system in the mediastinum region, without relying on data augmentation and requiring significantly fewer training samples.

1 Introduction

Quantitative assessment of lymph nodes (LNs) is routine in the daily radiological workflow. When measuring greater than 10 mm in short-axis diameter on an axial computed tomography (CT) slice, LNs are generally considered clinically relevant or actionable [13], indicative of diseases such as lung cancer, lymphoma, or inflammation. Manual detection of enlarged LNs, critical to determining disease progression and treatment response, is a time-consuming and error-prone process. Thus, there has been active research in recent years to develop accurate computer-aided lymph node detection (CADe) systems. A challenging object class for recognition, LNs exhibit substantial variation in appearance/location/pose as well as low contrast with surrounding anatomy on

---

* The rights of this work are transferred to the extent transferable according to title 17 § 105 U.S.C.

© Springer International Publishing Switzerland 2015 (outside the US)
N. Navab et al. (Eds.): MICCAI 2015, Part II, LNCS 9350, pp. 53–61, 2015.
DOI: 10.1007/978-3-319-24571-3_7

CT scans. Recent work on LN CADe has varied according to the feature types and learning algorithms used for training. [1, 8] utilize direct 3D information from CT scans, performing boosting-based feature selection over a pool of 50–60 thousand 3D Haar wavelet features. Due to the curse of dimensionality (analyzed in [14]), such approaches can result in systems with limited sensitivity (e.g. 60.9% at 6.1 FP/scan for mediastinal LNs in [8]). Circumventing 3D feature computation during LN classification, [14] implements a shallow hierarchy of linear models operating on 2D slices or views of LN candidate volumes of interest (VOIs) with histograms of oriented gradients (HOG) [3] features. Also using 2D (or 2.5D) views, the state-of-the-art performance is reported by [12] via a 5-layer, deep convolutional neural network (70% and 83% sensitivity at 3 FP/scan for mediastinal and abdominal LNs respectively).

In computer vision, edge detection serves as a valuable component in object detection tasks. Originally developed for use with natural images, the state-of-the-art edge detection methods [5,9] exploit the typical structures found in small edge patches such as straight lines and Y-junctions. [5] treats edge detection as a structured learning problem, using a random forest to predict a local edge annotation for each extracted patch from input images. While also using a random forest, [9] instead develops a multi-class classification approach, first clustering patches of ground truth edge annotations to define distinct classes of contours and then attempting to predict the cluster membership of input patches. In this work, our core hypothesis is that we can leverage the output response of semantic LN contour detection (built upon [9]) as mid-level object boundary maps, serving as enhanced input for HOG computation. By linking LN contour detection with LN detection itself, our proposed system will improve as the accuracy of state-of-the-art object contour detection methods improves.

Operating on 2D views (orthogonally sampled slices) of LN candidate volumes of interest (VOIs), our proposed method utilizes radiologist-annotated LN boundaries to first cluster small patches centered on LN boundaries into distinct contour classes. We then train a random forest [2] to classify the contour class membership of extracted LN candidate patches using sketch tokens [9]. Hybrid, mid-level feature maps are constructed by taking the per-voxel sums and maximums of the resulting contour class probabilities. In this manner, HOG is computed both on hybrid feature maps, which contain enhanced semantic objectness cues, and the CT intensity channel. A mixture-of-templates model (separate templates for modeling LNs of different size ranges) is efficiently implemented via a linear SVM, and the resulting 2D view confidence scores are averaged to obtain candidate-level classifications. Our experiments demonstrate that our new method leads to substantially improved performance over intensity-based HOG alone [14] and outperforms the state-of-the-art deep CNN system [12] on mediastinal LN detection, e.g. 78% vs. 70% recall at 3 FP/scan evaluated on the same benchmark data set. Our empirical study shows that HOG, when coupled with enriched hybrid image feature maps, can surprisingly be as effective as deep CNN. To the best of our knowledge, leveraging semantic object-label boundary cues for computer-aided diagnosis has not been previously studied.

2 Methods

Our lymph node detection system assumes we have a set of LN candidates generated within each target region. To facilitate benchmarking, we employ the publicly available LN detection datasets [12, 14]. There are 90 CT scans with ~1,000/3,200 true/false positive (TP/FP) mediastinal LNs and 86 scans with ~1,000/3,500 TP/FP abdominal LNs. Multiple TPs may correspond to the same LN. We also follow the view sampling procedure from [14]. For each generated candidate V, we extract 2D views or slices $\{v_i\}$ of size 45×45 voxels, sufficient to cover the size of most LNs with additional spatial context. Sampling at 0, 1, 2, 3, and 4 voxels away from the candidate centroid bi-directionally in each of the three orthogonal coordinate planes (axial, coronal, and sagittal) yields 27 views $\{v_i\}$ per V. To label the views, we simply transfer the label of V to each v_i: +1 if located inside any LN ground truth segmentation, -1 otherwise.

Defining Lymph Node Contour Classes. Computing our hybrid image feature maps (which will serve as input to HOG) begins with developing a lymph node contour detection system. To this end, we adapt the recent work on sketch tokens [9] to our CT imaging domain. However, in contrast to that work, where the objective is to detect the contours of any object category in natural images, we aim to identify semantic LN boundary contours. The substantial variation of LN shapes implies a wide spectrum of boundary contour appearances. Seeking to capture this wide distribution, we first cluster local LN edge patches into distinct sketch token contour classes. The CT scans in each target region's dataset were examined by a board-certified radiologist[1], who manually segmented any enlarged LNs encountered. Thus for each 2D slice of a CT scan, we have corresponding ground truth tracings of any LN boundaries present (Fig. 1).

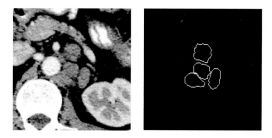

Fig. 1. Manual annotation of four abdominal lymph nodes on an axial CT slice.

After VOI decomposition of every LN candidate into 2D views of size 45×45 voxels, we have a corresponding set of binary images $\{S\}$ delineating the manually labeled LN boundaries. Following the notation of [9], we extract patches s of size 15×15 voxels from the images $\in \{S\}$. A patch s_i is extracted if its center

---

[1] The LN 3D segmentation mask datasets will be made publicly available. Visit
http://www.ariseff.com for info

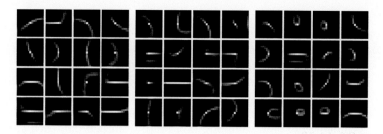

Fig. 2. Examples of sketch tokens learned from the manual tracings by radiologists for mediastinal LNs (left), abdominal LNs (middle), and colon polyps (right).

voxel is labeled as LN boundary. Approximately 1.7 million such patches are extracted in the training folds during our cross-validation experiments. Daisy descriptors [16] are then computed to compensate for subtle shifts in the manual boundary label placements across CT slices. Next, we perform k-means clustering on the Daisy descriptors, leading to $k = 150$ sketch token classes. Fig. 2 displays example patch cluster means for contours from LNs and colon polyps [15] (shown for comparison). Large variation in the sketch tokens is evident across LNs as well as colon polyps, a smaller-sized object class. Clustering-based labeling attempts to assign LN boundary patches into k classes for better detection.

Contour Detection. After defining the LN contour classes, we aim to detect their presence on candidate LN 2D views. Training labels for 15×15 patches are assigned as follows: If centered on a boundary pixel, patches are labeled according to their sketch token cluster membership (out of k choices); otherwise, they are labeled as negative. Similarly to [9], we compute multiple feature channels per patch [4]. These include 3 gradient magnitude channels using Gaussian blurs of $\sigma = 0$, 1.5 and 5 pixels and 8 oriented gradient channels. Because CT images are grayscale, we refrain from computing the CIE-LUV color space channels which would be relevant for natural images. Self-similarity features, useful for detecting texture-based contours, are computed on each gradient channel over a 5×5 grid leading to $\binom{5 \cdot 5}{2} = 300$ features per channel. Thus, for a 15×15 patch, we have $15 \cdot 15 \cdot 11 = 2475$ channel features and $300 \cdot 11 = 3300$ self-similarity features for a total of 5775 features per patch.

We train a random forest, an efficient method for multi-class classification, to detect the $k + 1$ LN contour classes [2]. Randomly sampling 1,000 patches per positive sketch token class and 2 negative patches per training image provides a decent balance between positive and negative training samples for each decision tree. 25 trees are trained whose leaf nodes denote the probability of a patch belonging to each class. Each tree uses a randomly selected subset of size $\sqrt{F}$ from F total available features for training.

Classification Using Boundary Input for HOG. A set of k sketch token class probability values are evaluated at every pixel for each 2D CT view. We construct the following mid-level, semantic representations as subsequent input for HOG computation. The first representation we compute is the sum of the

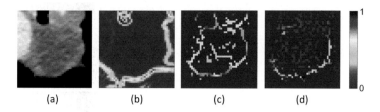

(a)   (b)   (c)   (d)

Fig. 3. (a) CT 2D View, (b) gradient transform, (c) *SumMap*, and (d) *MaxMap* (scaled for illustration), for a true mediastinal LN candidate. Note how the simple gradient transform (b) does not delineate the boundaries of the LN as strongly as the *SumMap* (c) derived from the supervisedly learned mid-level contour detection.

sketch token probabilities at each pixel in an image. Such a map can be interpreted as the total positive probability of each pixel residing on a true lymph node boundary. We also compute a map representing the maximum sketch token probability at each pixel because any true boundary pixel should fit well into at least one of the 150 contour classes (the reason for clustering positives into $k = 150$ classes in a "divide and conquer" manner). Letting t_{ij} denote the probability that a patch centered at pixel i belongs to a particular contour class j, and t_{i0} the probability of the negative background class, we derive the following two boundary probability cue maps: $SumMap_i = \sum_{j=1}^{k} t_{ij} = 1 - t_{i0}$; $MaxMap_i = \max_{1 \leq j \leq k} t_{ij}$ where k is the number of sketch token classes. Fig. 3 shows these learned feature maps for a mediastinal LN candidate. Compared to a simple image gradient transform, *SumMap* more accurately highlights the LN's boundary.

HOG can now be computed on each derived feature map in addition to the raw intensity CT image. The HOG descriptor divides an input image into square cells and delineates the quantized distribution of local intensity gradient magnitudes and orientations for each cell. 31 features are calculated per cell [7], which are then normalized within blocks of adjacent cells. Using the same parameters as [14], the 45×45-pixel 2D views are divided into square 5×5-pixel cells, yielding 25 cells and $25 \cdot 31 = 775$ features for each map. We test various concatenations of these feature sets in Sec. 3 for performance evaluation. For robust linear clas-

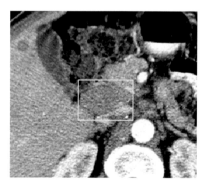

Fig. 4. A large abdominal lymph node that the single template model misses, but the mixture model detects. Larger LNs are especially clinically relevant.

sification (non-linear kernels exhibit poor generalization with limited datasets), we train an L2-regularized, L2-loss linear SVM [6], treating each 2D view as an independent instance and averaging their confidence scores to obtain the candidate-level predictions.

58   A. Seff et al.

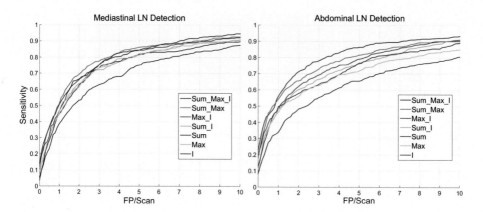

Fig. 5. Performance comparison of LN detection models trained on the seven integrated feature sets. For example, "Sum_Max_I" indicates the model trained on concatenated $HOG(SumMap)$, $HOG(MaxMap)$ and $HOG(Intensity)$ features. Six-fold cross-validation FROC curves are shown for both the mediastinal (left) and abdominal (right) target regions.

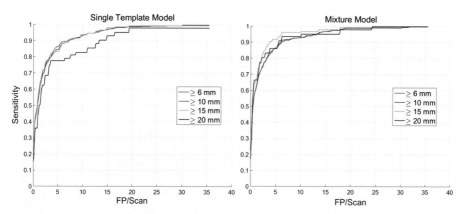

Fig. 6. Performance comparison of the single template model (left) and mixture-of-templates model (right) on abdominal LN detection. Note the substantially improved detection of malignant LNs greater than 20 mm in short-axis diameter by the mixture model.

Mixture-of-Templates Model by Size Gating. Enlarged LNs can vary greatly in size, reaching as large as 55 mm in short-axis diameter in the abdominal LN dataset. Although increasingly rare above 20 mm, very large LNs are especially clinically relevant. Thus it is crucial that LN CADe accurately identifies them. A single template of "HOG + Hybrid input" approach (modeling all LNs of varying sizes) will favor the detection of moderately enlarged LNs which are more common. Fig. 4 shows a typical large abdominal LN missed by a single template approach. Addressing this imbalance in the training/testing datasets, we extend our model by training two classifiers via a variation of size gating [11]. With a 15 mm size threshold (calibrated as the median ground truth LN size), one classifier is trained using all positives linked to LNs $\geq$ 15 mm and another is trained with the rest. The negative candidate set does not change. In testing, confidence scores output by each size-gated SVM are first scaled according to the corresponding range of training scores, making the classifiers' scores more comparable. For any instance, the mixture-of-templates model then reassigns the maximum of the two scaled scores as its final confidence. No LN size information is required in testing.

3   Evaluation and Discussion

Data and Protocol. To facilitate comparisons with other work, we evaluate our methods on the publicly available lymph node CT datasets used by [12,14]. There are 90 patients with 389 mediastinal LNs, and 86 patients with 595 abdominal LNs. We train and test models for each target region separately. Performing a six-fold cross-validation for the combined LN contour detection/LN detection, we randomly split each group of patients into 6 disjoint sets. For each fold, models are trained on five sets and and tested on the remaining set. Training the contour detection random forest (trees are parallelized) and subsequent linear SVM for a single fold takes $\sim$ 40 minutes. Testing on a single patient scan, including 2D view sampling and feature computation (not counting candidate generation), takes less than 5 seconds.

Performance. The three feature sets, $HOG(SumMap)$, $HOG(MaxMap)$ and $HOG(Intensity)$, are evaluated as single template models using all seven possible feature set integrations (Fig. 5) with the free-response operating characteristic (FROC). All six feature integrations that include at least one boundary cue map outperform HOG on raw intensity alone, in the full range of the FROC curves. The top performing integrations at low FP rates, Sum_Max for the mediastinum and Sum_Max_I for the abdomen, exhibit 24%–39% greater recall than the baseline HOG (e.g. 78% versus 63% at 3 FP/scan for mediastinal LNs; 78% versus 56% at 3 FP/scan for abdominal LNs). Furthermore, this performance is comparable to the state-of-the-art deep learning results [12], moderately outperforming in the mediastinum while only slightly lower for the abdomen. In detail, comparing with [12], we achieve sensitivities of 78% vs. 70% at 3 FP/scan and 88% vs. 84% at 6 FP/scan in the mediastinum, and sensitivities of 78% vs. 83% at 3 FP/scan and 89% vs. 90% at 6 FP/scan in the abdomen. The mixture-of-templates models are also evaluated using the top performing feature sets calibrated from the single template models. Fig. 6 shows the improvement in large malignant LN detection when the mixture model is used in the abdomen, e.g., 94% vs. 78% sensitivity at 6 FP/scan for LNs > 20 mm. We observe similar performance improvement for large mediastinal LNs when the mixture-of-templates model is employed.

Discussion. The proposed method significantly outperforms the recent work using HOG with a CT intensity map alone [14] which clearly demonstrates the merits of utilizing semantic object-level boundary cues for automated LN detection. This improvement is at the cost of annotated LN segmentation, required only at training and not in testing. The sketch tokens object boundary detector [9] is very robust and generalizable at a 15×15-pixel patch scale. The more recent structured forest edge detector [5] can be exploited as well. Comparing with the state-of-the-art deep CNN representation [12], our overall system is also a multi-layer pipeline with comparable/moderately better FROC curves in abdominal/mediastinal LN detection, respectively. The dense pixel-level semantic object boundary response map is especially critical for the performance gain over [12,14], but is non-trivial for a deep CNN, trained for direct LN recognition, to implement. CNNs are still mostly decision/classification models. While the newest fully convolutional neural networks can compute the output class support probability map, it is at a coarse (10–$20\times$ downsampled) spatial resolution [10] (thus not sufficient in our scenario). Instead we plan to investigate the feasibility of using our multi-channel hybrid image feature maps for direct CNN training as future work.

4   Conclusion

We propose a novel method to leverage hybrid image feature maps based on mid-level object boundary cues for computer-aided lymph node detection. The learned maps can be used in place of or in addition to raw CT intensity images as input to HOG feature computation. Evaluation of our approach for LN detection in two target regions demonstrates that the mid-level information supplied by the new representations both enhances and complements typical intensity-based HOG for this complex object recognition task. Our method achieves substantially improved results over baseline HOG systems [14] and moderately outperforms the state-of-the-art deep CNN system [12] in mediastinal LN detection.

Acknowledgments. This work was supported by the Intramural Research Program of the National Institutes of Health Clinical Center.

References

1. Barbu, A., Suehling, M., Xu, X., Liu, D., Zhou, S.K., Comaniciu, D.: Automatic detection and segmentation of lymph nodes from CT data. IEEE Trans. Med. Imaging 31(2), 240–250 (2012)
2. Breiman, L.: Random forests. Machine Learning 45(1), 5–32 (2001)
3. Dalal, N., Triggs, B.: Histograms of oriented gradients for human detection. In: CVPR, vol. 1, pp. 886–893 (2005)
4. Dollar, P., Tu, Z., Perona, P., Belongie, S.: Integral channel features. In: Proc. BMVC, pp. 1–11 (2009). doi:10.5244/C.23.91
5. Dollár, P., Zitnick, C.L.: Structured forests for fast edge detection. In: ICCV, pp. 1841–1848. IEEE (2013)

6. Fan, R.-E., Chang, K.-W., Hsieh, C.-J., Wang, X.-R., Lin, C.-J.: Liblinear: A library for large linear classification. Journal of Machine Learning Research 9, 1871–1874 (2008)
7. Felzenszwalb, P.F., Girshick, R.B., McAllester, D., Ramanan, D.: Object detection with discriminatively trained part-based models. IEEE Trans. on Pat. Ana. and Mach. Intell. 32(9), 1627–1645 (2010)
8. Feulner, J., Zhou, S.K., Hammon, M., Hornegger, J., Comaniciu, D.: Lymph node detection and segmentation in chest CT data using discriminative learning and a spatial prior. Medical Image Analysis 17(2), 254–270 (2013)
9. Lim, J.J., Zitnick, C.L., Dollár, P.: Sketch tokens: A learned mid-level representation for contour and object detection. In: CVPR, pp. 3158–3165. IEEE (2013)
10. Long, J., Shelhamer, E., Darrell, T.: Fully convolutional networks for semantic segmentation. In: CoRR abs/1411.4038 (2014)
11. Lu, L., Bi, J., Wolf, M., Salganicoff, M.: Effective 3D object detection and regression using probabilistic segmentation features in ct images. In: CVPR, pp. 1049–1056. IEEE (2011)
12. Roth, H., et al.: A new 2.5D representation for lymph node detection using random sets of deep convolutional neural network observations. In: Golland, P., Hata, N., Barillot, C., Hornegger, J., Howe, R. (eds.) MICCAI 2014, Part I. LNCS, vol. 8673, pp. 520–527. Springer, Heidelberg (2014)
13. Schwartz, L., Bogaerts, J., Ford, R., Shankar, L., Therasse, P., Gwyther, S., Eisenhauer, E.A.: Evaluation of lymph nodes with recist 1.1. Euro. J. of Cancer 45(2), 261–267 (2009)
14. Seff, A., et al.: 2D view aggregation for lymph node detection using a shallow hierarchy of linear classifiers. In: Golland, P., Hata, N., Barillot, C., Hornegger, J., Howe, R. (eds.) MICCAI 2014, Part I. LNCS, vol. 8673, pp. 544–552. Springer, Heidelberg (2014)
15. Summers, R.M., Yao, J., Pickhardt, P.J., Franaszek, M., Bitter, I., Brickman, D., Krishna, V., Choi, J.R.: Computed tomographic virtual colonoscopy computer-aided polyp detection in a screening population. Gastroenterology 129, 1832–1844 (2005)
16. Tola, E., Lepetit, V., Fua, P.: DAISY: An Efficient Dense Descriptor Applied to Wide Baseline Stereo. IEEE Trans. on Pat. Ana. and Mach. Intell. 32(5), 815–830 (2010)

Computer-Aided Pulmonary Embolism Detection Using a Novel Vessel-Aligned Multi-planar Image Representation and Convolutional Neural Networks

Nima Tajbakhsh[1], Michael B. Gotway[2], and Jianming Liang[1]

[1] Department of Biomedical Informatics, Arizona State University, Scottsdale, AZ, USA
{Nima.Tajbakhsh,Jianming.Liang}@asu.edu
[2] Department of Radiology, Mayo Clinic, Scottsdale, AZ, USA
Gotway.Michael@mayo.edu

Abstract. Computer-aided detection (CAD) can play a major role in diagnosing pulmonary embolism (PE) at CT pulmonary angiography (CTPA). However, despite their demonstrated utility, to achieve a clinically acceptable sensitivity, existing PE CAD systems generate a high number of false positives, imposing extra burdens on radiologists to adjudicate these superfluous CAD findings. In this study, we investigate the feasibility of convolutional neural networks (CNNs) as an effective mechanism for eliminating false positives. A critical issue in successfully utilizing CNNs for detecting an object in 3D images is to develop a "right" image representation for the object. Toward this end, we have developed a vessel-aligned multi-planar image representation of emboli. Our image representation offers three advantages: (1) efficiency and compactness—concisely summarizing the 3D contextual information around an embolus in only 2 image channels, (2) consistency—automatically aligning the embolus in the 2-channel images according to the orientation of the affected vessel, and (3) expandability—naturally supporting data augmentation for training CNNs. We have evaluated our CAD approach using 121 CTPA datasets with a total of 326 emboli, achieving a sensitivity of 83% at 2 false positives per volume. This performance is superior to the best performing CAD system in the literature, which achieves a sensitivity of 71% at the same level of false positives. We have further evaluated our system using the entire 20 CTPA test datasets from the PE challenge. Our system outperforms the winning system from the challenge at 0mm localization error but is outperformed by it at 2mm and 5mm localization errors. In our view, the performance at 0mm localization error is more important than those at 2mm and 5mm localization errors.

Keywords: Computer-aided detection, pulmonary embolism, convolutional neural networks, vessel-aligned image representation.

1 Introduction

Pulmonary embolism (PE) is a thrombus, occasionally colloquially referred to as a blood clot, that travels from the legs, or rarely other parts of the body, to the lungs where it obstructs central, lobar, segmental, or subsegmental pulmonary arteries depending on the size of the embolus. The untreated mortality rate of PE may approach

© Springer International Publishing Switzerland 2015
N. Navab et al. (Eds.): MICCAI 2015, Part II, LNCS 9350, pp. 62–69, 2015.
DOI: 10.1007/978-3-319-24571-3_8

30%. However, with early diagnosis and treatment, the mortality rate decreases to as low as 2% to 11%. CT pulmonary angiography (CTPA) is the primary means for the evaluation of suspected PE. At CTPA, an embolus appears as a dark region surrounded by the brighter, contrast-enhanced vessel lumen. CTPA dataset interpretation demands a radiologist to carefully trace each branch of the pulmonary artery for any suspected PEs. Therefore, PE diagnosis often requires extensive reading time, and the accuracy of CTPA interpretation depends on the radiologists' experience, attention span, eye fatigue, and their sensitivity to visual characteristics of PEs.

Computer-aided detection (CAD) can play a major role in detecting and diagnosing PEs. Recent clinical studies have shown that CAD systems can help radiologists increase their sensitivity for PE detection [3]. However, despite their demonstrated utility, existing CAD systems still require a relatively high false positive rate in order to achieve a clinically acceptable PE sensitivity. The false positives generated by CAD systems prolong the reading time of CTPA studies, because each CAD finding must be examined by a radiologist and adjudicated. It is therefore highly desirable to develop a CAD system that can achieve higher sensitivity while maintaining a clinically acceptable false positive range (between 1 to 5 false positives per CTPA study).

This paper investigates the feasibility of convolutional neural networks (CNNs) as an effective tool for eliminating false positive detections. We have found that the effective utilization of CNNs for detecting PEs and removing false detections in 3D CTPA datasets is contingent on an effective image representation of PEs. As such, a key finding from our work is a vessel-aligned multi-planar image representation of emboli that offers three advantages: (1) our proposed image representation is *efficient* and *compact* because it concisely summarizes the 3D contextual information around an embolus in only 2 image channels; (2) our proposed image representation is *consistent* because it automatically aligns the embolus in the 2-channel images according to the orientation of the affected vessel; and (3) our proposed image representation is *expandable* because it naturally supports data augmentation for training a CNN. We have evaluated our CAD system using 121 CTPA datasets containing a total of 326 emboli, achieving a sensitivity of 83% at 2 false positives per volume. This performance is superior to the best performing CAD system in the literature, which achieves a sensitivity of 71% at the same level of false positives. We have further evaluated our system with the entire 20 CTPA test datasets from the PE challenge [1]. Our system outperforms MeVis', the best reported system, at 0mm localization error but is outperformed by MeVis' at 2mm and 5mm localization errors. In our view, the performance at 0mm localization error is more important than those at 2mm and 5mm localization errors.

2   Related Work

CAD systems for PE typically consist of four stages: 1) extracting a volume of interest (VOI) from the original dataset by performing lung segmentation [5,11,8] or vessel segmentation [7,11,2]; 2) generating a set of PE candidates within the VOI using algorithms such as tobogganing [5]; 3) extracting hand-crafted features from each PE candidate (e.g., [6]), and 4) computing a confidence score for each of the candidates using a rule based classifier [7], neural networks and a nearest neighbor classifier [11,8], or a multi-instance classifier [5]. However, current CAD systems either produce many false positives to achieve a high detection sensitivity [7], or yield acceptable false positive rates but with only limited sensitivity levels [8,2,11] (see Table 1 for a detailed performance comparison). We hypothesize that inadequate modeling of PEs based on hand-crafted features results in suboptimal CAD performance, and therefore investigate the use of a new image representation for PEs, coupled with CNNs, to improve state-of-the-art performance.

3   Proposed Method

Given a CTPA dataset, our method first segments lungs and then generates a set of PE candidates within the lung area using the tobogganing algorithm [5]. Our method then uses our vessel-aligned multi-planar image representation to produce a 2-channel image representation for each PE candidate. The resulting 2-channel patches are then fed to a CNN to classify the underlying candidates into PE or non-PE categories. Please refer to [5] for the tobogganing algorithm and to [4] for the CNN. In the following, we shall focus on our suggested vessel-aligned multi-planar image representation.

3.1   Vessel-Aligned Multi-planar Image Representation

The success of CNNs for object detection in 3D volumetric datasets such as CT images heavily relies on the representation of the object of interest [9,10]. We have experimentally found that a suitable 3D image representation for CNNs must meet three requirements: (1) compactness and efficiency, (2) consistency across instances, and (3) expandability for data augmentation. With these requirements in mind, we propose an image representation, called vessel-aligned multi-planar image representation, for PE, which has these three critical properties. In the following, we first describe our unique image representation and then explain how it meets the above requirements.

To obtain our image representation, we first estimate the orientation of the vessel that contains the candidate. For this purpose, a 15x15x15mm neighborhood is extracted around the PE candidate. In the resulting subvolume, the PE appears as a filling defect, because PEs are relatively darker than the contrast-enhanced vessel. To minimize the influence of the filling defect on vessel orientation estimation, the vessel-like intensity value of 100 HU (Hounsfield units) is assigned to the PE voxels within the subvolume. Note that the tobogganing algorithm [4] has already labeled the PE voxels associated with each candidate. Next, a principle component analysis is performed in the connected component ($\geq$ 100 HU) that contains the PE. If v_1, v_2, v_3 denote the eigen vectors of the analyzed component ($\lambda_1 \geq \lambda_2 \geq \lambda_3$), then interpolating the volume along $\{v_1, v_2\}$ or $\{v_1, v_3\}$ results in the longitudinal view of the PE (the first channel of our image representation) and interpolating the volume along $\{v_2, v_3\}$ results in the cross-sectional view of the PE (the second channel of our image representation).

Our image representation is compact because it concisely summarizes the 3D contextual information around PEs in only 2 image channels. While it is theoretically possible to train a CNN using subvolumes with an arbitrary number of slices, the performance of such networks have been reported to be inferior to the CNNs that have been trained

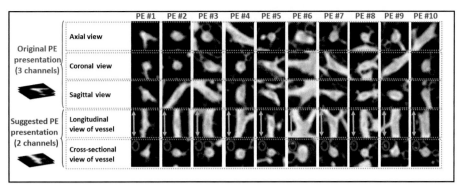

Fig. 1. The suggested 2-channel image representation characterizes emboli more consistently than the original axial, sagittal, and coronal views. As seen, in nearly all cases, the suggested scheme consistently captures PEs within the containing vessel as elongated and circular structures in the first and second channels, respectively. The three standard views do not provide this property given the varying orientation of the containing vessels. A consistent image appearance is the key to training an accurate image classifier.

using samples with a fewer number of slices [9]. In fact, the information embedded in the additional image slices has been shown to degrade classification performance [9]. This phenomenon is attributed to the curse of dimensionality, where a large number of image channels corresponds to learning a far larger number of network parameters, which in turn leads to over-fitting to the training samples and thus poor generalization performance. It is therefore desirable to efficiently represent the 3D context around the object of interest using a low dimensional image representation.

Our image representation consistently describes PEs and the containing vessels. In general, emboli can can affect pulmonary arteries in any orientation. As a result, images extracted from the axial, sagittal, coronal planes exhibit a significant variation in the appearance of emboli. This in turn complicates the classification task and hinders effective utilization of CNNs. With the benefit of vessel alignment, our image representation allows for a consistent image representation whereby emboli consistently appear as elongated structures in the longitudinal vessel view and as circular structures in the cross-sectional vessel view. Fig. 1 illustrates variations in PE appearances using the suggested vessel-aligned image representation and a standard image representation based on sagittal, coronal and axial views.

Our image representation amenably supports data augmentation, which is essential for effective training and testing of CNNs. In 2D applications, data augmentation is performed by applying arbitrary in-plane rotations and then collecting samples at multiple scales and translations. A 3D representation must also support the above operations to enable data augmentation. While it is straightforward to extend translation and scale to a 3D space, the rotation operation can be problematic. Our image representation is based on longitudinal and cross-sectionals planes; however, rotating such planes along a random axis will result in the arbitrary appearance of the same PE in the resulting 2-channel images (Fig. 2(a)). The major challenge is how to perform 3D rotation such that the PE representation remains consistent. Our image representation accommodates this need by rotating the planes around the vessel axis v_1. By doing so, we obtain two

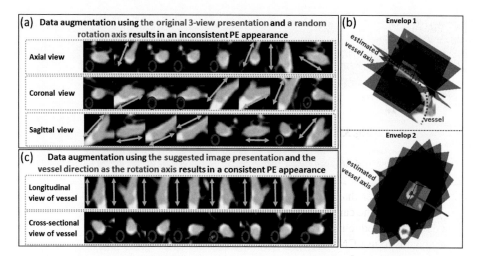

Fig. 2. (a) Data augmentation using random rotation axes, as suggested in [10], results in inconsistent PE appearance. (b) The suggested image representation uses two envelopes of planes to achieve consistency for data augmentation. (c) Consistent PE appearance after data augmentation using the suggested envelopes of planes. The green double arrows and red ellipses represent the shapes of PEs and the containing vessels.

envelopes of image planes (see Fig. 2(b)) where the first envelope contains the planes that all intersect at the vessel axis and the second envelope contains the image planes whose normals are the vessel axis. By selecting any pairs of planes from the two envelopes, one can generate a new PE instance while retaining the consistency. Fig. 2(c) illustrates consistency in appearance of PEs after data augmentation using the suggested envelopes of planes.

3.2 Convolutional Neural Networks (CNNs)

CNNs are deep learning machines that can potentially eliminate the need for designing hand-crafted features—they learn the features and train the classifier simultaneously. CNNs are so-named for their convolutional layers that learn discriminative patterns of the training samples at multiple scales. In this work, we employ the GPU-based open-source implementation of CNNs [4] and use the layout shown in Fig. 3. We have experimented with more sophisticated network architectures but observed no significant performance gain.

4   Experiments

We have evaluated our CAD system using 2 databases: (1) our private database consisting of 121 CTPA datasets with a total of 326 emboli, and (2) the test datasets from the PE challenge [1] consisting of 20 CTPA datasets with a total of 133 emboli.

Evaluations Using Our Database. The candidate generation module of our CAD system produces a total of 8585 PE candidates in the 121 CTPA datasets, of which 7722

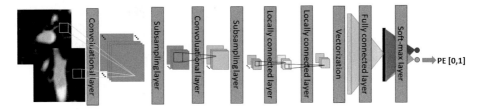

Fig. 3. The layout of the CNN used in our experiments.

are false positives and 863 are true positives. It is possible for a CAD system to produce multiple detections for a single large PE and that explains why the number of our true detections is greater than the number of PEs in the database. According to the available ground truth, the candidate generation module achieves a sensitivity of 93% for PE detection while producing, on average, 65.8 false positives per patient.

Our goal is to use CNNs to minimize the number of false positives while maintaining a high sensitivity for PE detection. To train CNNs, we randomly split the collected detections at the patient level into 3 groups, enabling a 3-fold cross validation of our CAD system. We then used the false positive detections as negative candidates and the true detections as positive candidates. Given the limited number of candidates, we formed the training set by performing data augmentation. For this purpose, we collected $N = N_r \times N_t \times N_s$ samples from each candidate location based on our vessel-aligned multi-planar PE representation, where N_r is the number of rotations, N_t is the number of translations, and N_s is the number of image scaling. To produce rotated patches, we rotated the longitudinal and cross-sectional vessel planes around the vessel axis $N_r = 5$ times. For scaling, we extracted patches at $N_s = 3$ different scales, resulting in 10mm, 15mm, and 20mm wide patches. In each scale, we have performed image interpolation so that the resulting patches are all 32x32 pixels. For translation, we shifted the candidate location along the vessel direction $N_t = 3$ times, up to 20% of the physical width of the patches. With data augmentation, we can increase the size of the training set by a factor of $N = 45$, which is sufficiently large to train CNNs. Given a test CTPA dataset, we first obtain a set of candidates, and then apply the trained CNN on N 2-channel image patches extracted from each candidate location. The confidence values for the underlying candidate is then computed as the average of the resulting N confidence values. Once all the test candidates are processed, we obtain an FROC curve by changing a threshold on the corresponding confidence values.

Fig. 4 shows the FROC curve of the suggested system. For comparison, we have computed the FROC curve of [5] using the prediction results provided by the corresponding author. We have chosen [5] for performance comparison because their suggested system has achieved the best performance reported in the literature on a reasonably large CTPA database (see Table 1). For further comparison, we have replaced our suggested image presentation with a 2.5D image representation as suggested in [10]. For fair comparisons, we have kept all the other stages the same. As seen in Fig. 4, our system outperforms [5], which is a CAD system based on a carefully designed set of hand-crafted features [6] and a multi-instance classifier. In addition, we observed that the CNN trained using a 2.5D image representation results in a performance which is not only inferior to our suggested image representation but also to the hand-crafted approach, demonstrating the

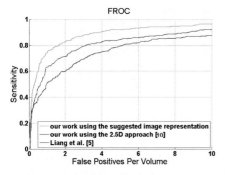

Fig. 4. Our CAD system using the suggested image representation outperforms the best hand-crafted approach [5] and also a CNN powered by a 2.5D approach [10].

Method	Sensitivity	FPs/vol	#datasets	#PEs
Liang et al. [5]	70.0%	2.0	132	716
Bouma et al. [2]	58%	4.0	19	116
Park et al. [8]	63.2	18.4	20	44
Ozkan et al. [7]	61%	8.2	33	450
Wang et al. [11]	62%	17.1	12	24
This work	83.4%	2.0	121	326
This work (2.5D)	60.4%	2.0	121	326
Liang et al. [5]	71.7%	2.0	121	326

Table 1. (top) Performance of the existing PE CAD systems obtained through different datasets. (bottom) Performance comparison based on our database of 121 CTPA datasets. Operating points are taken from Fig. 4.

significant contribution of our effective image representation in achieving the improved performance. Table 1 contrasts the performance of our proposed CAD system with that of the other CAD systems suggested in the literature.

Evaluations Using PE Challenge Database. We have further trained a CNN, powered by our unique image representation, using all 121 CTPA datasets from our database and then evaluated our CAD system using the test database from the PE challenge [1]. Since the ground-truth was not available on the website, our detection results were evaluated by the organizers. At 0mm localization error, our CAD system achieves a sensitivity of 34.6% at 2 FPs/vol, which outperforms the winning team (a commercial CAD system designed MeVis Medical Solutions) with a sensitivity of 28.4% at the same false positive rate. Our CAD system is, however, outperformed by MeVis' at 2mm and 5mm localization errors. For more detailed comparisons, please refer to [1]. Despite the demonstrated superiority at 0mm localization error, our CAD system exhibits a notable performance degradation compared to the results obtained using our database. We attribute this to faulty lung segmentation, which results in many PE candidates in the colon and diaphragm. Since such false positives had not been observed in our training sets, the trained CNN did not perform optimally in removing such false positives.

5   Conclusions and Discussions

In this work, we investigated the possibility of a unique PE representation, coupled with CNNs, to produce a more accurate PE CAD system. Our system contrasts with existing systems, wherein a traditional hand-crafted feature design is used for characterizing PEs. We evaluated our system in comparison with the most robust hand-crafted approach [5] and a learning-based approach using CNNs powered by a 2.5D PE representation, demonstrating a marked performance improvement. Our method was also tested using the test database from the PE challenge where it outperformed the academic systems at the three localization errors and also outperformed a commercial CAD system at 0mm localization error. Moving forward, we intend to improve the accuracy of our CAD system using additional training cases to address the issue of faulty lung segmentation resulting from non-pulmonary candidates.

Acknowledgment. This project is supported by a seed grant awarded by Arizona State University and Mayo Clinic. We thank German Gonzalez, the organizer of the CAD PE challenge, for evaluating our results with the test datasets from the challenge.

References

1. http://www.cad-pe.org
2. Bouma, H., Sonnemans, J.J., Vilanova, A., Gerritsen, F.A.: Automatic detection of pulmonary embolism in cta images. IEEE Transactions on Medical Imaging 28(8), 1223–1230 (2009)
3. Das, M., Mühlenbruch, G., Helm, A., Bakai, A., Salganicoff, M., Stanzel, S., Liang, J., Wolf, M., Günther, R.W., Wildberger, J.E.: Computer-aided detection of pulmonary embolism: influence on radiologists detection performance with respect to vessel segments. European Radiology 18(7), 1350–1355 (2008)
4. Krizhevsky, A., Sutskever, I., Hinton, G.E.: Imagenet classification with deep convolutional neural networks. In: Advances in Neural Information Processing Systems, pp. 1097–1105 (2012)
5. Liang, J., Bi, J.: Computer aided detection of pulmonary embolism with tobogganing and mutiple instance classification in CT pulmonary angiography. In: Karssemeijer, N., Lelieveldt, B. (eds.) IPMI 2007. LNCS, vol. 4584, pp. 630–641. Springer, Heidelberg (2007)
6. Liang, J., Bi, J.: Local characteristic features for computer aided detection of pulmonary embolism in ct angiography. In: Proceedings of the First MICCAI Workshop on Pulmonary Image Analysis, pp. 263–272 (2008)
7. Özkan, H., Osman, O., Şahin, S., Boz, A.F.: A novel method for pulmonary embolism detection in cta images. Computer Methods and Programs in Biomedicine 113(3), 757–766 (2014)
8. Park, S.C., Chapman, B.E., Zheng, B.: A multistage approach to improve performance of computer-aided detection of pulmonary embolisms depicted on CT images: Preliminary investigation. IEEE Transactions on Biomedical Engineering 58(6), 1519–1527 (2011)
9. Prasoon, A., Petersen, K., Igel, C., Lauze, F., Dam, E., Nielsen, M.: Deep feature learning for knee cartilage segmentation using a triplanar convolutional neural network. In: Mori, K., Sakuma, I., Sato, Y., Barillot, C., Navab, N. (eds.) MICCAI 2013, Part II. LNCS, vol. 8150, pp. 246–253. Springer, Heidelberg (2013)
10. Roth, H.R., et al.: A new 2.5D representation for lymph node detection using random sets of deep convolutional neural network observations. In: Golland, P., Hata, N., Barillot, C., Hornegger, J., Howe, R. (eds.) MICCAI 2014, Part I. LNCS, vol. 8673, pp. 520–527. Springer, Heidelberg (2014)
11. Wang, X., Song, X., Chapman, B.E., Zheng, B.: Improving performance of computer-aided detection of pulmonary embolisms by incorporating a new pulmonary vascular-tree segmentation algorithm. In: SPIE Medical Imaging, pp. 83152U–83152U. International Society for Optics and Photonics (2012)

Ultrasound-Based Detection of Prostate Cancer Using Automatic Feature Selection with Deep Belief Networks

Shekoofeh Azizi[1], Farhad Imani[1], Bo Zhuang[1], Amir Tahmasebi[2],
Jin Tae Kwak[3], Sheng Xu[3], Nishant Uniyal[1], Baris Turkbey[4], Peter Choyke[4],
Peter Pinto[4], Bradford Wood[4], Mehdi Moradi[5], Parvin Mousavi[6],
and Purang Abolmaesumi[1]

[1] The University of British Columbia, Vancouver, BC, Canada
[2] Philips Research North America, Briarcliff Manor, NY, USA
[3] National Institutes of Health, Bethesda, MD, USA
[4] National Cancer Institute, Bethesda, MD, USA
[5] IBM Almaden Research Center, San Jose, CA, USA
[6] Queen's University, Kingston, ON, Canada

Abstract. We propose an automatic feature selection framework for analyzing temporal ultrasound signals of prostate tissue. The framework consists of: 1) an unsupervised feature reduction step that uses Deep Belief Network (DBN) on spectral components of the temporal ultrasound data; 2) a supervised fine-tuning step that uses the histopathology of the tissue samples to further optimize the DBN; 3) a Support Vector Machine (SVM) classifier that uses the activation of the DBN as input and outputs a likelihood for the cancer. In leave-one-core-out cross-validation experiments using 35 biopsy cores, an area under the curve of 0.91 is obtained for cancer prediction. Subsequently, an independent group of 36 biopsy cores was used for validation of the model. The results show that the framework can predict 22 out of 23 benign, and all of cancerous cores correctly. We conclude that temporal analysis of ultrasound data can potentially complement multi-parametric Magnetic Resonance Imaging (mp-MRI) by improving the differentiation of benign and cancerous prostate tissue.

Keywords: Temporal ultrasound data, deep learning, deep belief network, cancer diagnosis, prostate cancer, feature selection, classification.

1 Introduction

The early diagnosis of prostate cancer, as the most common type of diagnosed malignancy in North American men, plays an important role in the choice and the success of treatments [8]. The definitive diagnosis of prostate cancer is histopathological analysis of biopsy tissue samples, which is typically guided under Transrectal Ultrasound (TRUS). However, conventional systematic biopsy under TRUS guidance does not have high sensitivity and specificity. Recently,

© Springer International Publishing Switzerland 2015
N. Navab et al. (Eds.): MICCAI 2015, Part II, LNCS 9350, pp. 70–77, 2015.
DOI: 10.1007/978-3-319-24571-3_9

fusion of multi-parametric MRI (mp-MRI) with TRUS has shown significant potential for improved cancer yield [7]. A meta-analysis of seven mp-MRI studies with 526 patients show specificity of 0.88 and sensitivity of 0.74, with negative predictive values ranging from 0.65 to 0.94 [9]. mp-MRI suffers from several limitations including low sensitivity for detection of small lesions and low grade cancer. Hence, there is a need to develop new imaging techniques that can complement mp-MRI for prostate cancer diagnosis.

Over the past two decades, several ultrasound-based techniques have been proposed for characterizing cancerous tissue [8]. The clinical uptake of these methods has been slow, mainly due to the large variability of the tissue characterization results. The primary sources of such variability are the heterogeneous patient population and cancer grades. Moreover, these methods do not generally report clinically sufficient specificity and sensitivity to ensure that all aggressive cancer cases can be captured by ultrasound analysis.

Ultrasound-based tissue typing techniques to-date mainly rely on spectral analysis of a single ultrasound image, or alternative modalities such as elastography and Doppler, that are not commonly used during prostate biopsy. Recently, analysis of temporal ultrasound data obtained from a fixed tissue location has been proposed to complement other ultrasound-based tissue typing techniques [4]. The key advantage of this technique is that it relies on conventional ultrasound imaging data, without the need to change the clinical scanning protocol. It has been shown that temporal changes in the ultrasound signal backscattered from the tissue varies across tissue types. Several hypotheses have been explored to determine the physical phenomenon governing the approach. It has been proposed that the acoustic radiation force of the transmit ultrasound signal increases the tissue temperature, and changes the speed of sound [2]. Another hypothesis indicates that micro-vibration of acoustic scatterers, contribute to tissue typing in this approach. Previous works [4,5,12] utilize a machine learning framework to determine the correlation between features extracted from the temporal ultrasound data and cancer presence or grade provided by histopathology. In these methods, features were heuristically determined from the spectral/wavelet analysis of the ultrasound data. In addition to challenges associated with defining features that are correlated with the underlying tissue properties, it is also difficult to determine the best combination of those features for effective tissue typing as the number of features increases. The lack of a systematic approach for feature selection can lead to a so-called "cherry picking" of the features [4,5,12].

Deep learning approaches have gained significant attention for capturing abstract representations of input data [1], and have been successfully used in medical image analysis [6,11]. In this paper, we exploit Deep Belief Networks (DBN) [1] to automatically learn a high-level feature representation of the temporal ultrasound data that can detect prostate cancer. Subsequently, we use the high-level features in a supervised classification step based on Support Vector Machines (SVM) to generate a cancer likelihood. In a study consisting of 71 biopsy cores obtained from 62 subjects, we demonstrate that the approach is effective in identifying both benign and cancerous biopsy cores in TRUS-guided biopsy, and can complement mp-MRI to further improve the cancer yield.

2   Materials

Temporal ultrasound Radio-Frequency (RF) data was acquired with a Philips iU22 ultrasound scanner during MRI-guided targeted TRUS biopsies using the Philips UroNav platform at the National Institutes of Health Clinical Center (NIH-CC), Bethesda, MD. Prior to the biopsy session, mp-MR images including T2-weighted, Diffusion Weighted Images (DWI), and Dynamic Contrast En- hanced (DCE) images were acquired for each subject. Two independent radiolo- gists identified and scored suspicious lesions in MR images based on a standard protocol, ranging from 1 (no cancer) to 5 (aggressive cancer) and assigned grades: low (2 or less), moderate (3) and high (4 or more). The desired biopsy targets were delineated on the T2-weighted MR image based on these scores. In the beginning of the procedure, a 3D ultrasound volume of the prostate was recon- structed by acquiring a series of electromagnetically (EM) tracked 2D TRUS images. For targeted biopsy, T2-weighted MR images were automatically fused with the 3D US volume of the prostate using the UroNav platform. Follow- ing the registration of ultrasound and MR volumes, the targeted locations for biopsy were transformed to the EM coordinate frame. During biopsy, the clini- cian navigates through the prostate volume to reach the desired target location for acquiring a core. The clinician then holds the TRUS transducer fixed for about 5 seconds to acquire 100 frames of ultrasound time series data. Temporal ultrasound data is collected from at most two MR-identified targets per subject. Tissue biopsy is then followed by histopathology analysis and results are used as the ground-truth labels for evaluation of cancer detection. The level of ab- normality for each biopsy core is described using Gleason Score (GS). Data is obtained from 71 biopsy cores of 62 subjects; among them 45 are benign while 26 other cores are cancerous. The data was divided into two independent data sets for training, D_1, and validation, D_2. For building the model, we need to use homogeneous tissue regions. Given potential mis-registration errors between MR and ultrasound images, we only include biopsy cores with at least 7.2 mm of cancer for a typical core length of 18 mm. We also add benign cases to the training data set.

The training dataset, D_1, consists of 35 biopsy cores obtained from 31 patients with the following histopathology label distribution: Benign: 22; GS 3+3: 0; GS 3+4: 5; GS 4+3: 2; GS 4+4: 4; and, GS 4+5: 2 cores. The validation data set, D_2, contains another 36 biopsy cores obtained from 31 patients with the following histopathology label distribution: Benign: 23; GS 3+3: 4; GS 3+4: 3; GS 4+3: 0; GS 4+4: 4; and, GS 4+5: 2 cores.

We extract features from temporal ultrasound data over 20 equally-sized Re- gions of Interest (ROI) of size 1 mm^2 for each biopsy core. For each biopsy target, we analyze an area of 2×10 mm^2 in the lateral and axial directions, respectively, along the projected needle path in the ultrasound image, and centered on the

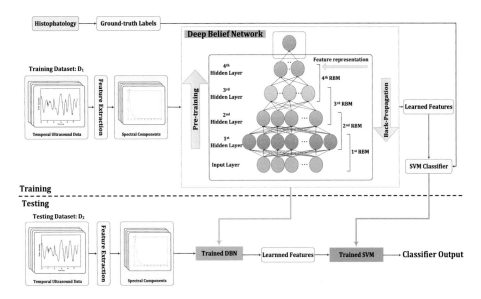

Fig. 1. An illustration of the proposed method for prostate cancer detection. Our DBN has a layer of real-valued visible units of dimension 50 and four hidden layers with 100, 50, 45 and 6 hidden units. The red box contains the pre-trained DBN, and the blue box containing one neuron is added for the fine-tuning step. The latent features are the output of the last layer of DBN.

target. The width of this area is close to the width of the biopsy core, but the length of the biopsy core is typically 18 mm. To generate the features of temporal ultrasound data, we take the Fourier transform of the entire time series, normalized to the frame rate. For each ROI, we generate 50 spectral features by averaging the absolute values of the Discrete Fourier Transform (DFT) of the zero-mean ultrasound time series for 50 positive frequency components. Due to symmetry, only the positive frequency components of the spectrum are used.

3   Methods

Fig. 1 illustrates a schematic diagram of the proposed method. Using D_1, we derive high level - latent- feature representation from the 50 extracted features using DBN. Then, we use the learned feature information along with ground-truth labels to train a Support Vector Machine (SVM). To verify the generated model, we extract the features for data set D_2. Then, we use the activations of the trained DBN and SVM to derive the tissue type labels for each ROI.

3.1   Deep Belief Networks

DBN, as a generative probabilistic model, can be trained to extract a deep hierarchical representation of the input data. We construct a DBN by stacking many layers of Restricted Boltzmann Machines (RBMs), each of which consists of a visible layer and a hidden layer of neurons. The two layers are connected by a matrix of weighted connections and there are no connections within a layer. RBMs can be stacked by linking the hidden layer of one RBM to the visible layer of the next RBM. A schematic representation is shown in Fig. 1. The role of a RBM is to model the distribution of its input and capturing patterns in the visible units. Thus, DBNs offer an unsupervised way to learn multi-layer probabilistic representations of data that are progressively *deeper* with each successive layer. Utilizing this representational power, we can find a latent representation of the original low-level features extracted from temporal ultrasound data.

We perform the contrast divergence approximation [1] to update the weights during training. The DBN can be trained by performing a greedy layer-wise unsupervised *pre-training* phase [1]. In a greedy layer-wise learning, we train one layer at a time and use the representation of the previous hidden layer as input for the next hidden layer. In order to capture a higher level representation of input features, we stack another output layer on top of the DBN. This layer is used to represent the class label of an input data. Therefore, by back-propagation and having parameters initialized by the pre-training, we can optimize the weights of the deep network. This supervised optimization step is called *fine-tuning* [1].

3.2   Feature Learning

The model architecture of the DBN is shown in Fig. 1. Training of the DBN requires trial and error to determine various parameters, such as the learning rate, the momentum, the weight-cost, the initial values of the weights, the number of hidden units and the size of each mini-batch [3]. We used the MATLAB library of Tanaka *et al.* [10] to build and train the DBN. We started with the default values for all parameters as it was suggested in this library. In the first step, we heuristically searched for the number of hidden layers and the number of neurons in each layer, within the layer-wise greedy training framework [1], so that lowest errors with the default library parameters were obtained in the the training data, D_1. Next, we followed the guidelines given by Hinton [3] to adjust the learning rate, the momentum and the weight-cost to achieve lower error in the training data. The pre-trained DBN was finalized with 100 passes (epochs), a fixed learning rate of 0.001 and batch size of 5, and has a layer of real-valued visible units of dimension 50, and four hidden layers, consisting of 100, 50, 45 and 6 hidden units. The last hidden layer produces the latent features. To further reduce the error, we then proceeded to a fine-tuning step using the same training set. We ran 70 epochs with a fixed learning rate of 0.01. During both pre-training and fine-tuning, a small weight-cost of 0.0002 was used and the learning was accelerated by using a momentum of 0.9. To mitigate the risk of over-fitting the model during training, all the parameters stated above were only tuned based on data set D_1. The classification performance reported in the paper is only associated with the independent data set D_2.

3.3   Classification

We use the latent features as input for the SVM classifier[1] with the Radial Basis Function (RBF) kernel in the final stage. The parameters of SVM were determined using a grid-search algorithm which uses leave-one-core-out cross-validation on latent features obtained from D_1. In addition to the binary output of the classifier, we estimate the likelihood of the ROIs to be cancerous by using the approach presented in [12]. Finally, the classification model developed using data set D_1, was validated with the data set D_2 in the testing step (See Fig. 1).

4   Results

In order to identify the consistency of learnt features in the training set D_1, we follow a cross-validation strategy. In leave-one-core-out cross-validation experiments, an area under Receiver Operating Characteristics (ROC) curve of 0.91 is obtained for cancer prediction in the biopsy cores. The result of validation of our classification framework on data set D_2 is shown in Fig. 2. Using a threshold of 55% for the model output, 22 out of 23 benign cores can be labeled correctly. Furthermore, all cancerous cores can be identified correctly. Finally, we compare the model output against the grade assigned to each biopsy core in MRI. As shown in Fig. 2(b), the majority of MRI grades are moderate and our method can detect all of cores with moderate MRI grade correctly. Moreover, except one benign case with low MRI grade, the model correctly predicts the label of all High MRI grade biopsy cores.

   We also performed an additional experiment by permuting the training and testing data. To create new training and test sets, in each permutation, we exchanged a randomly selected cancerous core larger than 1.5 mm between D1 and D2. Similarly, we exchanged a randomly selected benign core between the two data sets. This resulted in five different permutations given the distribution of large cancer cores in our data. One average, we achieved accuracy, sensitivity, and specificity of 93%, 98%, and 90%, respectively. In four out of five permutations, all cancer cores were correctly identified.

5   Discussion and Conclusion

We utilized a machine learning framework for analysing temporal ultrasound data to accurately predict prostate cancer in MRI-TRUS guided targeted prostate biopsy. A deep learning approach was used for automatic feature selection and learning of the high-level features from temporal ultrasound signals. We automatically reduced the dimensionality of the temporal ultrasound features using a DBN followed by supervised fine-tuning. Then, we used an SVM classifier along with the activation of the trained DBN to characterize the prostate tissue. The proposed approach systematically learned discriminant features from high-dimensional temporal ultrasound features to detect prostate cancer.

---

[1] A Library for SVMs: http://www.csie.ntu.edu.tw/~cjlin/libsvm/

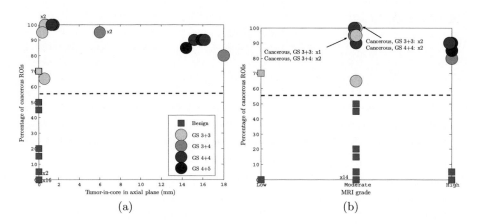

Fig. 2. Percentage of cancerous ROIs with a likelihood of more than 50% in the model output in each core: (a) The model output versus tumor-in-core-length for the validation data. (b) The model output versus MRI grade for the validation data. Cancer cores and benign cores are shown as circles and squares, respectively.

While our results with DBN are highly promising, DBN is a computationally expensive method that performs best on very large data sets. The greedy training algorithm [1] ensures that the parameters of the model can be tuned layer-by-layer, reducing the need for large sample sizes to a certain extent. We compare our approach with standard SVM and random forests implementations using the same input. In our data set, random forests outperforms SVM, and achieves sensitivity of 69% and specificity of 78%.

We built our model using a training data set consisting of temporal ultrasound data of 35 biopsy cores. The model was validated on an independent set of 36 biopsy cores. The results indicate that latent feature selection with DBN can improve the tissue typing capabilities of temporal ultrasound data analysis, which can potentially complement mp-MRI for TRUS-guided biopsy. Specifically, since all patients in our study were originally labeled as suspicious for cancer in mp-MRI, our results indicate that with a subsequent analysis of temporal ultrasound data, it might be possible to further improve the differentiation of benign and cancerous cases, hence reducing the need for unnecessary biopsy. This can be a powerful tool for surveillance of patients.

Acknowledgments. The authors would like to acknowledge the help of Dr. Jochen Kruecker and Dr. Pingkun Yan for assisting with the experiments. This work was supported in part by the Natural Sciences and Engineering Research Council of Canada (NSERC) and the Canadian Institutes of Health Research (CIHR).

References

1. Bengio, Y., Lamblin, P., Popovici, D., et al.: Greedy layer-wise training of deep networks. Advances in Neural Information Processing Systems 19, 153 (2007)
2. Daoud, M.I., Mousavi, P., Imani, F., Rohling, R., Abolmaesumi, P.: Tissue classification using ultrasound-induced variations in acoustic backscattering features. IEEE Transactions on Biomedical Engineering 60(2), 310–320 (2013)
3. Hinton, G.: A practical guide to training RBM. Momentum 9(1), 926 (2010)
4. Imani, F., et al.: Ultrasound-based characterization of prostate cancer: An *in vivo* clinical feasibility study. In: Mori, K., Sakuma, I., Sato, Y., Barillot, C., Navab, N. (eds.) MICCAI 2013, Part II. LNCS, vol. 8150, pp. 279–286. Springer, Heidelberg (2013)
5. Khojaste, A., Imani, F., Moradi, M., Berman, D., et al.: Characterization of aggressive prostate cancer using ultrasound RF time series. SPIE Medical Imaging (2015)
6. Liao, S., Gao, Y., Oto, A., Shen, D.: Representation learning: A unified deep learning framework for automatic prostate MR segmentation. In: Mori, K., Sakuma, I., Sato, Y., Barillot, C., Navab, N. (eds.) MICCAI 2013, Part II. LNCS, vol. 8150, pp. 254–261. Springer, Heidelberg (2013)
7. Margel, D., Yap, S.A., Lawrentschuk, N., Klotz, L., et al.: Impact of multiparametric endorectal coil prostate magnetic resonance imaging on disease reclassification among active surveillance candidates: a prospective cohort study. The Journal of Urology 187(4), 1247–1252 (2012)
8. Moradi, M., Mousavi, P., Boag, A., Sauerbrei, E.E., Siemens, D., Abolmaesumi, P.: Augmenting detection of prostate cancer in transrectal ultrasound images using SVM and RF time series. IEEE Transactions on Biomedical Engineering 56(9), 2214–2224 (2009)
9. de Rooij, M., Hamoen, E.H., Fütterer, J.J., Barentsz, J.O., Rovers, M.M.: Accuracy of multiparametric MRI for prostate cancer detection: a meta-analysis. American Journal of Roentgenology 202(2), 343–351 (2014)
10. Tanaka, M., Okutomi, M.: A novel inference of a restricted boltzmann machine. In: International Conference on Pattern Recognition, pp. 1526–1531. IEEE (2014)
11. van Tulder, G., de Bruijne, M.: Learning features for tissue classification with the classification restricted boltzmann machine. In: Menze, B., Langs, G., Montillo, A., Kelm, M., Müller, H., Zhang, S., Cai, W(T.), Metaxas, D. (eds.) MCV 2014. LNCS, vol. 8848, pp. 47–58. Springer, Heidelberg (2014)
12. Uniyal, N., et al.: Ultrasound-based predication of prostate cancer in MRI-guided biopsy. In: Linguraru, M.G., Laura, C.O., Shekhar, R., Wesarg, S., Ballester, M.Á.G., Drechsler, K., Sato, Y., Erdt, M. (eds.) CLIP 2014. LNCS, vol. 8680, pp. 142–150. Springer, Heidelberg (2017)

MCI Identification by Joint Learning
on Multiple MRI Data

Yue Gao[1], Chong-Yaw Wee[1], Minjeong Kim[1], Panteleimon Giannakopoulos[2],
Marie-Louise Montandon[3], Sven Haller[3], and Dinggang Shen[1]

[1] Department of Radiology and BRIC,
University of North Carolina at Chapel Hill, NC 27599, USA
[2] Division of Psychiatry, Geneva University Hospitals, Switzerland
[3] Department of Neuroradiology, University Hospitals of Geneva
and Faculty of Medicine of the University of Geneva, Switzerland

Abstract. The identification of subtle brain changes that are associated with mild cognitive impairment (MCI), the at-risk stage of Alzheimer's disease, is still a challenging task. Different from existing works, which employ multimodal data (e.g., MRI, PET or CSF) to identify MCI subjects from normal elderly controls, we use four MRI sequences, including T1-weighted MRI (T1), Diffusion Tensor Imaging (DTI), Resting-State functional MRI (RS-fMRI) and Arterial Spin Labeling (ASL) perfusion imaging. Since these MRI sequences simultaneously capture various aspects of brain structure and function during clinical routine scan, it simplifies finding the relationship between subjects by incorporating the mutual information among them. To this end, we devise a hypergraph-based semi-supervised learning algorithm. In particular, we first construct a hypergraph for each of MRI sequences separately using a star expansion method with both the training and testing data. A centralized learning is then performed to model the optimal relevance between subjects by incorporating mutual information between different MRI sequences. We then combine all centralized hypergraphs by learning the optimal weight of each hypergraph based on the minimum Laplacian. We apply our proposed method on a cohort of 41 consecutive MCI subjects and 63 age-and-gender matched controls with four MRI sequences. Our method achieves at least a 7.61% improvement in classification accuracy compared to state-of-the-art methods using multiple MRI data.

1 Introduction

Alzheimer's disease (AD) is the most common form of dementia in elderly over 65 years of age. The number of AD patients has reached 26.6 million in nowadays and is expected to double within the next 20 years, leading to 1 in every 85 people worldwide being affected by AD by 2050. Therefore, the diagnosis of AD at its at-risk stage of mild cognitive impairment (MCI) [7] becomes extremely essential and has attracted extensive research efforts in recent years [11, 9]. Previous studies [10] have shown that structural and functional brain changes may start before clinically converted to AD and can be used as potential biomarkers for MCI identification.

Recent studies [4, 11] show great promises for integrating multiple modalities, e.g., MRI, PET and CSF, for improving AD/MCI diagnosis accuracy, and semi-supervised

© Springer International Publishing Switzerland 2015
N. Navab et al. (Eds.): MICCAI 2015, Part II, LNCS 9350, pp. 78–85, 2015.
DOI: 10.1007/978-3-319-24571-3_10

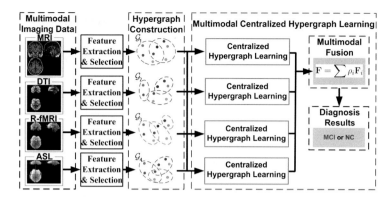

Fig. 1. An overview of the proposed centralized hypergraph learning for MCI diagnosis.

learning for multimodal data has also been investigated [2]. However, in most previous works, modeling the relationship among subjects is often performed separately for each modality, ignoring the crucial mutual information between different modalities. In practice, integrating the information acquired from different modalities is a challenging task, since the relationship among subjects may differ for different modalities.

On the other hand, multiple MR sequences, e.g., T1-weighted (T1), Diffusion Tensor Imaging (DTI) and Resting-State functional MRI (RS-fMRI), can be used in clinical routine scans to capture different aspects of the brain structures and functions. For instance, T1 provides the tissue type information of the brain, DTI measures macroscopic axonal organization in nervous system tissues, and RS-fMRI provides the regional interactions that take place when the subject in the absence of an explicit task. As a relatively new technique, Arterial Spin Labeling (ASL) [1] perfusion imaging is introduced to measure brain perfusion without any injection of a contrast agent and demonstrated consistent reduction in basal perfusion notably in the posterior cingulate cortex in MCI and AD [1]. More recently, ASL was even able to predict very early cognitive decline in healthy elderly controls, *i.e.*, the earliest stage of neurodegeneration. Multiple MRI sequences can be easily and simultaneously captured during clinical routine scans.

In this work, we propose a centralized hypergraph learning method (CHL) to better model relationship among subjects with multiple MRIs for the purpose of MCI diagnosis. The basic idea of the proposed method is to estimate the relevance between different subjects that reflects how likely two subjects belong to the same category by integrating multiple imaging data in a semi-supervised manner. Then, the relationship information among subjects is represented by a hypergraph structure that connects all subjects in both training and testing sets. Compared to the simple graph, in which an edge can only link two vertices, hypergraph [12] conveys more information through a set of hyperedges that connects more than two vertices at the same occasion. It has been successfully applied to various applications, such as image and object retrieval [3]. In this way, a hypergraph structure is able to capture the higher-order relationship among different subjects, i.e., whether a group of subjects share similar content. Then, MCI diagnosis is formulated as a binary classification task in the hypergraph structure to classify each subject as MCI patient or normal control (NC). Figure 1 presents the schematic diagram of the proposed framework. We first construct a hypergraph using both the training and testing data for each of multiple MRIs separately to reflect the higher-order relationship among subjects. In hypergraph construction, each time one subject is selected as a centroid. It is then connected to its K nearest subjects in the feature space via a hyperedge. We then conduct a centralized hypergraph learning to explore the underneath relationship of a set of samples, where the relevance among subjects and the hyperedge weights are optimized simultaneously via an alternating optimization approach. Specifically, each time one hypergraph is first selected as the core and the rest as auxiliary information in the learning process. This procedure is repeated for each hypergraph, producing a set of relevance scores for each subject for classification. To obtain the final decision, we assemble the relevance scores based on the optimal weights learned by minimizing the overall hypergraph Laplacian. Note that, for the training subjects, we just use their imaging features to construct hypergraphs. Therefore, the relevance scores are conveyed globally, leading to a semi-supervised learning model, and better avoiding over-fitting to the training set.

2   Method

Data and Preprocessing - A dataset containing T1, DTI, RS-fMRI and ASL from 41 MCI patients and 63 normal controls was collected through the University Hospital of Geneva in Switzerland. The T1 images were preprocessed by skull stripping, cerebellum removal, and tissue segmentation [6]. The anatomical automatic labeling (AAL) atlas, parcellated with 90 predefined regions-of-interest (ROIs) in cerebrum area, are aligned to the native space of each subject using a deformable registration algorithm. For T1 data, WM and GM tissue volumes in each region are computed and further normalized to generate a 180-dimensional feature vector, i.e., 90 WM and 90 GM features.

The DTI were first parcellated into 90 regions by propagating the AAL ROIs to each image using a deformable DTI registration algorithm. Whole-brain streamline fiber tractography was performed on each DTI image. The number of fibers passing through each pair of regions was counted and the averages of on-fiber fractional anisotropy (FA) for each ROI pair were computed to form a structural connectivity matrix.

For RS-fMRI, a 9min ON-OFF CO_2 challenge was employed, *i.e.*,1 min OFF, 2 min ON, 2 min OFF, 2 min ON, 2 min OFF, during data acquisition. Slice timing correction and head-motion correction were performed using the Statistical Parametric Mapping software package. To ensure magnetization equilibrium, the first 10 acquired RS-fMRI images of each subject were discarded. The remaining 170 images were first corrected for acquisition time delays among different slices before they were realigned to the first volume of the remaining images for head-motion corrections. A Pearson correlation-based connectivity matrix of dimension 90×90 based on AAL atlas was constructed for each subject.

Preprocessing of ASL images was performed using ASLtbx. Similar to RS-fMRI, a symmetric connectivity matrix of dimension 90×90 was constructed for each subject.

For DTI, RS-fMRI and ASL, the local clustering coefficients, which quantify the cliquishness of the nodes [8], are computed for the connectivity networks. For these three MRI sequences, both the raw feature (8100-D) and the clustering coefficients-based feature (90-D) are employed.

Hypergraph Construction - For each type of multiple imaging data, a hypergraph is constructed. For the i-th imaging with N subjects, a hypergraph $\mathcal{G}_i = (\mathcal{V}_i, \mathcal{E}_i, \mathbf{W}_i)$ with N vertices is constructed where each subject is represented by a vertex. Here, $\mathcal{V}_i$ is the vertex set, $\mathcal{E}_i$ is the hyperedge set, and $\mathbf{W}_i$ is the corresponding weight for the hyperedges. A star expansion method is employed to generate a set of hyperedges among vertices. Specifically, in each feature space, a vertex is selected as the centroid vertex and then a hyperedge is developed by connecting to its nearest neighbors within $\varphi\bar{d}$ distance, where $\bar{d}$ is the average distance between subjects in the feature space and φ is set as 1 in our experiment. Incidence matrix of the hypergraph is then generated to represent the relationship among different vertices. The (v, e)-th entry of the incidence matrix indicates whether the vertex v is connected via the hyperedge e to other vertices. The incidence matrix $\mathbf{H}_i$ of hypergraph $\mathcal{G}_i = (\mathcal{V}_i, \mathcal{E}_i, \mathbf{W}_i)$ is generated as

$$
\mathbf{H}_i(v, e) = \begin{cases} \exp\left(-\frac{d_i(v, v_c)}{0.1\bar{d}_i}\right) & \text{if } v \in e \\ 0 & \text{if } v \notin e \end{cases}, \tag{1}
$$

where $d_i(v, v_c)$ is the distance for the i-th imaging data between a vertex v and its corresponding centroid vertex v_c in hyperedge e, and $\hat{d}_i$ is the average pairwise subject distance for the i-th imaging data. Accordingly, the vertex degree of the vertex $v \in \mathcal{V}_i$ and hyperedge degree of the hyperedge $e \in \mathcal{E}_i$ are calculated, respectively, as $d_i(v) = \sum_{e \in \mathcal{E}_i} \mathbf{W}_i(e) \mathbf{H}_i(v, e)$ and $\delta_i(e) = \sum_{v \in \mathcal{V}_i} \mathbf{H}_i(v, e)$. Thus, we can define $\mathbf{D}_i^v$ and $\mathbf{D}_i^e$ as diagonal matrices representing vertex degrees and hyperedge degrees, respectively. Note that all the hyperedges are initialized with an equal weight, *e.g.*, 1.

Centralized Hypergraph Learning - To model the relationship of subjects with multiple imaging data, we propose a centralized hypergraph learning method. MCI diagnosis is formulated as a binary classification task in the hypergraph structure. Given four hypergraphs, at each stage one hypergraph is selected as the core hypergraph, while the rest are used to provide extra guidance for updating the hypergraphs.

During centralized learning, hypergraphs are assigned with different weights according to their influences on the structure of the core hypergraph. The core hypergraph is assigned with a weight of α_1, while the other hypergraphs are assigned with an equal weight, α_2. Assume the j-th hypergraph is selected as the core hypergraph, we can have the j-th centralized hypergraph. To learn the relevance among vertices and improve the structure of the j-th centralized hypergraph, we optimize the following objective function including the weights of hyperedges by imposing an ℓ_2-norm regularizer on $\mathbf{W}_{i\,(i=1,2,3,4)}$ as

$$
\underset{\mathbf{F}_j, \mathbf{W}_{i\,(i=1,2,3,4)}}{\arg\min} \left\{ \Omega_j^c(\mathbf{F}_j) + \lambda \mathcal{R}_{emp}(\mathbf{F}_j) + \mu \sum_i \sum_{e \in \mathcal{E}_i} \mathbf{W}_i(e)^2 \right\}, \tag{2}
$$
$$
\text{s.t.} \quad \mathbf{H}_i diag(\mathbf{W}_i) = diag(\mathbf{D}_i^v), \ diag(\mathbf{W}_i) \geq 0
$$

where $\Omega_j^c(\mathbf{F}_j)$ is the regularizer for the j-th centralized hypergraph, aiming to smooth the relationship among vertices on the hypergraph structure, $\mathbf{W}_i(e)$ is the weight of the hyperedge $e \in \mathcal{E}_i$, $\mathbf{F}_j$ is the to-be-learned relevance matrix, and $\mathcal{R}_{emp}(\mathbf{F}_j)$ is the empirical loss, and $\sum_i \sum_{e \in \mathcal{E}_i} \mathbf{W}_i(e)^2$ is the ℓ_2 regularizer term to learn the weights of hyperedges. The two constraints guarantee that the vertex degree is not changed during the learning process and all the weights are non-negative, respectively. $\Omega_j^c(\mathbf{F}_j)$ is defined as

$$\Omega_j^c(\mathbf{F}_j) = \alpha_1 \Omega_j(\mathbf{F}_j) + \sum_{i \neq j} \alpha_2 \Omega_i(\mathbf{F}_j), \tag{3}$$

where the first term is the regularizer for the core hypergraph and the second term is the regularizer for the other hypergraphs. We define the regularizer term $\Omega_i(\mathbf{F}_j)$ as

$$\Omega_i(\mathbf{F}_j) = \frac{1}{2} \sum_{k=1}^{2} \sum_{e \in \mathcal{E}_i} \sum_{u,v \in \mathcal{V}_i} \frac{\mathbf{W}_i(e)\mathbf{H}_i(u,e)\mathbf{H}_i(v,e)}{\delta_i(e)} \left(\frac{\mathbf{F}_j(u,k)}{\sqrt{d_i(u)}} - \frac{\mathbf{F}_j(v,k)}{\sqrt{d_i(v)}} \right)^2$$

$$= \mathbf{F}_j^{\mathrm{T}}(\mathbf{I} - \mathbf{\Theta}_i)\mathbf{F}_j, \tag{4}$$

where $\mathbf{\Theta}_i = \mathbf{D}_i^{e-\frac{1}{2}}\mathbf{H}_i\mathbf{W}_i\mathbf{D}_i^{e-1}\mathbf{H}_i^{\mathrm{T}}\mathbf{D}_i^{v-\frac{1}{2}}$. $\Omega_j(\mathbf{F}_j)$ can be accordingly obtained by $\Omega_j(\mathbf{F}_j) = \mathbf{F}_j^{\mathrm{T}}(\mathbf{I} - \mathbf{\Theta}_j)\mathbf{F}_j$. Then, $\Omega_j^c(\mathbf{F}_j)$ can be simplified as

$$\Omega_j^c(\mathbf{F}_j) = \mathbf{F}_j^{\mathrm{T}}\left(\mathbf{I} - (\alpha_1\mathbf{\Theta}_j + \alpha_2\sum_{i \neq j}\mathbf{\Theta}_i)\right)\mathbf{F}_j = \mathbf{F}_j^{\mathrm{T}}\mathbf{\Delta}_j^c\mathbf{F}_j, \tag{5}$$

where $\mathbf{\Delta}_j^c = \mathbf{I} - (\alpha_1\mathbf{\Theta}_j + \alpha_2\sum_{i \neq j}\mathbf{\Theta}_i)$ is the j-th centralized hypergraph Laplacian.

The empirical loss $\mathcal{R}_{emp}(\mathbf{F}_j)$ is defined as

$$\mathcal{R}_{emp}(\mathbf{F}_j) = \sum_{k=1}^{2} \|\mathbf{F}_j(:,k) - \mathbf{Y}(:,k)\|^2, \tag{6}$$

where $\mathbf{Y} \in \mathbb{R}^{n \times 2}$ is the label matrix and each of its entry denotes the category a subject belongs to. $\mathbf{Y}(:,k)$ is the k-th column of $\mathbf{Y}$. If the vertex v belongs to the first category, then the $(v,1)$-th and $(v,2)$-th entries in $\mathbf{Y}$ are set to 1 and 0, respectively.

Solution: To solve the optimization problem in Eq. (2), we employ an alternating optimization approach. We first fix $\mathbf{W}_i$ and optimize $\mathbf{F}_j$ as follows

$$\arg\min_{\mathbf{F}_j} \left\{ \Omega_j^c(\mathbf{F}_j) + \lambda\mathcal{R}_{emp}(\mathbf{F}_j) \right\}, \tag{7}$$

which leads to the following closed-form solution for

$$\mathbf{F}_j = \frac{\lambda}{1+\lambda}\left(\mathbf{I} - \frac{1}{1+\lambda}(\alpha_1\mathbf{\Theta}_j + \alpha_2\sum_{i \neq j}\mathbf{\Theta}_i)\right)^{-1}\mathbf{Y}. \tag{8}$$

We then fix $\mathbf{F}_j$ and optimize $\mathbf{W}_i$ as follows

$$\arg\min_{\mathbf{W}_i \ (i=1,2,3,4)} \left\{ \Omega_j^c(\mathbf{F}_j) + \mu\sum_{i}\sum_{e \in \mathcal{E}_i}\mathbf{W}_i(e)^2 \right\} \tag{9}$$

$$\text{s.t.} \quad \mathbf{H}_i diag(\mathbf{W}_i) = diag(\mathbf{D}_i^v), \ diag(\mathbf{W}_i) \geq 0.$$

The above optimization task is convex on $\mathbf{W}_i$ and can be solved via quadratic programming. The learning process is repeated several times, once for each of the hypergraphs as the core hypergraph, to generate a centralized relevance matrix for each imaging modality.

2.1 Relevance Matrices Fusion

To optimally integrate information from multiple MRIs, we learn the weights of each hypergraph by minimizing the overall hypergraph Laplacian. Let ρ_i be the weight for the i-th centralized hypergraph, we impose an ℓ_2-norm penalization on the weights of all centralized hypergraphs as follows

$$\arg\min_{\rho_i} \left\{ \sum \rho_i \mathbf{\Omega}_i^c (\mathbf{F}_i) + \eta \sum \rho_i^2 \right\} \quad \text{s.t.} \quad \sum \rho_i = 1, \tag{10}$$

where η is to balance the Laplacian and the weight regularizer. Eq. (10) can be solved using the Lagrangian method. The final relevance matrix is then computed as $\mathbf{F} = \sum \rho_i \mathbf{F}_i$. Classification of a subject could therefore be determined by its corresponding value in the final relevance matrix. If the relevance score to MCI is larger than that to NC, a subject is classified as MCI, and vice versa.

3 Experiments

Experimental Settings - To evaluate the performance of the proposed CHL method, a 10-fold cross-validation strategy is used in our experiments. Specifically, we randomly partition the subjects in the MCI and NC groups into 10 non-overlapping approximately equal sets. One set is first left out as testing set and the rest sets are used as the training set. The training set is further divided into 5 subsets for a 5-fold inner cross-validation to learn the optimal parameters. This procedure is repeated 10 times, once for each of the 10 sets, to compute the overall cross-validation classification performance. Six statistical measures are used for performance evaluation, which include accuracy (ACC), sensitivity (SEN), specificity (SPEC), balance accuracy (BAC), positive predictive value (PPV), and negative predictive value (NPV).

Results - We compare the proposed method with two state-of-the-art methods: 1) Multimodal multitask learning (M3T) [11], which employs multimodal imaging data for MCI classification, and 2) Manifold regularized multitask feature learning (M2TFS) [5], which is another semi-supervised method on MCI classification. We further compare with two simplified versions of the proposed method: 1) centralized simple graph learning (CSL), in which only simple graphs are employed instead of hypergraphs in our method, and 2) Multi-hypergraph learning (MHL) [3] without centralized learning.

Figure 2 shows the MCI classification results of all compared methods using different imaging data individually and together. The proposed method (CHL) outperforms all competing state-of-the-arts methods. Specifically, by using four types of imaging data, CHL achieves an improvement of $8.65 \pm 2.50\%$ and $7.61 \pm 1.92\%$, in terms of ACC, compared with M3T and M2TFS, respectively. Better performance of our method

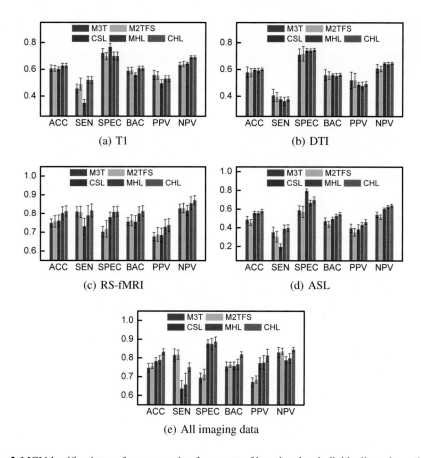

Fig. 2. MCI identification performance using four types of imaging data individually and together.

is attributed to the following aspects. First, different from existing methods that employ the labeled samples to train classifiers, the proposed method employs both the labeled and unlabeled samples to explore the underlying relationships among different subjects in a semi-supervised learning way, leading to a more general model that is not over-fitted to the training data. Second, the employed hypergraph structure [12] is superior in formulating the joint relationship among multiple vertices compared with simple graph. As shown in the results, CHL achieves an improvement of $5.10 \pm 2.13\%$ in terms of ACC compared with CSL when all four imaging data are employed. Third, the proposed method employs a centralized learning approach to model the subject relationship by using one of multiple imaging data with the guidance from others, enabling more accurate modeling of underlying relationships among samples.

Compared with MHL, the proposed CHL demonstrates better performance, especially when multiple types of imaging data are utilized. More specifically, CHL achieves an improvement of $4.42 \pm 1.57\%$ in terms of ACC compared with MHL by using four types of imaging data. This result demonstrates that the proposed centralized method can better explore the relationship underlying the multiple imaging data.

4   Conclusion

In this paper, we proposed a centralized hypergraph learning method to model the relationship among subjects with multiple MRIs for MCI identification. In our method, this relationship is encoded by the structure and the weights of hyperedges in a hypergraph. Multiple hypergraphs are constructed using multiple MRIs, respectively. In the learning process, each time one hypergraph is selected as the core and the relationships among subjects from other hypergraphs help to provide extra guidance to meliorate the structure of the core hypergraph. Integrating hypergraphs with different weights enables optimal utilization of supplementary information conveyed by different imaging data. Our findings demonstrate the effectiveness of the CHL method on MCI diagnosis.

References

[1] Binnewijzend, M.A., Kuijer, J.P., Benedictus, M.R., van der Flier, W.M., Wink, A.M., Wattjes, M.P., van Berckel, B.N., Scheltens, P., Barkhof, F.: Cerebral blood flow measured with 3D pseudocontinuous arterial spin-labeling MR imaging in alzheimer disease and mild cognitive impairment: a marker for disease severity. Radiology 267(1), 221–230 (2013)

[2] Cai, X., Nie, F., Cai, W., Huang, H.: Heterogeneous image features integration via multimodal semi-supervised learning model. In: IEEE International Conference on Computer Vision, pp. 1737–1744 (2013)

[3] Gao, Y., Wang, M., Tao, D., Ji, R., Dai, Q.: 3-D object retrieval and recognition with hypergraph analysis. IEEE Transactions on Image Processing 21(9), 4290–4303 (2012)

[4] Hinrichs, C., Singh, V., Xu, G., Johnson, S.C., Initiative, A.D.N., et al.: Predictive markers for AD in a multi-modality framework: an analysis of MCI progression in the ADNI population. NeuroImage 55(2), 574–589 (2011)

[5] Jie, B., Zhang, D., Cheng, B., Shen, D.: Manifold regularized multi-task feature selection for multi-modality classification in alzheimer's disease. In: Mori, K., Sakuma, I., Sato, Y., Barillot, C., Navab, N. (eds.) MICCAI 2013, Part I. LNCS, vol. 8149, pp. 275–283. Springer, Heidelberg (2013)

[6] Lim, K.O., Pfefferbaum, A.: Segmentation of mr brain images into cerebrospinal fluid spaces, white and gray matter. Journal of Computer Assisted Tomography 13(4), 588–593 (1989)

[7] Richiardi, J., Monsch, A.U., Haas, T., Barkhof, F., Van de Ville, D., Radü, E.W., Kressig, R.W., Haller, S.: Altered cerebrovascular reactivity velocity in mild cognitive impairment and Alzheimer's disease. Neurobiology of Aging (2014)

[8] Rubinov, M., Sporns, O.: Complex network measures of brain connectivity: uses and interpretations. NeuroImage 52(3), 1059–1069 (2010)

[9] Wang, H., Nie, F., Huang, H., Risacher, S.L., Saykin, A.J., Shen, L., et al.: Identifying disease sensitive and quantitative trait-relevant biomarkers from multidimensional heterogeneous imaging genetics data via sparse multimodal multitask learning. Bioinformatics 28(12), i127–i136 (2012)

[10] Ye, J., Wu, T., Li, J., Chen, K.: Machine learning approaches for the neuroimaging study of Alzheimer's disease. Computer 44(4), 99–101 (2011)

[11] Zhang, D., Shen, D.: Multi-modal multi-task learning for joint prediction of multiple regression and classification variables in Alzheimer's disease. NeuroImage 59(2), 895–907 (2012)

[12] Zhou, D., Huang, J., Schokopf, B.: Learning with hypergraphs: Clustering, classification, and embedding. In: Proceedings of Advances in Neural Information Processing Systems. pp. 1601–1608 (2006)

Medical Image Retrieval Using Multi-graph Learning for MCI Diagnostic Assistance

Yue Gao[1], Ehsan Adeli-M.[1], Minjeong Kim[1],
Panteleimon Giannakopoulos[2], Sven Haller[3], and Dinggang Shen[1]

[1] Department of Radiology and BRIC,
University of North Carolina at Chapel Hill, NC 27599, USA
[2] Division of Psychiatry, Geneva University Hospitals, Switzerland
[3] Department of Neuroradiology, University Hospitals of Geneva
and Faculty of Medicine of the University of Geneva, Switzerland

Abstract. Alzheimer's disease (AD) is an irreversible neurodegenerative disorder that can lead to progressive memory loss and cognition impairment. Therefore, diagnosing AD during the risk stage, a.k.a. Mild Cognitive Impairment (MCI), has attracted ever increasing interest. Besides the automated diagnosis of MCI, it is important to provide physicians with related MCI cases with visually similar imaging data for case-based reasoning or evidence-based medicine in clinical practices. To this end, we propose a multi-graph learning based medical image retrieval technique for MCI diagnostic assistance. Our method is comprised of two stages, the query category prediction and ranking. In the first stage, the query is formulated into a multi-graph structure with a set of selected subjects in the database to learn the relevance between the query subject and the existing subject categories through learning the multi-graph combination weights. This predicts the category that the query belongs to, based on which a set of subjects in the database are selected as candidate retrieval results. In the second stage, the relationship between these candidates and the query is further learned with a new multi-graph, which is used to rank the candidates. The returned subjects can be demonstrated to physicians as reference cases for MCI diagnosing. We evaluated the proposed method on a cohort of 60 consecutive MCI subjects and 350 normal controls with MRI data under three imaging parameters: T1 weighted imaging (T1), Diffusion Tensor Imaging (DTI) and Arterial Spin Labeling (ASL). The proposed method can achieve average 3.45 relevant samples in top 5 returned results, which significantly outperforms the baseline methods compared.

1 Introduction

Alzheimer's disease (AD) is an irreversible neurodegenerative disorder found in elderly over 65 years of age, accounts for 60% to 80% of age-related dementia cases [10]. AD can lead to progressive memory loss and cognition impairment. The number of AD patients has reached 26.6 million and is expected to double in the next two decades [1]. Therefore, accurate diagnosis of AD during the risk stage, a.k.a. Mild Cognitive Impairment (MCI), is important. In recent years, extensive research efforts have been dedicated to MCI identification using different imaging data, such as MRI [2], positron emission tomography (PET) [5], and Cerebrospinal fluid (CSF) [3], which aims to

© Springer International Publishing Switzerland 2015
N. Navab et al. (Eds.): MICCAI 2015, Part II, LNCS 9350, pp. 86–93, 2015.
DOI: 10.1007/978-3-319-24571-3_11

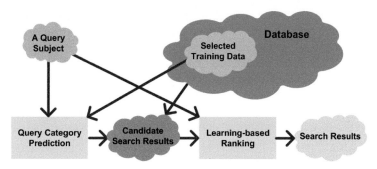

Fig. 1. The framework of the proposed medical image retrieval method for MCI diagnostic aid.

provide the physicians with brain structural and functional information of the brain for the patient's condition.

In addition to automatic MCI classification based on imaging data, providing physicians with cases of similar visual appearances and corresponding treatment records can indeed facilitate clinical decisions. It can supply references for physicians to perform case-based reasoning or evidence-based medicine with even more confidence. Therefore, medical image retrieval has attracted much more attention in recent years [11, 12, 7, 4]. We notice that most works target at retrieving similar objects in image content [11, 12] or the same imaging modalities [7, 4] for a given query image. However, for the purpose of MCI diagnostic aid, it should retrieve subjects from the database with similar brain patterns across all the imaging modalities. To assist MCI diagnosis, our goal is to identify similar brain patterns from imaging data. Given a **query**, as a set of imaging data belonging to one subject, our goal is to find the subjects with similar brain patterns from a **database**. The database contains subjects with clinical treatment records and the same imaging data types as the query.

Thus, in this work, we propose a medical image retrieval technique for application to MCI diagnosis assistance. The proposed method is composed of two main stages: *query category prediction* for candidate selection and *ranking*, as shown in Figure 1. In the first stage, we locate the most relevant subjects from the database to the query subject. In this step, a group of subjects from the database[1] are selected and then used to predict the category of the query subject, in a supervised manner. In this case, the categories are MCI and NC, while this framework could be adopted for all other neurodegenerative brain diseases. Given the selected supervised data from the database, for each imaging data modality, a graph is constructed based on the pair-wise subject distances. Then, graphs from different imaging data are combined into a single multi-graph to formulate the overall similarity, which includes both the selected subjects and the query. A learning procedure is conducted on the multi-graph to jointly estimate the relevance of the query subject to all predefined categories and to learn the optimal combination weights of the multiple graphs, which leads to a category prediction for the query subject. Then, all the subjects belonging to the same category are selected as candidate subjects.

---

[1] Note that, for all the subjects in the database, we have their medical records and therefore the category information for these subjects are available.

In the second stage, all these candidate subjects and the query subject are again modeled in a new multi-graph, which is built by combining the obtained weights from the previous stage of query category prediction, but only on the selected candidate subjects. A learning procedure on the graph reveals the relevance of these candidates to the query subject, which would lead to a ranking of candidate subjects from the database on how relevant they are compared to the query subject. The proposed method is evaluated on a cohort of 60 consecutive MCI subjects and 350 normal controls (NC) containing MRI data with three imaging parameters, including T1 weighted imaging (T1), Diffusion Tensor Imaging (DTI), and Arterial Spin Labeling (ASL).

2   The Method

In principle, our methods works in two-stage, i.e., a query category prediction stage to select the potential candidates along with the original query for retrieval and the ranking stage built based upon a multi-graph ranking scheme to find similar brain patterns to the query.

Query Category Prediction: Given the query imaging data, the first step is to predict the query category, which estimates the relevant data category in the database.

Graph Construction- Here, a group of subjects with annotations from the database are selected, for the purpose of query category prediction. Let $\mathcal{Q}$ denote the query subject and $\mathcal{M} = \{M_1, M_2, \ldots, M_N\}$ denote the N selected training subjects in the database (N is set equal to 100 in our experiments). The relationship among these subjects (with multimodal imaging data) could be formulated in a multi-graph structure as below. Let N_{Mod} denote the number of imaging modalities in total. For the ith imaging data, a graph $\mathcal{G}_i = \{\mathcal{V}_i, \mathcal{E}_i, \mathbf{W}_i\}_{N+1}$ is constructed by using all the N annotated subjects and the query $\mathcal{Q}$, where $\mathcal{V}_i$ is the vertex set containing $N + 1$ samples, and $\mathcal{E}_i$ is the edge set. $\mathcal{E}_i(v_s, v_t)$ is the edge connecting the sth and the tth vertices in $\mathcal{G}_i$ corresponding to the edge weight $\mathbf{W}_i(v_s, v_t)$. Here, $\mathbf{W}_i(v_s, v_t)$ is defined as:

$$\mathbf{W}_i(v_s, v_t) = \exp\left(-\frac{d^2(v_s, v_t)}{\sigma_i^2}\right),\tag{1}$$

where $d(v_s, v_t)$ is the distance between v_s and v_t, which is calculated as the Euclidean distance between two corresponding features (feature extraction will be introduced in Section 3). Let $\boldsymbol{\Theta}_i = \mathbf{D}_i^{-1/2}\mathbf{W}_i\mathbf{D}_i^{-1/2}$ denote the normalized weight matrix of the graph $\mathcal{G}_i$, where $\mathbf{D}_i$ is a diagonal matrix defined as $\mathbf{D}_i(s, s) = \sum_{v_t} \mathbf{W}_i(v_s, v_t)$.

Objective Function and Solution- Multi-graph learning has been applied in many applications, such as video annotation [9] and affective image analysis [13]. Given the N_{Mod} graphs generated from multimodal data, the query category prediction task can be formulated as a multi-graph learning framework, where the cost function is:

$$\mathcal{Q}(\mathbf{F}, \boldsymbol{\omega}) = \left\{\sum_{i=1}^{N_{\mathrm{Mod}}} \omega_i \boldsymbol{\Omega}_i(\mathbf{F}) + \mu\mathcal{R}(\mathbf{F}) + \eta\|\boldsymbol{\omega}\|_2^2\right\} \quad s.t. \sum_{i=1}^{N_{\mathrm{Mod}}} \omega_i = 1,\tag{2}$$

where $\boldsymbol{\omega} = \{\omega_1, \omega_2, \ldots, \omega_{\mathrm{Mod}}\}$ is the weighting parameter for each graph, $\boldsymbol{\Omega}_i$ is the regularizer on the ith graph, $\mathbf{F}$ is the relevance matrix, $\mathcal{R}(\mathbf{F})$ is the empirical loss,

$\|\boldsymbol{\omega}\|_2^2 = \sum_{i=1}^{N_{\text{Mod}}} w_i^2$ is the squared ℓ_2 norm of $\boldsymbol{\omega}$, and μ and η are the parameters to balance different components in the cost function. w_i can be initialized as $1/N_{\text{Mod}}$. We define the regularizer term, $\boldsymbol{\Omega}_i$, as:

$$\boldsymbol{\Omega}_i = \frac{1}{2} \sum_{v_s, v_t} \mathbf{W}_i \left(v_s, v_t \right) \left\| \frac{\mathbf{F}(v_s, \cdot)}{\sqrt{\mathbf{D}_i \left(v_s, v_s \right)}} - \frac{\mathbf{F}(v_t, \cdot)}{\sqrt{\mathbf{D}_i \left(v_t, v_t \right)}} \right\|^2. \tag{3}$$

$\mathcal{R}\left(\mathbf{F}\right)$ is defined as $\mathcal{R}\left(\mathbf{F}\right) = \sum \|\mathbf{F}_i - \mathbf{Y}_i\|^2$, where $\mathbf{Y} \in \mathbb{R}^{n \times 2}$ is the labeled matrix and initialized as follows. If the ath vertex belongs to the kth category, $\mathbf{Y}(a, k) = 1$; otherwise $\mathbf{Y}(a, k) = 0$.

The learning task on $\mathbf{F}$ and $\boldsymbol{\omega}$ can be written as

$$\arg\min_{\mathbf{F}, \, \boldsymbol{\omega}} \mathcal{Q}(\mathbf{F}, \boldsymbol{\omega}), \quad s.t. \sum_{i=1}^{N_{\text{Mod}}} w_i = 1. \tag{4}$$

where the relevance among vertices and the multi-graph combination weights can be simultaneously optimized.

To solve the above optimization task, we alternately optimize $\mathbf{F}$ and $\boldsymbol{\omega}$, respectively. In the first step, $\boldsymbol{\omega}$ is fixed and $\mathbf{F}$ is optimized, which leads to the following problem:

$$\arg\min_{\mathbf{F}} \left\{ \sum_{i=1}^{N_{\text{Mod}}} w_i \boldsymbol{\Omega}_i \left(\mathbf{F}\right) + \mu \mathcal{R}\left(\mathbf{F}\right) \right\}. \tag{5}$$

According to [14], it can be efficiently solved in an iterative procedure by

$$\mathbf{F}(t + 1) = \frac{1}{1 + \mu} \sum_{i=1}^{N_{\text{Mod}}} w_i \boldsymbol{\Theta}_i \mathbf{F}(t) + \frac{\mu}{1 + \mu} \mathbf{Y}, \tag{6}$$

where $\mathbf{F}(t + 1)$ is the $\mathbf{F}$ in the $(t + 1)^{th}$ iteration and $\mathbf{F}(0) = \mathbf{Y}$. This procedure is iterated until the convergence.

In the second step, $\mathbf{F}$ is fixed and $\boldsymbol{\omega}$ is optimized. The objective function in Eq. (4) can be rewritten as:

$$\arg\min_{\boldsymbol{\omega}} \left\{ \sum_{i=1}^{N_{\text{Mod}}} w_i \boldsymbol{\Omega}_i \left(\mathbf{F}\right) + \eta \|\boldsymbol{\omega}\|_2^2 \right\}, \quad s.t. \sum_{i=1}^{N_{\text{Mod}}} w_i = 1. \tag{7}$$

which can be solved using the Lagrangian method.

The above alternating optimization process is repeated until convergence. Here let $\mathbf{F}(q, :)$ denote the corresponding relevance vector of $\mathcal{Q}$. Then, $\mathcal{Q}$ can be classified into a predefined category by $\arg\max(\mathbf{F}(q, :))$. Then, all the data belonging to the same category in the database are selected as the candidate retrieval results, denoted by $\boldsymbol{\Gamma} = \{S_1, S_2, \ldots, S_{N_c}\}$. Here, each S_i is one candidate subject belonging to the query's category and N_c is the number of candidates.

Learning-based Ranking: Although the subjects in $\boldsymbol{\Gamma}$ are relevant to the query based on the category information, they could still be different from the point-of-view of imaging appearance or patterns present in the image. In this step, we need to rank all these selected candidates based on the imaging data to retrieve the most relevant subjects. Here, the N_c candidates $\mathbf{\Gamma}$ and the query $\mathcal{Q}$ are formulated in a new multi-graph structure and N_{Mod} graphs $\{\hat{\mathcal{G}}_1, \hat{\mathcal{G}}_2, \ldots, \hat{\mathcal{G}}_{N_{\mathrm{Mod}}}\}$ are generated, using these $N_c + 1$ subjects in a similar way as in the query category prediction step. Since the optimized combination weights ω are previously learned, in this step we only need to estimate the relevance between each subject in the candidate set and the query. So, the the optimization task on $\hat{\mathbf{f}}$ can be written as

$$\arg\min_{\hat{\mathbf{f}}} \hat{\mathcal{Q}}(\hat{\mathbf{f}}) = \arg\min_{\hat{\mathbf{f}}} \left\{ \sum_{i=1}^{N_{\mathrm{Mod}}} \omega_i \hat{\mathbf{\Omega}}_i(\hat{\mathbf{f}}) + \hat{\lambda}\hat{\mathcal{R}}(\hat{\mathbf{f}}) \right\}, \tag{8}$$

where $\hat{\mathbf{f}}$ is the to-be-learned relevance vector, $\hat{\mathbf{\Omega}}_i$ is the graph regularizer on the ith graph $\hat{\mathcal{G}}_i$, $\hat{\mathcal{R}}(\hat{\mathbf{f}}) = \|\hat{\mathbf{f}} - \hat{\mathbf{y}}\|^2$ is the empirical loss, and $\hat{\lambda}$ is the parameter to balance the graph regularizer and the empirical loss. Here, $\hat{\mathbf{y}}$ is the labeled vector, in which all the elements are 0 except that the value corresponding to the query is 1. Similar to the solution of Eq. (5), we can solve $\hat{\mathbf{f}}$ by iterating Eq. (9) until convergence, where $\hat{\mathbf{f}}(0) = \mathbf{y}$ and $\hat{\mathbf{\Theta}}_i = \hat{\mathbf{D}}_i^{-1/2} \hat{\mathbf{W}}_i \hat{\mathbf{D}}_i^{-1/2}$ is the normalized graph Laplacian of $\hat{\mathcal{G}}_i$.

$$\hat{\mathbf{f}}(t+1) = \frac{1}{1+\hat{\lambda}} \sum_{i=1}^{N_{\mathrm{Mod}}} \omega_i \hat{\mathbf{\Theta}}_i \mathbf{f}(t) + \frac{\hat{\lambda}}{1+\hat{\lambda}} \hat{\mathbf{y}}. \tag{9}$$

Based on $\hat{\mathbf{f}}$, all the candidates can be ranked in a descending order to demonstrate the retrieval results.

3   Validation

Experimental Settings: To evaluate the performance of the proposed medical imaging retrieval approach for MCI diagnosis assistance, a dataset containing 60 MCI patients and 350 normal controls was collected. Generally, T1, DTI and ASL were collected for each subject. For T1, the anatomical automatic labeling atlas, which are parcellated with 90 predefined regions-of-interest (ROIs), was registered to the native space of each subject. The white matter (WM) and gray matter (GM) tissue volumes in these ROIs are calculated to generate a 180-dimensional feature vector, (i.e., 90 WM and 90 GM features). For DTI and ASL, after the 90 ROIs parcellatation, two 90×90 connectivity matrices are computed. Then, the local clustering coefficients are calculated to quantify the cliquishness of the nodes [8], which generate two 90-dimensional feature vectors for these two types of imaging data, respectively. In the retrieval task, 50 MCI patients and 50 NCs are employed as the queries. In the query category prediction procedure, the training samples are randomly selected. The parameters in the proposed method are selected by a grid search via a 5-fold cross validation in the category prediction stage, and kept consistent in the ranking stage.

The evaluation criteria include #Correct@K and Normalized discounted cumulative gain value in the top K results (NDCG@K) [6]. Here, #Correct@K measures the average number of correct results in top K returned results. NDCG measures the performance of a ranking list based on the graded relevance of the results and ranges from

0 to 1. Generally, the most relevant results should be ranked at top-most positions leading to a higher NDCG value. NDCG has been commonly used in information retrieval to evaluate the performance of web search engines. In our experiments, the Mini Mental State Examination (MMSE) score, the most commonly used test for complaints of memory problems and dementia diagnosis in clinical practice, is used as the criteria to define the subject relevance. Generally, closer MMSE scores indicate high similarity between two subjects. Given a query $\mathcal{Q}$, the relevance of $\mathcal{T}$ to $\mathcal{Q}$ is generated by:

$$r(\mathcal{Q},\mathcal{T}) = \begin{cases} 3 & \text{if } \mathcal{Q} \text{ and } \mathcal{T} \text{ belong to the same category and } dif_{MMSE}(\mathcal{Q},\mathcal{T}) = 0 \\ 2 & \text{if } \mathcal{Q} \text{ and } \mathcal{T} \text{ belong to the same category and } dif_{MMSE}(\mathcal{Q},\mathcal{T}) = 1 \\ 1 & \text{if } \mathcal{Q} \text{ and } \mathcal{T} \text{ belong to the same category and } dif_{MMSE}(\mathcal{Q},\mathcal{T}) > 1 \\ 0 & \text{if } \mathcal{Q} \text{ and } \mathcal{T} \text{ do not belong to the same category} \end{cases},$$

where $dif_{MMSE}(\mathcal{Q},\mathcal{T})$ is the difference between the MMSE scores of $\mathcal{Q}$ and $\mathcal{T}$.

Three baseline methods are implemented for comparison:

- Mean distance. To compare two subjects, the distances by using different imaging modalities are calculated first, and the mean distance is used.
- Minimal distance. To compare two subjects, the distances by using different imaging modalities between these two subjects are calculated and the minimal distance is selected as the pair-wise subject similarity.
- Graph learning fusion. In this method, a graph is first constructed for each imaging modality, using all the subjects in the database together with the query, based on the distances from that imaging modality. The learning is conducted on each graph to estimate the pair-wise subject relevance. The relevance from different modalities are combined together as the similarity between the two subjects. In this method, the category information in the database is not used.

Experimental Results: Figure 2 shows the performance comparisons of different methods, when using different imaging data and all the three types of imaging data in terms of #Correct@K and NDCG@K, respectively. It is noted that in many cases, the performance curves of the three baseline methods overlap each other, such as in all the #Correct@K curves. We can observe from the results that the proposed method can achieve better results compared to three baseline methods. For example, when all the three imaging data are employed, the proposed method can return 3.45 relevant subjects in top 5 returned results and 6.90 relevant subjects in top 10 returned results. The proposed method can improve #Correct@10 by 1.90 ($p = 1.2e^{-5}$), 1.89 ($p = 4.5e^{-5}$), and 1.84 ($p = 1.6e^{-5}$) compared with the three baseline methods, respectively. The improvements on NDCG@10 are 0.10 ($p = 9.5e^{-3}$), 0.10 ($p = 2.0e^{-2}$), and 0.12 ($p = 1.6e^{-3}$), respectively. The better performance on #Correct@K indicates that the proposed method is able to return more relevant medical records, and a higher NDCG@K value means that highly relevant subjects are located at top-most positions. The better performance comes from the accurate query category prediction and the following ranking procedure, which can precisely locate possible relevant subjects and then finally provide a fine ranking list. It is possible for the physicians to obtain useful reference from existing patient's database given the imaging data of the query subject.

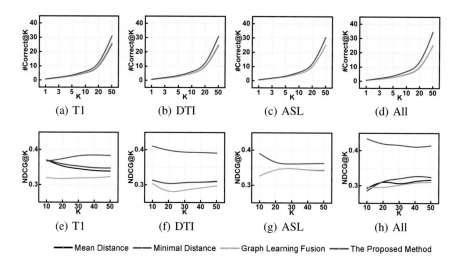

Fig. 2. The retrieval results comparison among different methods using different modalities in terms of #Correct@K and NDCG@K, where (d) and (h) refer to the using of all the three types of imaging data.

Table 1. The comparison among the proposed method using different data combinations.

Data Combination	#Correct@3	#Correct@5	#Correct@10	NDCG@10	NDCG@20
T1	1.830	3.050	6.100	0.390	0.361
DTI	1.860	3.100	6.200	0.367	0.373
ASL	1.860	3.100	6.200	0.410	0.397
T1+DTI	1.830	3.050	6.100	0.350	0.368
T1+ASL	1.650	2.750	5.500	0.337	0.346
DTI+ASL	1.860	3.100	6.200	0.340	0.334
T1+DTI+ASL	2.070	3.450	6.900	0.417	0.417

We further investigate the impact of multimodal data in the retrieval task. Table 1 demonstrates the comparisons of our method when different multimodal data combinations are employed. We can observe from the results that more imaging data from the query can lead to better results. The best performance comes from the using of T1, DTI and ASL together, which can be dedicated to the fact that different imaging data can represent the subject through different views and can be complementary for each other. This result also suggests that having more imaging data for a patient can be helpful for diagnosis assistance.

4   Conclusion

In this paper, we proposed to retrieve relevant medical records using imaging data to assist MCI diagnosis. Different from existing medical image retrieval tasks, which focus on similar image object content or the same type of imaging modalities as the retrieval target, our objective is to find disease-related imaging data, with similar brain patterns in the same imaging modalities. Our two-stage retrieval method is able to locate candidate results and then rank them to obtain relevant imaging data for the query. The results show that the top returned subjects are highly relevant to the query, which demonstrates the effectiveness of the proposed method on MCI diagnosis assistance.

References

[1] Brookmeyer, R., Johnson, E., Ziegler-Graham, K., Arrighi, M.H.: Forecasting the global burden of Alzheimer's disease. Alzheimer's & Dementia: the Journal of the Alzheimer's Association 3(3), 186–191 (2007)

[2] Cuingnet, R., Gerardin, E., Tessieras, J., Auzias, G., Lehéricy, S., Habert, M.O., Chupin, M., Benali, H., Colliot, O.: Automatic classification of patients with Alzheimer's disease from structural MRI: a comparison of ten methods using the ADNI database. NeuroImage 56(2), 766–781 (2011)

[3] Fjell, A.M., Walhovd, K.B., Fennema-Notestine, C., McEvoy, L.K., Hagler, D.J., Holland, D., Brewer, J.B., Dale, A.M.: The Alzheimer's Disease Neuroimaging Initiative: CSF biomarkers in prediction of cerebral and clinical change in mild cognitive impairment and Alzheimer's disease. The Journal of Neuroscience 30(6), 2088–2101 (2010)

[4] de Herrera, A.G.S., Kalpathy-Cramer, J., Fushman, D.D., Antani, S., Müller, H.: Overview of the imageclef 2013 medical tasks. In: Working Notes of CLEF 2013, pp. 1–15 (2013)

[5] Hinrichs, C., Singh, V., Mukherjee, L., Xu, G., Chung, M.K., Johnson, S.C.: Spatially augmented lpboosting for AD classification with evaluations on the ADNI dataset. NeuroImage 48(1), 138–149 (2009)

[6] Järvelin, K., Kekäläinen, J.: Ir evaluation methods for retrieving highly relevant documents. In: ACM SIGIR Conference on Research and Development in Information Retrieval, pp. 41–48. ACM (2000)

[7] Müller, H., de Herrera, A.G.S., Kalpathy-Cramer, J., Demner-Fushman, D., Antani, S., Eggel, I.: Overview of the imageclef 2012 medical image retrieval and classification tasks. In: CLEF (Online Working Notes/Labs/Workshop), pp. 1–16 (2012)

[8] Rubinov, M., Sporns, O.: Complex network measures of brain connectivity: uses and interpretations. NeuroImage 52(3), 1059–1069 (2010)

[9] Wang, M., Hua, X.S., Hong, R., Tang, J., Qi, G.J., Song, Y.: Unified video annotation via multigraph learning. IEEE Transactions on Circuits and Systems for Video Technology 19(5), 733–746 (2009)

[10] Ye, J., Wu, T., Li, J., Chen, K.: Machine learning approaches for the neuroimaging study of Alzheimer's disease. Computer 44(4), 99–101 (2011)

[11] Zhang, X., Liu, W., Dundar, M., Badve, S., Zhang, S.: Towards large-scale histopathological image analysis: Hashing-based image retrieval. IEEE Transactions on Medical Imaging 34(2), 496–506 (2015)

[12] Zhang, X., Yang, L., Liu, W., Su, H., Zhang, S.: Mining histopathological images via composite hashing and online learning. In: Golland, P., Hata, N., Barillot, C., Hornegger, J., Howe, R. (eds.) MICCAI 2014, Part II. LNCS, vol. 8674, pp. 479–486. Springer, Heidelberg (2014)

[13] Zhao, S., Yao, H., Yang, Y., Zhang, Y.: Affective image retrieval via multi-graph learning. In: ACM International Conference on Multimedia, pp. 1025–1028. ACM (2014)

[14] Zhou, D., Bousquet, O., Lal, T.N., Weston, J., Schölkopf, B.: Learning with local and global consistency. Advances in Neural Information Processing Systems 16(16), 321–328 (2004)

Regenerative Random Forest with Automatic Feature Selection to Detect Mitosis in Histopathological Breast Cancer Images

Angshuman Paul[1], Anisha Dey[2], Dipti Prasad Mukherjee[1],
Jayanthi Sivaswamy[2], and Vijaya Tourani[3]

[1] Indian Statistical Institute, Kolkata, India,
[2] Center for Visual Information Technology, International Institute of Information Technology, Hyderabad, India,
[3] CARE Hospital, Hyderabad, India

Abstract. We propose a fast and accurate method for counting the mitotic figures from histopathological slides using regenerative random forest. Our method performs automatic feature selection in an integrated manner with classification. The proposed random forest assigns a weight to each feature (dimension) of the feature vector in a novel manner based on the importance of the feature (dimension). The forest also assigns a misclassification-based penalty term to each tree in the forest. The trees are then regenerated to make a new population of trees (new forest) and only the more important features survive in the new forest. The feature vector is constructed from domain knowledge using the intensity features of nucleus, features of nuclear membrane and features of the possible stroma region surrounding the cell. The use of domain knowledge improves the classification performance. Experiments show at least 4% improvement in F-measure with an improvement in time complexity on the MITOS dataset from ICPR 2012 grand challenge.

Keywords: Breast cancer grading, random forest, weighted voting, tree penalty, forest regeneration, feature selection

1 Introduction

Detecting and counting of mitotic cells from histopathological images are key steps in breast cancer diagnosis as mitosis signals cell division. Interest in automating this process is driven from the arduous and error-prone nature of the manual detection. Research in this area has received much interest after the launch of mitosis detection as a challenge in ICPR 2012. The images that need to be analyzed are obtained with Hematoxylin & Eosin ($H\&E$) staining which render the cell nuclei dark blue against pinkish background (see Fig. 1).

Early solutions proposed for this problem include Gamma-Gaussian mixture modeling [7] and independent component analysis [6]. The difficulty in identifying appropriate features has been addressed by augmenting handcrafted features with those learnt by a convolutional neural network [9] or using only features

© Springer International Publishing Switzerland 2015
N. Navab et al. (Eds.): MICCAI 2015, Part II, LNCS 9350, pp. 94–102, 2015.
DOI: 10.1007/978-3-319-24571-3_12

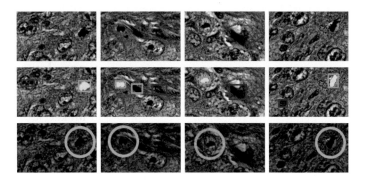

Fig. 1. Sample results: Row 1: Original sub-images , Row 2: Mitosis detection with proposed method (green/blue boxes indicate true/false positive) and Row 3: Mitosis detection with IDSIA [4] (green/cyan circles indicate true positive/false negative). Ground truth provided by [1] are shown as yellow regions in the middle row.

learnt with a deep neural network [4]. But this benefit of neural networks comes at a cost of tuning effort and training time for optimal performance. For instance, [4] reports a training time of 1 day on a GPU and processing time of 8 minutes per image. The latter poses a major deterrent for considering automated mitosis detection with high throughput processing of tissue microarrays. More extensive review can be found in [11]. Recently, random forests with population update [10] have been tried for mitosis detection where tree weights are changed based on classification performance. An in-depth biological study of the breast cancer tissues reveal that key factors in mitosis detection are: color of the nucleus, shape of the nuclear membrane and texture of the surrounding region. Presence of nucleus in a stromal region rules out the possibility of it being mitotic, while the absence or rupture of the nuclear membrane signals mitosis. Hence, we propose a fast mitosis detection method with the following contributions (i) new features based on domain knowledge mentioned above and (ii) regenerative random forest-based classification *with* automatic feature selection, unlike [10]. Automatic feature selection is achieved using a novel feature weighting scheme. Feature weights are based on the importance of a feature and we reject features with low weights. A new generation of forest (new population of trees) is created which operates on a reduced feature set. During the test phase, each tree of the trained forest votes with its corresponding weights to perform the classification.

The rest of the paper is organized as follows: section 2 describes our proposed method and proves that the process of forest regeneration converges with maximum classification accuracy with the training data. We present the experimental results in section 3 and the paper concludes in section 4.

2   Methods

We focus on several important biological cues for mitosis detection. First, after chromosomal condensation in interphase, the nucleolus disappears and the nuclear envelope breaks down during prophase. Consequently, most of the liquid contents of the nucleus is released into the cytoplasm making the nucleus denser with darker appearance compared to non-mitotic nucleus [2] after $H\&E$ staining. This intensity pattern of mitotic nuclei remains almost phase invariant during mitosis. Thus, the nuclear intensity pattern provides discriminative features between mitotic and non-mitotic cells. Second, it has been observed that the stroma or the connecting tissues contain non-cancerous fibroadenomas and a large number of non-mitotic cells. Thus, if stroma is found surrounding an unknown cell, the cell can be classified as non-mitotic. Hence, we evaluate the texture features of the regions surrounding the cell to find whether the cell belong to stroma or not. Further, after the nuclear membrane breaks down during mitosis, the nuclear contour of a mitotic cell becomes irregular compared to the contour of a non-mitotic cell with nuclear membrane. Thus, the pattern of the contour of nucleus also provides useful information in categorizing the mitotic and the non-mitotic cells. But the above features can be correctly evaluated and used for classification only if the nuclei are accurately segmented. So, the proposed method consists of three steps, namely: nuclei segmentation, feature extraction, classification. We segment the nuclei using [10]. These nuclei are used for feature extraction. In the next few paragraphs we discuss the feature extraction and classification steps in detail.

2.1   Feature Extraction

The blue channels of the $H\&E$ stained images lack useful information since both mitotic and non-mitotic nuclei are almost uniformly stained in blue [8]. Hence, we use only the red and green channel images for feature extraction. First, we extract the red and green channel histograms of the segmented nuclei. Next we look for the features of stroma by taking a region with 3 times the area enclosing the nucleus. In each such area, we evaluate the Haralick texture feature [5] of the region excluding pixels representing nuclei. We further detect the features associated with nuclear membrane. Here, we rely on the fact that a detected object (nucleus) with nuclear membrane has smooth and almost circular boundary whereas the mitotic nucleus with ruptured nuclear membrane generally has a rough boundary with non-circular shape. In order to characterize the detected object contour (whether the contour is circular or not) we evaluate the solidity, extent and lengths of major and minor axes of an ellipse equivalent to the detected object. This yields a 604-dimensional feature vector for each of the detected object (nucleus). Let the feature vector of kth nucleus be denoted as $\mathcal{F}(k)$. Intensity histogram of nucleus, stromal texture and nuclear membrane contribute 512, 88 and 4 features respectively. We use these feature vectors in the next step for classification of the nuclei in mitotic and non-mitotic category.

2.2   Classification

Our training dataset relies on manual ground truth [1] which inherently includes observer bias. Further a wide variation of feature magnitudes among the nuclei of same category (mitotic or non-mitotic) dictates the use of an ensemble classifier rather than a single classifier. Further, the variability in class-specific signatures in this problem precludes an explicit feature initialization in the classifier. All these prompt us to use random forest classifier [3] which is an ensemble classifier without the requirement for explicit feature initialization. A random forest is constructed of T trees each of which is grown using a bootstrap sample [3] from the training dataset. While splitting a node in each such tree, a subset of f number of features from $\mathcal{F}(k)$ are chosen. The best out of these f features is used for splitting the node. But, all of the features (dimensions) of $\mathcal{F}(k)$ may not have class-discriminative information. So, we propose a novel regenerative random forest that keeps on improving its classification performance by eliminating less discriminative features (dimensions) as the new populations of trees (new forest) are produced and thus performs feature selection and classification in an integrated manner.

Regenerative Random Forest: Our present aim is to classify the detected nuclei into two classes: mitotic and non-mitotic. For this, let S be the training dataset with s number of training data. A feature vector $\mathcal{F}(k)$ of dimension 604 is associated with k^{th} such data. During first step of training, we build T number of binary trees. For each tree τ, we construct a subset of training feature vectors Ψ^τ (with $\#\Psi^\tau = s$) by selecting s number of training feature vectors randomly with replacement from S. At each node of tree τ, we randomly choose a set (Λ) of f number of features (dimensions) from each training feature vector $F(k) \in \Psi^\tau$ without replacement for splitting the node into its two child nodes. Now, for selecting the split point, we consider the fact that an ideal split should result in child nodes each of which contains training data of exactly one class. Let a node u be composed of ξ_f^u number of training feature vectors and the class label of jth feature vector be denoted by c_j. We indicate the probability of class c_j in node u by $p(u, c_j)$. Then the total entropy of node u is defined as: $H(u) = \sum_{c_j} p(u, c_j) \log \frac{1}{p(u,c_j)}; \forall j \in \xi_f^u$. So, the total entropy of two child nodes after a split from parent node v using feature (dimension) f_l is:

$$E(v, f_l) = \sum_{u=1}^{2} H(u) = \sum_{u=1}^{2} \sum_{c_j} p(u, c_j) \log \frac{1}{p(u, c_j)}; \forall j \in \xi_f^u. \qquad (1)$$

In case of an ideal split from parent node v, $p(u, c_j) = 1$ making $H(u) = 0; \forall u$, where u is a child node of v. Thus, from (1), we get $E(v) = \sum_{u=1}^{2} H(u) = 0$ which indicates that the best split should result in minimum total entropy of the child nodes. Hence we look for the split point in node v based on a feature (dimension) $f_\chi \in f$ that minimizes the total entropy of its child nodes. So,

$$f_\chi = \underbrace{argmin}_{f_l} \{E(v, f_l)\} = \underbrace{argmin}_{f_l} \left\{ \sum_{u=1}^{2} \sum_{\forall j \in \xi_f^u} p(u, c_j) \log \frac{1}{p(u, c_j)} \right\}. \qquad (2)$$

We continue splitting a node u until u has a very small value (δ) of entropy. So, we split a node u only if $H(u) > \delta$. Now, suppose the ground truth class label of jth training feature vector is given by c_j and tree τ predicts the proper class label with probability $q_\tau^0(j, c_j)$ [3]. Then, probability of misclassification on j^{th} training feature vector by tree τ is $1 - q_\tau^0(j, c_j)$. Once all the trees are grown, we calculate weight (importance) of each tree in a novel manner based on tree's classification performance on the labeled training data. Initially, each tree τ is assigned a weight $w_\tau^0 = 1$. Now, we propose a penalty for each tree on the basis of above misclassification probabilities. The normalized penalty of tree τ is given by: $\Upsilon_\tau^0 = \frac{1}{s} \sum_{\forall j \in \Psi^\tau} (1 - q_\tau^0(j, c_j))$. Consequently, the weight of a tree after the first population (first phase of training) is given by: $w_\tau = w_\tau^0 - \kappa \Upsilon_\tau^0 = w_\tau^0 - \frac{\kappa}{s} \sum_{\forall j \in \Psi^\tau} (1 - q_\tau^0(j, c_j))$,

where κ is a constant in $(0, 1]$. Subsequently, we assign weight to each feature of the feature vector $\mathcal{F}$. Consider a tree τ where feature x has been selected $\alpha_\tau(x)$ times in Λ, out of which it has been used $\beta_\tau(x)$ times for node splitting. Then we define the importance of feature x in tree τ as $\gamma_\tau(x) = \frac{\beta_\tau(x)}{\alpha_\tau(x)}$ and the global importance (weight) of feature x is defined as: $\eta(x) = \frac{1}{T} \sum_{\tau=1}^{T} \hat{w}_\tau \gamma_\tau(x)$,

where $\hat{w}_\tau$ is the value of w_τ, normalized w.r.t. $max(w_\tau), \forall \tau \in T$. Note that $\alpha_\tau(x) = 0 \Rightarrow \beta_\tau(x) = 0$. So, if $\alpha_\tau(x) = 0$, we take $\gamma_\tau(x) = 1$. Clearly, the feature (dimension) that provides more class-discriminative information will be used for splitting more number of times as evident from (1) and (2) yielding high value of $\gamma_\tau(x)$ in each tree. Thus a more class-discriminative feature (dimension) x will have higher value of weight $\eta(x)$. Let μ and σ be the mean and standard deviation of feature weights $\eta(x), \forall x$. Also, let $\mathcal{L}$ be the set of features that has weight $\eta(x) < (\mu - \sigma)$. Clearly, the features in $\mathcal{L}$ are the redundant features with low weights. So, we remove the features in $\mathcal{L}$ and make $\mathcal{F} = \mathcal{F} - \mathcal{L}$. Then we create a new population of trees (new forest) which are trained with a subset of training data Ψ^τ. Ψ^τ is composed of s number of training feature vectors randomly selected with replacement from $\mathcal{S}$. Thus, the weight of tree τ in $(n+1)^{th}$ population is given by: $w_\tau^{n+1} = w_\tau^n - \kappa \Upsilon_\tau^n = w_\tau^n - \frac{\kappa}{s} \sum_{\forall j \in \Psi^\tau} (1 - q_\tau^n(j, c_j))$. Let $\mathcal{F}^n$ be the set of features in n^{th} population and $\mathcal{L}^n$ be the set of features to be removed from $\mathcal{F}^n$. Then the reduced feature set in $(n + 1)^{th}$ population is given by: $\mathcal{F}^{n+1} = \mathcal{F}^n - \mathcal{L}^n$. Thus, our approach performs automatic selection of features that provide more class-discriminative information. Next, we show that the proposed approach results in maximization of classification performance of the forest on training data.

Maximization of Forest Classification Performance: Let the relative weight of rth feature (dimension) be $\hat{\eta}(r) = \eta(r)/max(\eta(r))$. We consider an empirical dependence that the accurate classification probability by the forest Φ in the nth population (P_Φ^n) depends on the relative weight of true discriminative features (dimensions). The relative weight $\hat{\eta}(r)$ indicates the probability of rth feature (dimension) to be selected as the feature for splitting a node, given that the feature is there in Λ of the corresponding node. Consequently, P_Φ^n also depends on the probability that the above mentioned true discriminative feature is chosen in Λ. Let there be d number of true discriminative features in $\mathcal{F}$. Also, let the subset of features to be considered for node splitting in tree τ in the nth population be Λ_n^τ. Given this, we obtain the probability that r^{th} true discriminative feature is selected in Λ_n^τ ($\#\Lambda_n^\tau = f$) is given by $\rho_n^\tau(r) = \binom{\#\mathcal{F}-1}{f-1}/\binom{\#\mathcal{F}}{f}$. Now, if the weight of the rth discriminative feature is $\eta(r)$, then, we consider the empirical function Π that relates P_Φ^n and $\rho_n^\tau(r), \eta(r)$ as: $P_\Phi^n = \Pi\left(\sum_{r=1}^{d} \rho_n^\tau(r)\hat{\eta}(r)\right)$. So, if we go on removing redundant features using the equation $\mathcal{F}^{n+1} = \mathcal{F}^n - \mathcal{L}^n$, $\#\mathcal{F}$ will decrease. Thus, from straightforward observation, for every infinitesimal change in iteration (population number) $\frac{\Delta\rho_n^\tau(r)}{\Delta n} > 0$. Now, if we take sufficient training data, the relative weight of the features can be considered to be statistically independent of the subset of data chosen for training each tree. So, using the expression of P_Φ, we can write $\frac{\Delta P_\Phi^n}{\Delta n} > 0$ until we remove any important feature.

Forest Convergence: Increase in ΔP_Φ^n corresponds to decrease in misclassification probability of the forest on training data [3]. So, we conclude that our proposed approach converges with minimum misclassification probability. We terminate the population update when misclassification probability starts increasing after attaining a minima. This situation corresponds to removal of discriminative feature from the feature vector. Finally we discard the current population and select the trees of previous population (that attained misclassification minima). We compute the weights of the selected trees and use a weighted voting from these tress to classify test data. At this point, we discuss two situations that may arise during training. First, at some iteration number (population) n^*, the feature vector may have all the features with weight $\eta(x) \geq (\mu - \sigma)$, indicating that all the features now present in feature vector are important (class-discriminative). In this condition we terminate the regeneration process and go for testing. Fig. 2(a)-(b) shows a typical situation where convergence is achieved based on misclassification probability and as many as 96% of the features are above $(\mu - \sigma)$ limit at the convergence point. Second, as we go on reducing the features, at some population, although very rare, it may happen that $\#\mathcal{F} < f$. To avoid this, we terminate the training procedure pre-matured when $\#\mathcal{F} = f$. In the next section, we present and analyze the experimental results.

3 Experimental Results

3.1 Dataset and Parameters

We use the MITOS dataset [1] for our experiments. The training data contains 35 images with 233 mitotic cells and the test data contains 15 images with 103 mitotic cells. During classification, our forest is composed of $T = 1000$ trees and the initial feature vector contains 604 features. We take $f = 15$ for each node. When the proposed forest tends to misclassification minima, the tree weights have a high mean value and a low value of standard deviation as evident from previous discussions. In this near minima situation, the rate of change of tree

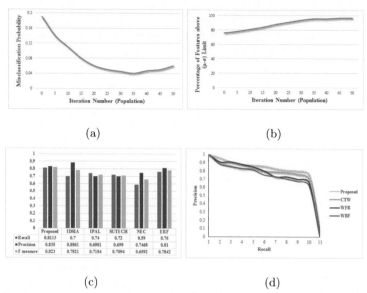

Fig. 2. Performance of proposed method: (a) Probability of misclassification, (b) percentage of features above $(\mu - \sigma)$ limit, (c) classification performances of different methods, (d) P-R curves for different methods (proposed, CTW, WFR and WBF).

weights (and consequently κ) should be low so that the forest does not cross the minima. Hence, we take $\kappa = \sigma_\tau^n(1 - \mu_\tau^n)$ where μ_τ^n and σ_τ^n are mean and standard deviation of tree weights in the nth population.

3.2 Performance Measures and Comparisons

Following [1] we evaluate recall, precision and F-measures on the test data. We obtain recall and precision values of 0.8113 and 0.8350, respectively, yielding an F-measure of 0.823. We compare our classification performance with the four best results reported for MITOS dataset [1] and the result using the method proposed in [10] (abbreviated as ERF). The four best results are from groups IDSIA, IPAL, SUTECH and NEC respectively [1]. We show the comparative results in Fig. 2(c) where the proposed method is found to outperform other competing methods in terms of F-measure. Note that the ranking of the groups in [1] are performed in terms of F-measure. However, it can be observed that the precision value in the proposed method is less compared to IDSIA. The reason is imbalance in the number of dense non-mitotic nuclei in the training dataset due to which the forest did not properly learn the corresponding signature. The precision-recall (P-R) curves obtained by varying the number of features selected for each node (f) are shown in Fig. 2(d). We also examined the performance of the method a) while keeping constant tree weight (CTW) of value 1 across all generations (populations), b) without feature reduction (WFR) (by updating only the tree weights) and c) using the proposed random forest without using biological (stroma and nuclear membrane) features (WBF). The P-R curves for each of these experiments are also presented in Fig. 2(d). We find that the area under the curve of the proposed method is the largest which indicates that both feature reductions and tree weights play significant roles in classification performances. It also indicates the importance of using the biological features. Some sample sub-images are shown in Fig. 1 along with classification results of our method and IDSIA [4]. It is notable that there is significant improvement in training and testing times compared to [4]. The training time for the proposed method is 12 minutes and the average testing time per image is 22 sec using a PC with 3.2 GHz intel Xeon processor and 16 GB memory.

4   Conclusions

We propose a novel approach for mitosis detection utilizing domain knowledge. Intensity features of the nucleus, texture features of possible stroma and features of nuclear membrane are classified with a novel regenerative random forest that performs automatic feature selection. We prove that the regeneration process converges producing maximum classification accuracy during training. We achieve lower time complexity comp ared to state-of-the-art techniques. In future, we want to use more biological features to further improve the classification performance. A generalized regenerative random forest will also be a significant direction of future research.

References

1. (2012). http://ipal.cnrs.fr/ICPR2012/?q=node/5 Available as on (February 18, 2015)
2. Barlow, P.W.: Changes in chromatin structure during the mitotic cycle. Protoplasma 91(2), 207–211 (1977)
3. Breiman, L.: Random forests. Machine Learning 45(1), 5–32 (2001)
4. Cireşan, D.C., Giusti, A., Gambardella, L.M., Schmidhuber, J.: Mitosis detection in breast cancer histology images with deep neural networks. In: Mori, K., Sakuma, I., Sato, Y., Barillot, C., Navab, N. (eds.) MICCAI 2013, Part II. LNCS, vol. 8150, pp. 411–418. Springer, Heidelberg (2013)
5. Haralick, R.M., Shanmugam, K., Dinstein, I.H.: Textural features for image classification. IEEE Transactions on Systems, Man and Cybernetics (6), 610–621 (1973)
6. Huang, C.H., et al.: Automated mitosis detection based on exclusive independent component analysis. In: 21st ICPR, pp. 1856–1859. IEEE (2012)
7. Khan, A.M., et al.: A gamma-gaussian mixture model for detection of mitotic cells in breast cancer histopathology images. Journal of Pathology Informatics 4 (2013)
8. Kuru, K.: Optimization and enhancement of h&e stained microscopical images by applying bilinear interpolation method on lab color mode. Theoretical Biology and Medical Modelling 11(1), 9 (2014)

9. Malon, C.D., Cosatto, E.: Classification of mitotic figures with convolutional neural networks and seeded blob features. Journal of Pathology Informatics 4 (2013)
10. Paul, A., Mukherjee, D.P.: Enhanced random forest for mitosis detection. In: Proceedings of the 2014 Indian Conference on Computer Vision Graphics and Image Processing, p. 85. ACM (2014)
11. Veta, M., et al.: Breast cancer histopathology image analysis: a review. IEEE Trans. Biomed. Engineering 61(5), 1400–1411 (2014)

HoTPiG: A Novel Geometrical Feature
for Vessel Morphometry and Its Application
to Cerebral Aneurysm Detection

Shouhei Hanaoka[1,2], Yukihiro Nomura[3], Mitsutaka Nemoto[3], Soichiro Miki[3],
Takeharu Yoshikawa[3], Naoto Hayashi[3], Kuni Ohtomo[1,3],
Yoshitaka Masutani[4], and Akinobu Shimizu[2]

[1] Department of Radiology, The University of Tokyo Hospital, 7-3-1 Hongo,
Bunkyo-ku, Tokyo, Japan
[2] Tokyo University of Agriculture and Technology,
2-24-16 Nakamachi, Koganei, Tokyo, Japan
[3] Department of Computational Diagnostic Radiology and Preventive Medicine,
The University of Tokyo Hospital, 7-3-1 Hongo, Bunkyo-ku, Tokyo, Japan
[4] Department of Intelligent Systems, Graduate School of Information Sciences,
Hiroshima City University, 3-4-1 Otsuka-higashi, Asaminami-ku, Hiroshima, Japan
hanaoka-tky@umin.ac.jp

Abstract. A novel feature set for medical image analysis, named HoTPiG (Histogram of Triangular Paths in Graph), is presented. The feature set is designed to detect morphologically abnormal lesions in branching tree-like structures such as vessels. Given a graph structure extracted from a binarized volume, the proposed feature extraction algorithm can effectively encode both the morphological characteristics and the local branching pattern of the structure around each graph node (e.g., each voxel in the vessel). The features are derived from a 3-D histogram whose bins represent a triplet of shortest path distances between the target node and all possible node pairs near the target node. The extracted feature set is a vector with a fixed length and is readily applicable to state-of-the-art machine learning methods. Furthermore, since our method can handle vessel-like structures without thinning or centerline extraction processes, it is free from the "short-hair" problem and local features of vessels such as caliper changes and bumps are also encoded as a whole. Using the proposed feature set, a cerebral aneurysm detection application for clinical magnetic resonance angiography (MRA) images was implemented. In an evaluation with 300 datasets, the sensitivities of aneurysm detection were 81.8% and 89.2% when the numbers of false positives were 3 and 10 per case, respectively, thus validating the effectiveness of the proposed feature set.

Keywords: graph feature, computer-assisted detection, MR arteriography, cerebral aneurysm, support vector machine.

1 Introduction

A branching treelike structure is one of the major types of structure in the human body. For example, a wide variety of vessels (blood vessels, bronchi, bile ducts, etc.)

© Springer International Publishing Switzerland 2015
N. Navab et al. (Eds.): MICCAI 2015, Part II, LNCS 9350, pp. 103–110, 2015.
DOI: 10.1007/978-3-319-24571-3_13

have a treelike structure. Quite a large number of diseases affect these vascular structures and cause pathological shape changes including narrowing, occlusion, and dilation. Vascular diseases, including cerebral infarction and coronary occlusive disease, are one of the major causes of death in advanced nations. Since precise evaluation of the shape of vessels is essential in diagnosing these diseases, computer-assisted detection/diagnosis (CAD) of these treelike structures is required.

Among the vascular diseases, cerebral aneurysm has been one of the targets of CAD applications [1-3]. Although unruptured cerebral aneurysms are generally asymptomatic, they rupture in approximately 1% of patients per year, leading to high rates of mortality and disability [2]. This is why the early detection of cerebral aneurysms is needed. In clinical practice, noninvasive magnetic resonance arteriography (MRA) examination is most frequently used for screening, in which diagnostic radiologists search for abnormal structures (i.e., saccular protuberances and fusiform dilation). However, it is known that a normal arterial system may include pseudo-lesions such as infundibular dilatations. CAD applications for detecting cerebral aneurysm also have to distinguish abnormal aneurysmal structures from normal ones, including branching sites of small cerebral arteries and tightly curving carotid siphons.

In previous studies, two approaches to searching for aneurysms have generally been used: (1) voxel-by-voxel evaluation using Hessian matrix-derived features, and (2) three-dimensional (3-D) thinning of a presegmented arterial region and branching pattern analysis. In the first approach, a Hessian-based filter emphasizes spherical structures with various sizes. For example, Arimura et al. [3] used a dot enhancement filter that outputs a high value when all three eigenvalues of the Hessian matrix have large negative values. Nomura et al. [2] used a similarity index that can distinguish spherelike aneurisms from ridgelike vessels. Although their approach usually works well, the detected candidates inevitably include a large number of false positives, especially at vessel bifurcations. Therefore, subsequent processes to eliminate false positives are required, greatly affecting the overall performance.

The other approach is to find an abnormal arterial branching pattern from the graph structure of an extracted artery. After segmentation of the artery voxels, a 3-D thinning algorithm is applied to extract the centerlines. Then the centerlines are analyzed to find any suspicious points, such as end points of centerlines [4], short branches, or points with a locally maximal vascular radius [1]. In contrast to the curvature approach, the centerline approach can utilize branching pattern information to discriminate aneurysms from bifurcations. On the other hand, the 3-D thinning process has the "short hair" problem, i.e., a large number of false short branches where the arterial wall has small "lumps." Therefore, a postprocess to remove [5] or classify [1, 3] short hairs is indispensable. Another problem is how to represent local morphological and topological changes in the graph in the context of machine learning. A large number of studies on the analysis of whole graph structures have been conducted in which the graph structure is embedded into a vector field (graph embedding) or evaluated by kernel methods (graph kernel) [6].

In this study, we propose a novel feature set named HoTPiG (Histogram of Triangular Paths in Graph). It is defined at each node in a given graph based on a 3-D histogram of shortest path distances between the node of interest and each of its neighboring node pairs. The feature vector efficiently encodes the local graph network pattern around the node. The graph structure can be determined directly from a binary label volume. Since the thickness of the vessel is naturally encoded without any centerline extraction process, the "short hair" problem caused by the thinning algorithm does not occur. Furthermore, the proposed feature is essentially robust to nonrigid deformations under the assumption that the graph structure extracted from the original image is not significantly changed by the deformation. The proposed feature set is sufficiently effective for aneurysms in MRA images to be accurately classified by a support vector machine (SVM) without any complicated pre- or postprocesses. The contributions of this study are as follows: (1) A novel vector representation of a local graph structure for detecting abnormalities is presented, (2) a CAD application for detecting aneurysms in MRA images is implemented using the proposed graph feature and a state-of-the-art SVM classifier with explicit feature mapping, and (3) the usefulness of the proposed method is experimentally validated using a large dataset with 300 clinical MRA images, and high performance comparable to that of other state-of-the-art methods is demonstrated.

2   HoTPiG

The proposed HoTPiG feature is defined for any arbitrary undirected graph based on bin counts of a 3-D histogram of shortest path lengths (Fig. 1). One feature vector is determined for each node in the graph and can be readily used to classify the corresponding node as positive (e.g., aneurysm) or negative. The 3-D histogram accumulates counts of each triplet of distances between the target node and its two neighbor nodes as well as between the two neighbor nodes.

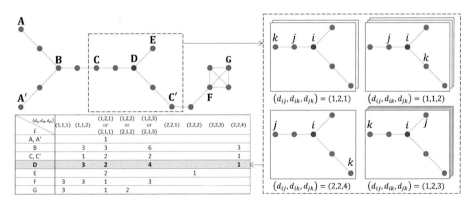

$\begin{array}{c}(d_{ij}, d_{ik}, d_{jk})\\ i\end{array}$	(1,1,1)	(1,1,2)	(1,2,1) or (2,1,1)	(1,2,2) or (2,1,2)	(1,2,3) or (2,1,3)	(2,2,1)	(2,2,2)	(2,2,3)	(2,2,4)
A, A'				1					
B			3	3			6		3
C, C'			1	2			2		1
D			3	2			4		1
E				2				1	
F			3	3	1		3		
G			3		1	2			

Fig. 1. Example of calculation of HoTPiG features (with $d_{max} = 2$).

Suppose that the graph includes $|U|$ nodes, and each node in the graph has an integer index $l \in U = \{1,2,3, \dots, |U|\}$. Also suppose that the feature vector of node i is to be calculated. First, the shortest path distances from i to all other nodes are calculated (by a breadth first search). Here, the shortest path distance is the number of steps (edges) along the shortest path between the pair of nodes. Let the distance between nodes a and b be $dist(a, b)$. We define the *neighborhood* of i, N_i, as the set of nodes whose distances from i are no more than a predefined integer d_{max}. That means $N_i = \{l \in U | 0 < dist(i, l) \leq d_{max} \}$.

Then, for any triplet of distances (d_{ij}, d_{ik}, d_{jk}), the value of the 3-D histogram $H_i(d_{ij}, d_{ik}, d_{jk})$ is defined as the number of node pairs (j, k) that satisfy the following conditions

$$j \in N_i, k \in N_i, dist(i, j) = d_{ij}, dist(i, k) = d_{ik}, dist(j, k) = d_{jk}. \tag{1}$$

In practice, the two bins (d_{ij}, d_{ik}, d_{jk}) and (d_{ik}, d_{ij}, d_{jk}) are simply those with neighbor nodes j and k swapped. Thus, these two bins are considered to be the same and only one count is incremented for such pairs of distance triplets.

The counts of bins in histogram H_i are used as the feature vector of node i. As shown in Fig. 1, the feature vector tends to vary widely among different nodes and is sensitive to topological changes in the local graph structure. Note that the extent of the locality can be controlled via the parameter d_{max}.

The calculation cost for the proposed method is estimated as follows. The breadth-first search algorithm can calculate all the shortest path distances by performing $O(|U| \cdot E(|N_i|))$ calculations, where $E(|N_i|)$ is the mean size of the neighborhoods. On the other hand, the histogram counting requires $O(|U| \cdot E(|N_i|)^2)$ count increment calculations. Therefore, most of the calculation cost is for histogram counting.

3   Computer-Assisted Detection of Aneurysms

As an application of the proposed HoTPiG feature, we have developed CAD software for aneurysm detection in MRA images. The proposed CAD application is composed of four steps: (1) extraction of the binary label volume of arteries from MRA images, (2) calculation of graph structure features, (3) voxel-based classification by SVM, and (4) a thresholding and labeling process.

3.1   Artery Region Extraction and HoTPiG Feature Calculation

Firstly, the artery region is extracted by a conventional region growing method. The average $\bar{I}$ and standard deviation σ_I of the brain region are estimated by sampling voxel values from a predefined mid-central subregion, that is, a horizontal rectangular plane with half the width and height placed at the center of the volume. Then, the initial artery region is extracted by region growing, where the seed threshold and growing threshold are $> \bar{I} + 3\sigma_I$ and $> \bar{I} + 2.5\sigma_I$, respectively.

After the artery region is extracted, an undirected graph is composed. We choose a simple graph structure whose nodes are all foreground (i.e., intra-arterial) voxels, and the edges connect all 18-neighbor voxel pairs (Fig. 2). Here, an 18-neighborhood is chosen because it is more similar to the Euclidean distance than 6- and 26-neighborhoods.

Using this graph, the HoTPiG feature is calculated at each foreground voxel. The maximum distance used is $d_{max} = 11$, considering the balance between the performance and the calculation cost. Two modifications are applied to the method described in Section 2. Firstly, a 1-D histogram with $d_{max} = 11$ bins whose distances are $\{1, 2, 3, ..., 11\}$ may be too sparse when it is used as part of a 3-D histogram. To cope with this, some distances are grouped into one bin and only six bins $\{1, 2, 3, [4, 5], [6, 7], [8, 11]\}$ are used. These bins are determined so that their upper bounds are the geometric series $1.5^n, n = 1,2,3,4,5,6$. Applying this bin set to each of three distances (d_{ij}, d_{ik}, d_{jk}), the entire 3-D histogram has $6 \cdot_6 C_2 = 126$ bins. However, some bins never have a count because the corresponding distance triplet does not satisfy the triangle inequality. After removing such bins, a total of 85 bins are included in the 3-D histogram in this study.

Additionally, a multidimensional approach is added to analyze gross vascular structures. After downsampling the artery binary volume to half and a quarter of its original size, the graph structure features are extracted in the same manner. After feature extraction, each feature is upsampled by nearest neighbor interpolation and all the features of the three scales are merged voxel by voxel. Therefore, a total of $85 \times 3 = 255$ features are calculated for each voxel.

Prior to the classification process, each feature is normalized by dividing by the standard deviation estimated from training datasets.

3.2 Voxel-Based Classification by SVM

Using the extracted features, each voxel is classified as positive (aneurysm) or negative (normal artery) by a an SVM classifier [7]. The exponential-χ^2 kernel $K(\mathbf{x}, \mathbf{y}) = \exp\left(-\frac{1}{2\sigma^2} \cdot \frac{1}{2} \sum_l \frac{(x_l - y_l)^2}{x_l + y_l}\right)$ [8], which is designed specifically for histogram comparison, is used in this study. The classifier is trained using manually inputted aneurysm voxels in the training datasets as positive samples and other arterial voxels as negative samples. Here, one of the difficulties is the huge number ($> 10^8$) of training samples, because one MRA volume has approximately 10^6 artery voxels. It is known that the computational cost of kernel SVM is of order $O(dM^2) \sim O(dM^3)$, where d and M are the data dimensionality and number of samples, respectively. To solve this problem, we utilized a feature map of the exponential-χ^2 kernel [8] to reduce the original problem to a linear SVM whose computational cost is $O(dM)$. The feature map is a function that *explicitly* maps the original feature vector of each sample to a higher-dimensional space, in contrast to the conventional kernel method, in which a vector is *implicitly* mapped to a higher-dimensional space. Using this feature map and the random reduction of negative samples (to 3% of the original number), the training task was calculated in approximately 20 min for 2×10^8 original samples.

In addition to the classifier with the HoTPiG feature set only, another classifier is also trained by adding two sets of Hessian-derived features (the dot enhancement filter [3] and shape index [2]) to evaluate the cooperativity of both types of features. The two Hessian-derived features are calculated with six different scales; thus, a total of 12 features are added to the HoTPiG features.

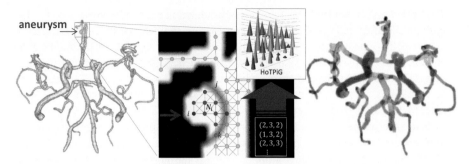

Fig. 2. (Left) Example of cerebral arteries in a volume. (Middle) HoTPiG feature calculation for a voxel in an aneurysm. (Right) Result of voxelwise clustering of HoTPiG features into 20 clusters (displayed by their colors) by a k-means method. Note that the vessel thickness and branching pattern can be clearly distinguished. Furthermore, the mirror symmetry of the clustering result implies its robustness against local deformations and sensitivity to caliper changes.

In this study, the parameters of feature mapping are set to $m = 5000$, $n = 2$, and $L = 0.6$, referring to [8]. The parameters of the kernel σ and the linear SVM C are experimentally optimized (as described later in the next section).

Using the output values of the SVM, candidate aneurysm lesions and their lesionwise likelihoods are determined as follows. Firstly, the SVM outputs are thresholded by zero and all nonpositive voxels are discarded. Then, the positive voxels are labeled by connected component analysis and all connected components are outputted as candidate lesions. The likelihood of each lesion is determined as the maximal value of SVM-derived likelihoods of the voxels in the lesion. The representative point of each lesion is defined as this maximal value point.

4   Experimental Results

This study was approved by the ethical review board of our institution. A total of 300 time-of-flight cerebral MRA volumes with 333 aneurysms were used in the experiment. The voxel size was 0.469×0.469×0.6 mm. Two board-certified radiologists diagnosed all images and manually inputted aneurysm regions.

The proposed method was evaluated using 3-fold cross-validation. Before the actual training, a hyperparameter optimization was performed in each fold using another nested 3-fold cross validation. The optimal values of the two parameters σ and C were searched for from the search space $\sigma \in \{20,30,40\}$ and $C \in \{10,20,30\}$ by performing a grid search. After optimization, the actual training was performed using all training datasets. The calculation of HoTPiG features took approximately 3 min per case using a workstation with 2 ×6 core Intel Xeon processers and 72 GB memory.

The overall performance of the method was evaluated using the free receiver operating characteristic (FROC) curve. Each outputted lesion was determined as a successful detection if the representative point of the lesion was no more than 3 mm from the center of gravity of the ground truth region.

Figure 3 shows the FROC curves of the proposed method with and without additional Hessian features, as well as the one with Hessian features only. The sensitivities with only HoTPiG features were 76.6% and 86.5% when the numbers of false positives (FPs) were 3 and 10 per case, respectively. When combined with Hessian features, the sensitivities increased to 81.8% and 89.2% for 3 and 10 FPs/case, respectively. Although a strict comparison cannot be made owing to the different datasets used, the sensitivity of 81.8% is superior to that reported by Yang et al. [1], whose detection sensitivity was 80% for 3 FPs/case. On the other hand, Nomura et al. [2] reported sensitivities of 81.5% and 89.5% when the training dataset sizes were 181 and 500 (also for 3 FPs/case), respectively. Since we used 200 datasets to train each SVM, we conclude that the performance of our CAD is comparable to that of Nomura et al. when the dataset size is equal. Note that Nomura et al. did not use any objective criterion (e.g., maximum acceptable error distance) to judge lesions outputted by CAD as true positives or false positives; instead, radiologists subjectively decided whether or not each CAD-outputted lesion corresponded to an aneurysm.

Figure 3 also shows the sensitivity for each aneurysm size (maximized by using 21 FPs/case). Most detection failures occurred when the size of the aneurysms was less than 4 mm. On the other hand, our method failed to detect two large aneurysms whose sizes were 6 mm and 13 mm. This was very likely to have been due to a shortage of large aneurysms (only 19 with sizes $\geq$ 6 mm) in our dataset.

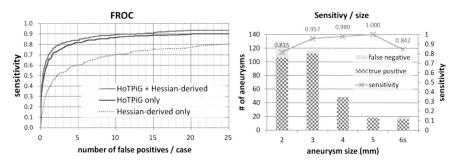

Fig. 3. (Left) FROC curves for the proposed method with and without additional Hessian-derived features. (Right) Sensitivities (with Hessian features) for each aneurysm size.

5   Discussion and Conclusion

Among the various vascular diseases that involve the human body, aneurysms are characterized by their particular protuberant shape. This study was inspired by the fact that many radiologists rely on 3-D reconstructed vascular images to find aneurysms and other diseases in daily image interpretation. This implies that only the shape of the tissue can be sufficient to detect such abnormalities. The HoTPiG feature is designed to evaluate only the shape of the tissue and discard all image intensity information including image gradations and textures. This can be both a disadvantage and an advantage of HoTPiG. On the one hand, it can only utilize a small part of the information provided by the original image. On the other hand, HoTPiG can reveal image characteristics very different from those collected by most other image features based on image intensity information. Indeed, HoTPiG showed cooperativity with existing Hessian-based features which has a weakness at branching sites of vessels. The effectiveness of HoTPiG shown in this study may also be owing to the robustness of HoTPiG against local deformations. Therefore, we believe that HoTPiG will be a powerful alternative tool for vectorizing shape characteristics of vessel-like organs.

In conclusion, a novel HoTPiG feature set for evaluating vessel-like shapes was presented. It showed high performance for detecting cerebral aneurysms and cooperativity with existing image features. Our future works may include the application of HoTPiG to other applications such as lung nodule detection, in which discrimination between lesions and vascular bifurcations has similar importance.

Acknowledgement. This study is a part of the research project "Multidisciplinary Computational Anatomy", which is financially supported by the grant-in-aid for scientific research on innovative areas MEXT, Japan.

References

1. Yang, X., Blezek, D.J., Cheng, L.T., Ryan, W.J., Kallmes, D.F., Erickson, B.J.: Computer-aided detection of intracranial aneurysms in MR angiography. Journal of Digital Imaging 24, 86–95 (2011)
2. Nomura, Y., Masutani, Y., Miki, S., Nemoto, M., Hanaoka, S., Yoshikawa, T., Hayashi, N., Ohtomo, K.: Performance improvement in computerized detection of cerebral aneurysms by retraining classifier using feedback data collected in routine reading environment. Journal of Biomedical Graphics and Computing 4, 12 (2014)
3. Arimura, H., Katsuragawa, S., Suzuki, K., Li, F., Shiraishi, J., Sone, S., Doi, K.: Computerized scheme for automated detection of lung nodules in low-dose computed tomography images for lung cancer screening 1. Academic Radiology 11, 617–629 (2004)
4. Suniaga, S., Werner, R., Kemmling, A., Groth, M., Fiehler, J., Forkert, N.D.: Computer-aided detection of aneurysms in 3D time-of-flight MRA datasets. In: Wang, F., Shen, D., Yan, P., Suzuki, K. (eds.) MLMI 2012. LNCS, vol. 7588, pp. 63–69. Springer, Heidelberg (2012)
5. Kobashi, S., Kondo, K., Yutaka, H.: Computer-aided diagnosis of intracranial aneurysms in MRA images with case-based reasoning. IEICE Transactions on Information and Systems 89, 340–350 (2006)
6. Suard, F., Guigue, V., Rakotomamonjy, A., Benshrair, A.: Pedestrian detection using stereo-vision and graph kernels. In: Proceedings of the IEEE Intelligent Vehicles Symposium, pp. 267–272. IEEE (2005)
7. Fan, R.-E., Chang, K.-W., Hsieh, C.-J., Wang, X.-R., Lin, C.-J.: LIBLINEAR: A library for large linear classification. The Journal of Machine Learning Research 9, 1871–1874 (2008)
8. Sreekanth, V., Vedaldi, A., Zisserman, A., Jawahar, C.: Generalized RBF feature maps for efficient detection. In: Proceedings of the British Machine Vision Conference (BMVC), Aberystwyth, 31 August - 3 September, pp. 1–11 (2010)

Robust Segmentation of Various Anatomies in 3D Ultrasound Using Hough Forests and Learned Data Representations

Fausto Milletari[1], Seyed-Ahmad Ahmadi[3], Christine Kroll[1],
Christoph Hennersperger[1], Federico Tombari[1], Amit Shah[1], Annika Plate[3],
Kai Boetzel[3], and Nassir Navab[1,2]

[1] Computer Aided Medical Procedures, Technische Universität München, Germany
[2] Computer Aided Medical Procedures, Johns Hopkins University, Baltimore, USA
[3] Department of Neurology, Klinikum Grosshadern, Ludwig-Maximilians-Universität München, Germany

Abstract. 3D ultrasound segmentation is a challenging task due to image artefacts, low signal-to-noise ratio and lack of contrast at anatomical boundaries. Current solutions usually rely on complex, anatomy-specific regularization methods to improve segmentation accuracy. In this work, we propose a highly adaptive learning-based method for fully automatic segmentation of ultrasound volumes. During training, anatomy-specific features are obtained through a sparse auto-encoder. The extracted features are employed in a Hough Forest based framework to retrieve the position of the target anatomy and its segmentation contour. The resulting method is fully automatic, i.e. it does not require any human interaction, and can robustly and automatically adapt to different anatomies yet enforcing appearance and shape constraints. We demonstrate the performance of the method for three different applications: segmentation of midbrain, left ventricle of the heart and prostate.

1 Introduction and Related Work

Manual segmentation of ultrasound volumes is tedious, time consuming and subjective. In the attempt to produce results that are invariant to the presence of noise, drop-out regions and poorly distinguishable boundaries, current computer-aided approaches either use complex cost functions, often regularized by statistical prior models, or require extensive user interaction. Many optimization-based methods utilize cost functions based on local gradients, texture, region intensities or speckle statistics [10]. Methods employing shape and appearance models often require a difficult and time-consuming training stage where the annotated data must be carefully aligned to establish correspondence across shapes in order to ensure the correctness of the extracted statistics. Learning approaches have been successfully proposed to solve localization and segmentation tasks both in computer vision [7,12] and medical image analysis [6]. Handcrafted features which exhibit robustness towards the presence of noise and artefacts have been often

© Springer International Publishing Switzerland 2015
N. Navab et al. (Eds.): MICCAI 2015, Part II, LNCS 9350, pp. 111–118, 2015.
DOI: 10.1007/978-3-319-24571-3_14

employed to deliver automatic segmentations [8]. Recent work [3] in the machine learning community focused on approaches leveraging single [5] or multi-layer [9] auto-encoders to discover features from large amount of data. In particular, sparse auto-encoders with a single-layer have been proven to learn more discriminative features compared to multi-layer ones [5] when a sufficiently large number of hidden units is chosen. In the medical community, recent approaches [4] have employed deep neural networks to solve segmentation tasks, despite their computational burden due to the presence of cascaded 3D convolutions when dealing with volumes.

The segmentation method proposed in this paper is (i) fully automatic, (ii) highly adaptive to different kinds of anatomies, and (iii) capable of enforcing shape and appearance constraints to ensure sufficient robustness. A sparse auto-encoder is trained from a set of ultrasound volumes in order to create a bank of 3D features, which are specific and discriminative to the anatomy at hand. Through a voting strategy, the position of the region to be segmented is assessed and a contour is obtained by patch-wise projection of appropriate portions of a multi-atlas. Differently from [12], each contribution to the contour is weighted by a factor dependent on the appearance pattern of the region that it was collected from. In this way, we effectively enforce shape *and* appearance constraints.

We demonstrate the performance of our method by segmenting three different and challenging anatomies: left ventricle of the heart, prostate and midbrain. The experiments show that our approach is competitive compared to state-of-the-art anatomy specific methods and that, in most cases, the quality of our segmentations lies within the expected inter-expert variability for the particular dataset.

2   Method

Our approach comprises a training and a test phase. During training, we discover anatomy-specific features that are employed to learn a Hough Forest. During testing, we perform simultaneous object localization and segmentation.

2.1   Feature Learning

Sparse Auto-Encoders are feed-forward neural networks designed to produce close approximations of the input signals as output (Fig. 1 - a). By employing a limited number of neurons in the hidden layer and imposing a sparsity constraint through the Kullback-Leibler (KL) divergence, the network is forced to learn a sparse lower-dimensional representation of the training signals [5,9].

The network has N inputs, K neurons in the hidden layer and N outputs. The biases $b_i^{(1,2)}$ are integrated in the network through the presence of two additional neurons in the input and hidden layer having a constant value of 1. The weights of the connections between the j-th neuron in one layer and the i-th neuron in the next are represented by $w_{ij}^{(1,2)} \in \mathbb{R}$, that are grouped in the matrices $\mathbf{W}_1 \in \mathbb{R}^{K \times (N+1)}$ and $\mathbf{W}_2^\top \in \mathbb{R}^{N \times (K+1)}$. Network outputs can

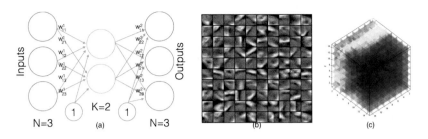

Fig. 1. a) Schematic Illustration of a Sparse Auto-Encoder (SAE); b) Bank of filter obtained from 2D ultrasound images of the midbrain; c) One filter obtained from 3D echocardiographical data through the SAE.

be written as $h_{\mathbf{W}^{(1,2)}}(\mathbf{X}) = f\left(\mathbf{W}_2^\top f\left(\mathbf{W}_1\mathbf{X}\right)\right)$, where $f(z) = \frac{1}{1+exp(-z)}$ is the sigmoid activation function.

The matrix $\mathbf{X}$ is filled with M unlabeled ultrasound training patches arranged column-wise. After a normalization step to compensate for illumination variations through the dataset, the network is trained via back-propagation. The network weights are initialized with random values. The objective function to be minimized comprises of three terms, enforcing the fidelity of the reconstructions, small weights magnitude and sparsity respectively:

$$C(\mathbf{X}, \mathbf{W}_{1,2}) = \frac{1}{2}\left\|h_{\mathbf{W}^{(1,2)}}(\mathbf{X}) - \mathbf{X}\right\|^2 + \frac{\lambda}{2}\sum_{l=1}^{2}\sum_{k=1}^{K}\sum_{n=1}^{N}\left(w_{nk}^{(l)}\right)^2 + \beta\sum_{j=1}^{K}KL(\rho\|\rho_j). \quad (1)$$

In the third term, we indicate as $\rho_j = \frac{1}{M}\left(\mathbf{1}^\top f\left(\mathbf{W}_1\mathbf{X}\right)\right)$ the average firing rate of the j-th hidden neuron, and we define the KL divergence, which enforces the sparsity constraint by penalizing deviations of ρ_j from ρ, as:

$$KL(\rho\|\rho_j) = \rho\,log\left(\frac{\rho}{\rho_j}\right) + (1-\rho)log\left(\frac{1-\rho}{1-\rho_j}\right). \quad (2)$$

The parameter ρ represents the desired firing rate of the neurons of the hidden layer, and must be set prior to training together with λ, β and K, which control the weight of the two regularization terms and the number of neurons of the hidden layer respectively.

After optimization, the rows of the weight matrix $\mathbf{W}_1$ can be re-arranged to form a set of 3D filters $\varXi = \{\xi_1...\xi_K\}$ having the same size as the ultrasound patches collected during training (Fig. 1 - b,c).

2.2 Training the Hough Forest

Our implementation of Hough Forests (HF) combines the classification performance of Random Forests (RF) with the capability of carrying out organ localization and segmentation. Differently from the classical Hough Forest framework [7], our method retrieves segmentations enforcing shape and appearance constraints.

We consider a training set composed of N data samples, $\mathbf{d}_{1...N}$, where each sample $\mathbf{d}_i = [d_x, d_y, d_z]^\top$ corresponds to a voxel element of an annotated volume V_t belonging to the training set T. Each data point is described by K features $F_{1...K}$, which are computed by applying one of the filters ξ from the set Ξ obtained via Sparse Auto-Encoders as described in the previous step. Specifically, we write

$$F_k(\mathbf{d}) = \sum_{i=-r_x}^{r_x} \sum_{j=-r_y}^{r_y} \sum_{k=-r_z}^{r_z} V_t(d_x + i, d_y + j, d_z + k) * \xi(i, j, k). \tag{3}$$

The annotation G_t, obtained in the form of a 3D binary mask associated with the volume V_t, determines the binary labels $l_i = \{f, b\}$ that characterize each data-point as belonging to the foreground or to the background. Foreground data-points are associated with a vote $\mathbf{v}_i = \mathbf{c}_t - \mathbf{d}_i$, which is expressed as a displacement vector connecting $\mathbf{d}_i$ to the centroid of the annotated anatomy $\mathbf{c}_t = [c_x, c_y, c_z]^\top$, obtained from G_t.

During training, the best binary decision is selected in each node of the Hough Forest, either maximizing the Information Gain (IG) or maximizing the Vote Uniformity (VU). In each node, we compute M random features and we determine S candidate splits through the thresholds $\tau_{1...S}$. Each split determines a partitioning of the data D_p reaching the parent node in two subsets $D_l = \{\mathbf{d}_i \in D_p : F_k(\mathbf{d}_i) \leq \tau_s\}$ and $D_r = \{\mathbf{d}_i \in D_p : F_k(\mathbf{d}_i) > \tau_s\}$ reaching the left and right child nodes, respectively. The Information Gain is obtained as:

$$IG(D_p, D_l, D_r) = H(D_p) - \sum_{i \in \{l,r\}} \frac{|D_i|}{|\bar{D}|} H(D_i), \tag{4}$$

where the Shannon entropy $H(D) = \sum_{c \in \{f,b\}} -p_c log\,(p_c)$ is obtained through the empirical probability $p_c = \frac{|D_c|}{|D|}$ using $D_c = \{d_i \in D : l_i = c\}$.

The Vote Uniformity criterion requires the votes $\mathbf{v}_j^{\{l,r\}}$ contained in D_l and D_r to be optimally clustered around their respective means $\bar{\mathbf{v}}^{\{l,r\}}$:

$$VU(D_l, D_r) = \sum_{i \in \{l,r\}} \sum_{\mathbf{v}_j} \left\| \mathbf{v}_j^i - \bar{\mathbf{v}}^i \right\|. \tag{5}$$

Once (i) the maximum tree depth has been reached or (ii) the number of data points reaching the node is below a certain threshold or (iii) the Information Gain is zero, the recursion terminates and a leaf is instantiated. The proportion of foreground versus background points $p_{\{f,b\}}$ is stored together with the votes $\mathbf{v}_i$ and the associated original positions $\mathbf{d}_i$. The coordinates $\mathbf{d}_i$, in particular, refer to training volumes which will be used as atlases during segmentation.

2.3 Segmentation via Hough Forests

Given an ultrasound volume I of the test set, we first classify it into foreground and background, then we allow foreground data-points to cast votes in order to

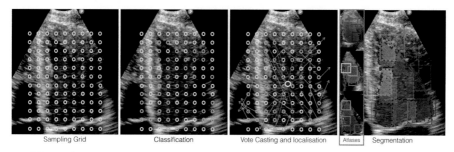

Fig. 2. Schematic representation of our segmentation approach shown in 2D.

localize the target anatomy, and finally, we obtain the contour by projecting 3D segmentation patches from the atlases associated with each vote that correctly contributed to localization (Fig. 2).

The data-points processed in the Hough Forest are obtained through a regular grid of sampling coordinates $S = \{s_1...s_{N_d}\}$. In this way, we can reduce the computational load during testing without significantly deteriorating the results. Each data-point s_i classified as foreground in a specific leaf l of the Hough trees is allowed to cast the n_v^l votes $v_{1...n_v^l}$ stored in that leaf during training.

Each vote determines a contribution, weighted by the classification confidence, at the location $s_i + v_j$ of a volume C having the same size as I and whose content is initially set to zero.

The target anatomy is localized retrieving the position of the highest peak in the vote map. All the votes $\hat{v}_j$ falling within a radius r around the peak are traced back to the coordinates $\hat{s}_i$ of the data-points that cast them. Each vote $\hat{v}_j$ is associated with the coordinates $\hat{d}_j$ of a specific annotated training volume.

We retrieve the 3D appearance patch A_j and the segmentation patch P_j associated to each vote by using the coordinates $\hat{d}_j$ to sample the appropriate training volume and its annotation. The segmentation patches are projected at the positions $\hat{s}_i$ after being weighted by the Normalized Cross Correlation (NCC) between the patch A_j and the corresponding intensity patterns around $\hat{s}_i$ in the test volume. The fusion of all the reprojected segmentation patches forms the final contour, which implicitly enforces shape and appearance constraints.

3   Results

We demonstrate the segmentation accuracy and the flexibility of our algorithm using three datasets of different anatomies comprising in total 87 ultrasound volumes. A brief description of each dataset and the relative state-of-the-art segmentation approach being used for comparison is provided below.

1. The left ventricle of the heart is segmented and traced in [2] using an elliptical shape constraint and a B-Spline Explicit Active Surface model. The dataset employed for our tests, comprising 60 cases, was published during

the MICCAI 2014 "CETUS" challenge. Evaluations were performed using the MIDAS platform[1].

2. The prostate segmentation method proposed in [11] requires manual initialization. Its contour is retrieved using a min-cut formulation on intensity profiles regularized with a volumetric size-preserving prior. We test on a self-acquired trans-rectal ultrasound (TRUS) dataset comprising 15 subjects. All the volumes were manually segmented by one expert clinician via 'TurtleSeg'. Our results are obtained via cross-validation.

3. Segmentation of the midbrain in transcranial ultrasound (TCUS) is valuable for Parkinson's Disease diagnosis. In [1], the authors employed a discrete active surface method enforcing shape and local appearance constraints. We test the methods on 12 ultrasound volumes annotated by one expert using 'ITK snap' and acquired through one of the skull bones of the patients. Our results are obtained via cross-validation.

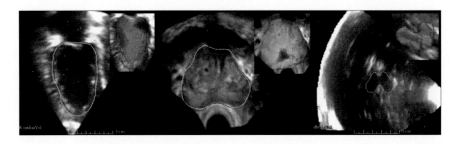

Fig. 3. Exemplary segmentation results (green curves) Vs. ground-truth (red curves). Mesh color encodes distances from ground truth in the range −3mm (red) to +3mm (blue), with green indicating perfect overlap.

Table 1 shows the performance of our method in comparison to the other state-of-the-art approaches on the three datasets. Results are expressed in terms of Dice coefficients and mean absolute distance (MAD) from ground truth annotation. Typical inter-expert annotation variability is also shown for each anatomy.

3.1   Parameters of the Model

The Sparse Auto-Encoder was trained to obtain $K = 300$ 3D filters having size $15 \times 15 \times 15$ pixels, with parameters $\lambda = 10^{-4}$, $\beta = 10$ and $\rho = 10^{-3}$. The Hough Forest includes 12 trees with at most 35 decision levels and leafs that contain at least 25 data-points. During testing, the images were uniformly sampled every 3 voxels. All the votes accumulating in a radius of 3 voxels from the object centroid were reprojected. The size of the segmentation and intensity patches employed for reprojection during segmentation was different for the three datasets due to

---

[1] Documentation under: http://www.creatis.insa-lyon.fr/Challenge/CETUS

Table 1. Overview of Dice coefficients and mean absolute distance (MAD) achieved during testing. Inter-expert-variabilities (IEV) are also reported. MAD was not provided by the authors of the algorithms used for comparison.

Dataset	Avg. our approach	MAD	Avg.state-of-the-art	IEV(Dice)
Left Ventricle	0.87 ± 0.08 *Dice*	2.90 ± 1.87 *mm*	0.89 ± 0.03 *Dice*	86.1%[2]
Prostate	0.83 ± 0.06 *Dice*	2.37 ± 0.95 *mm*	0.89 ± 0.02 *Dice*	83.8%[11]
Midbrain	0.85 ± 0.03 *Dice*	1.18 ± 0.24 *mm*	0.83 ± 0.06 *Dice*	85.0%[1]

the variable size the object of interest. Values for left ventricle, prostate and midbrain were $35 \times 35 \times 35$, $30 \times 30 \times 30$ and $15 \times 15 \times 15$ pixels respectively.

Training time for the Auto-Encoder was approximately 24 hours per dataset, with 500,000 patches. The training time for the forest ranged from 20 minutes to 5 hours. The processing time during testing was always below 40sec. per volume.

3.2   Experimental Evaluation

In Fig. 4 we show the histogram of Dice scores observed during our tests. Its resolution is 0.05 Dice. Additional results can be found in Table 1 and Fig. 3.

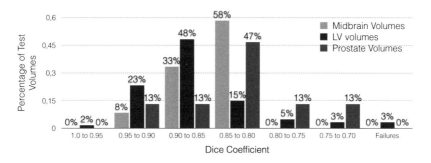

Fig. 4. Percentage of test volumes vs. Dice coefficient. This histogram shows the percentage of test volumes falling in each Dice bin on the horizontal axis.

3.3   Discussion

Localization of the target anatomy through a voting strategy, removes the need for user interaction while being very efficient in rejecting false positive datapoints, whose votes could not accumulate in the vicinity of the true anatomy centroid. During our tests, only one out of 87 localizations failed, resulting in a wrong contour. A trade-off between appearance and shape constraints can be set choosing the size of the segmentation patches. Bigger patches force smoother contours, while smaller ones lead to more adaptation to local volume contents. The method is not suited for segmentation of elongated structures (eg. vessels).

4   Conclusion and Acknowledgement

In this work, we presented a learning-based method for fully automatic localization and segmentation of various anatomies in 3D ultrasound. The method learns an optimal representation of the data and implicitly encodes a prior on shape and appearance. We apply the method on three clinical 3D ultrasound datasets of challenging anatomies, with results comparable to the state-of-the-art. This work was founded by DFG BO 1895/4-1 and ICT FP7 270460 (ACTIVE).

References

1. Ahmadi, S.A., Baust, M., Karamalis, A., Plate, A., Boetzel, K., Klein, T., Navab, N.: Midbrain segmentation in transcranial 3D ultrasound for Parkinson diagnosis. Med. Image Comput. Comput. Assist. Interv. 14(Pt 3), 362–369 (2011)
2. Barbosa, D., Heyde, B., Dietenbeck, T., Houle, H., Friboulet, D., Bernard, O., D'hooge, J.: Quantification of left ventricular volume and global function using a fast automated segmentation tool: validation in a clinical setting. Int. J.Cardiovasc. Imaging 29(2), 309–316 (2013)
3. Bengio, Y., Courville, A., Vincent, P.: Representation learning: A review and new perspectives. IEEE Transactions on Pattern Analysis and Machine Intelligence 35(8), 1798–1828 (2013)
4. Carneiro, G., Nascimento, J., Freitas, A.: Robust left ventricle segmentation from ultrasound data using deep neural networks and efficient search methods. In: 2010 IEEE International Symposium on Biomedical Imaging: From Nano to Macro, pp. 1085–1088. IEEE (2010)
5. Coates, A., Ng, A.Y., Lee, H.: An analysis of single-layer networks in unsupervised feature learning. In: International Conference on Artificial Intelligence and Statistics, pp. 215–223 (2011)
6. Donner, R., Menze, B.H., Bischof, H., Langs, G.: Global localization of 3D anatomical structures by pre-filtered hough forests and discrete optimization. Medical Image Analysis 17(8), 1304–1314 (2013)
7. Gall, J., Yao, A., Razavi, N., Van Gool, L., Lempitsky, V.: Hough forests for object detection, tracking, and action recognition. IEEE Transactions on Pattern Analysis and Machine Intelligence 33(11), 2188–2202 (2011)
8. Ionasec, R.I., Voigt, I., Georgescu, B., Wang, Y., Houle, H., Vega-Higuera, F., Navab, N., Comaniciu, D.: Patient-specific modeling and quantification of the aortic and mitral valves from 4-D cardiac CT and TEE. IEEE Trans. Med. Imaging 29(9), 1636–1651 (2010)
9. Le, Q.V.: Building high-level features using large scale unsupervised learning. In: 2013 IEEE International Conference on Acoustics, Speech and Signal Processing (ICASSP), pp. 8595–8598. IEEE (2013)
10. Noble, J.A., Boukerroui, D.: Ultrasound image segmentation: a survey. IEEE Trans. Med. Imaging 25(8), 987–1010 (2006)
11. Qiu, W., Rajchl, M., Guo, F., Sun, Y., Ukwatta, E., Fenster, A., Yuan, J.: 3D prostate TRUS segmentation using globally optimized volume-preserving prior. Med. Image Comput. Comput. Assist. Interv. 17(Pt 1), 796–803 (2014)
12. Rematas, K., Leibe, B.: Efficient object detection and segmentation with a cascaded hough forest ISM. In: 2011 IEEE International Conference on Computer Vision Workshops (ICCV Workshops), pp. 966–973, November 2011

Improved Parkinson's Disease Classification from Diffusion MRI Data by Fisher Vector Descriptors

Luis Salamanca[1], Nikos Vlassis[2], Nico Diederich[1,3], Florian Bernard[1,3,4], and Alexander Skupin[1]

[1] Luxembourg Centre for Systems Biomedicine, University of Luxembourg, Esch-sur-Alzette, Luxembourg
[2] Adobe Research, San Jose, CA, USA
[3] Centre Hospitalier de Luxembourg, Luxembourg City, Luxembourg
[4] Trier University of Applied Sciences, Trier, Germany

Abstract. Due to the complex clinical picture of Parkinson's disease (PD), the reliable diagnosis of patients is still challenging. A promising approach is the structural characterization of brain areas affected in PD by diffusion magnetic resonance imaging (dMRI). Standard classification methods depend on an accurate non-linear alignment of all images to a common reference template, and are challenged by the resulting huge dimensionality of the extracted feature space. Here, we propose a novel diagnosis pipeline based on the Fisher vector algorithm. This technique allows for a precise encoding into a high-level descriptor of standard diffusion measures like the fractional anisotropy and the mean diffusivity, extracted from the regions of interest (ROIs) typically involved in PD. The obtained low dimensional, fixed-length descriptors are independent of the image alignment and boost the linear separability of the problem in the description space, leading to more efficient and accurate diagnosis. In a test cohort of 50 PD patients and 50 controls, the implemented methodology outperforms previous methods when using a logistic linear regressor for classification of each ROI independently, which are subsequently combined into a single classification decision.

Keywords: neurodegenerative diseases, diagnosis, diffusion magnetic resonance imaging, machine learning, feature extraction.

1 Introduction

Magnetic resonance imaging (MRI) has become a well-known useful and established technique for the diagnosis and progression monitoring of neurodegenerative diseases. Recent developments on MRI allow for capturing different properties of brain tissues, like the structural integrity by diffusion MRI (dMRI), or the activation and interaction between different brain regions when performing a task or in resting-state by functional MRI. To extract diagnostic parameters, traditional approaches for the statistical analysis of these images rely on

© Springer International Publishing Switzerland 2015
N. Navab et al. (Eds.): MICCAI 2015, Part II, LNCS 9350, pp. 119–126, 2015.
DOI: 10.1007/978-3-319-24571-3_15

a group-level, voxel-wise comparison of the extracted measures by using univariate statistical tools such as the t-test, χ^2-test, etc. Common techniques like voxel-based morphometry [1] can provide good insights in the pathological involvement of different brain regions, but lack the ability of fully integrate the extracted features.

Currently, more advanced machine learning methodologies are being used to fully integrate the data and provide results at the level of the individual [11]. The typically small sample size and the high-dimensionality of the data pose major problems when using these methods. Although a step of feature selection may alleviate the problem, there is still a huge risk of overfitting that may obscure the results' validity [11]. Additionally, the considered features are, most presumably, non-linearly separable, what restrains the ability of linear classifiers, and even more advanced kernel-based methods, for obtaining optimal decision thresholds.

In this paper we propose a novel pipeline for the diagnosis of Parkinson's disease (PD). Our methodology utilizes the advantages of the Fisher vector (FV) algorithm [14] to regionally encode the data in high-level descriptors. This way, and in contrast to standard approaches, we get rid of the necessity of a fine alignment between different subjects' brains, since a voxel-wise comparison is not required. Therefore, the step of non-linear registration of all images to a reference template can be skipped, excluding artefacts or undesired corruption of the subject data due to under- or over-alignments. Further, thanks to representing the distribution of the data captured from all voxels of each region of interest (ROI) as a fixed-length high-level descriptor, we lead to an immense reduction of the dimensionality of the problem. Finally, since the FV algorithm is based on the Fisher Kernel (FK) principle [8], we can understand the process of computing the FV descriptor as an embedding of the extracted features into a higher-dimensional space, more suitable to linear classification. This strategy directly supports the last stage of classification and crucially improves the diagnosis results.

Although the diagnosis of PD remains as a challenging problem, especially in the early stages when there is not clear evidence of brain atrophy, there have been already promising machine learning approaches in the literature [10,13]. However, these previous studies lack a sufficient number of subjects. In the current paper, we apply the proposed methodology to the dMRI data of a test cohort of 50 PD patients and 50 healthy controls, chosen from the PPMI consortium database [12]. In our test scenario we show that our approach reaches a global accuracy of 77%, outperforming other machine learning strategies on the same data set by at least 5%.

2   Methods

In this section we provide a brief overview of the Fisher vector algorithm, and how the high-level descriptor is obtained from the raw neuroimaging data. We also describe in detail the developed pipeline, from the preprocessing of the data to the last step of classification.

2.1 Fisher Vector Algorithm

Given the measures extracted from all the subjects for a specific brain ROI, we define the sample $\mathbf{X} = \{\mathbf{x}_n : n = 1, \ldots, N\}$ of D-dimensional observations $\mathbf{x}_n \in \mathcal{X}$, with N the total number of voxels and D the number of extracted features. Let's consider a generative process defined by the probability density function (p.d.f.) u_θ, which models the generation of the elements in $\mathcal{X}$. The p.d.f. u_θ is defined by the set of parameters $\theta = \{\theta_m : m = 1, \ldots, M\}$, where $\theta \in \mathbb{R}^M$. To measure the similarity between two samples $\mathbf{X}$ and $\mathbf{Y}$, the authors in [8] use the Fisher Kernel, which is defined as follows:

$$K_{\text{FK}}(\mathbf{X}, \mathbf{Y}) = G_\theta^{\mathbf{X}'} F_\theta^{-1} G_\theta^{\mathbf{Y}} = G_\theta^{\mathbf{X}'} L_\theta' L_\theta G_\theta^{\mathbf{Y}} = \mathcal{G}_\theta^{\mathbf{X}'} \mathcal{G}_\theta^{\mathbf{Y}}, \tag{1}$$

where F_θ is the Fisher information matrix (FIM), factorized into terms L_θ through Cholesky decomposition, and $G_\theta^{\mathbf{X}}$ is the score function. This function, defined as $G_\theta^{\mathbf{X}} = \nabla_\theta \log u_\theta(\mathbf{X})$, measures how the parameters θ of the generative model u_θ should be modified to better fit $\mathbf{X}$. The Cholesky decomposition of the FIM allows to re-write the FK as the dot-product of the gradient statistics $\mathcal{G}_\theta$, as we observe in Eq. (1).

In [14], the authors choose a Gaussian mixture model (GMM) as the generative model u_θ, due to it can accurately capture any continuous distribution [15]. Thus, the p.d.f. u_θ is defined by K Gaussian components as follows:

$$u_\theta(\mathbf{x}) = \sum_{k=1}^{K} w_k u_k(\mathbf{x}) \quad \text{with} \quad u_k \sim \mathcal{N}(\mu_k, \sigma_k \mathbf{I}), \tag{2}$$

where $\mu_k \in \mathbb{R}^D$ is the mean and $\sigma_k \in \mathbb{R}^D$ is the diagonal of the covariance matrix for the k-th Gaussian component. The restrictions $w_k \geq 0 \,\forall\, k$ and $\sum_{k=1}^{K} w_k = 1$ over the mixture weights w_k can be implicitly included in the auxiliary parameter $\alpha_k \in \mathbb{R}$ [14]. Therefore, the set of parameters results in $\theta = \{\alpha_k, \mu_k, \sigma_k : k = 1, \ldots, K\}$. Given $\mathbf{X}$, they can be computed by using the expectation-maximization (EM) algorithm [5].

Now, let us define $\mathbf{X}_\ell = \{\mathbf{x}_{n_\ell} : n_\ell = 1, \ldots, N_\ell\}$ as the subset of observations $\mathbf{X}_\ell \subset \mathbf{X}$ for subject ℓ. Given the set of parameters θ computed using the whole sample $\mathbf{X}$, and assuming independence between observations in $\mathbf{X}_\ell$, the gradient statistics in Eq. (1) can be obtained as [14]:

$$\mathcal{G}_\theta^{\mathbf{X}_\ell} = \sum_{n_\ell=1}^{N_\ell} L_\theta \nabla_\theta \log u_\theta(\mathbf{x}_{n_\ell}) \tag{3}$$

Thanks to considering a GMM as the generative model, and by assuming the FIM to be diagonal, analytic expressions can be derived for each parameters θ_m, as detailed in [14]. Through these expressions, we readily calculate the gradients $\mathcal{G}_{\mu_k}^{\mathbf{X}_\ell}$, $\mathcal{G}_{\sigma_k}^{\mathbf{X}_\ell}$ and $\mathcal{G}_{\alpha_k}^{\mathbf{X}_\ell}$ for each Gaussian component k, which are stacked together to form the Fisher vector (FV) for each subject ℓ, hereafter denoted as $\mathbf{F}_\ell$. The gradient statistics $\mathcal{G}_{\theta_m}^{\mathbf{X}_\ell}$ measure the deviation of the subject data $\mathbf{X}_\ell$ from the distribution of the generative model, fitted for all data $\mathbf{X}$. This way, the FV descriptor captures the slight variations in each subject's data distribution with respect to the distribution for all samples. Now, since $\mathcal{G}_{\alpha_k}^{\mathbf{X}_\ell}$ is scalar, and $\mathcal{G}_{\mu_k}^{\mathbf{X}_\ell}$ and $\mathcal{G}_{\sigma_k}^{\mathbf{X}_\ell}$ are D-dimensional vectors, the dimension of $\mathbf{F}_\ell$ is $(2D+1)K$, therefore depending only on the parameters of the generative model, and not on the size of the ROI described. Finally, given that the Fisher kernel is equivalent to the dot product of the gradient statistics, Eq. (1), using the FV descriptor as input to a linear classifier is equivalent to directly feeding the original features to a non-linear classifier using the Fisher kernel. Therefore, the description space of the Fisher vector is a more amenable representation of the extracted measures.

2.2   Pipeline for dMRI Analysis

To conveniently illustrate the proposed methodology, we depict in Fig. 1 the flow diagram of the pipeline. The input data required is:

- The diffusion weighted image (DWI) of each subject. Through *eddy*, included in the FMRIB Software Library (FSL) [9], we first correct the eddy current and head motion. Then, the brain is extracted from the T2-weighted b0 volume, contained in the DWI tensor, using *bet*, also included in FSL.
- A reference template to align the subjects to.
- Masks for the ROIs considered, in the same space as the reference template.

Given this data, we first use FLIRT (FMRIB's Linear Image Registration Tool) to linearly align the DWI volume to the reference template, by using an affine transformation with 12 degrees of freedom and the T2-weighted b0 volume as the moving image. Then, the reference template is non-linearly aligned to each subject's space, using the symmetric image normalisation method (SyN) contained in the ANTS package [2], considering cross-correlation as the image metric. The transformations obtained are used to warp the masks of all the selected ROIs to each subject space. Thanks to this strategy of registration, already used before in the literature, the patient images are not deformed, and therefore the risk of corrupting the data is minimised, in contrast to approaches where patient images are non-linearly aligned to the reference template.

Using the warped masks of the ROIs for all the subjects, we subdivide each ROI in different subROIs in the x, y and z directions according to some given minimum and maximum voxel sizes for the resulting subdivisions. It is important to note that, although for every ROI all the subjects will have the same number of subROIs and the same scheme of division in every direction, each subROI will have a particular voxel size because the subjects' brains are not non-linearly aligned to a common template. Then, by using the *DTIfit* tool included in FSL, we apply diffusion tensor imaging (DTI) method on the DWI data to extract the diffusion tensor and related diffusion measures. With the subROIs indices obtained from the masks, we extract a matrix $\mathbf{X}_\ell^r$ of diffusion features for every subject ℓ and subROI r.

Finally, for each r, we fit the GMM to the data $\mathbf{X}^r = [\mathbf{X}_1^r; \ldots; \mathbf{X}_L^r]$ using the EM algorithm [5]. The parameters obtained, together with each subROI data

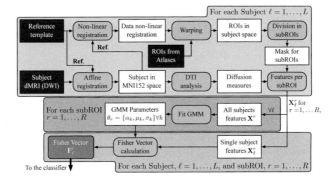

Fig. 1. Flow diagram for the proposed pipeline.

$\mathbf{X}_\ell^r$, allow to finally compute the fixed-length Fisher vector descriptor $\mathbf{F}_\ell^r$ for every subROI and subject, as described in Section 2.1.

2.3 Classification

To show the enhanced separability of the problem in the description space, we consider a logistic linear regressor as classifier, with an $L2$ regularizer. Since this classifier can easily handle thousands of features, we first perform the training and classification for all the ROIs. Additionally, we also provide the performance for each ROI separately. These individual predictions are combined to provide a single diagnosis for each subject, by using a polling procedure, i.e. the decision chosen is the one taken by the majority of the ROIs. Additionally, and for the sake of comparison, we also consider a support vector machine (SVM) classifier, with a radial-basis function (RBF) kernel. This will allow to compare the performance of using the FV descriptors as input to a linear classifier, against the performance of more powerful kernel methods using directly the diffusion measures. But the FV descriptors are not fed to the SVM because we just want to show their potential when using linear classifiers. The software packages *liblinear* and *libSVM* are used to run the experiments [3,6].

3 Experiments

The data used in the preparation of this article was obtained from the Parkinson's Progression Markers Initiative (PPMI) database (www.ppmi-info.org/data). For up-to-date information on the study, visit www.ppmi-info.org. From the whole database, we initially chose only the baseline data of those subjects with DTI-gated images, resulting a total of 185 subjects, 131 PD patients and 54 controls. We visually inspected all the images, and excluded 10 of them due to noticeable imaging artefacts. Then, we select 50 PD patients and 50 controls by using the following criteria: we first select the 50 PD cases that minimize the deviation from the mean disease duration, from the date of diagnosis. Then, the control group is chosen such that we match the mean age of the PD group. The ages (mean $\pm$ standard deviation) of the PD and controls groups are 60.21 $\pm$ 10.23 and 61.00 $\pm$ 10.74, respectively, and the disease duration 4.56 $\pm$ 1.73 months.

The DWI images from the PPMI database have a resolution of 1.98 $\times$ 1.98 $\times$ 2mm. Thus, from the MNI-ICBM152 symmetric template [7], we obtain a T2 reference image with resolution 2 $\times$ 2 $\times$ 2mm. For the analyses we initially selected 14 ROIs usually related with the disease pathology: *superior and middle cerebellar penduncle, internal and external capsule, gyrus rectus, caudate body, dentate nucleus, pons, sub-thalamic nucleus, red nucleus, globus pallidus externa and interna, putamen* and *substantia nigra*. From them, only the most discriminative ones were selected, as we observe in Table 1. The atlases considered to extract these ROIs are the MNI, JHU and Talairach, all included in FSL. From the set of orthogonal diffusion measures obtained through DTI, we just consider the FA and MD, as they are the most extended ones in the neuroimaging literature [4]. Any linear correlation of these measures with the age and/or gender is regressed out before computing the FV descriptors.

The algorithm implemented for dividing the ROIs tries to bound the size of each subROI between some minimum and maximum number of voxels, whenever possible. After testing different configurations, a size from 48 to 64 voxels has been chosen. This range results in a good trade-off between having enough samples to conveniently approximate the data distribution of each subROI, and enough subROIs for encoding in detail the regional information of each ROI. Then, once obtained $\mathbf{X}_\ell^r$ for all subjects and subROIs, instead of jointly considering the FA and MD, we fit a GMM for each measure in order to provide independent scores, showing the different sensibility of each ROI to the brain alterations caused by the disease. The number of components K for the GMM is set to 6, which allows to precisely fit the data distribution without excessively increasing the model complexity.

To show the performance of the proposed methodology, we compare it against an approach that directly uses the diffusion measures as inputs to a linear or an SVM-RBF classifier. For each of these schemes, we adjust separately the regularization parameter. We perform 100 experiments of 10-fold cross-validation to obtain an average accuracy score. A mean prediction is also obtained for each ROI by averaging the results of each experiment, which are then use to obtain a combined score for each subject. As we can observe in Table 1, when comparing separately each of the ROIs, the proposed methodology allows to moderately enhance the accuracy of the classifier, and remarkably in the case of the *putamen*, brain region critically involved in the disease. However, sometimes the methodology is not able to correctly capture the distribution of the data through the FV descriptor, reducing its informativeness, as with the *gyrus rectus*, which performs better in the traditional schemes. But in general, the individual scores for all the ROIs are better than those provided by the other schemes, slight improvements that are crucial when computing the combined score. For the case of the accuracy score for all the ROIs, the proposed methodology also outperform standard approaches, but with a decrease on the performance.

Table 1. Rate of correct classification for the different experiments performed.

	FA and MD			FA			MD		
Input Data	FV Desc.	Diff. Feat.	Diff. Feat.	FV Desc.	Diff. Feat.	Diff. Feat.	FV Desc.	Diff. Feat.	Diff. Feat.
Classifier	Log. Reg.	Log. Reg.	SVM-RBF	Log. Reg.	Log. Reg.	SVM-RBF	Log. Reg.	Log. Reg.	SVM-RBF
Internal Caps.	**63.98%**	56.26%	61.08%	**64.06%**	62.19%	60.98%	**61.16%**	55.34%	60.72%
External Caps.	**63.41%**	60.13%	61.15%	**67.30%**	51.24%	61.18%	63.15%	**65.42%**	60.78%
Middle Cer. Pend.	57.78%	57.11%	**61.20%**	52.74%	55.67%	**61.50%**	54.87%	48.04%	**61.13%**
Gyrus rectus	50.63%	60.49%	**61.62%**	52.30%	**68.61%**	61.51%	50.36%	59.01%	**61.52%**
Caudate	**61.96%**	56.66%	61.46%	**64.17%**	52.61%	60.74%	54.04%	50.13%	**61.54%**
Dentate	**65.36%**	56.26%	61.66%	58.65%	58.13%	**60.90%**	59.02%	50.42%	**61.74%**
Putamen	**77.18%**	63.45%	60.76%	**74.91%**	51.32%	60.40%	60.01%	**63.53%**	60.95%
Combined score	**77%**	66%	60%	**74%**	64%	69%	**65%**	61%	61%
All ROIs	**70.34%**	59.58%	60.66%	**72.90%**	61.58%	61.06%	**62.24%**	58.00%	59.84%

4   Discussion and Future Work

In the present paper we have proposed a novel pipeline for the diagnosis of PD through dMRI data. By using the FV algorithm, we accurately encode the regional information of the diffusion measures extracted, obtaining a more amenable descriptor for the classifier, as well as alleviating the problem of dimensionality. We have reported an accuracy of 77%, outperforming equivalent approaches when either considering all the ROIs as inputs to the classifier or each of them separately. Besides, and in contrast to voxel-based morphometry approaches, where the accuracy of the non-linear transformation from the subjects' images to a common template plays a major role, the combination of the registration strategy from the template image to the patient image and the use of high-level FV descriptors allows to reduce the influence of the non-linear registration accuracy on the outcome. Furthermore, despite we have focused on the problem of PD diagnosis through dMRI, we can equally apply the current pipeline for the diagnosis of other diseases, as well as make use of other imaging modalities. In these other cases, due to the general nature of our approach, it can be expected that the proposed methodology will outperform more naive approaches, specially considering the higher sensibility other modalities may have to the alterations caused by the disease.

Whilst there is room for improvements in our methodology, for example in the way of combining the individual ROI classification results to obtain a single score, or in tuning parameters, we were able to demonstrate the validity of using high-level description techniques for the classification of neuroimaging data. Future work will tackle these potential weaknesses by, for example: considering more involved approaches for the combination of the class probabilities in order to provide a better prediction; exploring the advantages of using a single GMM for all the extracted features; and defining optimal methods to select the number of GMM components. Together with all these potential improvements, we will lead then to a more robust and generalisable diagnostic methodology.

Acknowledgements. Supported by the Fonds National de la Recherche, Lux-embourg, and cofunded by the Marie Curie Actions of the European

Commission (FP7-COFUND) (9169303), and (6538106). PPMI -a public-private partnership- is funded by the Michael J. Fox Foundation for Parkinsons Research and funding partners, including Abbott, Avid, Biogen Idec, Bristol-Myers Squibb, Covance, Elan, GE Healthcare, Genentech, GlaxoSmithKline, Lilly, Merck, MesoScaleDiscovery, Pfizer, Roche, Piramal, AbbVie, and UCB.

References

1. Ashburner, J., Friston, K.J.: Voxel-based morphometry–the methods. NeuroImage 11(6 Pt 1), 805–821 (2000)
2. Avants, B.B., Epstein, C.L., Grossman, M., Gee, J.C.: Symmetric diffeomorphic image registration with cross-correlation: evaluating automated labeling of elderly and neurodegenerative brain. Medical Image Analysis 12(1), 26–41 (2008)
3. Chang, C.C., Lin, C.J.: LIBSVM: A library for support vector machines. ACM Transactions on Intelligent Systems and Technology 2, 27:1–27:27 (2011)
4. Cochrane, C.J., Ebmeier, K.P.: Diffusion tensor imaging in parkinsonian syndromes: a systematic review and meta-analysis. Neurology 80(9), 857–864 (2013)
5. Dempster, A.P., Laird, N.M., Rubin, D.B.: Maximum likelihood from incomplete data via the EM algorithm. Journal of the Royal Society, Series B 39(1), 1–38 (1977)
6. Fan, R.E., Chang, K.W., Hsieh, C.J., Wang, X.R., Lin, C.J.: LIBLINEAR: A library for large linear classification. The Journal of Machine Learning Research 9, 1871–1874 (2008)
7. Fonov, V., Evans, A., McKinstry, R., Almli, C., Collins, D.: Unbiased nonlinear average age-appropriate brain templates from birth to adulthood. NeuroImage 47(S1), S102 (2009)
8. Jaakkola, T.S., Haussler, D.: Exploiting generative models in discriminative classifiers. In: Proc. of the 1998 Conf. on Advances in Neural Information Processing Systems II, pp. 487–493. MIT Press, Cambridge (1999)
9. Jenkinson, M., Beckmann, C.F., Behrens, T.E., Woolrich, M.W., Smith, S.M.: FSL. Neuroimage 62(2), 782–790 (2012)
10. Long, D., Wang, J., Xuan, M., Gu, Q., Xu, X., Kong, D., Zhang, M.: Automatic classification of early Parkinson's disease with multi-modal MR imaging. PLOS ONE 7(11), e47714 (2012)
11. Orrù, G., Pettersson-Yeo, W., Marquand, A.F., Sartori, G., Mechelli, A.: Using support vector machine to identify imaging biomarkers of neurological and psychiatric disease: a critical review. Neuroscience & Biobehavioral Reviews 36(4), 1140–1152 (2012)
12. Parkinson Progression Marker Initiative: The Parkinson Progression Marker Initiative (PPMI). Progress in Neurobiology 95(4), 629–635 (2011)
13. Salvatore, C., Cerasa, A., Castiglioni, I., Gallivanone, F., Augimeri, A., Lopez, M., Arabia, G., Morelli, M., Gilardi, M.C., Quattrone, A.: Machine learning on brain MRI data for differential diagnosis of Parkinson's disease and progressive supranuclear palsy. Journal of Neuroscience Methods 222, 230–237 (2014)
14. Sánchez, J., Perronnin, F., Mensink, T., Verbeek, J.: Image classification with the Fisher vector: Theory and practice. International Journal of Computer Vision 105(3), 222–245 (2013)
15. Titterington, D., Smith, A., Makov, U.: Statistical Analysis of Finite Mixture Distributions. John Wiley (1985)

Automated Shape and Texture Analysis for Detection of Osteoarthritis from Radiographs of the Knee

Jessie Thomson[1,2], Terence O'Neill[2,3], David Felson[2,3,4], and Tim Cootes[1]

[1] Centre for Imaging Sciences, University of Manchester, UK
[2] NIHR Manchester Musculoskeletal BRU, Central Manchester NHS Foundation Trust, MAHSC, UK
[3] Arthritis Research UK Centre for Epidemiology, University of Manchester, UK
[4] Boston University, Boston, Massachusetts, USA

Abstract. Osteoarthritis (OA) is considered to be one of the leading causes of disability, however clinical detection relies heavily on subjective experience to condense the continuous features into discrete grades. We present a fully automated method to standardise the measurement of OA features in the knee used to diagnose disease grade. Our approach combines features derived from both bone shape (obtained from an automated bone segmentation system) and image texture in the tibia. A simple weighted sum of the outputs of two Random Forest classifiers (one trained on shape features, the other on texture features) is sufficient to improve performance over either method on its own. We also demonstrate that Random Forests trained on simple pixel ratio features are as effective as the best previously reported texture measures on this task. We demonstrate the performance of the system on 500 knee radiographs from the OAI study.

Keywords: Computer-aided diagnosis, Quantitative Image Analysis, X-ray Imaging, Imaging Biomarkers, Computer Vision.

1 Introduction

Osteoarthritis is considered to be one of the leading causes of disability today. It is a degenerative disease that effects the entire joint, degrading articular cartilage and deforming the surrounding bones and tissue of the affected joint. The disease is associated with pain, disability and substantial care costs each year [1]. Experienced clinicians currently perform the clinical grading of x-ray images. However, the features involved in OA are continuous, so the classification into the distinctive grades (normal, doubtful, minimal, moderate and severe) is often left to the subjective opinion of the grader. This quantisation and the uncertainties in assigning a grade make it hard to detect changes. Clinical trials thus require large numbers of subjects to identify effects of interventions reliably. There is a need for automated methods to make measurements and classifications to remove subjectivity. Work in the area of OA classification on radiographs is still limited.

© Springer International Publishing Switzerland 2015
N. Navab et al. (Eds.): MICCAI 2015, Part II, LNCS 9350, pp. 127–134, 2015.
DOI: 10.1007/978-3-319-24571-3_16

The most significant approaches [2] and [4] include analysing textural information across the joint using image processing techniques. These methods look at
the texture across the overall joint, with implicit shape information gathered
from the radiographic images. However, from the pathophysiological properties
of the progression of the disease, it is apparent that both shape and texture are
useful for describing OA.

Recent work has shown quantification of the changes in texture and shape
of Osteoarthritic knees. For instance [13] examines the correlation found between the Trabecular Bone fractal signature, seen in the texture under the tibial
plateaus and the progression of OA [11]. [12] use statistical shape models to
quantify changes in shape.

We describe a fully automated system which accurately identifies the outlines
of the bones of the knee joint and combines both shape and texture features
to better identify signs of disease. We use a Random Forest Regression Voting
Constrained Local Model (RFCLM) (described comprehensively in [8]) to detect
the position of the bones and to accurately locate a set of key landmarks across
the tibia and femur. As well as giving a way of quantifying the shape of the bones
this also allows us to define a consistent region of interest in the tibia in which
to perform texture analysis. We train separate classifiers to distinguish between
OA and non-OA, and demonstrate that a combination of the two independent
measures leads to better overall discrimination.

2 Background

2.1 Fractal Signature

We use a method similar to that in [13]. This creates a set of features based on
mean absolute pixel differences. The pixels are sampled using a circular region
R_{xy}, where all pixels are compared against the central pixel (x, y). All pixels
must lie at a Euclidean distance d_j between $4 \leq d_j \leq 16$ pixels (to reduce
artefact errors). For each new pixel $(x_{ij}, y_{ij}) \in R_{xy}$, where $(x_{ij}, y_{ij}) \neq (x, y)$
and $i = 1, 2, ..., N_\theta$, $j = 1, 2, ..., N_d$, the absolute intensity difference is calculated
$abs(I(x_{ij}, y_{ij}) - I(x, y))$, see Fig. (1), where N_θ is the number of angles considered
and N_d is the max distance along the direction θ. These intensity differences are
stored in a table $R(\theta, d)$ with θ corresponding to the direction, and d the distance.
This is applied to each image patch over the region of interest. The differences at
each direction and distance are summed and a mean calculated of the absolute
differences across the texture region. This gives a representation of the texture
changes at different angles across the region, a property found to be correlated
to the progression of OA [11].

2.2 Statistical Shape Model

A linear statistical shape model [6] is learned from a set of aligned shapes by
applying principal component analysis, leading to a model with the form

$$x = \hat{x} + Pb \tag{1}$$

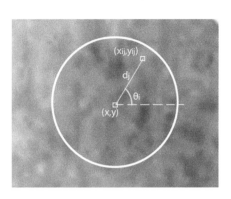 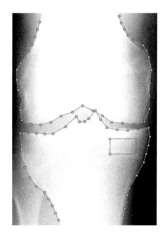

Fig. 1. Example of the circular region sampling to calculate Fractal Signature (left). Example of the 74 landmark points and 4 points computed from them outlining the ROI used for evaluating tibial texture (right).

where x is a vector representing the shape in a reference frame, $\hat{x}$ is the mean shape, P is the set of eigenvectors corresponding to the t highest eigenvalues, which describe different modes of variation, and b is a set of parameter values.

3   Method

3.1   Data

We use radiographic images from the OsteoArthritis Initiative [5], a longitudinal, prospective study of knee OA in the USA. The cohort has a collection of data from 4796 participants (men and women ages 45-79) taking scans annually across 8 years. The images have all been independently graded with Kellgren-Lawrence (KL) [7] grades 0 to 4, indicating the disease groups: normal, doubtful, minimal, moderate and severe. For the purpose of this study the grades have been split to distinguish either OA or non-OA. The non-OA class contains KL 0 and KL 1, whilst the OA class contains KL grades 2, 3 and 4. This distinction has been used in other OA classification studies, where KL1 is considered non-OA due to the features often described as doubtful. 500 AP knee images were selected from the cohort, based solely on the KL and Joint Space Narrowing (JSN) scores. The number of images within each grade are: KL0 - 110 (22%), KL1 - 142 (28.2%), KL2 - 87 (17.4%), KL3 - 118 (23.6%), KL4 - 43 (8.6%).

Knee Annotations: Each of the knees was annotated with 74 landmark points (Fig. 1). These annotations were then used to train a statistical shape model and an RFCLM object detection algorithm. The data was randomly split into two sets, one for training, one for evaluation. The manual annotations also provided an initial estimate of the OA classification performance to optimise training and analysis parameters.

3.2   Shape Model Matching

Using the set of 500 images a RFCLM model was trained and tested on halves of the data, producing shape model points on the test sets to use in the fully automated analysis. The RFCLM construction follows a similar process to that in [9], with a single global model to find the initial 2 points central to the joint, and 4 local RFCLM models built to iterate through increasing resolutions of the image, fitting the points to the best location at each stage. The accuracy of the algorithm was tested by comparing the detected point locations against the gold standard of the manually annotated points.

3.3   Classification Using Texture Information

The texture in regions of the tibia is known to change in knees with OA. We thus train two different classifiers to distinguish between the texture in knees with signs of OA and those without. As features we either use the data used to calculate fractal signature, or simple pixel ratios.

Region Selection: The region was defined under the medial tibial plateau. The analysis can be performed using both sides, however, to remove confounding effects from the fibula and due to the typically high prevalence of medial OA, only the side shown was analysed. This region was selected using two of the landmark points described in Sec. (3.1) along the sides of the tibia as guide points. Projecting a vector between the points a reference frame relative to the orientation, location and scale of the bone object can be made. From this the four points to make up the rectangle of the ROI can be found relative to the reference frame (see Fig. 1). The region within this rectangle is analysed to compute two different texture measures.

Fractal Signature: Using the method described in Sec. (2.1), we then made a slight alteration to the original method - collecting pixels outside of the set directions. For each pixel pair, the angle is rounded to the nearest fraction of the search region i.e. if 24 directions wanted; each angle is rounded to the nearest multiple of 15°. This is to collect an average of pixel differences across a wider section of each search region. Due to time constraints in computation, the data used to originally compute Fractal Dimensions was omitted, instead all the data was used to train the Random Forest. The pixel samples were gathered from a region under the medial tibial plateau similar to that used in previous studies [11] and [13] that quantified fractal signatures of tibial texture.

Simple Pixel Features: As an alternative measure of texture we trained a Random Forest using pixel ratios as features in 32x32 pixel patches. For each image we randomly sampled 670 patches from the region on the tibia described above. A random forest was trained in which the decision at each node is a threshold on the ratio between intensities at two pixels from the patch. In this case when testing on new images we again extract 670 random 32x32 patches. We then compute the classifier response as the average of the RF response on each individual patch.

3.4 Shape Information

A Statistical Shape Model (described in section 2.2) was trained on a 74 point shape model, with 37 points per bone (tibia and femur). The shape model had 19 modes, sufficient to explain 90% of the variation in the training set. The shape parameter vectors, corresponding to b in Eq.(1), were then used to train a Random Forest classifier.

4 Results

4.1 Accuracy of Automatic Segmentation

We used two-fold cross validation (training on half the data, testing on the other half then swapping the sets) on 500 annotated images to evaluate the accuracy of the RFCLM when detecting the outline of the femur and tibia. Following [14] the mean point-to-curve distance was recorded as a percentage of a reference width across the tibial plateau, then converted to mm by assuming a mean width of 75mm. Results were: mean: 0.39% (0.29mm)±0.14mm, median: 0.34% (0.26mm) and 95th percentile: 0.72% (0.54mm). These results are similar to those presented by [14], though on a different dataset.

4.2 Classification Experiments

To test the accuracy of each of the features, Random Forest [10] classifiers were trained on even splits of the 500 x-ray images taken from the OAI data. This classification was trained and tested on the clinically given KL grades, described in Sec. (3.1). The 500 images contained 244 OA and 256 non-OA. When split in half (250 train, 250 test images) the split to OA / non-OA was 120 /129 training, 127 / 122 testing.

4.3 Fractal Signature and Pixel Ratio Features

Fig. (2) shows the classification performance of the two texture based methods as ROC curves. Both methods have similar Area Under the Curve (AUC), with 0.74 for the Fractal Signature method and 0.75 for the pixel ratios. This suggests that the Random Forest is able to learn relevant features directly from the pixel ratios, avoiding the need to calculate more complex fractal texture signature. In the following we use the RF trained on pixel ratios to analyse the texture information.

Table 1. The AUC for each multi-feature analysis.

	Area Under ROC	
Analysis Method	Manual	Automated
Texture	0.745	0.754
Shape	0.796	0.789
Combined	0.844	0.845

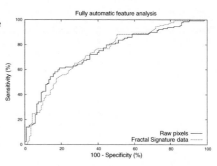

Fig. 2. The ROC curves for raw pixel ratio and Fractal Signature analysis.

4.4 Comparing Shape and Texture

Experiments were performed to compare the classifiers using (i) shape information, (ii) texture information (iii) both shape and texture.

Experiments were performed twice, once using the manually annotated landmark points (which define the shape and the region of interest for the texture analysis) and once using the results of the automated search (points for each image were generated by searching with a model trained on a different half of the data). The evaluation of each classifier was done by computing an ROC curve on the original train/test split, computing the AUC for each, and then finally an overall measure of accuracy was taken by using 5-fold cross-validation, repeated twice over all 500 images. The results for each stage can be seen in Table (1).

The two Random Forests trained independently on the separate features were then combined, with varying weights of the classification. The data was trained on two separate classifiers to allow more flexibility in the weight of classification from each model, and also to allow multiple texture samples per each image to be analysed. The optimal weighted combination of the two classifiers was found to be weighting by 2:1 in favour of the shape classification score, showing an

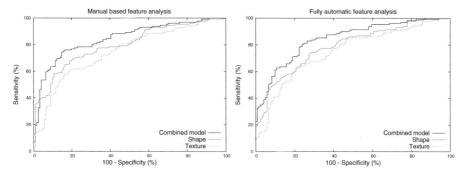

Fig. 3. ROC curves of classifiers using points from manual annotation (left), and fully automated approach (right)

accuracy of 0.84 in the fully automated annotations. The manual based and fully automated results for the 250/250 split in the data can be seen in Fig. (3).

5   Discussion and Conclusion

The experiments show that combining the results of the shape and texture based classifiers leads to a considerable improvement in overall classification performance, with an AUC of 0.849 compared to 0.789 for shape alone in the automated case.

The fully automatic system works as well as that based on manual annotation of the landmarks, due to the robustness and accuracy of the RFCLM matching algorithm. These results show that the combination of independently measured features of texture and shape create a stronger classifier when distinguishing Osteoarthritic knees. This study also looked at the classification comparison between Random Forests using the popular Fractal Signature and simple ratios pixel features. There is very little difference between the two when comparing AUC, suggesting that during training the Random Forest is learning appropriate combinations of pixel pairs to capture information encoded in the fractal signature in a different way.

Shamir *et al.* [2] reported obtaining classification rates of 86.1% distinguishing between OA and non-OA on a set of 350 images. They also distribute their OA classification software online (WND-CHARM). This algorithm was tested on the current dataset, achieving an AUC of 0.82, which is marginally less than our combined model. [3] focuses on using medial tibial texture to detect OA from a set of 102 images, also reporting a higher classification accuracy in comparison to WND-CHARM. Their model obtained a classification accuracy of 77.1%, which is higher than WND-CHARM (64.2%) and our own texture classification (69.2%). However, this was tested on a different dataset to that which we use.

In this paper we have focused on simple diagnosis (OA vs non-OA). In future work we will expand the classification to distinguish between separate KL grades, to determine the accuracy across each of the Osteoarthritic groups. The shape features were found to mainly separate the classes using the size of the joint space, in future work we will expand our method to analyse Osteophytes and bone remodelling. We will also investigate the effects of expanding the texture analysis to take more textural information from the images, from both the lateral tibial plateau, as well as sections of the femur, to determine whether including more information across both bones will increase the overall accuracy. Finally a regressor will be trained to give a continuous score (rather than a discrete value) to quantify the severity of disease. Since the process is completely automatic, it will be possible to apply the system to very large databases of images. We will examine the correlation between the results of our system and other clinical symptoms, and study how the response changes at different time-points as the disease progresses.

Acknowledgements. This report includes independent research funded by the National Institute for Health Research Biomedical Research Unit Funding Scheme. The views expressed in this publication are those of the author(s) and not necessarily those of the NHS, the NIHR or the Department of Health.

References

1. Chen, A., Gupte, C., Akhtar, K., Smith, P., Cobb, J.: The global economic cost of Osteoarthritis: How the UK compares. Arthritis, vol. 2012 (2012)
2. Shamir, L., Ling, S.M., Scott, W.W., Bos, A., Orlov, N.: Knee X-ray image analysis method for automated detection of Osteoarthritis. IEEE Trans. Biomed. Eng. 56(2), 407–415 (2009)
3. Woloszynski, T., Podsiadlo, P., Stachowiak, G.W., Kurzynski, M.: A signature dissimilarity measure for trabecular bone texture in knee radiographs. Med. Phys. 37(5), 2030–2042 (2010)
4. Anifah, L., Purnama, I.K.E., Hariadi, M., Purnomo, M.H.: Osteoarthritis classification using self organizing map based on gabor kernel and contrast-limited adaptive histogram equalization. Open Biomed. Eng. J. 7, 18–28 (2013)
5. Lester, G.: Clinical research in OA. The NIH Osteoarthritis Initiative. J. Musculoskelet. Neuronal. Interact. 8(4), 313–314 (2008)
6. Cootes, T.F., Taylor, C.J.: Statistical Models of Appearance for Computer Vision. Technical report, University of Manchester (2004)
7. Kellgren, J.H., Lawrence, J.S.: Radiological assessment of Osteo-Arthrosis. Annals of the Rheumatic Diseases 16(4), 494–502 (1957)
8. Cootes, T.F., Ionita, M.C., Lindner, C., Sauer, P.: Robust and accurate shape model fitting using random forest regression voting. In: Fitzgibbon, A., Lazebnik, S., Perona, P., Sato, Y., Schmid, C. (eds.) ECCV 2012, Part VII. LNCS, vol. 7578, pp. 278–291. Springer, Heidelberg (2012)
9. Lindner, C., Wilkinson, J.M., Consortium, T.A., Wallis, G.A., Cootes, T.F.: Fully automatic segmentation of the proximal femur using random forest regression voting. IEEE Trans. on Med. Imaging 32(8), 1462–1472 (2013)
10. Breiman, L.: Random Forests. Machine Learning 45(1), 5–32 (2001)
11. Podsiadlo, P., Stachowiak, G.W.: Analysis of shape wear particles found in synovial joints. J. Orthop. Rheumatol. 8, 155–160 (1995)
12. Lee, H., Lee, J., Lin, M. C., Wu, C., Sun, Y.: Automatic assessment of knee Osteoarthritis parameters from two-dimensional X-ray images. In: First International Conference on ICICIC 2006, vol. 2, pp. 673–676 (2006)
13. Wolski, M., Podsiadlo, P., Stachowiak, G. W.: Directional fractal signature analysis of trabecular bone: Evaluation of different methods to detect early Osteoarthritis in knee radiographs. In: Proc. IMechE, vol. 223(2), Part H: J. Eng. Med. pp. 211–236 (2009)
14. Lindner, C., Thiagarajah, S., Wilkinson, J.M., arcOGEN Consortium, Wallis, G.A., Cootes, T.F.: Accurate bone segmentation in 2D radiographs using fully automatic shape model matching based on regression-voting. In: Mori, K., Sakuma, I., Sato, Y., Barillot, C., Navab, N. (eds.) MICCAI 2013, Part II. LNCS, vol. 8150, pp. 181–189. Springer, Heidelberg (2013)

Hashing Forests for Morphological Search and Retrieval in Neuroscientific Image Databases

Sepideh Mesbah[1,2,*], Sailesh Conjeti[1,*], Ajayrama Kumaraswamy[3],
Philipp Rautenberg[2,3], Nassir Navab[1,4], and Amin Katouzian[1]

[1] Computer Aided Medical Procedures, Technische Universität München, Germany
[2] Max Plank Digital Library, München, Germany
[3] Computational Neuroscience, Ludwigs Maximillian Universität München, Germany
[4] Computer Aided Medical Procedures, Johns Hopkins University, USA

Abstract. In this paper, for the first time, we propose a data-driven
search and retrieval (hashing) technique for large neuron image databases.
The presented method is established upon hashing forests, where multiple unsupervised random trees are used to encode neurons by parsing the
neuromorphological feature space into balanced subspaces. We introduce
an inverse coding formulation for retrieval of relevant neurons to effectively mitigate the need for pairwise comparisons across the database.
Experimental validations show the superiority of our proposed technique
over the state-of-the art methods, in terms of precision-recall trade off for
a particular code size. This demonstrates the potential of this approach
for effective morphology preserving encoding and retrieval in large neuron databases.

1 Introduction

Neuroscientists often analyze the 3D neuromorphology of neurons to understand
neuronal network connectivity and how neural information is processed for evaluating brain functionality [1, 2]. Of late, there is a deluge of publicly available neuroscientific databases (especially 3D digital reconstructions of neurons),
which consist of heterogeneous multi-institutional neuron collection, acquired
from different species, brain regions, and experimental settings [3, 4]. Finding
relevant neurons within such databases is important for comparative morphological analyses which are used to study age related changes and the relationship
between structure and function [1].

Recently, the concept of the neuromorphological space has been introduced
where each neuron is represented by a set of morphological and topological measures [1]. Authors in [1] used this feature space for multidimensional analysis of
neuronal shape and showed that the cells of the same brain regions, types, or
species tend to cluster together in such a space. This motivated us to leverage
this space for evaluating inter-neuron similarity and propose a data-driven retrieval (hashing) system for large neuron databases. Recently, a neuron search

---

* S. Mesbah and S. Conjeti contributed equally towards the work.

© Springer International Publishing Switzerland 2015
N. Navab et al. (Eds.): MICCAI 2015, Part II, LNCS 9350, pp. 135–143, 2015.
DOI: 10.1007/978-3-319-24571-3_17

algorithm was proposed by [2], where pairwise $3D$ structural alignment was employed to find similar neurons. In another approach, authors in [5] focused on the evaluation of morphological similarities and dissimilarities between groups of neurons deploying clustering technique using expert-labeled metadata (like species, brain region, cell type, and archive). These existing neuronal search and retrieval systems are either too broad (*lacking specificity in search*) or too restrictive (*dependent on exact expert-defined values/meta information*) and thus not suitable for reference-based hashing in large scale neuron databases.

Several efficient encoding and searching approaches have been proposed for large scale retrieval in machine learning and medical image computing, including **(1)** generalized hashing methods like data independent methods (*e.g.* Locality Sensitive Hashing (LSH) [6]), data-driven methods (*e.g.* Spectral Hashing (SH), and Self Taught Hashing (STH) [7, 8]); and **(2)** application-specific methods including composite hashing for histopathological image search [9] and on finding similar coronary angiograms in $2D$ X-ray database [10].

The LSH generates binary encoding by partitioning feature space with randomly generated hyperplanes [6]. Unlike LSH, instead of working on the original feature space, the SH generates hash codes using low dimensional representation obtained using Laplacian Eigenmaps (LEM) [7]. Later, Zhang *et al.* [8] introduced self-learnt hashing functions by median-thresholding the low dimensional embedding from LEM and training a support vector machine (SVM) classifier as the hash function for encoding new input data. Data independent methods like LSH require large code words to efficiently parse the feature space as they rely on their asymptotic nature for convergence [11]. For similar code lengths, SH and STH can provide better retrieval as the hashing function is based on the data distribution. However, these data driven methods are mainly challenged by their restricted scalability in code size and lack of independence of the hashing functions. It has also been observed that increasing code length in such data driven methods may not necessarily improve performance, depending on the data characteristics. Redressing these issues are crucial for fast growing heterogeneous database like neuroscientific databases, where both scalability and sensitivity are important.

In this paper, we propose a data-driven hashing scheme for large neuron databases called hashing forests (HF). These are established upon unsupervised random forests trained to parse the neuromorphological space in a hierarchical fashion. We demonstrate that HF can generate more sensitive code words than LSH, SH or STH by effectively utilizing its tree-structure and ensemble nature. Trees in HF are trained independently and they are more easily scalable to larger code lengths than SH and STH. In comparison to random forest hashing method proposed in [11], we introduce an inverse coding scheme which effectively mitigates database-wide pairwise comparisons, which is better suited for fast large-scale hashing. We formulate tree-traversal path based coding scheme for more efficient hierarchical parsing of the neuromorphological space. Further, to the best of our knowledge, this is the first work that focuses in entirety on hashing in large neuroscientific databases.

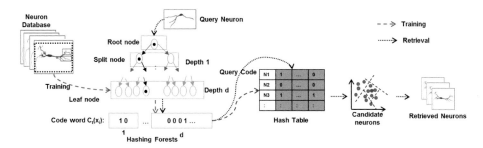

Fig. 1. Schematic of proposed search and retrieval scheme using Hashing Forests.

2   Methodology

Ideally, the hashing method should generate compact, similarity-preserving and easy to compute representations (called *code words*), which can be used for accurate search and fast retrieval [7]. In the context of neuroscientific databases, the desired similarity preserving aspect of the hashing function implies that *morphologically similar neurons are encoded with similar binary codes*. In the neuromorphological space, the normalized Euclidean distance defined between neurons correlates well with the inter-neuron morphological similarity. However, it is not desirable for hashing in large neuron databases owing to high memory expenditure in addition to increased computational time complexity. Consider the neuromorphological feature vector of a neuron n_i, say $\mathbf{x}_i := \{\mathbf{x}_1, .., \mathbf{x}_k, .., \mathbf{x}_n\} \in \mathbb{R}^N$, were N is the space dimensionality. A detailed description of the feature extraction and biological significance is presented in [12]. We model hashing functions through *unsupervised* randomized forest (called hashing forests $\mathcal{H}$) which parse and encode the neuromorphological subspaces in similarity-preserving binary codes. Fig. 1 illustrates the schematic of the overall hashing process, which is discussed in following section.

Training Phase: Hashing forest ($\mathcal{H}$) is an ensemble of binary decision trees which partitions the feature space hierarchically based on learnt binary split functions. A forest of T binary trees with maximum depth of d, requires $(T \times d)$ bits to encode each neuron. Each tree is grown in an *unsupervised* fashion by recursively partitioning the selected feature sub-space (*say into left and right with s_l and s_r samples respectively*) at each node. This is based on a univariate split function (*say ϕ*) which optimizes tree balance by minimizing $\mathcal{E}(\phi)$ ($\mathcal{E}(\phi) = max\{(s_l/s_r) - 1, (s_r/s_l) - 1\}$) [13] . The splitting continues until the maximum defined tree-depth d is reached. The time complexities to grow a tree and ensemble a forest are tabulated in Table 1 (S1-S2).

Hash Table Generation: Given a trained tree (t) of the hashing forest $\mathcal{H}$, each neuron n_i (*characterized by* $\mathbf{x}_i$) in the database is passed through it till it reaches the leaf node. We propose to use the neuron's traversal path to generate the tree-specific code word $C_t(\mathbf{x}_i)$, instead of just the leaf indices. For a tree t of depth d, the split and the leaf nodes are assigned breadth-first order indices

Table 1. Time Complexity Analysis

S1	Building tree	$O(\sqrt{N} * M * d)$ [13]	
S2	Building forests	$O(T * \sqrt{N} * M * d)$	Training
S3	Generating hash table	$O(T * d) + O(M * S)$	
S4	Generating Single Query Code	$O(T * d)$	
S5	Retrieving with Forward Code	$O(M * S)$	
S6	Retrieving with Inverse Code	$O(T * d) + O(T * (d - 1))$	Retrieval
S7	Quick sort	$O(M \log M)$	

Symbols: Code word Size $S = T(2^{d+1} - 2)$); Number of Trees T; Number of Features N; Tree Depth d; Retrieval Database Size M.

(say k_t) which are associated with binary bit b_{k_t} in the code word $C_t(\mathbf{x}_i)$. For a particular neuron, if node k_t is part of its path, then b_{k_t} is set to 1, otherwise its set to 0. This leads to a $(2^{d+1} - 2)$ bit sparse code word $C_t(\mathbf{x}_i)$ with (d) ones. It must however be noted that only d bits are required to generate $C_t(\mathbf{x}_i)$ as there are only 2^d possible traversal paths, each leading to a unique leaf node. We repeat the same process for every other tree in the forest to generate the sparse code block $C_{\mathcal{H}}(\mathbf{x}_i)$ of size $(T * (2^{d+1} - 2))$ for each neuron. The time complexity of this step is shown in Table 1 (S3). For faster retrieval, we pre-compute the code blocks for all M neurons in retrieval/training database $\mathcal{D}$ and generate a hash table of size $M \times (T * (2^{d+1} - 2))$. This is stored using $(M * T * d)$ bits along with traversal paths saved in a $(2^d * (2^{d+1} - 2))$ binary look-up table.

Inverse Coding: Each bit b_{k_t} in $C_{\mathcal{H}}$ encodes a unique neuromorphological subspace, which is constrained by the split functions of t leading to node k_t. In order to avoid pair-wise comparisons between the neurons during retrieval in large databases, we formulate an inverse coding scheme. We transpose the hash table to generate the inverted hash table $\mathcal{I}$ which is a sparse $((T*(2^{d+1}-2)) \times M)$ dimensional matrix. This implies that for feature vector $\mathbf{x}_i$, if bit b_{k_t} in $C_t(\mathbf{x}_i)$ is 1, then $\mathcal{I}(k_t, i) = 1$, and it belongs to the feature subspace encoded by b_{k_t}.

Testing Phase: For a given *query* neuron n_q (with feature vector $\mathbf{x}_q$), the corresponding code block $C_{\mathcal{H}}(\mathbf{x}_q)$ is generated in a similar fashion to the Hash Table Generation phase. In the direct retrieval formulation, pairwise comparisons (*through hamming distance*) between $C_{\mathcal{H}}(\mathbf{x}_q)$ and code blocks of neurons (say $C_{\mathcal{H}}(\mathbf{x}_i)$ for neuron n_i) in the retrieval database $\mathcal{D}$ are made to evaluate inter-neuron similarity $\mathcal{S}(n_q, n_i)$ *i.e.*

$$\mathcal{S}(n_q, n_i) = \frac{1}{(T * (2^{d+1} - 2))} \sum_{\forall bits} (C_{\mathcal{H}}(\mathbf{x}_q) == C_{\mathcal{H}}(\mathbf{x}_i)) \tag{1}$$

If n_q generates the same code block as a neuron in $\mathcal{D}$ (*i.e. both belong to the same neuromorphological subspace*), we assign perfect similarity to them ($S = 1$). However, the pairwise comparison for large scale databases is computationally expensive as seen from its time complexity in Table 1 (S5). To mitigate this, in the inverse coding, we formulate the similarity function as $T*(d-1)$ dimensional similarity accumulator cell $\mathcal{A}_{n_q}$. Given the code block $C_{\mathcal{H}}(\mathbf{x}_q)$ for the query neuron n_q, $\mathcal{A}_{n_q}$ is calculated as:

$$\mathcal{A}_{n_q}(i) = \frac{1}{T*(d-1)} \sum_{\forall k_t} \mathcal{I}(k_t, i) \text{ if bit } b_{k_t} \text{ in } C_{\mathcal{H}}(\mathbf{x}_q) = 1 \qquad (2)$$

The inter-neuron similarity $\mathcal{S}(n_q, n_i)$ is related to $\mathcal{A}_{n_q}$ as $\mathcal{S}(n_q, n_i) = \mathcal{A}_{n_q}(i)$. Such an inverse formulation is computationally more efficient for large databases(as seen from the order complexity in Table 1 (S6)), than the forward scheme (Table 1 (S5)). In the task of retrieving an ordered set of K most morphologically similar neurons from $\mathcal{D}$, we dynamically generate a set of candidate neurons (say size of $2K$) from $\mathcal{D}$ by using quick sort on the hashing forest similarity (Table 1 (S7)). We further sort them by using normalized Euclidean distance between the neurons in this set and the *query* neuron for more morphologically consistent ranking. The additional computational expense due to this refinement step is low as $K << M$. (For validation purposes, this refinement using normalized Euclidean distance is performed on all the comparative methods considered in Section 3)

3   Experiments and Observations

Database: We used 18106 publicly available 3D reconstructions of neurons (extracted from [3, 15–23]). We employed Lmeasure toolbox [12] to extract 3D neuromorphological features, which characterize different aspects of neuron structure including whole neuron morphology, bifurcation features, and neuron compartment level features [1]. Successful morphology-preserving hashing in neuroscientific databases depends on the efficacy of the code word to compactly represent this neuromorphological space as well as efficiently compute interneuron similarity using the code word.

Experiment 1: *Effective Neighbourhood Approximation with fixed codesize* We introduce the *Neighbourhood Approximation* (NA) graph which models how close the neighbourhood estimated using code words (*from the hashing method*), approximates the true neighbourhood around a neuron in the neuromorphological space. For a particular hashing method, NA for the jth neighbour is defined as the average of the normalized Euclidean distance between the neurons and retrieved j^{th} neighbour for all neurons in $\mathcal{D}$. Let, for neuron n_i (with feature vector $\mathbf{x}_i^0$), the jth neighbour have a feature vector $\mathbf{x}_i^j$, then NA$(j) =$ $\frac{1}{M}\left(\sum_{i=1}^{M} \varepsilon(\mathbf{x}_i^0, \mathbf{x}_i^j)\right)$ where $\varepsilon(\mathbf{x}_i^0, \mathbf{x}_i^j) = \left(\sqrt{\frac{1}{N}\sum_{a=1}^{N}\frac{(x_{ia}^0 - x_{ia}^j)^2}{s_a}}\right)$. $\varepsilon(\mathbf{x}_i^0, \mathbf{x}_i^j)$ is the

normalized Euclidean distance between $\mathbf{x}_i^0$ and its jth neighbour $\mathbf{x}_i^j$ with a^{th} feature standard deviation s_a estimated over the whole database which is chosen for invariance to scales of different features. We use the NA graph calculated using neighbourhood based on normalized Euclidean distance (NA$_{EUC}$) as the benchmark and the hashing method which performs closest to it is considered as

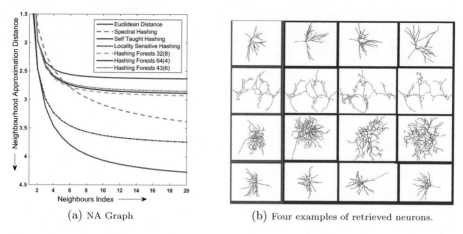

(a) NA Graph   (b) Four examples of retrieved neurons.

Fig. 2. Evaluation of the proposed retrieval system. **Fig. 2a:** Neighborhood Approximation (NA) graph for the comparative methods and configurations of hashing forests for fixed codeword size (256 bits). **Fig. 2b:** For each query neuron on the left (pink), the three best matches are shown on the right (blue). (*High resolution images are provided in the supplementary material.*)

to have the best neighbourhood approximation in comparison. NA graph is evaluated over the target database and the results for all the comparative methods are reported in Fig. 2a. For fair validation, we keep the size of the code-block fixed at 256 bits for this experiment. Further, to examine the sensitivity of HF parameters (number of trees (T) vs. depth (d)) towards neighbourhood approximation, we tested three different configurations varying tree depths: $T = 32$ trees with $d = 8$ ($32 * 8 = 256$ bits); $T = 64$ trees with $d = 4$ ($64 * 4 = 256$ bits); and $T = 43$ trees with $d = 6$ ($43 * 6 = 258$ bits(~ 256 bits))

Observations on Experiment 1: Fig. 2a demonstrates that for a fixed code size, HF approximates neighbourhood better than the comparative LSH, SH and STH methods. Further, analysis of the sensitivity of HF parameters (T vs. d) towards NA, demonstrated that HF with 43 trees and depth 6 performs better than other shallower and deeper tree configurations. Thus, we infer that there exists an optimal depth for a given codesize, where HF optimally parses the neuromorphological space. Fig. 2b demonstrates the performance for 4 distinct neurons with the closest neighbours retrieved using HF and shows close morphological similarity amongst the neurons and the neighbours.

Experiment 2: *Hashing retrieval precision vs. Code block size.* We evaluate the retrieval performance by computing the $F1_{score}$ as follows:

$$F1_{score} = \sqrt{Precision \times Recall} = \sqrt{\frac{|\mathcal{N}_\varepsilon(n_i) \bigcap \mathcal{N}_{\mathcal{H}}(n_i)|^2}{|\mathcal{N}_{\mathcal{H}}(n_i)| \times |\mathcal{N}_\varepsilon(n_i)|}}.$$

This measure is often used in information retrieval algorithms to better understand the tradeoff between precision and recall. The $\mathcal{N}_\varepsilon(n_i)$ represents the set

Table 2. Experiment 2: $F1_{score}$ (in %) vs. Code Size (in *bytes*)

Code Size	Case 10				Case 25			
(*in bytes*)	LSH	SH	STH	HF	LSH	SH	STH	HF
8	6.0	14.0	**16.2**	7.2	5.06	13.03	**14.55**	8.98
16	13.4	23.6	18.6	**37.0**	11.26	22.01	17.46	**39.21**
32	17.8	34.4	19.6	**51.2**	16.32	33.39	17.46	**51.86**
64	27.8	40.4	19.6	**69.2**	26.31	35.92	17.58	**60.59**
128	37.4	26.2	12.4	**79.0**	35.80	22.77	10.12	**63.12**

Note: The best performance for a fixed code size is shown in **boldface**. and the best result amongst all the comparative methods is framed boxed .

of neurons 'relevant' to the query neuron, which is the top K nearest neighbours depined upon the normalized Euclidean distance in the neuromorphological space and $\mathcal{N}_{\mathcal{H}}(n_i)$ represents the retrieved neurons through hashing as a set of k morphologically similar neurons. We measeur the $F1_{score}$ for all comparative methods by varying the codeblock size from 8 bytes to 128 bytes in geometric order of 2. We cmopare the performance for two cases of top 10 and 25 retrieved neurons, as tabulated in Table 2.

Observations on Experiment 2: Table 2 demonstrates the superiority of proposed retrieval technique over comparative methods for both cases (10 NN and 25NN), when sufficient code size was chosen (> 8 bytes). It must be noted that we chose larger code sizes over conventional code sizes (> 16 bytes), as it was observed that precision-recall performances for HF and comparative methods for smaller code sizes were not sufficient enough for the application at hand. HF is able to encode distinct subspaces of the neuromorphological space better due to its hierarchical tree structure. It must also be noted that for larger code sizes, the retrieval performance of both SH and STH significantly decreases (from 64 to 128 bytes), as noisy eigenvectors corresponding to higher eigenvalues are increasingly used in encoding. For comparable performance, LSH needs a large code size to achieve high performance which is computationally expensive (corroborates observations reported by [11]). We also observe that there is no significant improvement in the performance of STH with increasing code size, though it outperforms all methods for small code size (8 bytes). We further infer that increasing code size rather augments HF performance, thus HF is more scalable towards large code sizes than the comparative methods.

4   Conclusions

In this paper, we present hashing forests as an effective approach for accurate retrieval of morphologically similar neurons in large neuroscientific image databases. HF uses unsupervised random forests to extract compact representation of neuron morphological features that enables efficient query, retrieve and analysis of neurons. The use of ensemble of trees and hierarchical tree-structure makes hashing forests more robust to noisy neuromorphological features (observed due to inconsistent 3D digital reconstruction of neuron). Due to independent training, HF is easily scalable to large code sizes as the database size and heterogeneity increases. To the best of our knowledge, this is the first paper to present hashing in neuroscientific databases and demonstrates higher flexibility for reference-based retrieval over existing alternative methods [14]. HF is established to preserve morphological similarity while encoding extracts has better precision and recall *per* bit than the comparative methods. The formulation for HF is generic and it can be easily leveraged for other large-scale reference based retrieval systems. The proposed formulation utilizes inverse coding in HF which helps avoid pairwise comparisons across the database while retrieving, without compromising on retrieval performance.

References

1. Costa, L.D.F., et al.: Unveiling the neuromorphological space. Front. Comput. Neurosci. 4, 150 (2010)
2. Costa, M., et al.: NBLAST: Rapid, sensitive comparison of neuronal structure and construction of neuron family databases. bioRxiv, 006346 (2014)
3. Ascoli, G.A., et al.: NeuroMorpho. Org: a central resource for neuronal morphologies. J. Neurosci. 27(35), 9247–9251 (2007)
4. Rautenberg, P.L., et al.: NeuronDepot: keeping your colleagues in sync by combining modern cloud storage services, the local file system, and simple web applications. Front. Neuroinform. 8, 55 (2014)
5. Polavaram, S., et al.: Statistical analysis and data mining of digital reconstructions of dendritic morphologies. Front. Neuroanat. 8, 138 (2014)
6. Slaney, M., et al.: Locality-sensitive hashing for finding nearest neighbors. IEEE Signal Process. Mag. 25(2), 128–131 (2008)
7. Weiss, Y., et al.: Spectral hashing. In: NIPS, pp. 1753–1760 (2009)
8. Zhang, D., et al.: Self-taught hashing for fast similarity search. In: ACM SIGIR 2010, vol. 33, pp. 18–25 (2010)
9. Zhang, X., et al.: Towards Large-Scale Histopathological Image Analysis: Hashing-Based Image Retrieval. IEEE Trans. Med. Imaging 34(2), 496–506 (2015)
10. Syeda-Mahmood, T., Wang, F., Kumar, R., Beymer, D., Zhang, Y., Lundstrom, R., McNulty, E.: Finding similar 2D X-ray coronary angiograms. In: Ayache, N., Delingette, H., Golland, P., Mori, K. (eds.) MICCAI 2012, Part III. LNCS, vol. 7512, pp. 501–508. Springer, Heidelberg (2012)
11. Yu, G., et al.: Scalable forest hashing for fast similarity search. In: IEEE ICME 2014, pp. 1–6 (2014)
12. Scorcioni, R., et al.: L-Measure: a web-accessible tool for the analysis, comparison and search of digital reconstructions of neuronal morphologies. Nat. Protoc. 3(5), 866–876 (2008), http://cng.gmu.edu:8080/Lm/
13. Moosmann, F., et al.: Fast discriminative visual codebooks using randomized clustering forests. In: NIPS, pp. 985–992 (2007)
14. Neuromorpho, http://neuromorpho.org/neuroMorpho/MorphometrySearch.jsp
15. Neuromorpho Search, http://neuromorpho.org/neuroMorpho/index.jsp

16. Jacobs, B., et al.: Regional dendritic and spine variation in human cerebral cortex: a quantitative golgi study. Cereb. Cortex (2001)
17. Anderson, K., et al.: The morphology of supragranular pyramidal neurons in the human insular cortex: a quantitative Golgi study. Cereb. Cortex 19, 2131–2144 (2009)
18. Kong, J.H., et al.: Diversity of ganglion cells in the mouse retina: unsupervised morphological classification and its limits. J. Comp. Neurol. 489(3), 293–310 (2005)
19. Coombs, J., et al.: Morphological properties of mouse retinal ganglion cells. Neuroscience 140(1), 123–136 (2012)
20. Rodger, J., et al.: Long-term gene therapy causes transgene-specific changes in the morphology of regenerating retinal ganglion cells. PLoS One 7(2), e31061 (2012)
21. Chiang, A.S., et al.: Three-dimensional reconstruction of brain-wide wiring networks in Drosophila at single-cell resolution. Curr. Biol., 1–11 (2011)
22. Jacobs, B., et al.: Neuronal morphology in the African elephant (Loxodonta africana) neocortex. Brain Struct. Funct. 215, 273–298 (2010)
23. Jacobs, B., et al.: Life-span dendritic and spine changes in areas 10 and 18 of human cortex: a quantitative Golgi study. J. Comp. Neurol. 386(4), 661–680 (1997)

Computer-Aided Infarction Identification from Cardiac CT Images: A Biomechanical Approach with SVM[*]

Ken C.L. Wong[1], Michael Tee[1,3], Marcus Chen[2], David A. Bluemke[1],
Ronald M. Summers[1], and Jianhua Yao[1]

[1] Radiology and Imaging Sciences, Clinical Center, NIH, Bethesda, MD, USA
[2] Cardiovascular and Pulmonary Branch, NHLBI, NIH, Bethesda, MD, USA
[3] Institute of Biomedical Engineering, University of Oxford, Oxford, UK

Abstract. Compared with global measurements such as ejection fraction, regional myocardial deformation can better aid detection of cardiac dysfunction. Although tagged and strain-encoded MR images can provide such regional information, they are uncommon in clinical routine. In contrast, cardiac CT images are more common with lower cost, but only provide motion of cardiac boundaries and additional constraints are required to obtain the myocardial strains. To verify the potential of contrast-enhanced CT images on computer-aided infarction identification, we propose a biomechanical approach combined with the support vector machine (SVM). A biomechanical model is used with deformable image registration to estimate 3D myocardial strains from CT images, and the regional strains and CT image intensities are input to the SVM classifier for regional infarction identification. Cross-validations on ten canine image sequences with artificially induced infarctions showed that the normalized radial and first principal strains were the most discriminative features, with respective classification accuracies of $87\pm13\%$ and $84\pm10\%$ when used with the normalized CT image intensity.

1 Introduction

Compared with global cardiac measurements such as wall thickening or ejection fraction, regional myocardial deformation has the potential for early quantification and identification of cardiac dysfunction, especially for myocardial infarction [4]. Cardiac magnetic resonance (MR) imaging techniques such as tagged and strain-encoded imaging are useful in this aspect as they can reveal local myocardial deformation [13], but they are uncommon in clinical routine and relatively expensive. Furthermore, the long breath-hold acquisition time also limits the image quality. In contrast, cardiac computed tomographic (CT) images are more commonly available with lower cost, and a high-resolution image sequence can be produced in just a single heartbeat [8]. However, CT imaging associates with potential radiation risks. Moreover, as CT images can only provide motion of salient features such as the cardiac boundaries, additional constraints are required to estimate the myocardial deformation [13].

Despite the extensive studies of cardiac images in disease diagnosis [4], [9], [6], there are only limited frameworks proposed for computer-aided infarction identification, and most of them are for MR images. In [12], regional 2D myocardial strains and rotation

---

[*] The rights of this work are transferred to the extent transferable according to title 17 § 105 U.S.C.

© Springer International Publishing Switzerland 2015 (outside the US)
N. Navab et al. (Eds.): MICCAI 2015, Part II, LNCS 9350, pp. 144–151, 2015.
DOI: 10.1007/978-3-319-24571-3_18

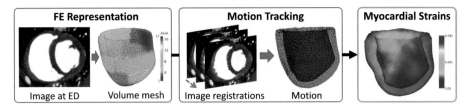

Fig. 1. Biomechanics-based myocardial strain estimation.

angles were estimated from each 2D tagged MR image sequence using nontracking-based estimation. By combining these spatiotemporal measurements into a matrix, a tensor-based linear discriminant analysis framework was proposed to verify whether a heart is normal or diseased. In [11], spatiotemporal measurements of the endocardium and epicardium were extracted from each 2D cine MR image sequence at different ventricular levels using image registration. By using the Shannon's differential entropies of these patterns, a naive Bayes classifier was used to identify regional infarction. To the best of our knowledge, there are currently no computer-aided infarction identification frameworks specifically proposed for CT images.

To study the potential of the clinically more common contrast-enhanced CT images on computer-aided regional infarction identification, we propose a biomechanical approach combined with the support vector machine (SVM) as the classifier. To estimate 3D myocardial strains, displacements of the cardiac boundaries are computed using deformable image registration. By applying these boundary displacements to a finite element (FE) heart representation with hyperelastic and isotropic material properties, the strains are computed by solving the cardiac system dynamics. Apart from strains, CT image intensity which has been shown to be correlated to infarction is also utilized [9]. For regional identification, the left ventricle is divided into 17 zones of the American Heart Association (AHA) nomenclature [1], and the zonal strains and image intensities are input to the SVM classifier. To assess the identification capability, leave-one-subject-out (LOSO) cross-validations were performed on ten canine cardiac image sequences with artificially induced infarctions, and the performances of using different feature combinations were studied.

2   Myocardial Strain Estimation from CT Images

Myocardial strain estimation can be achieved through biomechanics and deformable image registration (Fig. 1). To obtain the FE heart representation, manual segmentation is performed on the end-diastolic image to provide the tetrahedral mesh of the left ventricle which is partitioned into the 17 zones of the AHA nomenclature [1]. With the displacement boundary conditions from image registration, the FE mesh is deformed through the biomechanical model to estimate the myocardial strains.

2.1   Displacement Boundary Conditions by Deformable Image Registration

Image-derived displacement boundary conditions are required to deform the FE mesh. Because of the high image quality of single-heartbeat contrast-enhanced CT images, motion tracking algorithms developed for cine MR images can be adopted [13]. During the initial framework development, the block-matching method which compares local image blocks between consecutive images was used. Without additional constraints, the resulting displacement fields are unsmooth and physically unrealistic deformation may occur, and thus filtering techniques or manual adjustments are required. In consequence, to facilitate clinical applications, B-spline deformable image registration is used instead [10]. This approach provides smooth deformation fields because of the nature of the B-spline interpolation, and its ITK implementation can provide robust inputs to our biomechanics-based strain estimation.

2.2 Biomechanics-Based Myocardial Strain Estimation

As the displacement fields from image registration can only provide useful information of the salient features such as the cardiac boundaries, to estimate the myocardial strains, deformable models are required. Among different algorithms [13], biomechanics-based approaches have shown promising performance because of the physically realistic constraints such as smooth deformation and tissue incompressibility. Although the heart tissue is known to be orthotropic [3], we use the isotropic material property because subject-specific tissue structures are clinically unavailable. Furthermore, the hyperelastic material property is used as it is more realistic for soft tissues which undergo large deformation [3]. For simplicity, we use the modified Saint-Venant-Kirchhoff constitutive law to model the tissue as nearly incompressible and isotropic material [7]:

$$\psi(\epsilon) = \frac{1}{2}\lambda(J-1)^2 + \mu\mathrm{Tr}(\bar{\epsilon}^2) \tag{1}$$

where $J = \det \mathbf{F}$, with $\mathbf{F}$ the deformation gradient tensor. $\bar{\epsilon}$ is the isovolumetric part of the Green-Lagrange strain tensor $\epsilon = \frac{1}{2}(\mathbf{F}^\mathrm{T}\mathbf{F} - \mathbf{I})$. λ and μ are the bulk and shear modulus, respectively. With (1), the second Piola-Kirchhoff stress tensor $(\frac{\partial\psi}{\partial\epsilon})$ and the elasticity tensor $(\frac{\partial^2\psi}{\partial\epsilon^2})$ can be computed, which are embedded to the FE-based total-Lagrangian cardiac system dynamics for the myocardial deformation [14]:

$$\mathbf{M\ddot{U}} + \mathbf{C\dot{U}} + \mathbf{K}\Delta\mathbf{U} = \mathbf{F}_b - \mathbf{F}_t \tag{2}$$

with $\mathbf{M}$, $\mathbf{C}$, and $\mathbf{K}$ the mass, damping, and stiffness matrix, respectively. $\Delta\mathbf{U}$, $\dot{\mathbf{U}}$, and $\ddot{\mathbf{U}}$ contain the nodal incremental displacements, velocities, and accelerations, respectively. $\mathbf{F}_b$ contains the displacement boundary conditions from image registration, and $\mathbf{F}_t$ contains the internal stresses. By solving (2), the nodal displacements and thus strains can be estimated from the image-derived motion. At each node, the three principal strains $(\epsilon_1 > \epsilon_2 > \epsilon_3)$ and the six cylindrical strains with respect to the long-axis of the left ventricle $(\epsilon_{rr}, \epsilon_{\theta\theta}, \epsilon_{zz}, \epsilon_{r\theta}, \epsilon_{rz}, \epsilon_{\theta z}$, with r, θ, and z the radial, circumferential, and longitudinal direction, respectively) are computed for the whole cardiac cycle.

3   Infarction Identification Using SVM

SVM is used to identify infarction from the image-derived features [2]. SVM is a supervised learning algorithm frequently used in medical image analysis because of its

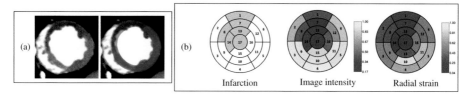

Infarction   Image intensity   Radial strain

Fig. 2. Data example. (a) Short-axis slice and expert-identified infarction in red (zone 7 and 8). (b) Expert-identified infarction, normalized image intensity, and normalized radial strain (ϵ_{rr}) in terms of AHA zones.

accuracy and flexibility in adapting different sources of data. In a binary classification problem, given training feature vectors with known labels, the SVM classifier constructs a hyperplane whose distances to the nearest training vectors of each class are maximized. Experimentally verified features are used, which include myocardial strains and contrast-enhanced CT image intensity.

3.1 Contrast-Enhanced CT Image Intensity

The capability of using contrast-enhanced CT image intensity to depict myocardial infarction has been verified through experiments [9]. To obtain contrast-enhanced CT images, an iodine-based contrast agent which causes greater absorption and scattering of X-ray radiation is injected into the subject, which leads to an increase in CT attenuation and thus contrast enhancement. As infarction reduces myocardial blood supply, hypo-enhancement can be observed (e.g. Fig. 2(a)). The correlation between the hypo-enhanced and infarcted regions was validated through porcine data with postmortem TTC staining [9]. As hypo-enhancement lasts for several cardiac cycles, it can be a robust feature for infarction identification. In our framework, as regional infarction is of interest, the average value of the image intensities at the bottom 10th percentile of each AHA zone at end-diastole is used (Fig. 2(b)). To alleviate the effects of inter-subject variability and to facilitate the accuracy and stability of the SVM classifier, the AHA zonal intensities are normalized (divided) by the largest zonal intensity of each subject.

3.2 Myocardial Strains

The capability of using strains to identify infarction has been verified from animal and human data, with the strain magnitude inversely proportional to the infarction severity [4], [6]. Strains estimated from tagged MR images show their superiority to wall thickening [4], and strains estimated by speckle tracking echocardiography correlate well with the normal and abnormal cardiac functions including infarction [6]. In our framework, the AHA zonal strains estimated by the biomechanical model are used, which are computed as the average nodal strains of the zones. For each strain type (e.g. ϵ_{rr}) in each zone, the zonal strain with the largest magnitude in the whole cardiac cycle is used as a SVM instance. To alleviate the effects of inter-subject variability, for each strain type, the zonal strains are normalized (divided) by the largest zonal strain magnitude among all zones in the whole cardiac cycle of each subject (Fig. 2(b)). The differences between using normalized and unnormalized strains are presented in Section 4.

Table 1. F-scores of normalized and unnormalized features.

	ϵ_{rr}	$\epsilon_{\theta\theta}$	ϵ_{zz}	$\epsilon_{r\theta}$	ϵ_{rz}	$\epsilon_{\theta z}$	ϵ_1	ϵ_2	ϵ_3	Intensity
Normalized	0.79	0.42	0.06	0.00	0.11	0.00	0.59	0.07	0.17	0.48
Unnormalized	0.36	0.37	0.05	0.00	0.13	0.00	0.21	0.05	0.07	0.29

3.3 SVM and Cross-Validations

The SVM C-support vector classification which is less sensitive to outliers is utilized
[2]. We use the linear kernel because it gave similar results as the nonlinear kernels in
our experiments but was more computationally efficient. Grid search is used to select
the optimal regularization parameter C using the training data.

To verify the capabilities of different feature combinations on infarction identification, LOSO cross-validations are used. Let n be the number of subjects. In each test,
the zonal features of $n-1$ subjects are used to train the classifier, which is then used to
classify the zonal infarction of the left-out subject. The average performance can then
be obtained after the n tests. The classification accuracy ($\in [0,1]$) of each LOSO test is
defined as (# of correctly identified zones) / (# of zones). For the inter-rater agreement
between the ground truth and the classification, the Gwet's AC1 coefficient ($\in [-1,1]$),
which has been shown to be more reliable than the Cohen's kappa, is used [5].

Moreover, to measure feature discrimination, a variant of Fisher score is used [2]:

$$\text{F-score} = \frac{\left(\bar{x}^{(+)} - \bar{x}\right)^2 + \left(\bar{x}^{(-)} - \bar{x}\right)^2}{\frac{1}{n_+ - 1}\sum_{i=1}^{n_+}\left(x_i^{(+)} - \bar{x}^{(+)}\right)^2 + \frac{1}{n_- - 1}\sum_{i=1}^{n_-}\left(x_i^{(-)} - \bar{x}^{(-)}\right)^2} \quad (3)$$

with $\bar{x}$, $\bar{x}^{(+)}$, and $\bar{x}^{(-)}$ the average value of the whole, positive-labeled (infarct), and
negative-labeled (normal) instances of a feature, respectively. n_+ and n_- are the numbers of positive and negative instances, and $x_i^{(+)}$ and $x_i^{(-)}$ are the ith positive and negative instances. Therefore, a larger F-score means a more discriminative feature.

4 Experiments

4.1 Experimental Setups

Ten single-heartbeat contrast-enhanced CT image sequences of ten canines with artificially induced myocardial infarctions were acquired by the Toshiba Aquilion ONE CT
system, with the infarctions caused by left anterior descending artery blockages. Each
cardiac cycle (0.52-0.96s) had 20 frames, with voxel size of $0.28 \times 0.28 \times 1.00$ mm^3.
The infarcted regions were identified by experts using dynamic perfusion CT images in
terms of AHA zones, with 110 normal and 60 infarcted zones in total. Different feature
combinations were studied, including using the strains separately (single-strain) or altogether (all-strain), and with or without using normalization and image intensity. As
the control group without infarction was unavailable, the capability of the framework
on discriminating between infarcted and non-infarcted hearts could not be studied.

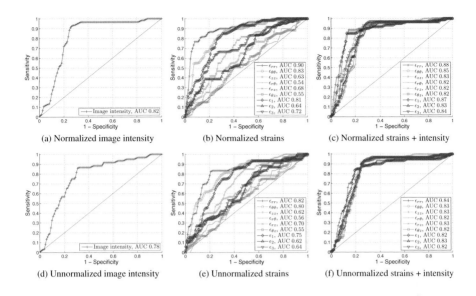

Fig. 3. Single-strain features. Average ROC curves of LOSO cross-validations. Each curve was constructed from the SVM decision values of all tests in a cross-validation. In (c) and (f), only the normalized image intensity was used with the strains.

Table 2. Single-strain features. Results of LOSO cross-validations. For normalized image intensity, accuracy = $81\pm16\%$ and AC1 = $63\pm32\%$. For unnormalized image intensity, accuracy = $74\pm24\%$ and AC1 = $52\pm44\%$. Only the normalized image intensity was used with the strains.

		ϵ_{rr}	$\epsilon_{\theta\theta}$	ϵ_{zz}	$\epsilon_{r\theta}$	ϵ_{rz}	$\epsilon_{\theta z}$	ϵ_1	ϵ_2	ϵ_3
Normalized strains										
Strains	Accuracy (%)	84 ± 11	79 ± 9	66 ± 14	58 ± 15	66 ± 8	56 ± 16	72 ± 15	58 ± 15	71 ± 10
	AC1 (%)	71 ± 20	65 ± 14	40 ± 28	34 ± 30	37 ± 17	30 ± 37	47 ± 30	34 ± 30	45 ± 21
Strains + intensity	Accuracy (%)	87 ± 13	80 ± 14	80 ± 16	80 ± 16	79 ± 17	80 ± 16	84 ± 10	79 ± 18	77 ± 15
	AC1 (%)	75 ± 25	61 ± 28	62 ± 32	62 ± 31	61 ± 32	62 ± 32	69 ± 20	60 ± 33	56 ± 30
Unnormalized strains										
Strains	Accuracy (%)	76 ± 17	75 ± 10	64 ± 11	58 ± 15	65 ± 10	57 ± 15	68 ± 20	58 ± 15	59 ± 14
	AC1 (%)	54 ± 34	57 ± 21	36 ± 22	34 ± 30	33 ± 21	31 ± 35	40 ± 36	34 ± 30	36 ± 29
Strains + intensity	Accuracy (%)	80 ± 20	81 ± 17	80 ± 16	80 ± 16	80 ± 16	79 ± 16	80 ± 20	80 ± 16	79 ± 16
	AC1 (%)	62 ± 38	64 ± 32	62 ± 32	62 ± 31	62 ± 32	61 ± 31	62 ± 37	62 ± 31	61 ± 31

4.2   Results

Table 1 shows the F-scores of the normalized and unnormalized features. The radial (ϵ_{rr}), circumferential ($\epsilon_{\theta\theta}$), and first principal (ϵ_1) strains were more discriminative than the other strains, regardless of normalization. This finding is consistent with the literature [4], [6]. With normalization, the F-scores were improved in general and those of ϵ_{rr} and ϵ_1 were more than doubled. The small F-scores of the shear and longitudinal strains are consistent with the fact that twisting and long-axis motions cannot be properly revealed by CT images. The F-score of the normalized image intensity (0.48)

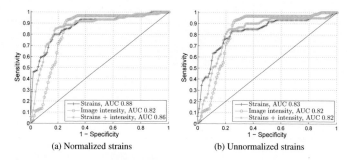

(a) Normalized strains   (b) Unnormalized strains

Fig. 4. All-strain features. Average ROC curves of LOSO cross-validations. Each curve was constructed from the SVM decision values of all tests in a cross-validation. Only the normalized image intensity was used.

Table 3. All-strain features. Results of LOSO cross-validations. For the normalized image intensity, accuracy = 81±16% and AC1 = 63±32%. Only the normalized image intensity was used.

		Normalized strains	Unnormalized strains
Strains	Accuracy (%)	79±10	74±18
	AC1 (%)	61±19	50±34
Strains + intensity	Accuracy (%)	83±12	80±17
	AC1 (%)	67±24	63±32

was larger than the unnormalized one (0.29), and it was also larger than those of the unnormalized strains but comparable to those of the more discriminative normalized strains. These show that the proposed feature normalization in Section 3 for alleviating inter-subject variability can improve the identification performance.

Fig. 3 and Table 2 show the results of using the single-strain features. The classification capabilities were consistent with the F-scores. The capability of the normalized image intensity was better than those of the unnormalized strains as indicated by the area under curve (AUC) (Fig. 3(a) and (e)) and other measures (Table 2). When using the normalized image intensity with the unnormalized strains (Fig. 3(f)), the normalized image intensity was dominant and thus the unnormalized strains were unnecessary. On the other hand, the normalized ϵ_{rr} (Fig. 3(b)) outperformed the normalized image intensity. When combining with the normalized image intensity (Fig. 3(c)), both the normalized ϵ_{rr} and the normalized ϵ_1 outperformed themselves and the normalized image intensity alone, and the performance of the normalized ϵ_1 became similar to that of the normalized ϵ_{rr}. This is an important observation as ϵ_1 is simpler to compute and is more robust without the need to define the long-axis of the left ventricle.

Fig. 4 and Table 3 show the results of using the all-strain features. Similar to the single-strain features, the normalized strains outperformed the unnormalized ones. The combination of the normalized image intensity and the unnormalized strains was similar to using the normalized image intensity alone. The combination of the normalized image intensity and the normalized strains gave the best results, however, its performance (Table 3) was worse than those using the normalized ϵ_{rr} or the normalized ϵ_1 with image intensity (Table 2). These show that the use of all strains is unnecessary.

5   Conclusion

We have presented a biomechanics-based computer-aided framework to identify myocardial infarction from cardiac CT images. Regional CT image intensities and myocardial strains, whose correlations with infarction have been experimentally verified, are used with SVM to achieve promising identification performance. Experimental results showed that the normalized features outperformed the unnormalized ones, and the normalized radial strain and the normalized first principal strain were the most discriminative strain features when combined with the normalized image intensity.

References

1. Cerqueira, M.D., Weissman, N.J., Dilsizian, V., Jacobs, A.K., Kaul, S., Laskey, W.K., Pennell, D.J., Rumberger, J.A., Ryan, T., Verani, M.S.: Standardized myocardial segmentation and nomenclature for tomographic imaging of the heart: a statement for healthcare professionals from the cardiac imaging committee of the Council on Clinical Cardiology of the American Heart Association. Circulation 105(4), 539–542 (2002)
2. Chen, Y.W., Lin, C.J.: Combining SVMs with various feature selection strategies. In: Guyon, I., Nikravesh, M., Gunn, S., Zadeh, L.A. (eds.) Combining SVMs with Various Feature Selection Strategies. STUDFUZZ, vol. 207, pp. 315–324. Springer, Heidelberg (2006)
3. Glass, L., Hunter, P., McCulloch, A. (eds.): Theory of Heart: Biomechanics, Biophysics, and Nonlinear Dynamics of Cardiac Function. Springer (1991)
4. Götte, M.J.W., van Rossum, A.C., Twisk, J.W.R., Kuijer, J.P.A., Tim Marcus, J., Visser, C.A.: Quantification of regional contractile function after infarction: strain analysis superior to wall thickening analysis in discriminating infarct from remote myocardium. Journal of the American College of Cardiology 37(3), 808–817 (2001)
5. Gwet, K.L.: Computing inter-rater reliability and its variance in the presence of high agreement. British Journal of Mathematical and Statistical Psychology 61(1), 29–48 (2008)
6. Hoit, B.D.: Strain and strain rate echocardiography and coronary artery disease. Circulation: Cardiovascular Imaging 4(2), 179–190 (2011)
7. Holzapfel, G.A.: Nonlinear Solid Mechanics: A Continuum Approach for Engineering. John Wiley & Sons, Inc. (2000)
8. Hsiao, E.M., Rybicki, F.J., Steigner, M.: CT coronary angiography: 256-slice and 320-detector row scanners. Current Cardiology Reports 12(1), 68–75 (2010)
9. Mahnken, A.H., Bruners, P., Katoh, M., Wildberger, J.E., Günther, R.W., Buecker, A.: Dynamic multi-section CT imaging in acute myocardial infarction: preliminary animal experience. European Radiology 16(3), 746–752 (2006)
10. Pluim, J.P.W., Maintz, J.B.A., Viergever, M.A.: Mutual-information-based registration of medical images: a survey. IEEE Transactions on Medical Imaging 22(8), 986–1004 (2003)
11. Punithakumar, K., Ayed, I.B., Islam, A., Goela, A., Ross, I.G., Chong, J., Li, S.: Regional heart motion abnormality detection: an information theoretic approach. Medical Image Analysis 17(3), 311–324 (2013)
12. Qian, Z., Liu, Q., Metaxas, D.N., Axel, L.: Identifying regional cardiac abnormalities from myocardial strains using nontracking-based strain estimation and spatio-temporal tensor analysis. IEEE Transactions on Medical Imaging 30(12), 2017–2029 (2011)
13. Wang, H., Amini, A.A.: Cardiac motion and deformation recovery from MRI: a review. IEEE Transactions on Medical Imaging 31(2), 487–503 (2012)
14. Wong, K.C.L., Wang, L., Zhang, H., Liu, H., Shi, P.: Physiological fusion of functional and structural images for cardiac deformation recovery. IEEE Transactions on Medical Imaging 30(4), 990–1000 (2011)

Automatic Graph-Based Localization of Cochlear Implant Electrodes in CT

Jack H. Noble and Benoit M. Dawant

Dept. of Elect. Eng. and Comp. Sci., Vanderbilt University, Nashville, TN, USA

Abstract. Cochlear Implants (CIs) restore hearing using an electrode array that is surgically implanted into the cochlea. Research has indicated there is a link between electrode location within the cochlea and hearing outcomes, however, comprehensive analysis of this phenomenon has not been possible because techniques proposed for locating electrodes only work for specific implant models or are too labor intensive to be applied on large datasets. We present a general and automatic graph-based method for localizing electrode arrays in CTs that is effective for various implant models. It relies on a novel algorithm for finding an optimal path of fixed length in a graph and achieves maximum localization errors that are sub-voxel. These results indicate that our methods could be used on a large scale to study the link between electrode placement and outcome across electrode array types, which could lead to advances that improve hearing outcomes for CI users.

Keywords: cochlear implant, optimal path, graph, segmentation.

1 Introduction

Cochlear implants (CIs) are considered the standard of care treatment for profound hearing loss [1]. CIs use an array of electrodes surgically implanted into the cochlea to directly stimulate the auditory nerve, inducing the sensation of hearing. Although CIs have been remarkably successful, speech recognition ability remains highly variable across CI recipients. Research has indicated there is a strong link between electrode location within the cochlea and hearing outcomes [2-6]. However, comprehensive analysis of this phenomenon has not been possible because precise electrode position has been unknown. Electrode position is generally unknown in surgery because the array is blindly threaded into a small opening of the cochlea. To analyze the relationship between electrode position and outcome, several groups have proposed post-operative imaging techniques. This has included imprecise measures such as ones that can be visually assessed in CT images, e.g., is the array entirely within one internal cavity of the cochlea, the depth of insertion of the last electrode, etc. [2-6]. These studies have concluded that electrode position and outcomes are correlated but are conflicting or inconclusive regarding what specific factors are important because dataset sizes were limited and electrode positions were not precisely determined. Dataset size has been limited due in part to the amount of manual effort that must be undertaken to analyze the images. Another application where precise electrode

© Springer International Publishing Switzerland 2015
N. Navab et al. (Eds.): MICCAI 2015, Part II, LNCS 9350, pp. 152–159, 2015.
DOI: 10.1007/978-3-319-24571-3_19

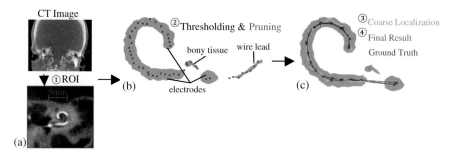

Fig. 1. Process flow chart. The ROI is shown in (a). In (b), example thresholding and pruning results are shown. In (c), coarse and refined electrode localization results are shown with the ground truth.

localization is important is for systems being developed that use electrode position to select better CI processor settings [7]. Such systems have been shown to significantly improve hearing outcomes compared to standard clinical results. In the current work, we propose a fully automatic approach for localizing CI electrodes in CT images. Such an approach could permit localizing electrodes on large numbers of datasets to better analyze the relationship between electrode position and outcome, which may lead to advances in implant design or surgical techniques. It could also automate the electrode localization process in systems designed to determine patient-customized CI settings, such as the one proposed in [7], reducing the technical expertise required to use such technologies and facilitating transition to large scale clinical use.

Figure 1 shows an example of an electrode array in CT. Localizing the electrodes in CT images is difficult because, as seen in figure 1b, finding a threshold to isolate the electrodes is not possible due to the presence of the connecting wires and because adjacent bony tissue voxels are assigned erroneously high intensity in image reconstruction due to beam hardening artifacts caused by the metallic electrodes. Another issue is that there is often no contrast between the electrodes, even when the CTs are acquired at very fine slice thickness and resolution. Where there is no contrast, the challenge is to identify the center of each of the contacts, and where the electrodes are separated, the challenge is to determine how the different groups of contacts are connected. Previous approaches [8,9] require electrodes to be grouped to determine their connectivity and thus are not applicable to many electrode types that have wider contact spacing. Our solution is to simultaneously identify the centers of the electrodes and their connectivity using a novel, graph-based path finding technique. Our approach can handle varying degrees of contrast between electrodes and thus is applicable to many electrode types. Our results, presented and discussed in Sections 3 and 4, will show that this fully automatic approach can reliably be applied to clinical images.

2   Methods

The automatic segmentation method we propose is outlined in Figure 1. As can be seen in the figure, the first step (1) involves coarsely estimating the location of the region of interest (ROI), which is a local region ~30 cm^3 around the cochlea. This is done through registration with a known volume. The subsequent processing steps are then performed solely within the ROI. The next step (2) is to identify a set of points in the ROI representing candidate electrode locations. This is required for the following coarse electrode localization step (3) in which a graph search technique is used to identify points corresponding to electrodes from among those candidates using an intensity and shape-based cost function. Once the electrodes are coarsely localized, the next step (4) is to refine their positions using a subsequent path finding step. The following subsections detail this approach.

2.1   Data

The images in our dataset include images from 20 subjects acquired with a Xoran xCAT®. The images have voxel size 0.4 x 0.4 x 0.4 mm³. Half of the subjects were implanted with Advanced Bionics Mid Scala arrays and the other half with Advanced Bionics 1J arrays. Since the Mid-Scala arrays have little contrast between electrodes in CT due to close electrode spacing (<1 mm) whereas the 1J arrays typically have strong contrast between electrodes in CT due to larger electrode spacing (>1 mm), these two array types are reasonably representative of the types of image contrast variations seen among the many FDA approved array models. Both Mid-Scala and 1J arrays are composed of 16 active contacts and 1 non-stimulating marker contact. The dataset of 20 subjects was subsequently divided into a training and testing set of 10 subjects each. The training and testing sets had equal number of each electrode type. The training set was used for parameter tuning and the algorithm was validated on the testing set with fixed parameters. A ground truth electrode localization solution for each dataset was created by manual localization of the contact positions by an expert. For the testing set, average contact positions from three manual localization sessions were used for ground truth.

2.2   Candidate Selection

After identifying the ROI, the first step in our approach is to select points that represent candidate electrode locations. The following process will select from among these candidates the points that coarsely correspond to the electrodes. To select the candidates, we first create a binary mask by thresholding the image at the intensity corresponding to the top $\alpha_1 = 0.08\%$ of the cumulative histogram of the ROI image. This threshold represents a value that is low enough to ensure no contacts are discarded from the result, which is vital for the success of the following procedures, but not so low that an excessively large volume of non-contact voxels are included in the result, which is also important to prevent the following steps from becoming too complex. An example result of this process is shown in transparent gray in Figure 1b. After thresholding, the set of connected components, each of which corresponds to one or multiple electrodes or background tissue, is voxel thinned by extracting its medial axis [10] to further prune the results. The set of candidate points are chosen as the voxels $\{v\}_1^V$ that compose this set of M medial axes $\{m\}_1^M$. This procedure typically results in $V = \sim 80$ candidate points. Example results of this process where medial axes were extracted from $M=4$ connected components are shown in red in Figure 1b.

2.3   Coarse Electrode Localization

After the candidates are selected, a graph-based procedure is used to localize the electrodes. Each candidate point is treated as a node in a graph, and the path finding algorithm aims to find the sequence of $L=17$ nodes, where L is the number of electrodes,
that obeys node neighbor constraints and minimizes an intensity and shape-based cost
function. The path finding algorithm pseudocode is shown in Algorithm 1. The algorithm begins with a seed node, chosen as discussed below, that represents the position
of the first electrode. Then, the L-1 remaining nodes are determined by growing a tree
of candidate paths $\{p\}$ that stem from the seed node. At each ith iteration in the main
for-loop, in the **Grow** stage, the set of new candidate paths $\{q\}$ of length $i+1$ are
found as the combination of all possible one-node extensions of the set of length i
candidate paths $\{p\}$ to their permissible child nodes $\{c\}$. This potentially large set of
candidate paths $\{q\}$ is then reduced in the **Prune** stage to keep for the next iteration
only the P candidate paths that correspond to the lowest cost. The output of the algorithm is the lowest cost length L path, p_1. While our technique provides no guarantee
of finding a global optimum, the advantage over techniques like Dijkstra's algorithm
[11] is that, as shown below, it permits non-local and shape-based constraints. Shape
constraint is needed because a path composed of electrodes will not generally optimize an intensity-only cost function due to electrode image intensity inhomogeneity.

The child nodes $\{c\}$ of a path p of length i are chosen to be the nodes that obey
reasonable constraints. First, they must obey the hard constraint

$$\frac{1}{\alpha_2} d_i < \|p_i - c\|_2 < \alpha_2 d_i, \tag{1}$$

where d_i is the *a priori* expected distance between electrodes i and $i+1$, which is
specific to the model of the array; and $\alpha_2 = 2.0$. This constraint only permits child
nodes with distance to the candidate path's endnode p_i that falls within bounds of the
expected distance between electrodes. The child nodes must obey further hard constraints that that $c \notin p$, i.e., c is not already in the path; $c \notin \{m\}$ ∀ medial axes m
that do not include p_i but do include any of the points in $\{p\}_1^{i-1}$, which is a constraint that prevents the path from containing disjoint groups of nodes that belong to
the same medial axis m (defined above in Section 2.2), i.e., a medial axis cannot be
revisited by a path; and a final constraint that if $c, p_i, p_{i-1} \in m$, then c is a valid
child node only if $c, p_i,$ and p_{i-1} are monotonically ordered in medial axis m, which
is a constraint that prohibits paths that are following a given medial axis from changing directions on that curve. The underlying assumption forming the basis for last two
medial axis-based constraints is that the ordering of electrodes belonging to the same
medial axis should match their order in the final path.

The cost function for a child node that obeys the above hard constraints is defined
as a combination of intensity and shape-based cost terms,

$$\text{Cost}_1(c, p) = C_I(c, p) + C_S(c, p), \tag{2}$$

where

$$C_I(c, p) = \frac{(I_{\max} - I(c))}{2000} \times \begin{cases} \alpha_3 & i \geq \alpha_4 \\ 1 & \text{else} \end{cases}, \tag{3}$$

Algorithm 1. Path finding algorithm

Input: s = seed node, L = # of nodes in final path, and P = maximum # of candidate paths
Initialize list of candidate paths $\{p\} = \{\{s, \text{Cost}(s)\}\}$
for L-1 iterations
  Grow
    Initialize new list of candidate paths $\{q\} = \{\ \}$
    for each candidate path in $\{p\}$
      Find child nodes of p, $\{c\} = \{n, \text{Cost}(n, p)\}$
      for each node in $\{c\}$
        Add new path to list $\{q\} = \{q\} \mid (p + c)$
      end
    end
  Prune
    Sort candidate paths in $\{q\}$ by increasing path cost
    Update $\{p\} = \{q\}_1^P$
end
Output: p_1

$$C_S(c, p) = \alpha_5 \left(1 - \begin{cases} \text{Cos}(c, p) & \text{Cos}(c, p) < 0.5 \\ 1 & \text{else} \end{cases}\right) + \begin{cases} -\alpha_6 \text{Dst}(c, p) & \text{Dst}(c, p) < 0 \\ \alpha_7 \text{Dst}(c, p) & \text{else} \end{cases}, \quad (4)$$

$$\text{Cos}(c, p) = \frac{(c - p_i) \cdot (p_i - p_{i-1})}{\|c - p_i\| \|p_i - p_{i-1}\|}, \quad \text{Dst}(c, p) = \|c - p_i\|_2 - d_i, \quad (5)$$

I_{max} is the maximum intensity of the ROI image, $I(c)$ is the intensity of the image at c, i is the length of path p, d_i is defined as in Eqn. (1), and α_{3-7} are set to 0.1, 14, 1.0, 5.2, and 2.0 after training. Eqn. (3) assigns lower cost to child nodes that correspond to higher image intensity. The conditional term decreases the importance of image intensity for the last $L + 1 - \alpha_4$ electrodes in the path. This term is included because the last few electrodes are typically less bright in CT because fewer internal wires extend to the end electrodes compared to those at the base. The first term in the shape cost function, Eqn. (4), is a smoothness term that punishes child nodes that would create a bend sharper than $45°$ if added to p. The second term punishes child nodes that are not the expected distance from p_i.

With the cost function and neighbor constraints defined, Algorithm 1 is executed (with $P = 500$) to locate the coarse position of each electrode. Each of the V candidate points in $\{v\}$ (see Section 2.2) could potentially correspond to electrode 1. Thus, we treat each point in $\{v\}$ as a seed node and execute Algorithm 1 V times in parallel, once for each of those seeds. Since the algorithm is pose invariant, there is potential to find low cost paths that are ordered undesirably from end to base. Such paths are detected using the orientation of the cochlea, which is known from the registration with the know volume, and these are discarded from the resulting set of V paths. The final path is then selected from among the remaining paths as the one with minimum cost.

2.4   Electrode Localization Refinement

The above process is able to only coarsely identify electrode location due to imperfect selection of candidate points $\{v\}$ and the fact that the above process does not permit sub-voxel precision. Thus, we use a secondary path finding procedure to refine the resulting coarse path. In this step, a set of nodes are defined by sampling a fine rectangular grid of points around each of the L coarse electrode estimates, $\{l_i\}_{i=1}^L$, as $\{n\}^i = \{l_i + \alpha_8[x, y, z]\}_{x,y,z \in [-\alpha_9, \alpha_9]}$, where $\alpha_8 = 0.12$ mm and $\alpha_9 = 3$. The path finding step aims to refine the estimated position l_i of each ith electrode with one of the nearby candidates $\{n\}^i$. The cost function is defined as

$$\text{Cost}_2(c, p) = -G_\sigma\big(I(c)\big) + \begin{cases} -\alpha_{10}\text{Dst}(c, p) & \text{Dst}(c, p) < 0 \\ \alpha_{11}\text{Dst}(c, p) & \text{else} \end{cases}, \qquad (6)$$

where $G_\sigma\big(I(c)\big)$ is the Gaussian filter response of the image at c with $\sigma = 0.3$ mm, $\text{Dst}(c, p)$ is defined as in Eqn. (5), $\alpha_{10} = 50$, and $\alpha_{11} = 20$. The first term in Eqn. (6) represents a scaled blob finding filter, and the second term applies the same geometric constraints on the spacing of the electrodes used in Section 2.3. The children nodes $\{c\}$ of each node in $\{n\}^i$ are simply defined as the set of all nodes in $\{n\}^{i+1}$. All nodes in $\{n\}^1$ are treated as seed nodes and Algorithm 1 is executed with $P = 500$. The resulting path refines the coarse electrode localization determined above and represents the automatically selected final position of the electrodes.

2.5   Parameter Selection and Validation

Initial values for all parameters were determined heuristically. Then, the parameters were optimized sequentially and iteratively until a solution was found where each parameter is locally optimal with respect to mean electrode localization error in the training dataset. The range around each value was updated when the selected value was changed. Step size was uniform over the range as shown in Fig2bc. The coarse localization step parameters were optimized first, followed by the refinement step parameters. After all parameters were fixed, the method was applied to the testing set and mean and max electrode localization errors were measured to validate the results.

3   Results

Figure 2 shows the results of the parameter tuning procedure. As can been seen in the figure, a local optimum of each parameter was successfully obtained on the training dataset. Several of the parameters in panel (b), $\alpha_2, \alpha_3, \alpha_5$, and P, and several parameters in (c), α_{10}, α_{11}, and P, were relatively insensitive around the minimum and their tuning curves have regions that are nearly flat and have high overlap. Selection of the other parameters was more crucial to obtaining the most accurate results.

Table 1 shows the overall segmentation error results. As shown, on our testing set our method is able to achieve mean electrode localization errors of 0.13 mm for Mid-Scala arrays and 0.09 mm for 1J arrays. These errors are slightly larger than intra-rater variability levels of 0.09 and 0.08 mm for Mid-Scala and 1J arrays. The maximum error in locating any electrode over all ten testing datasets was 0.33 mm. Given that the voxel size of these images is 0.4 x 0.4 x 0.4 mm^3, our worst electrode localization error was sub-voxel. An example Mid-Scala result is shown in Figure 1c.

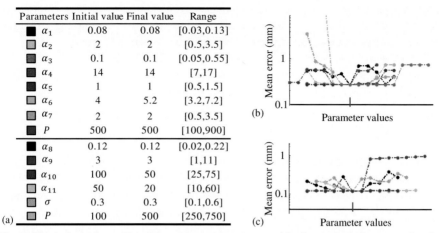

Parameters	Initial value	Final value	Range
■ α_1	0.08	0.08	[0.03,0.13]
□ α_2	2	2	[0.5,3.5]
■ α_3	0.1	0.1	[0.05,0.55]
■ α_4	14	14	[7,17]
■ α_5	1	1	[0.5,1.5]
□ α_6	4	5.2	[3.2,7.2]
□ α_7	2	2	[0.5,3.5]
■ P	500	500	[100,900]
■ α_8	0.12	0.12	[0.02,0.22]
■ α_9	3	3	[1,11]
■ α_{10}	100	50	[25,75]
□ α_{11}	50	20	[10,60]
■ σ	0.3	0.3	[0.1,0.6]
□ P	100	500	[250,750]

Fig. 2. Shown in (a) is a table of the various parameters used in the methods for coarse localization (top group) and refinement (bottom group). (b) and (c) show errors when testing each parameter (color-codes in (a)) over the range specified in (a). The red hash mark indicates the final parameter value.

Table 1. Automatic electrode localization results

Dataset	Array type	Coarse Localization Mean error (mm)	Coarse Localization Max error (mm)	Final Localization Mean error (mm)	Final Localization Max error (mm)
Training	Mid-Scala	0.27	0.67	0.12	0.31
	1J	0.26	0.72	0.12	0.27
Testing	Mid-Scala	0.26	0.72	**0.13**	**0.33**
	1J	0.28	0.62	0.09	0.19

4   Conclusions

In this work, we have proposed a novel and fully automatic cochlear implant electrode localization method. Our experiments show that our method is extremely accurate, even when applied to clinical images. Compared to previous electrode localization techniques that are only applicable to certain electrode models [8,9], the method we propose handles varying electrode array geometries and is generally applicable. Our approach is also fast, requiring only 3-5 seconds of processing time after a ~2 minute registration procedure is used to localize the ROI. The novel path finding algorithm we propose permits shape constraint and could be used for other applications.

Future studies will involve testing our method with images acquired with different scanners and of subjects with different implant models. We also plan to apply our method to large numbers of datasets to facilitate studying how the location of individual electrodes correlates with outcomes with the goal of developing technologies that can improve hearing outcomes with CIs.

Acknowledgements. This research has been supported by NIH grants R01DC014037 and R21DC012620 from the NIDCD. The content is solely the responsibility of the authors and does not necessarily represent the official views of this institute.

References

1. Cochlear Implants, National Institute on Deafness and Other Communication Disorders, No. 11-4798 (2011)
2. Verbist, B.M., Frijns, J.H.M., Geleijns, J., van Buchem, M.A.: Multisection CT as a Valua-ble Tool in the Postoperative Assessment of Cochlear Implant Patients. Am. J. Neuroradiol. 26, 424–429 (2005)
3. Aschendorff, A., Kubalek, R., Turowski, B., Zanella, F., Hochmuth, A., Schumacher, M., Klenzner, T., Laszig, R.: Quality control after cochlear implant surgery by means of rotational tomography. Otol. Neurotol. 26, 34–37 (2005)
4. Skinner, M.W., Holden, T.A., Whiting, B.R., Voie, A.H., Brundsen, B., Neely, G.J., Saxon, E.A., Hullar, T.E., Finley, C.C.: In vivo estimates of the position of advanced bionics electrode arrays in the human cochlea. Annals of Otology, Rhinology and Laryngology Supplement 197, 2–24 (2007)
5. Wanna, G.B., Noble, J.H., McRacken, T.R., Dawant, B.M., Dietrich, M.S., Watkins, L.D., Schuman, T.A., Labadie, R.F.: Assessment of electrode placement and audiologic outcomes in bilateral cochlear implantation. Otol. Neurotol. 32, 428–432 (2011)
6. Wanna, G.B., Noble, J.H., Carlson, M.L., Gifford, R.H., Dietrich, M.S., Haynes, D.S., Dawant, B.M., Labadie, R.F.: Impact of electrode design and surgical approach on scalar location and cochlear implant outcomes. Laryngoscope 124(S6), S1–S7 (2014)
7. Noble, J.H., Labadie, R.F., Gifford, R.H., Dawant, B.M.: Image-guidance enables new methods for customizing cochlear implant stimulation strategies. IEEE Trans. on Neural Systems and Rehabilitiation Engineering 21(5), 820–829 (2013)
8. Noble J.H., Schuman T.A., Wright C.G., Labadie R.F., Dawant B.M.: Automatic Identification of Cochlear Implant Electrode Arrays for Post-Operative Assessment. In: Dawant, B.M. and Haynor, D.R. (eds.) Medical Imaging 2011: Image Processing, Proc. of the SPIE conf. on Med. Imag., vol. 7962, p. 796217 (2011)
9. Zhao, Y., Dawant, B.M., Labadie, R.F., Noble, J.H.: Automatic localization of cochlear implant electrodes in CT. In: Golland, P., Hata, N., Barillot, C., Hornegger, J., Howe, R. (eds.) MICCAI 2014, Part I. LNCS, vol. 8673, pp. 331–338. Springer, Heidelberg (2014)
10. Bouix, S., Siddiqi, K., Tannenbaum, A.: Flux driven automatic centerline extraction. Medical Image Analysis 9, 209–221 (2005)
11. Dijkstra, E.W.: A note on two problems in connexion with graphs. Numerische Mathematik 1, 269–271 (1959)

Towards Non-invasive Image-Based Early Diagnosis of Autism

M. Mostapha[1], M. F. Casanova[2], G. Gimel'farb[3], and A. El-Baz[1,*]

[1] Bioengineering Department, University of Louisville, Louisville, KY, USA
aselba01@louisville.edu
[2] Department of Psychiatry and Behavioral Science, University of Louisville,
Louisville, KY, USA
[3] Department of Computer Science, University of Auckland, Auckland, New Zealand

Abstract. The ultimate goal of this paper is to develop a computer-aided diagnostic (CAD) system for the accurate and early diagnosis of autism spectrum disorders (ASDs) using diffusion tensor imaging (DTI). This CAD system consists of three main steps. First, the brain tissues are segmented based on three image descriptors: a visual appearance model that has the ability to model a large dimensional feature space, a shape model that is adapted during the segmentation process using first- and second-order visual appearance features, and a spatially invariant second-order homogeneity descriptor. Secondly, discriminatory features are extracted from the segmented brains. Cortex shape variability is assessed using shape construction methods, and white matter integrity is further examined through connectivity analysis. Finally, the diagnostic capabilities of these extracted features are investigated. The accuracy of the presented CAD system has been tested on 38 infants with a high risk of developing ASDs. The statistical analysis and the diagnostic results (87% accuracy and AUC of 0.96 using random forest classifier) confirm the high performance and the efficiency of the proposed CAD system.

Keywords: Infant, Tissue segmentation, DTI, Subject-specific atlas.

1 Introduction

Autism spectrum disorders (ASDs) are a group of lifetime developmental disabilities that are defined by significant social, communication, and behavioral challenges. Currently, ASDs denote a significant growing public health concern. According to the report issued by the Centers for Disease Control and Prevention (CDC) in 2014, one in 68 children has been diagnosed with ASDs in the United States, which is approximately 30% greater than previous estimates in 2012 of one in 88 children [1]. Thus, there is an urgent need for a non-invasive technology with the capability of providing new laboratory-based measures that confer an early and accurate diagnosis of ASDs.

Recent molecular and functional connectivity studies indicated that brain connectivity and the underlying white matter tracts might be impaired in patients

---

* Corresponding author.

© Springer International Publishing Switzerland 2015
N. Navab et al. (Eds.): MICCAI 2015, Part II, LNCS 9350, pp. 160–168, 2015.
DOI: 10.1007/978-3-319-24571-3_20

with ASDs, but these studies failed to provide sufficient information about the morphology characteristics of these white matter tracts [2]. On the other hand, structural studies were based on extracting volumetric [3] or shape [4] information from the brain to detect differences between control and autistic patients. However, most of these studies were age sensitive and failed to detect abnormalities in infant brains [5]. Fortunately, the recent advances in diffusion tensor imaging (DTI) has allowed researchers to study, in a noninvasive manner, both the macrostructure and microstructure of white matter tracts of the brain. These new advances have allowed the growth of DTI-based studies investigating ASDs in the last decade [2]. However, developing a noninvasive computer-aided diagnostic (CAD) system for the early detection of ASDs from DTI is still challenging. One of the major existing challenges is the segmentation of anatomical structures such as white matter (WM) and gray matter (GM) regions from infant DTI images. This is due to the fact that most of the current magnetic resonance (MR) infant segmentation techniques are dedicated to segment infant brains either in the early infantile stage (≤ 5 months) or early adult-like stage (≥ 12 months) by using a T1 or T2 scan or the combination of both [6,7]. However, these methods would fail in the case of infants in the isointense stage (6-12 months), which is the primary focus of this paper, because both WM and GM have roughly the same intensity levels [7]. Therefore, segmentation frameworks that integrate DTI image contrasts (e.g., fractional anistropy (FA) maps) would result in a better differentiation between WM and GM in the isointense stage [8,9]. However, none of these frameworks tried to integrate other DTI image contrasts in their segmentation procedure.

To overcome the limitations mentioned above, we propose a new CAD system that integrates both shape and connectivity extracted features in the classification process. Before describing the proposed methods, the basic notation used throughout this paper is presented, $\mathbf{R} = \{(x, y, z) : 0 \leq x \leq X - 1, 0 \leq y \leq Y - 1, 0 \leq z \leq Z - 1\}$ – a finite arithmetic lattice supporting digital images and their region maps, and a voxel $s = (x, y, z)$ is associated with its neighbors, $\{(x+\xi, y+\eta, z+\zeta) : (x+\xi, y+\eta, z+\zeta) \in \mathbf{R}; (\xi, \eta, \zeta) \in \nu_s\}$ where ν_s is the 26-neighbourhood defined by $\xi \in \{-1, 0, 1\}$, $\eta \in \{-1, 0, 1\}$, and $\zeta \in \{-1, 0, 1\}$; $\mathbf{g} = \{g_{x,y,z} : (x, y, z) \in \mathbf{R}; g_{x,y,z} \in \mathbf{Q}\}$ – a gray scale image taking values from a finite set of gray levels $\mathbf{Q} = \{0, 1, \ldots, Q-1\}$; $\mathbf{m} = \{m_{x,y,z} : (x, y, z) \in \mathbf{R}; m_{x,y,z} \in \mathbf{L}\}$ – a region map taking values from from a finite set $\mathbf{L} = \{0, \ldots, L\}$; $\mathbf{A} = \{a_{i,n} : i = 1, \ldots, I, n = 1, \ldots, XYZ; a_{i,n} \in \mathbf{Q}\}$ – a 2D matrix contains image features of all n voxels in a vector form, where i is the dimension size of image features; $\mathbf{W} = \{w_{i,j} : i = 1, \ldots, I, j = 1, \ldots, J; w_{i,j} \in \mathbb{R}^+\}$ – a 2D matrix contains J basis image features; $\mathbf{H} = \{h_{j,n} : j = 1, \ldots, J, n = 1, \ldots, XYZ; h_{i,j} \in \mathbb{R}^+\}$ – a 2D matrix contains n voxels in new feature space of size J.

2 Methods

The proposed CAD system consists of three main steps: *(i)* segmentation of the brain cortex and the WM tracts from DTI, *(ii)* extraction of discriminatory features from the segmented brain tissues, i.e., shape features from the brain cortex and connectivity features from the WM tracts, and *(iii)* classification of the input infant brain to autistic or control based on analyzing the extracted shape and connectivity features.

2.1   Segmentation

Infant Brain Extraction: In order to increase the segmentation accuracy, the brain is first extracted to minimize the overall intensity overlap and decrease the segmentation search space. To achieve this step, we developed a new stochastic brain extraction algorithm (see Algorithm 1).

Infant Brain Segmentation: To segment various brain structures, a co-aligned to the training database image $\mathbf{g}$ of the extracted infant brain and its region map, $\mathbf{m}$, are considered a sample of a 3D Markov Gibbs random field (MGRF) with a joint probability distribution: $P(\mathbf{g}, \mathbf{m}) = P(\mathbf{g}|\mathbf{m})P(\mathbf{m})$, which combines a conditional distribution of the images given the map $P(\mathbf{g}|\mathbf{m})$, and an unconditional probability distribution of maps $P(\mathbf{m}) = P_{\mathrm{sp}}(\mathbf{m})P_{\mathbf{V}}(\mathbf{m})$. Here, $P(\mathbf{g}|\mathbf{m})$ is a nonnegative matrix factorization (NMF) based visual appearance model, $P_{\mathrm{sp}}(\mathbf{m})$ is an adaptive shape model, and $P_{\mathbf{V}}(\mathbf{m})$ is a Gibbs probability distribution with potentials $\mathbf{V}$, which specifies an MGRF model of spatially homogeneous maps $\mathbf{m}$.

1- NMF-Based Visual Appearance Model: Following DTI estimation, five different DTI features were calculated using the 3D Slicer software [10], namely, mean diffusivity (MD), fractional anisotropy (FA), relative anisotropy (RA), axial diffusivity ($\lambda_{\parallel}$), and radial diffusivity ($\lambda_{\perp}$) [11]. To distinguish better between the brain structures, the high-dimensional space of these features is reduced with the NMF, which approximates the input $6 \times R$ matrix $\mathbf{A}$ containing all the voxelwise feature vectors from a given DWI/DTI (five DTI features and b0 volume) with a $J \times R$; $J < 6$ (determined experimentally by comparing segmentation accuracies), matrix of fused lower-dimensional voxel-wise features: $\mathbf{A} \approx \mathbf{WH}$ where $\mathbf{W}$ is the $6 \times J$ basis matrix performing the fusion [12]. The non-negative matrices $\mathbf{W}$ and $\mathbf{H}$ are obtained by constrained minimization of the squared approximation error:

$$\min_{\mathbf{W},\mathbf{H}} |\mathbf{A} - \mathbf{WH}|^2 \text{ subject to } \mathbf{W} \geq \mathbf{0}; \, \mathbf{H} \geq \mathbf{0} \tag{1}$$

using most often multiplicative matrix update, projected gradient descent, and alternating least square (ALS) iterative solutions [13]. Our framework employs the ALS owing to its higher speed and flexibility due to solving at each iteration two successive constrained convex minimization problems of finding the minimiser $\mathbf{W}$, given the fixed $\mathbf{H}$, and the minimiser $\mathbf{H}$, given the fixed $\mathbf{W}$.

In our framework, the input matrix $\mathbf{A}$ contains all voxel-wise 6-component vector-columns for all training volumes and the resulting J-component vector-columns; $J < 6$, of $\mathbf{H}$ are clustered to find centroids $\mathbf{c}_l$, one per each goal brain structure $l \in \mathbf{L}$, in the reduced J-dimensional feature space. Each new data matrix $\mathbf{B}$ with the same six voxel-wise feature vectors $\mathbf{b}_r$; $r \in \mathbf{R}$, is transformed using the pseudo-inverse of $\mathbf{W}$:

$$\mathbf{H}_B = \mathbf{W}^{\dagger}\mathbf{B} = (\mathbf{W}^{\mathsf{T}}\mathbf{W})^{-1}\mathbf{W}^{\mathsf{T}}\mathbf{B} \tag{2}$$

Algorithm 1. Steps of the Proposed Brain Extraction Approach

1. Approximate the empirical signal marginal for an input image $\mathbf{g}$ using a linear combination of discrete Gaussians (LCDG) with two dominant brain / non-brain modes and partition it into the LCDG models of both classes [14].
2. Determine the discriminant threshold, τ, giving the best separation of the brain and non-brain voxel-wise signals.
3. Smooth the image, $\mathbf{g} \to \widehat{\mathbf{g}}$, by the gradient descent minimization of the voxel-wise energy of Equation (4) for each voxel-wise signal $(q_s; s \in \mathbf{R}, q \in \mathbf{Q})$ to reduce $\mathbf{g}$ inhomogeneity:

$$\widehat{q}_s = \arg\min_{\widetilde{q}_s}[|q_s - \widetilde{q}_s|^\alpha + \rho^\alpha \lambda^\beta \sum_{r \in \nu_s} \eta_{s,r} |\widetilde{q}_s - q_r|^\beta], \qquad (4)$$

   where $\eta_{s,r}$ is the GGMRF potential, ρ and λ are scaling factors, β controls the level of smoothing, and α determines the prior distribution of the estimator.
4. Nudge $\widehat{q}_s$; $\mathbf{s} \in \mathbf{R}$, which may be close to the boundary between the two classes:

$$\widehat{q}_\mathbf{s} \leftarrow \widehat{q}_\mathbf{s} \begin{cases} +\epsilon \text{ if } \widehat{q}_\mathbf{s} \geq \tau \\ -\epsilon \text{ otherwise} \end{cases} \qquad (5)$$

   where τ is the threshold, obtained at Step 2, and ϵ is a preselected small bias.
5. Apply 3D region growing and connected component analysis to obtain final results.

where T denotes the matrix transposition. The learned centroids are used in a K-means classifier to assign each vector $\mathbf{h_r} = \mathbf{W}^\dagger \mathbf{b_r}$ of the reduced features to the closest, by the Euclidean distance d in the reduced feature space, brain structure. Marginal conditional probabilities of each reduced feature vector, $\mathbf{h_r} = [h_{1:r}, \ldots, h_{J:r}]^\mathsf{T}$; $\mathbf{r} \in \mathbf{R}$, characterising the J-dimensional brain appearance, are defined for each class $l \in \mathbf{L}$ as membership functions of soft clustering with the cluster centroids $\mathbf{c}_l = [c_{1:l}, \ldots, c_{J:l}]^\mathsf{T}$:

$$P_\mathbf{r}(h_\mathbf{r}|m_\mathbf{r} = \lambda) = \frac{d^{-1}(\mathbf{h_r}, \mathbf{c}_\lambda)}{\sum_{l \in \mathbf{L}} d^{-1}(\mathbf{h_r}, \mathbf{c}_l)}. \qquad (3)$$

2- Adaptive Shape Model: To enhance the segmentation accuracy, expected shapes of each brain label are constrained with an adaptive probabilistic shape prior. To create the shape (atlas) database, a training set of images are collected for different subjects (10 datasets) with their new NMF fused features. They are co-aligned by 3D affine transformations with 12 degrees of freedom in a way that maximizes their mutual information. The shape priors are spatially variant independent random fields of region labels for the co-aligned data:

$$P_{\mathrm{sp}}(\mathbf{m}) = \prod_{r \in \mathbf{R}} p_{\mathrm{sp}:\mathbf{r}}(m_\mathbf{r}), \qquad (6)$$

where $p_{\mathrm{sp}:\mathbf{r}}(l)$ refers to the voxel-wise empirical probabilities for each brain label $l \in \mathbf{L}$. To generate the ground truth labels for the atlas, the infant tissue probability maps provided by IDEA lab [15] were used with the unified segmentation algorithm, implemented in the statistical parametric mapping (SPM) software, to segment the non-diffusion (b0) scans of the training datasets [15]. Then, an MR expert refined the generated initial segmentation to produce the final brain labels. For each input subject data to be segmented, the shape prior is constructed by an adaptive process guided by the visual appearance of its NMF fused features as described in [16].

Algorithm 2. Steps for the Proposed Segmentation Approach

---

1. Detect artifacts, correct motion and eddy current distortions using DTIprep [17].
2. Derive DTI from DWI using the weighted linear least square (WLLS) method, and extract five DTI features (MD, FA, RA, $\lambda_{\parallel}$, $\lambda_{\perp}$) using 3D Slicer [10].
3. Remove any non-brain tissues from DWI brain images by applying the proposed automated brain extraction approach to the b0 volumes (Algorithm 1).
4. Create a new NMF input data matrix **B** from the obtained DWI/DTI data.
5. Use the weight matrix **W** (calculated in the training phase) to transform **B** from the original space to the new J^{th}-dimensional space, according to Equation (2).
6. Create the subject-specific shape prior model as described in [16].
7. Form an initial region map **m** using the appearance and shape models.
8. Find the Gibbs potentials for the MGRF model from the initial map **m** [14].
9. Improve the region map **m** using voxel-wise Bayes classifier after integrating the three descriptors in the proposed joint MGRF model.

3- Spatial Interaction MGRF Model: In order to overcome noise effects and to ensure segmentation homogeneity, spatially homogeneous 3D pair-wise interactions between the region labels are additionally incorporated in the proposed segmentation model (extension to the 2D version in [14]). The utilized second-order 3D MGRF model of the region map **m** is defined as:

$$P_V(\mathbf{m}) = \frac{1}{Z_{\nu_s}} \exp \sum_{(x,\,y,\,z) \in \mathbf{R}} \sum_{(\xi,\,\eta,\,\zeta) \in \nu_s} \mathbf{V}(m_{x,y,z}, m_{x+\xi,y+\eta,z+\zeta}), \qquad (7)$$

where Z_{ν_s} is the normalization factor and **V** is the bi-valued Gibbs potential, which depends on whether the nearest pair of labels are equal or not. The initial region map results in an approximation with the following analytical maximum likelihood estimates of the potentials [14]:

$$v_{eq} = -v_{ne} \approx 2f_{eq}(\mathbf{m}) - 1, \qquad (8)$$

where $f_{eq}(\mathbf{m})$ is the relative frequency of equal labels in the voxel pairs $\{((x,y,z),(x+\xi,y+\eta,z+\zeta)): (x,y,z) \in \mathbf{R}; (x+\xi,y+\eta,z+\zeta) \in \mathbf{R}; (\xi,\eta,\zeta) \in \nu_s\}$. These estimates allow for computing the voxel-wise probabilities $p_{x,y,z}(m_{x,y,z} = l)$ of each brain label; $l \in \mathbf{L}$. In total, the complete segmentation steps of the proposed framework are summarized in Algorithm 2.

2.2   Feature Extraction

Shape Features: The shape analysis was based on spherical harmonic reconstruction [18], which considers 3D surface data (i.e., brain cortex) as a linear combination of specific basis functions, namely spherical harmonics (SHs). First, a 3D mesh model of the segmented brain cortex surface is generated from a re-sampled higher resolution version (1 mm^3) of the segmented DTI data using a Delaunay triangulated 3D mesh. Secondly, a smoothed version of the 3D mesh is created to ensure the uniqueness of each point in the given dataset. Then, the smoothed brain mesh is mapped to a unit sphere utilizing the attraction-repulsion mapping approach [19]. The SHs are produced by solving an isotropic heat equation for the brain cortex surface on the unit sphere [19]. A step-by-step of the proposed SH analysis is demonstrated in Figure 1. After SH reconstruction, two techniques for measuring the complexity of the cerebral cortex are proposed:

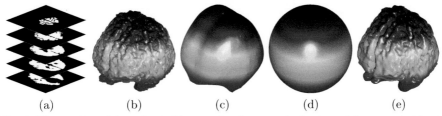

|(a)|(b)|(c)|(d)|(e)|

Fig. 1. Illustration of the spherical harmonics shape analysis steps: (a) segmented brain cortex, (b) original mesh, (c) smoothed mesh, (d) unit sphere mesh, and (e) the SHs reconstructed mesh.

1- SH Reconstruction Error (SHRE): Due to the unit sphere mapping, the original cortex mesh for each subject is inherently aligned with the SH approximated mesh. The error between the original cortex mesh nodes and the SH approximated cortex mesh nodes can be calculated in terms of the Euclidean distance. This error generates a reconstruction error curve that is unique to each subject, where the area under the curve is examined to provide a representative metric for the brain cortex [19].

2- Surface Complexity (SC): A new metric for examining the complexity of the brain using the SH coefficients is also proposed. For a unit sphere f, having an SH expansion, the surface complexity metric $S(f)$ is defined as:

$$S(f) = \sum_{N=0}^{\infty} \varepsilon_N^2 = \sum_{N=0}^{\infty} N B_N^2, \tag{9}$$

where N is the number of harmonics, and B are the previously calculated SH coefficients. The squared residual ε_N^2 is defined as:

$$\varepsilon_N^2 = \|f - f_N\|^2 = \|\sum_{n=N+1}^{\infty} \sum_{m=-n}^{n} b_{nm} Y_n^m\|^2 = \sum_{n=N+1}^{\infty} \sum_{m=-n}^{n} |b_{nm}|^2 = \sum_{n=N+1}^{\infty} B_n^2. \tag{10}$$

For use in 3D SH analysis there are three sets of coefficients for each direction, x, y and z. Hence, the surface complexity is expanded from Equation (9) to be defined as:

$$S(f) = \frac{\sum_{N=0}^{\infty} N(B_{N,x}^2 + B_{N,y}^2 + B_{N,z}^2)}{\|f_x\|^2 + \|f_y\|^2 + \|f_z\|^2}. \tag{11}$$

This metric generates a unique curve for each subject similar to the SH reconstruction error curves. Some of the advantages to this calculation are that it depends only on the SH coefficients, making it a self-contained metric, and it serves to represent the average degree of SH expansion. Also, it is considered as a convergent metric, and can be computed over the range of harmonics of interest.

Connectivity Features: In this paper, the obtained WM label maps were used as seeds to generate the required WM tracts according to existing tractography methods built in the 3D slicer software [10]. After WM fiber tracts were extracted, FA values were generated for each fiber tract to measure the degree of anisotropy of local diffusivity. In addition to the FA values, axial ($\lambda_{\|}$) and radial ($\lambda_{\perp}$) diffusivity values, which represent diffusion parallel and transverse to axonal directions, were also produced [11].

Table 1. Summary of the segmentation results using DSC(%), MHD(mm), and AVD(%).

	Brain Extraction			Brain Segmentation							
	Brain Mask			Brain Cortex				White Matter			
Metric	Prop.	BET	iBEAT	Prop.	[14]	FSL	iBEAT	Prop.	[14]	FSL	iBEAT
DSC	**96.96** ±**1.42**	91.16 ±0.77	93.15 ±2.40	**97.58** ±**3.60**	90.72 ±1.06	93.60 ±5.36	92.52 ±1.73	**95.11** ±**5.07**	95.23 ±1.18	79.49 ±4.69	88.85 ±0.84
p-value		0.0003	0.0001		0.0001	0.0191	0.0002		0.0001	0.0002	0.0001
MHD	**6.57** ±**4.08**	10.01 ±1.05	9.49 ±5.41	**2.71** ±**0.84**	14.79 ±1.25	4.66 ±1.91	6.46 ±2.06	**1.98** ±**0.55**	1.98 ±0.01	5.84 ±0.90	5.05 ±1.05
p-value		0.0067	0.0302		0.0001	0.0094	0.0001		0.0001	0.0009	0.0001
AVD	**2.46** ±**3.34**	4.09 ±2.10	3.96 ±2.97	**2.03** ±**0.82**	7.33 ±5.47	13.78 ±13.99	16.19 ±3.93	**5.19** ±**1.98**	5.15 ±2.03	51.76 ±16.68	25.10 ±2.12
p-value		0.3116	0.0480		0.0001	0.0001	0.0027		0.0001	0.0004	0.0008

3 Experimental Results and Conclusions

This paper included data from the Infant Brain Imaging Study (IBIS) [20]. The study participants are six-month-old infants with a high risk of developing ASDs. Based on an ASD cutoff threshold, the high-risk infants were divided into two groups: ASD negative (control) and ASD-positive (autistic). From the 280 subjects available, there were only 38 subjects with available final diagnosis provided to our group (19 autistic and 19 control). Diffusion weighted MR brain scans were acquired using the following parameters: field of view of: 190 mm, number of slices: 75–81, voxel resolution: $2 \times 2 \times 2$ mm^3, variable b values between 0 and 1,000 s/mm^2, and 25 gradient directions [20].

Since the segmentation accuracy significantly affects the diagnostic results, performance assessment of the segmentation results is necessary. This is achieved by applying the proposed segmentation techniques on all 38 diffusion weighted infant MR brain datasets, and evaluated on 10 training datasets with a manually segmented gold standard, using leave-one-out cross validation. Three performance metrics were used: *(i)* the Dice similarity coefficient (DSC), *(ii)* the 95-percentile modified Hausdorff distance (MHD), and *(iii)* the percentage absolute volume difference (AVD) [21]. The proposed brain extraction and brain segmentation frameworks were compared with the available software packages: the brain extraction tool (BET) [22], the FMRIB software library (FSL) [23], and the infant brain extraction and analysis toolbox (iBEAT) [24]. In order to highlight the usefulness of using the NMF to amplify the MGRF in [14], the accuracies of the NMF/non-NMF-based segmentation were also compared. Segmentation accuracies for each method using the DSC, MHD, and AVD are summarized in Table 1. The obtained results show the high accuracy of the proposed NMF-based segmentation approach compared to the state-of-the-art software packages as confirmed from the DSC paired t-test results (p-value<0.05). In addition, the proposed segmentation techniques show a particular advantage in terms of processing speed (<1 min) when compared to the competing techniques (iBeat >75 min and FSL >15 min).

Table 2. Statistical analysis results.

	Control	Autistic	p-value
SHRE	261.42±37.53	233.26±30.14	**0.0251**
SC	87.29±2.52	85.59±1.36	**0.0139**
FA	0.66±0.08	0.70±0.02	**0.0408**
$\lambda_{\parallel}$	4.55±4.01	5.87±3.07	0.2607
$\lambda_{\perp}$	1.09±0.54	1.77±1.06	**0.0166**

Table 3. Classification results.

Classifier	ACC	AUC
Naive Bayes	76.31%	0.864
KNN	86.84%	0.906
SVM	86.84%	0.868
Random Forest	**86.84%**	**0.960**

The statistical analysis results of the shape and connectivity features extracted from all available 19 autistic and 19 control sets, which reflects the variability of the healthy and autistic populations, are shown in Table 2. According to the unpaired t-test results, all shape features and two out of the three connectivity features (FA, $\lambda_{\perp}$) show statistically significant differences between control and autistic infant brains (p-value<0.05). These results encouraged us to explore the classification potential of those four statistically significant features. In this paper, random forest classifier was used, and its results were validated only by comparisons with other known classifiers (naïve Bayes Bayes, K-nearest neighbor (KNN), and support vector machine (SVM)) because no complete CAD system currently exists for detecting ASDs at early (infancy) stage. Table 3 provides a comparison between the performance of these classifiers in terms of the classification accuracy (ACC) and the area under the ROC curve (AUC) using leave-one-out cross validation. It is clear that the random forest classifier provides the best diagnostic results (ACC of 86.84% and AUC of 0.96), which confirms both the robustness and the accuracy of the random forest classifier.

To conclude, this paper presents a novel CAD system for diagnosing ASDs. The novelties are four-fold: *(i)* automatic removal of non-brain tissues to extract infant brains directly from input DTI (most existing techniques are designed to work primarily with T1 MRI); *(ii)* infant brain segmentation by image modelling with an MGRF, combining new NMF appearance, atlas-based shape, and 3D homogeneity descriptors; *(iii)* measuring the brain cortex variability (surface complexity) by analyzing shapes with spherical harmonics, and *(iv)* diagnosing ASDs using shape and connectivity features extracted from brain tissues, segmented using the same imaging modality to eliminate errors typical for the multi-modality CAD. The preliminary diagnostic results, based on the available dataset, are promising in identifying autistic from control patients. Our future work will include collecting more DTI data with better resolution to build a more powerful classifier, and to extend our work to involve advanced identification of brain regions that have significant group differences using constructed brain maps.

References

1. Wingate, M., et al.: Prevalence of autism spectrum disorder among children aged 8 years-autism and developmental disabilities monitoring network, 11 sites, united states, 2010. MMWR Surveillance Summaries 63(2) (2014)
2. Travers, B.G., et al.: Diffusion tensor imaging in autism spectrum disorder: a review. Autism Research 5(5), 289–313 (2012)

3. Aylward, E.H., et al.: Effects of age on brain volume and head circumference in autism. Neurology 59(2), 175–183 (2002)

4. El-Baz, A.S., Casanova, M.F., Gimel'farb, G.G., Mott, M., Switala, A.E.: Autism diagnostics by 3D texture analysis of cerebral white matter gyrifications. In: Ayache, N., Ourselin, S., Maeder, A. (eds.) MICCAI 2007, Part II. LNCS, vol. 4792, pp. 882–890. Springer, Heidelberg (2007)

5. Hazlett, H.C., et al.: Brain volume findings in 6-month-old infants at high familial risk for autism. American Journal of Psychiatry 169(6), 601–608 (2012)

6. Shi, F., et al.: Neonatal brain image segmentation in longitudinal MRI studies. Neuroimage 49(1), 391–400 (2010)

7. Xue, H., et al.: Automatic segmentation and reconstruction of the cortex from neonatal MRI. Neuroimage 38(3), 461–477 (2007)

8. Wang, L., et al.: Integration of sparse multi-modality representation and anatomical constraint for isointense infant brain MR image segmentation. NeuroImage 89, 152–164 (2014)

9. Wang, X., Wang, L., Suk, H.-I., Shen, D.: Online discriminative multi-atlas learning for isointense infant brain segmentation. In: Wu, G., Zhang, D., Zhou, L. (eds.) MLMI 2014. LNCS, vol. 8679, pp. 297–305. Springer, Heidelberg (2014)

10. Fedorov, A., et al.: 3d slicer as an image computing platform for the quantitative imaging network. Magnetic Resonance Imaging 30(9), 1323–1341 (2012)

11. Mori, S., et al.: Introduction to Diffusion Tensor Imaging 2e: And Higher Order Models (2013)

12. Lee, D.D., et al.: Learning the parts of objects by non-negative matrix factorization. Nature 401(6755), 788 791 (1999)

13. Berry, M.W., et al.: Algorithms and applications for approximate nonnegative matrix factorization. Computational Statistics & Data Analysis 52(1), 155–173 (2007)

14. Farag, A.A., et al.: Precise segmentation of multimodal images. IEEE Transactions on Image Processing 15(4), 952–968 (2006)

15. Shi, F., et al.: Infant brain atlases from neonates to 1-and 2-year-olds. PLoS One 6(4), e18746 (2011)

16. Mostapha, M., et al.: A statistical framework for the classification of infant dt images. In: ICIP, pp. 2222–2226. IEEE (2014)

17. Liu, Z., et al.: Quality control of diffusion weighted images. In: SPIE Medical Imaging, p. 76280J. International Society for Optics and Photonics (2010)

18. Gerig, G., et al.: Shape analysis of brain ventricles using spharm. In: IEEE Workshop on Mathematical Methods in Biomedical Image Analysis, MMBIA 2001, pp. 171–178. IEEE (2001)

19. Nitzken, M., et al.: 3d shape analysis of the brain cortex with application to autism. In: ISBI, pp. 1847–1850. IEEE (2011)

20. Wolff, J.J., et al.: Differences in white matter fiber tract development present from 6 to 24 months in infants with autism. American Journal of Psychiatry 169(6), 589–600 (2012)

21. Babalola, K.O., et al.: An evaluation of four automatic methods of segmenting the subcortical structures in the brain. Neuroimage 47(4), 1435–1447 (2009)

22. Smith, S.M.: Fast robust automated brain extraction. Human Brain Mapping 17(3), 143–155 (2002)

23. Jenkinson, M., et al.: Fsl. Neuroimage 62(2), 782–790 (2012)

24. Dai, Y., et al.: iBEAT: a toolbox for infant brain magnetic resonance image processing. Neuroinformatics 11(2), 211–225 (2013)

Identifying Connectome Module Patterns via New Balanced Multi-graph Normalized Cut⋆

Hongchang Gao[1], Chengtao Cai[2], Jingwen Yan[2], Lin Yan[3],
Joaquin Goni Cortes[2], Yang Wang[2], Feiping Nie[1], John West[2],
Andrew Saykin[2], Li Shen[2], and Heng Huang[1,⋆⋆]

[1] Computer Science and Engineering, University of Texas at Arlington, TX, USA
[2] Radiology and Imaging Sciences, Indiana University School of Medicine, IN, USA
[3] Department of Electronic Engineering, School of Electronic Information
and Electrical Engineering, Shanghai Jiao Tong University, Shanghai, China

Abstract. Computational tools for the analysis of complex biological
networks are lacking in human connectome research. Especially, how to
discover the brain network patterns shared by a group of subjects is
a challenging computational neuroscience problem. Although some single graph clustering methods can be extended to solve the multi-graph
cases, the discovered network patterns are often imbalanced, *e.g.* isolated points. To address these problems, we propose a novel indicator
constrained and balanced multi-graph normalized cut method to identify
the connectome module patterns from the connectivity brain networks
of the targeted subject group. We evaluated our method by analyzing
the weighted fiber connectivity networks.

1 Introduction

To understand the mechanisms of human brain comprehensively, it is important to reveal the functioning of the brain network [9]. The emerging human
connectome projects provide the fundamental insights into the organization and
integration of brain networks, and greatly support the studies of brain circuitry
and the understanding of human brain [9]. Each connectome is a comprehensive
description of the network elements and connections that form the brain. In order to discover the full potential patterns of the connectome, the graph theory
based models have been applied to reveal the architecture of the connectome
[4,11,7]. In such a graph, nodes are neuroanatomical regions and edges are the
density of the nerve fibers connecting the nodes. Analysis of the graph can dis-
close the topological structure, corresponding to a certain connectivity pattern
in the connectome, which helps to understand the mechanisms of human brain.

⋆ HG, FN, and HH were supported in part by IIS-1117965, IIS-1302675, IIS-1344152,
DBI-1356628. CC, JY, AS, and LS were supported in part by NSF IIS-1117335, NIH
UL1 RR025761, U01 AG024904, NIA RC2 AG036535, NIA R01 AG19771, NIH R01
LM011360, and NIA P30 AG1013318S1.
⋆⋆ Corresponding Author: heng@uta.edu

To understand the underlying structural and functional mechanisms of the human brain, we need to discover the connectome module patterns which are shared by a group of subjects under the same conditions. However, the existing methods mostly focus on analyzing the connectome of individual subject rather than unifying them together [1,8], which is not sufficient to find the shared network module patterns. The straightforward solution is to use the average connectivity networks of all subjects to detect the network module patterns. However, in such a method, some strong signals from individual networks could strongly influence the identified patterns. For example, if some networks have certain connections with high values, the average connectivity values of all networks will be dominated by these odd values and lead to the wrong patterns.

To address this challenging problem, we propose a new indicator constrained balanced multi-graph normalized cut method to identify the shared connectome module patterns from a group of subjects. The novelties of our proposed machine learning model are in three-fold: 1) The traditional normalized cut methods relax the discrete objectives to continuous formulation and require the k-means clustering as post-processing, which leads to sub-optimal results. We propose to utilize the clustering indicator matrix directly in our new objective such that the optimal results can be achieved; 2) Our new model can perform normalized cut on all connectivity networks simultaneously to identify the shared network patterns; 3) Because the connectivity networks are not fully connected graph, the naive multi-graph normalized cut model could find the biased patters, such as the isolated nodes. To tackle this problem, we introduce a new regularization term for balanced normalized cut. We apply the proposed method to study the connectivity networks of four different subject groups: Health Control (HC), Significant Memory Concern (SMC), Mild Cognitive Impairment (MCI), and Alzheimer Disease (AD). In all empirical results, the top network module patterns identified by our method are more significant than the top modules detected by other related methods.

2   Methodology

The brain connectivity network can be represented as a graph $G = \{X, E, W\}$ with node set X, edge set E, and connectivity matrix W. Each node in X denotes an ROI (Region of Interest) in human brain. Each edge in E means that the end nodes (ROIs) of the edge are connective to each other. Each element in W denotes the density of the nerve fibers between a pair of nodes. Given m subjects under the same condition with n ROIs, we get m graph with m weight matrices $W^1, W^2, ..., W^m$, where $W^k \in \Re^{n \times n}$, where W_{ij}^k is the density of nerve fibers between the i-th ROI and the j-th ROI in the k-th subject, where $k = 1, ..., m, 1 \le i \le n, 1 \le j \le n$. Our goal is to discover the connectivity network patterns shared by the brain networks of all/most subjects. Traditional graph clustering methods can only deal with single graph, thus, we propose a novel balanced multi-graph normalized cut with indicator constraint algorithm to identify the shared network module patterns.

2.1 Balanced Multi-graph Normalized Cut with Indicator Constraint

Given a connectivity matrix $W \in \Re^{n \times n}$, we can perform graph clustering on the network. Let $F = [f_1, f_2, ..., f_c] \in \Re^{n \times c}$ as the cluster indicator matrix. The normalized cut model is to minimize $Tr(F^T LF)$ with the constraint $f_k = (0, ..., 0, \frac{1}{\sqrt{f_k^T Df_k}}, \cdots, \frac{1}{\sqrt{f_k^T Df_k}}, 0, \cdots, 0)^T$ where $L = D - W$, and D is a diagonal matrix with $D_{ii} = \sum_j W_{ij}$. Minimizing this objective function with such constraint is an NP hard problem [3]. The traditional method is to relax the desired discrete values to the continuous ones and solve the following problem:

$$\min_{F^T DF = I} Tr(F^T LF) , \qquad (1)$$

where elements of F are not discrete. Eq. (1) can be solved by the eigenvalue decomposition of the matrix L. After that, the discrete solution can be obtained by performing k-means clustering as post-processing, which converges to a local minimum and leads to suboptimal results. To address this problem, we propose a novel normalized cut method with indicator constraint to get the graph clustering results directly.

The normalized cut with indicator constraint is to minimize the following objective function:

$$\min_{F \in Ind} Tr(F^T LF) , \qquad (2)$$

where $F = [f_1, f_2, ..., f_c] \in \Re^{n \times c}$ is the group indicator matrix and c is the number of groups. The i-th element of f_k is set to 1 if the i-th node belongs to k-th group, otherwise 0. Because our solutions are clustering indicators, the final clustering results can be achieved directly without any post-processing step.

To discover the connectome module patterns on multiple graphs, we need perform the normalized cut on multiple graphs simultaneously. When the graph clustering model is performed on all networks, the corresponding nodes in each network should appear in the same group [6]. Thus, we force the group indicator matrices of all the networks to be the same matrix F. As a result, our multi-graph normalized cut objective is to solve:

$$\min_{F \in Ind} \sum_{v=1}^{m} Tr(F^T L^v F) , \qquad (3)$$

where $F \in \Re^{n \times c}$ is the common group indicator matrix and m is the number of networks, L^v is the Laplacian matrix of the v-th connectivity network.

However, this model may identify isolated nodes as patterns, because many isolated nodes could be shared by all networks. Obviously, these isolated node patterns are not the correct ones. To avoid such a case, we introduce a new regularization term to guarantee a balanced multi-graph normalized cut as following:

$$\min_{F \in Ind} \sum_{v=1}^{m} Tr(F^T L^v F) + \gamma Tr(F^T 11^T F) , \qquad (4)$$

where $Tr(F^v 11^T F^v) = \sqrt{\sum_{j=1}^{c}(\sum_{i=1}^{n}||f_{ij}^v||)^2}$, which is the square-sum of the number of nodes in each group. To obtain the minimum of the square-sum of some numbers whose sum is fixed, these numbers should be equal to each other. Therefore, our proposed method combining both indicator constrained multi-graph normalize cut loss and balanced clustering regularization term, can achieve the balanced multi-graph clustering results.

2.2   Optimization Algorithm

In this paper, we solve the optimization problem via the Augmented Lagrangian Multiplier (ALM) method . We introduce an ancillary variable $G = F$ to obtain efficient updates on the optimization variables as following:

$$\min_{F \in Ind, G, F=G} Tr(F^T(\sum_{v=1}^{m} L^v + \gamma 11^T)G). \tag{5}$$

Next, we add a penalty term and a Lagrangian term to eliminate the constraints.

$$\min_{F \in Ind, G} Tr(F^T(\sum_{v=1}^{m} L^v + \gamma 11^T)G) + Tr(\Gamma^T(F - G)) + \frac{\mu}{2}||F - G||_F^2, \tag{6}$$

where $\Gamma \in \Re^{n \times c}$ is the Lagrangian multiplier and μ is the regularity coefficient. It is equivalent to the following problem, because they have the same derivatives.

$$\min_{F \in Ind, G} Tr(F^T(\sum_{v=1}^{m} L^v + \gamma 11^T)G) + \frac{\mu}{2}||F - G + \frac{1}{\mu}\Gamma||_F^2. \tag{7}$$

The updating rules for F, G, Γ and μ are as following:

Update F: Optimizing Eq. (7) with respect to F is equivalent to optimizing

$$\min_{F \in Ind} ||F - C + \frac{1}{\mu}B||_F^2. \tag{8}$$

where $B = AG$, $A = \sum_{v=1}^{m} L^v + \gamma 11^T$ and $C = G - \frac{1}{\mu}\Gamma$. Because each node belongs to only one group, there is only one element equal to one in each row. Thus, for i-th row, the solution of F_{ij} is:

$$F_{ij} = \begin{cases} 1 & \max_j(C_{ij} - \frac{1}{\mu}B_{ij}) \\ 0 & otherwise \end{cases} \tag{9}$$

Update G: Similar to optimize F, optimizing Eq. (7) with respect to G is equivalent to optimizing:

$$\min_G Tr(F^T AG) + \frac{\mu}{2}||F - G + \frac{1}{\mu}\Gamma||_F^2. \tag{10}$$

Taking the derivative w.r.t G and setting it equal to zero, we can get:

$$G = F - \frac{1}{\mu}(F^T A - \Gamma) \tag{11}$$

Update Γ and μ: At each iteration, we update μ and Γ as the following:

$$\Gamma = \Gamma + \mu(F - G), \mu = \rho\mu. \tag{12}$$

where ρ is a positive parameter to control the convergence speed. The above updating rules are repeated until convergence is achieved. Obviously, our proposed algorithm is convergent, because we divide the original optimization problem (7) into several subproblems and each of them is a convex optimization problem. Thus, by solving these subproblems alternatively, the proposed algorithm will guarantee the convergence.

3 Experiments and Discussions

3.1 Data Set and Network Construction

Data used in this work were obtained from the ADNI database (adni.loni.usc.edu). One goal of ADNI has been to test whether serial MRI, PET, other biological markers, and clinical and neuropsychological assessment can be combined to measure the progression of MCI and early AD. For up-to-date information, see www.adni-info.org. We downloaded baseline MRI and Diffusion Tensor Imaging (DTI) scans for 174 ADNI-GO/2 participants. Below we describe our method for constructing structural brain networks from MRI and DTI data.

1) ROI Generation: Anatomical parcellation was performed on the MRI scans using FreeSurfer 5.1 (http://surfer.nmr.mgh.harvard.edu/), coupled with Lausanne parcellation [5], to create 129 regions of interest (ROIs). Each MRI scan was registered to the low resolution b0 image of DTI data using the FLIRT toolbox in FSL (http://www.fmrib.ox.ac.uk/fsl.html), and the warping parameters were applied to the ROIs so that a new set of ROIs in the DTI image space were created. These new ROIs were used for constructing the structural network.

2) DTI Tractography: The DTI data were analyzed using FSL. Preprocessing included correction for motion and eddy current effects in DTI images. The processed images were then output to Diffusion Toolkit (http://trackvis.org/) for fiber tracking, using the streamline tractography algorithm called FACT (fiber assignment by continuous tracking). Quality control (QC) was performed via visual inspection, and 20 participants with questionable results were excluded.

3) Network Construction: The nodes were 129 ROIs obtained from parcellation. The edge weight is defined as the density of the fibers connecting the node pair, which is the number of tracks between two ROIs divided by the mean volume of two ROIs. A fiber is considered to connect two ROIs if and only if its end points fall in two ROIs respectively. The weighted network can be described by a matrix: The rows and columns correspond to the nodes, and matrix elements correspond to the edge weights.

3.2 Experiment Setup

Totally 154 participants (30 HC, 34 SMC, 62 MCI, and 28 AD) passed tractography QC and had networks constructed. We aimed to discover the connectome module patterns for each group. The scale of each network is 129×129. We set

Table 1. Connectivity measure on four types of subjects. SC denotes the results of spectral clustering on the average graph; MMSC denotes the results of multi-modal spectral clustering on all the graphs; MCC denotes the results of min-cut clustering on average graph; MGMC denotes the results of multi-graph minmax cut on all graphs.

(a) HC

#	Our	SC	MMSC	MCC	MGMC
1	**0.2557**	0.1411	0.1926	0.1926	0.2496
2	**0.1926**	0.1048	0.1639	0.1590	0.1781
3	**0.1777**	0.0890	0.1531	0.1242	0.1401
4	**0.1573**	0.0779	0.1422	0.0973	0.1399
5	**0.1428**	0.0766	0.1205	0.0964	0.1330
6	**0.1339**	0.0434	0.0964	0.0900	0.1315
avg	**0.1767**	0.0888	0.1448	0.1266	0.1620

(b) MCI

#	Our	SC	MMSC	MCC	MGMC
1	**0.2604**	0.1907	0.1675	0.1186	0.2462
2	**0.2388**	0.1578	0.1251	0.0998	0.1652
3	**0.2027**	0.1550	0.1224	0.0948	0.1440
4	**0.1988**	0.1309	0.1102	0.0909	0.1339
5	**0.1406**	0.1003	0.1005	0.0894	0.1335
6	0.0849	0.0899	0.0843	0.0825	**0.1297**
avg	**0.1877**	0.1375	0.1183	0.0960	0.1587

(c) AD

#	Our	SC	MMSC	MCC	MGMC
1	**0.2015**	0.1860	0.1649	0.1312	0.1879
2	**0.1796**	0.1296	0.1626	0.1024	0.1628
3	**0.1649**	0.1071	0.1280	0.0980	0.1412
4	**0.1612**	0.0921	0.1265	0.0950	0.1368
5	**0.1529**	0.0799	0.1233	0.0943	0.1346
6	0.1224	0.0659	0.1142	0.0811	**0.1337**
avg	**0.1638**	0.1101	0.1365	0.1003	0.1495

(d) SMC

#	Our	SC	MMSC	MCC	MGMC
1	**0.2791**	0.1882	0.1671	0.1773	0.1640
2	**0.1790**	0.0996	0.1668	0.1447	0.1494
3	**0.1783**	0.0993	0.1503	0.1306	0.1436
4	**0.1582**	0.0900	0.1399	0.1214	0.1425
5	**0.1487**	0.0821	0.1301	0.1060	0.1393
6	**0.1306**	0.0724	0.1266	0.0904	0.1292
avg	**0.1790**	0.1053	0.1468	0.1284	0.1447

the group number as 12. We used the normalized connectivity measure of connectome modules to evaluate the density of detected modules: $D_{tt} = \frac{\sum_{v=1}^{m} s_{tt}^v}{mn_t^2}$, where D_{tt} is the normalized connectivity of the t-th module, m is the number of networks, n_t is the number of ROI in the t-th module M_t, $s_{tt}^v = \sum_{i \in M_t, j \in M_t} W_{ij}^v$ is the connectivity of the t-th module in the v-th network.

Table 2. T-test between our method and other methods: p-values are shown.

Pair	HC	MCI	AD	SMC
Our-SC	0.00004	0.01060	0.00140	0.00002
Our-MMSC	0.00570	0.00940	0.00250	0.10500
Our-MCC	0.00010	0.00920	0.00006	0.00470
Our-MGMC	0.03510	0.17900	0.04550	0.09850

3.3 Comparison of Connectivity Measures

To evaluate the performance of our algorithm, we compared our algorithm with four other algorithms: (1) Spectral clustering on the average network (SC), performing the classical spectral clustering on the average of all the networks. (2) Multi-modal spectral clustering [2] (MMSC), which is to unify different networks from different subjects to perform spectral clustering. (3) Min-cut clustering (MCC), performing min-cut clustering on the average of all the networks. (4)

HC   SMC   MCI   AD

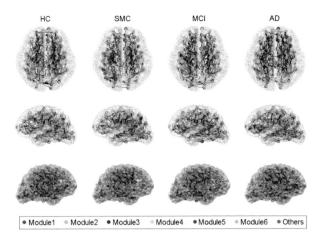

• Module1   • Module2   • Module3   • Module4   • Module5   • Module6   • Others

Fig. 1. Top 6 connectome modules identified for each type. These modules are color-coded and mapped to the group mean networks. Line widths are proportional to the edge weights, where the maximum edge weight corresponds to the line width value of 1. Lines with their width values less than 0.1 are not plotted. Each row shows a visualization from a specific viewing angle.

Multi-graph minmax cut [10] (MGMC), performing minmax cut on each network and then unifying them together.

The connectivity measures of top 6 groups are shown in Table 1. Because the other four methods are not balanced clustering methods, some isolated nodes are identified as clusters (its corresponding normalized connectivity measure value is extremely high), which are not the significant patterns we expected. We view them as outliers and remove them. Thus, the result in Table 1 is the evaluation of the cluster with more than one node. Our results have no such cluster with isolated point, thus our method creates balanced results. As shown in Table 1, our method outperforms the other four methods in most cases. We performed T-test on the connectivity measures to evaluate the difference between our method and the others. As shown in Table 2, almost p value is less than 0.05, showing our method differently outperforms the other four methods.

3.4   Visualization of Detected Modules

To illustrate the grouping result, we visualized the top 6 connectome modules in Fig. 1. We mapped the modules to the mean networks, and visualized those from three different angles. Module 1 of HC, SMC and MCI groups were all located on the right hemisphere, including paracentral lobule, superior frontal gyri, and precuneus. Module 1 of AD group was, however, located on the left caudate and thalamus. For Module 2, both the HC and SMC groups had the clusters on the left hemisphere, where the HC group showed the pattern on hippocampus, amygdala, parahippocampal gyri, and temporal pole, and SMC on accumbens, frontal pole, medial orbital frontal, rostral anterior cingulate thickness, and superior frontal gyri thickness. The MCI group shared a similar pattern to SMC but on the right hemisphere. The AD group had the pattern on the right side including lingual gyri, pericalcarine gyri and superior parietal gyri. For Module 3, HC, SMC and MCI all had the clusters on the left hemisphere, including posterior cingulate, precuneus, and middle temporal gyri. The pattern of AD group was located on the right frontal lobe, including superior frontal gyri, rostral middle frontal gyri and caudal middle frontal gyri.

4   Conclusion and Future Work

In this paper, we proposed a novel indicator constrained balanced multi-graph normalized cut method to detect the connectome module patterns shared by a group of subjects. We utilized a common indicator matrix to unify multiple graph clustering results directly, and introduced a new regularization term to make the graph clustering results balanced. Our method discovers the significant connectome modules for different brain disorder groups. These connectome modules can help other researchers on the variation studies of brain circuitries related to complex brain disorders. Our future work will also focus on identifying the genetic bases of these significant modules to enhance our understanding on the system biology of brain mechanism.

References

1. Bullmore, E., Sporns, O.: Complex brain networks: graph theoretical analysis of structural and functional systems. Nat. Rev. Neurosci. 10(3), 186–198 (2009)
2. Cai, X., Nie, F., Huang, H., Kamangar, F.: Heterogeneous image feature integration via multi-modal spectral clustering. In: 2011 IEEE Conference on Computer Vision and Pattern Recognition (CVPR), pp. 1977–1984. IEEE (2011)
3. Chan, P.K., Schlag, M.D., Zien, J.Y.: Spectral k-way ratio-cut partitioning and clustering. IEEE Transactions on Computer-Aided Design of Integrated Circuits and Systems 13(9), 1088–1096 (1994)
4. Fornito, A., Zalesky, A., Breakspear, M.: Graph analysis of the human connectome: promise, progress, and pitfalls. Neuroimage 80, 426–444 (2013)
5. Hagmann, P., Cammoun, L., Gigandet, X., Meuli, R., Honey, C.J., Wedeen, V.J., Sporns, O.: Mapping the structural core of human cerebral cortex. PLoS Biol. 6(7), e159 (2008)
6. Kumar, A., Rai, P., Daume, H.: Co-regularized multi-view spectral clustering. In: Advances in Neural Information Processing Systems, pp. 1413–1421 (2011)
7. Nakagawa, T., Jirsa, V., Spiegler, A., McIntosh, A., Deco, G.: Bottom up modeling of the connectome: linking structure and function in the resting brain and their changes in aging. Neuroimage 80, 318–329 (2013)
8. Rubinov, M., Sporns, O.: Complex network measures of brain connectivity: uses and interpretations. Neuroimage 52(3), 1059–1069 (2010)
9. Sporns, O., Tononi, G., Kötter, R.: The human connectome: a structural description of the human brain. PLoS Computational Biology 1(4), e42 (2005)
10. Wang, D., Wang, Y., Nie, F., Yan, J., Cai, W., Saykin, A.J., Shen, L., Huang, H.: Human connectome module pattern detection using a new multi-graph minMax cut model. In: Golland, P., Hata, N., Barillot, C., Hornegger, J., Howe, R. (eds.) MICCAI 2014, Part III. LNCS, vol. 8675, pp. 313–320. Springer, Heidelberg (2014)
11. Woolrich, M., Stephan, K.: Biophysical network models and the human connectome. Neuroimage 80, 330–338 (2013)

Semantic 3-D Labeling of Ear Implants Using a Global Parametric Transition Prior

Alexander Zouhar, Carsten Rother, and Siegfried Fuchs

University of Technology Dresden, Germany

Abstract. In this work we consider the problem of sematic part-labeling of 3-D meshesof ear implants. This is a challenging problem and automatic solutions are of high practical relevance, since they help to automate the design of hearing aids. The contribution of this work is a new framework which outperforms existing approaches for this task. To achieve the boost in performance we introduce the new concept of a global parametric transition prior. To our knowledge, this is the first time that such a generic prior is used for 3-D mesh processing, and it may be found useful for a large class of 3-D meshes. To foster more research on the important topic of ear implant labeling, we collected a large data set of 3-D meshes, with associated ground truth labels, which we will make publicly available.

1 Introduction

Semantic part-labeling of organic surfaces is an important task in computer-aided shape modeling and visualization. The problem is to partition a polygonal surface mesh into non overlapping subsurfaces each of which represents a semantic part of the underlying object. Such decomposition into parts is extremely challenging due to the anatomical variability. Moreover, it is typically not possible to consistently infer the transition boundaries between adjacent segments solely from geometric cues, and the need of strong boundary transition priors becomes immanent. Fig. 1 illustrates why this is the case in the personalized computer-aided shape modeling of ear implants. Input to the process is a polygonal surface mesh capturing a patient's outer ear geometry. The essence of the hearing aid design process is captured by a part-labeling of 6 anatomical surface regions and piecewise planar transition boundaries between the labeled segments. The ultimate goal is to minimize the user interactions and to maximize the label quality which involves the shape of the transition boundaries.

In standard 2-D labeling problems it is very common to employ shape priors to drive the segmentation towards a meaningful result. Existing region and boundary models over arbitrary shapes mainly use region and length priors. For example, in [6] the authors distinguish between regions being interior/exterior to each other along with preferred distances between their boundaries. In [7] the authors compute a globally optimal labeling for tiered scenes where the correct order between the objects and the parts is enforced.

© Springer International Publishing Switzerland 2015

N. Navab et al. (Eds.): MICCAI 2015, Part II, LNCS 9350, pp. 177–184, 2015.

DOI: 10.1007/978-3-319-24571-3_22

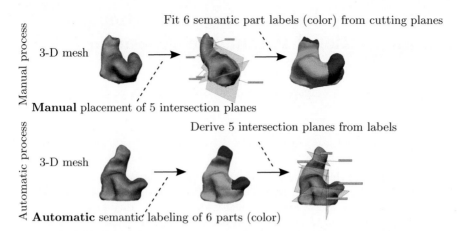

Fig. 1. Semantic 3-D labeling of ear implants in hearing aid (HA) design. **(Top row)**: A domain expert manually places 5 cutting planes along anatomical lines based on hearing aid design rules. This manual procedure is very cumbersome. Part labels (color) corresponding to 6 anatomical regions are derived from the cutting planes. Both, the cutting planes and the labeled regions play a key role in personalized hearing aid design. **(Bottom row)**: Part-labeling using our algorithm. Labels and transition boundaries between segments are optimized jointly (Bottom middle). Planes are derived from the labels (Bottom right).

The most recent state of the art approaches segment and label 3-D surface meshes jointly. The authors in [8], for example, collect statistics of neighboring surface features to learn a conditional random field (CRF) with local pairwise interactions. The prior model in [8], however, is not well suited to adequately constrain the transition boundaries between adjacent segments to an a-priori known parametric form. Consider, for example, the case of subtle shape variations in form of bends which are typical for organic surfaces. In this case the geometry dependent likelihood of a difference in labels, as proposed in [8], tends to be constant (or zero) across the surface.

Not much work exists on the labeling of ear shapes. Similar to [8] the authors in [12] use data dependent pairwise terms to penalize inconsistent labels based on local feature statistics. An alternative approach is presented in [13] where the authors employ multiple shape class specific CRFs with pairwise Potts interactions to overcome the large variability of the ear. While both methods achieve reasonable recognition rates the transition boundaries between adjacent segments tend to deviate significantly from the ground-truth. By comparison, the work in [1] firstly detects a set of generic features of the ear (concavities, elbows, ridges, bumps) which are then used to derive anatomical features of the ear including points, curves, areas and cutting planes. A part labeling may readily be derived from the cutting planes as illustrated in the top row in Fig. 1. Another completely different approach would be to build a human digital ear atlas and to propagate the labels from the atlas to the new data via surface registration (see e.g. [2]). However, due to the variability of the ear it is extremely challenging to consistently establish anatomical correspondence across individuals.

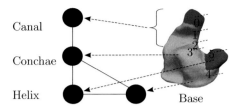

Fig. 2. Part adjacency graph of the human outer ear (courtesy [12]). Adjacent parts (black circles) in the graph are linked (solid line). The colors indicate the anatomical interpretation (dashed line) of the parts. The ear canal is composed of 3 subparts. Numbers represent anatomical part labels in the label set $\mathcal{L}$.

Inspired by the practical challenge of hearing aid design, we address the surface labeling problem by jointly optimizing the part-labels and the piecewise planar transition boundaries between labeled segments as illustrated in the bottom row in Fig. 1. For this we consider 3-D surface meshes of ear implants without additional appearance information, such as color or texture. The main idea in this paper is to model the label distribution as a CRF with local pairwise interactions between labels along with a consistency term that penalizes incompatible arrangements between labels and parametric representations of the segment transition boundaries thereby emphasizing on the global consistency of a labeling. This is why we refer to the latter term as *global parametric transition prior*. Incorporating such a prior into a CRF has several advantages. Firstly, the prior encourages long range compatibility between labels giving rise to a globally consistent part layout. Secondly, the desired shape of the transition boundaries is explicitly enforced. Thirdly, the underlying energy function may be optimized jointly with respect to the labels and to the transition boundaries. Providing that the global parametric transition prior is convex the underlying energy is guaranteed to decrease monotonically during iterative optimization.

2   Model

We consider the following model. A surface mesh $\mathcal{X} = (\mathcal{V}, \mathcal{E})$ consists of vertices $\mathcal{V}$, edges $\mathcal{E}$. A labeling $h : \mathcal{V} \to \mathcal{L}$ of $\mathcal{X}$ assigns a discrete label $h_i \in \mathcal{L} = \{0, 1, 2, 3, 4, 5\}$ to each vertex $i \in \mathcal{V}$. The hearing aid design process gives rise to $|\mathcal{L}| = 6$ anatomical parts as illustrated in figure 2.

The transition boundaries are induced by 5 cutting planes passing through the mesh. Let $b = (b_1, ..., b_B)$ denote a vector of transition boundaries between the adjacent segments with $b_\ell \in \mathbb{R}^4, 1 \le \ell \le B$ denoting a parametric representation of the ℓth boundary. Since the transition boundaries connecting red and green, and yellow and green are induced by the same cutting plane, we may think of these two transitions as one. This is why we have $B = 5$. Moreover, let $W_i(h_i, b, \mathcal{X}) \ge 0$ denote a function that penalizes inconsistent locations of a label h_i relative to all boundaries b_ℓ. We define the behavior of $W_i(h_i, b, \mathcal{X})$ as follows. If a label h_i resides on the *correct side* of all boundaries b_ℓ then $W_i(h_i, b, \mathcal{X}) = 0$ and $W_i(h_i, b, \mathcal{X}) > 0$ otherwise. We define the following energy function:

$$U(h,b,\mathcal{X},\theta) = \sum_{i\in\mathcal{V}} U_i(h_i,\mathcal{X}) + \sum_{\{i,j\}\in\mathcal{E}} U_{ij}(h_i,h_j,\theta_1) + \sum_{i\in\mathcal{V}} W_i(h_i,b,\mathcal{X},\theta_2), \quad (1)$$

where

$$U_i(h_i,\mathcal{X}) = -\log(p(h_i|\mathcal{X})), \quad (2)$$

$$U_{ij}(h_i,h_j,\theta_1) = \theta_1\delta(h_i,h_j), \quad (3)$$

$$W_i(h_i,b,\mathcal{X},\theta_2) = \theta_2\sum_{\ell=1}^{B}\max\{0; 1 - y_\ell(h_i)<b_\ell,z_i>\}. \quad (4)$$

Note that the weighting parameters $\theta_1,\theta_2 \geq 0$ regularize the influence of the individual terms. The variable z_i in Eqn. (4) denotes the homogeneous 3-D coordinates of a vertex $i \in \mathcal{V}$ and $y_\ell(h_i) \in \{-1,1\}$ indicates whether a label h_i is expected to be located above b_ℓ, $(y_\ell(h_i) = 1)$ or below b_ℓ, $(y_\ell(h_i) = -1)$. The expression $< \cdot,\cdot >$ denotes the dot product between two vectors. Eqn. (4) resembles the well known *hinge loss* function (see, e.g., [10]) which in our model gives rise to a convex global parametric transition prior. The function $\delta(h_i,h_j) \in \mathbb{N}$ in Eqn. (3) returns the smallest number of links connecting two nodes in the underlying part adjacency graph

$$\mathcal{G}_A = (\mathcal{L}, \{\{0,1\},\{1,2\},\{2,3\},\{3,4\},\{4,5\},\{3,5\}\}) \quad (5)$$

shown in figure 2, i.e., $\delta(h_i,h_j) = |h_i - h_j|$ if both labels h_i and h_j are in the set $\{4,5\}$ or if both labels are in the set $\{0,1,2,3,4\}$, otherwise we have $\delta(h_i,h_j) = |h_i - h_j| - 1$. While the classical Potts model enforces smoothness it does not prevent incompatible labels from being adjacent. This is achieved by the layout consistency function in Eqn. (3) which also forms a metric over $\mathcal{L}$. Since the part adjacency graph $\mathcal{G}_A$ contains a loop the energy (1) is not submodular. For the unary terms in Eqn. (2) we use a randomized decision forest (see, e.g., [5]) and 3-D shape contexts as local descriptors of the vertices $\mathcal{V}$. 3-D shape contexts [9] are rich, highly discriminative local representations of global shape which we found to work well for our data.

3   Optimization

We use the energy minimization framework to jointly derive an estimate of the labeling h and of the transition boundaries b. Minimizing Eqn. (1) with respect to h and b leads to an optimization problem of the form

$$\min_{h,b} U(h,b,\mathcal{X},\theta). \quad (6)$$

Given h, the problem (6) reduces to

$$\min_{b=(b_1,\dots,b_B)} \sum_{\ell=1}^{B}\sum_{i\in\mathcal{V}}\max\{0; 1 - y_\ell(h_i)<b_\ell,z_i>\}, \quad (7)$$

where we can drop the weighting parameter θ_2 in Eqn. (1) since it does not depend on b. Note, that we have 20 parameters, i.e., $b \in \mathbb{R}^{20}$. As Eqn. (7) is convex and is subdifferentiable a subgradient method [3] is well suited to solve the task. Given an estimate of b optimizing the energy (1) with respect to h may be carried out using the expansion move algorithm [4] since the pairwise terms in Eqn. (3) form a metric over the label set $\mathcal{L}$.

We get a very simple, iterative optimization schema. Given an estimate of h the problem (7) gives rise to a global solution since the transition prior in Eqn. (4) is convex. In turn, given an estimate of the transition boundaries b the expansion move algorithm is guaranteed to find a lower or equal energy labeling h. From this it follows that the energy in Eqn. (1) decreases monotonically. Moreover, the iterative optimization of Eqn. (6) converges more quickly if we initialize b with the least squares estimate of the cutting planes using the initial estimate of h. About 10 iterations are sufficient on our data which for a mesh with $|\mathcal{V}| \approx 20000$ vertices takes about 12s on a standard PC.

4   Learning

Given a labeled training set $\mathcal{T} = \{(\mathcal{X}, h, b)\}$ we use a supervised algorithm to learn the model parameters in Eqn. (1). The unary terms $U_i(h_i, \mathcal{X})$ comprise the decision forest structure as a parameter where we assume that the forest consists of binary trees. The parameters $\theta = (\theta_1, \theta_2)$ regularize the influence of the energy terms $U_{ij}(h_i, h_j, \theta_1)$ and $W_i(h_i, b, \mathcal{X}, \theta_2)$, respectively. Ideally, we would like to learn all model parameters jointly using a single objective function. However, whereas the weights θ_1, θ_2 are continuous variables, the random forest is a large combinatorial set. We therefore adopt a simple two-step heuristic: (1) learning of the decision forest using the labeled training data and the *information gain splitting criterion* and (2) estimation of the weights θ via cross-validation similar to [11]. To this end we allow θ to vary over a discrete possibly very large set. To keep the training process simple we follow the suggestion in [5] and proceed by growing full trees where each leaf contains only one training example.

5   Experiments

For a fair comparison of our method with prior work [1],[12],[13] we derive labels from the detected plane features in [1] as shown in the first row in Fig. 1 whereas for the methods in [12], [13] planes were fit to the inferred labels. We define a measure of label accuracy to compare the inferred labels with the ground-truth. To get a measure of label accuracy per surface we compute the *Dice* coefficient between the area of the estimated labels of the mth part ($m \in \mathcal{L}$) $\hat{\mathcal{A}}_m = \{i \in \mathcal{V} | \hat{h}_i = m\}$ and the area of the ground-truth labels $\mathcal{A}_m = \{i \in \mathcal{V} | h_i = m\}$:

$$\mathrm{LA}(\mathcal{X}, m) = \frac{2|\hat{\mathcal{A}}_m \cap \mathcal{A}_m|}{|\hat{\mathcal{A}}_m \cup \mathcal{A}_m|}, \qquad (8)$$

where $\hat{h}_i$ and h_i denote the estimated label and the ground-truth label of the ith vertex of $\mathcal{X}$, respectively. For a surface $\mathcal{X}$ the label accuracy $\mathrm{LA}(\mathcal{X})$ amounts to

$$\mathrm{LA}(\mathcal{X}) = \frac{1}{|\mathcal{V}|} \sum_{m=0}^{|\mathcal{L}|-1} \mathrm{LA}(\mathcal{X}, m). \tag{9}$$

The value $\mathrm{LA}(\mathcal{X}) \in [0,6]$ ranges between 0 and 6, where 6 is best. Note that in contrast to the classical Hamming loss the *Dice* coefficient avoids overemphasizing large area parts over small area parts. This is important, since the human ear involves regions with both large and small area segments.

We have a novel data set of 427 human outer ear impressions at our disposal which in turn were laser scanned to reconstruct 3-D triangular surface meshes. A typical 3-D mesh of the ear is composed of roughly 20000 vertices with an average resolution of 0.22 mm. Topologically, a reconstructed outer ear surface constitutes a compact, orientable 2-manifold with boundary.

We randomly pick 90% of the surfaces for training while setting the other 10% aside for testing. For model learning the training set was divided in two halves, and the weighting parameters θ_1, θ_2 were optimized against one half via cross-validation. The randomized decision forrest was then retrained using the entire training set. For the parameters we obtain $\theta_1 = 10, \theta_2 = 20$. Inference was carried out using the algorithm in section 3.

Fig. 3(a) shows a test surface labeled by our model (1) without regularization $(\theta_1, \theta_2 = 0)$ and in Fig. 3(b) without global parametric transition prior $(\theta_1 = 10, \theta_2 = 0)$. A visual comparison of the two results with the ground truth in Fig. 3(d) reveals several inaccuracies despite the overall consistent layout. Note, how the transition boundaries deviate from the ground-truth in Fig. 3(d). The label accuracy according to Eqn. (9) is depicted below the surfaces. In Fig. 3(c) we show the result after estimating planes from the label output in Fig. 3(a) via least squares fitting which slightly improves the label accuracy.

Next, in Fig. 4 (first row) we show the best test examples obtained by our competitors in [1], [12], [13] together with the result using our model (1) with

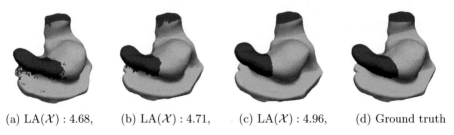

(a) LA($\mathcal{X}$) : 4.68,   (b) LA($\mathcal{X}$) : 4.71,   (c) LA($\mathcal{X}$) : 4.96,   (d) Ground truth

Fig. 3. Label example using (1): (a) without regularization, i.e., $\theta_1, \theta_2 = 0$, (b) without global parametric transition prior, i.e., $\theta_2 = 0$. Note, in (a–b) how the segment boundaries differ from the ground truth. In (c) we show the result after least squares fitting of planes to the labels in (b) and reassigning of misclassified labels after which the label accuracy LA($\mathcal{X}$) $\in [0,6]$ slightly increases (6 is best).

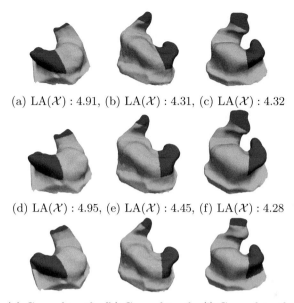

(a) LA($\mathcal{X}$) : 4.91, (b) LA($\mathcal{X}$) : 4.31, (c) LA($\mathcal{X}$) : 4.32

(d) LA($\mathcal{X}$) : 4.95, (e) LA($\mathcal{X}$) : 4.45, (f) LA($\mathcal{X}$) : 4.28

(g) Ground truth, (h) Ground truth, (i) Ground truth

Fig. 4. Most accurate label examples on our test data using (a): [1], (b): [12], (c): [13]. The 2nd row depicts the result using our model (1) with global parametric transition prior (d)-(f). In terms of label accuracy LA($\mathcal{X}$) $\in [0, 6]$ (6 is best) our model performs slightly better except for (f) when compared with (g)-(i).

Table 1. Various statistics computed over 43 test examples: $\overline{\text{LA}(\mathcal{X})}$ (average label accuracy), $\widetilde{\text{LA}(\mathcal{X})}$ (median label accuracy), $\sigma_{\text{LA}(\mathcal{X})}$ (standard deviation of label accuracy). The methods used for comparison were: our model (1) w/o global parametric transition prior ($\theta_2 = 0$), our model (1), the canonical ear signature (CES) [1], the layout CRF with spatial ordering constraints in [12], the joint shape classification and labeling (JSCL) model in [13].

	Our (Eqn. 1,$\theta_2 = 0$)	Our (Eqn. 1)	CES [1]	CRF [12]	JSCL [13]
$\overline{\text{LA}(\mathcal{X})}$	3.98	4.10	3.80	3.28	3.35
$\widetilde{\text{LA}(\mathcal{X})}$	4.00	4.10	3.79	3.27	3.31
$\sigma_{\text{LA}(\mathcal{X})}$	0.47	0.48	0.49	0.60	0.60

global parametric transition prior, i.e., $\theta_2 > 0$ (Fig. 4 (second row)). In terms of label accuracy LA($\mathcal{X}$) our algorithm performs slightly better when compared with the ground-truth in Fig. 4 (third row).

For a quantitative comparison of the methods several statistics were computed over the test data which we summarize in table 1. From the table one can see that on average our model (1) with global parametric transition prior performs best. While the methods [12], [13] perform equally well they were outperformed by [1]. Also note, that our model (1) without global parametric transition prior ($\theta_2 = 0$) achieves a higher label accuracy than [1] after least squares fitting of the planes as illustrated in Fig. 3.

6   Conclusions and Future Work

We have proposed a new framework for the semantic labeling of 3-D meshes of ear implants. Specifically, we incorporated a parametric representation of the transition boundaries into the labeling model which in the case of ear implants was used to enforce planar transitions between the parts. This combined model lead to a performance boost in label accuracy and outperformed previous methods for ear implant labeling. We will make our data set publicly available.

References

1. Baloch, S., Melkisetoglu, R., Flöry, S., Azernikov, S., Slabaugh, G., Zouhar, A., Fang, T.: Automatic detection of anatomical features on 3D ear impressions for canonical representation. In: Jiang, T., Navab, N., Pluim, J.P.W., Viergever, M.A. (eds.) MICCAI 2010, Part III. LNCS, vol. 6363, pp. 555–562. Springer, Heidelberg (2010)
2. Baloch, S., Zouhar, A., Fang, T.: Deformable registration of organic shapes via surface intrinsic integrals: application to outer ear surfaces. In: Menze, B., Langs, G., Tu, Z., Criminisi, A. (eds.) MICCAI 2010. LNCS, vol. 6533, pp. 11–20. Springer, Heidelberg (2011)
3. Boyd, S., Vandenberghe, L.: Convex Optimization. Cambridge Un. Press (2004)
4. Boykov, Y., Veksler, O., Zabih, R.: Fast approximate energy minimization via graph cuts. IEEE Trans. Pattern Analysis, and Machine Intelligence (2001)
5. Criminisi, A., Shotton, J.: Decision Forests for Computer Vision and Medical Image Analysis. Springer Publishing Company, Incorporated (2013)
6. Delong, A., Boykov, Y.: Globally optimal segmentation of multi-region objects. In: ICCV, pp. 285–292. IEEE (2009)
7. Felzenszwalb, P.F., Veksler, O.: Tiered scene labeling with dynamic programming. In: CVPR, pp. 3097–3104. IEEE (2010)
8. Kalogerakis, E., et al.: Learning 3D mesh segmentation and labeling. In: SIGG (2010)
9. Koertgen, M., Park, G.J., Novotni, M., Klein, R.: 3D shape matching with 3d shape contexts. In: Proc. 7th Central European Seminar on Comp. Graphics (2003)
10. Nello, C., Shawe-Taylor, J.: An Introduction to Support Vector Machines and Other Kernel-based Learning Methods, 1 edn. Cambridge University Press (2000)
11. Winn, J., Shotton, J.: The layout consistent random field for recognizing and segmenting partially occluded objects. In: CVPR (2006)
12. Zouhar, A., Baloch, S., Tsin, Y., Fang, T., Fuchs, S.: Layout consistent segmentation of 3-D meshes via conditional random fields and spatial ordering constraints. In: Jiang, T., Navab, N., Pluim, J.P.W., Viergever, M.A. (eds.) MICCAI 2010, Part III. LNCS, vol. 6363, pp. 113–120. Springer, Heidelberg (2010)
13. Zouhar, A., Schlesinger, D., Fuchs, S.: Joint shape classification and labeling of 3-D objects using the energy minimization framework. In: Weickert, J., Hein, M., Schiele, B. (eds.) GCPR 2013. LNCS, vol. 8142, pp. 71–80. Springer, Heidelberg (2013)

Learning the Correlation Between Images and Disease Labels Using Ambiguous Learning

Tanveer Syeda-Mahmood, Ritwik Kumar, and Colin Compas

IBM Almaden Research Center, San Jose, CA, USA

Abstract. In this paper, we present a novel approach to candidate ground truth label generation for large-scale medical image collections by combining clinically-relevant textual and visual analysis through the framework of ambiguous label learning. In particular, we present a novel string matching algorithm for extracting disease labels from patient reports associated with imaging studies. These are assigned as ambiguous labels to the images of the study. Visual analysis is then performed on the images of the study and diagnostically relevant features are extracted from relevant regions within images. Finally, we learn the correlation between the ambiguous disease labels and visual features through an ambiguous SVM learning framework. The approach was validated in a large Doppler image collection of over 7000 images showing a scalable way to semi-automatically ground truth large image collections.

1 Introduction

With big data becoming relevant to medical imaging community, there is a growing need to more easily label these images for disease occurrences in a semi-automatic fashion to ease the labeling burden of clinical experts. Often medical imaging studies have reports associated with them that mention the disease labels. However, due to the large variety in spoken utterances, spotting disease labels using known medical vocabularies is difficult. Diseases may be implicitly mentioned, occur in negative sense, or be denoted through abbreviations or synonyms. Table 2 illustrates this problem through sample sentences taken from actual reports (Column 2) and their corresponding medical vocabulary phrases (Column 1). Associating disease labels of reports with relevant images in the study is also a difficult problem ordinarily requiring clinical expertise to spot the anomaly within the images. Figure 1 shows three images within the same patient study. An excerpt from the corresponding report is shown in Table 1. It is not clear from this data, what labels should be assigned to these images.

The goal of this work is to address this problem by studying the correlation between anomaly depicting feature regions within images with potential disease labels through an ambiguous label learning formulation. Specifically, we extract disease depicting features from images and correlate with potentially ambiguous labels extracted from reports using a convex optimization learning formulation that minimizes a surrogate loss appropriate for the ambiguous labels. While the

© Springer International Publishing Switzerland 2015
N. Navab et al. (Eds.): MICCAI 2015, Part II, LNCS 9350, pp. 185–193, 2015.
DOI: 10.1007/978-3-319-24571-3_23

text-based disease label extraction method is generally applicable across modalities and specialties, disease-depicting visual features will need to be customized per modality and anatomical specialty. We illustrate this methodology, therefore, by restricting to images to cardiac Doppler ultrasound imaging. As shown in Figure 1, these images possess sufficient variety of disease-specific and localized velocity patterns to serve as a good case to validate this methodology.

2   Related Work

The work reported here overlaps with work in three inter-disciplinary fields. There is considerable work in the text mining literature on concept extraction including sentence extraction, stop-word removal, term spotting, and negation finding[10,8,6]. While these algorithms have reasonable precision, their recall rate is low due to low tolerance for deviations in spoken phrases during string matching. Similarly, the work in Doppler image analysis has mostly focused on extracting the Doppler envelope traces[13,15,14,4]. However, important disease-specific information is also available in the interior of the Doppler regions such as the left ventricular outflow tract (LVOT), which has not been addressed. Finally, the automatic labeling of ground truth data is being actively addressed through crowdsourcing[11] in social media, using textual annotations of photos [2] and learning to reduce the ambiguity in the associations between image and surrounding text[5]. However, these approaches have addressed the classification problem [5,7,1,3] rather than the training problem as in our case.

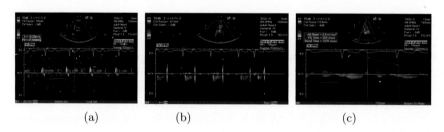

(a)   (b)   (c)

Fig. 1. Illustration of Doppler images from a single study. An extract of corresponding report shown in Table 1.

3   Extracting Disease Labels from Reports

Our approach to disease label detection in reports uses a vocabulary of disease terms from reference medical ontologies from UMLS. To spot the occurrence of the disease phrase within reports, we develop a new string matching algorithm called the *longest common suffix (LCF)* algorithm. Given a query vocabulary phrase$S = <s_1s_2...s_K>$ of K words and a candidate sentence $T = <t_1t_2...t_N>$ of N words, we define longest common suffix as $LCF(S,T) = <p_1p_2...p_L>$,

Table 1. Illustration of an extract of text report corresponding the study with images shown in Figure 1.

> Comparison: Prior examination reports are available and were reviewed for comparison purposes.Since the prior study, the mitral regurgitation is now moderate as opposed to mild. Summary: 1. Severe aortic stensosis.
> 2. The aortic valve is restricted, thickened and calcified.
> 3. Mildly dilated left atrium.
> 4. Normal left ventricular function.
> 5. Moderate mitral stenosis.

where L is the largest subset of words from S that found a partial match in T and p_i is a partial match of a word $s_i \in S$ to a word in T. A word s_i in S is said to partially match a word t_j in T if it shares a maximum length common prefix p_i such that $\frac{|p_i|}{\max\{|s_i|,|t_j|\}} > \tau$. If we make the threshold $\tau = 1.0$, this reduces to the case of finding exact matches to words of S. Note that this formulation is different from the conventional longest common subsequence (LCS) string matching as there is an emphasis on character grouping into words and the use of word prefixes to relate words in the English language. Using dynamic programming

Table 2. Disease label extraction from text results.

Disease Label	Sentence detected to contain the disease label
Aortic sclerosis,	Marked **aortic sclerosis** present with evidence of **stenosis**.
Aortic stenosis	
Fracture of clavicle	There is a transverse **fracture of** the mid left **clavicle** with mild superior angulation of the fracture fragment.
Perforation of Esophagus	A contrast esophagram shows **esophageal perforation** of the anterior left esophagus at C4-5 with extra-luminal contrast seen.
Edema of lower extremity	Extremities: **Lower extremity** trace pitting **edema** and bilateral lower extremity toe ulceration.
Atrial dilatation	Left atrium: Left **atrial** size is mildly **dilated**.
Abnormal findings in lung	**abn findings-lung** field.

to implement the longest common subfix algorithm, the best alignment between a vocabulary phrase S and candidate sentence T is found by keeping an array $C[i,j]$ to calculate the score of matching a fragment of S up to the ith word and fragment of T up to the jth word. We then update the dynamic programming matrix according to the algorithm shown in Algorithm 1. Here $p_{max}(i,j)$ is the longest prefix of the strings (s_i, t_j) and δ is a mismatch penalty, which controls the separation between matched words and prevents words that are too far apart in a sentence from being associated with the same vocabulary phrase. Using this algorithm, a vocabulary phrase S is said to be detected in a sentence T if

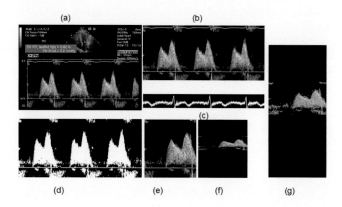

Fig. 2. Illustration of SIFT feature extraction from Doppler ultrasound images. (a) Original image. (c) Selected region of interest containing Doppler spectrum. (d) Detected EKG pattern in the image of (c) (shown expanded for clarity). (d) Doppler spectrum outlined by Otsu thresholding. (e) Single period Doppler spectrum extracted from the spectrum of (d) by detecting periodicities in the thresholded waveform and synchronizing with the R-wave of the EKG. (f) Scaled Doppler spectrum after converting to velocity coordinates. (g) SIFT features extracted in the scaled Doppler spectrum of (f).

$\frac{|LCF(S,T)|}{|S|} \geq \Gamma$ for some threshold Γ. The choice of τ and Γ affect precision and recall in matching and was chosen to meet specified criteria for precision and recall based on an ROC curve analysis on labeled collection. Using a pre-indexing step for large vocabularies, the LCF matching only needs to be invoked on likely phrases keeping the resulting $O(n^2)$ complexity still manageable for small n.

Table 2 shows the results of applying the longest common subfix algorithm on a variety of sentences found in textual reports. It can be seen that the algorithm spots multiple vocabulary word occurrences in a sentence and under considerable word distortions (e.g. dilatation versus dilated), even without a deep understanding of their linguistic origins. The algorithm uses other enhancements for negation pattern finding, abbreviation expansions and fast indexing of vocabularies which are skipped here for brevity.

4   Feature Extraction from Doppler Images

In Doppler echocardiography images, the clinically relevant region is known to be within the Doppler spectrum, contained in a rectangular region of interest as shown in Figure 1. The shape of the velocity envelope, its amplitude (scale), as well as its density within the envelope convey important discriminatory information about diseases[14]. Our method of extracting Doppler spectrum uses the same pre-processing steps of: region of interest detection, EKG extraction, periodicity detection, and envelope extraction as described in [14] but adds the

Algorithm 1. Longest Common Subfix Algorithm

LCF(S,T):
1: **Input/Output** Input: two strings (S,T). Output: an alignment score.
2: **Initialize** $c[i,0] = 0, c[0,j] = 0, 0 \le i \le K, 0 \le j \le N$.
3: **Iterate** for $(1 \le i \le K)$

    for $(1 \le j \le N)$

      $\rho_{ij} = \frac{|p_{max}(i,j)|}{\max\{|s_i|,|t_j|\}}$

      If $C[i-1, j-1] + \rho_{ij} > C[i-1, j]$ and

        $C[i-1, j-1] + \rho_{ij} > C[i, j-1]$

          $C[i,j] = C[i-1, j-1] + \rho_{ij}$

    else

      if $(C[i-1, j] + \rho_{ij} > C[i, j-1]$

        $C[i,j] = C[i-1, j] - \delta$

      else

        $C[i,j] = C[i, j-1] - \delta$

two enhancements below that are necessary to (a) translate the visual measurements to the more clinically relevant velocity measurements and, (b) produce more discriminable features that consider density of Doppler spectra in addition to their shape.

Table 3. Illustration of accuracy of disease label detection in textual reports.

Algorithms	Average Precision	Average Recall
LanguageWare	80.1%	48.1%
CTakes	34.03%	59.6%
LCF	89.2%	83.25%

4.1 Building a Common Doppler Reference Frame

Since the amplitude of Doppler velocity is important for disease discrimination, we recover the amplitude units from the text calibration markers on Doppler images using the open-source optical character recognition algorithm 'Tesseract'.

To render the recovered velocity values in a common reference frame for feature extraction and comparison, we transform the pixels in the Doppler spectrum region using a similarity transform to a reference image of fixed size (W_M x H_M) corresponding to the maximum range of velocities $V_M = V_{Ma} - V_{Mb}$. Then given any single period Doppler spectrum image of size (W_I x H_I) representing a range of velocities $= V_I = (V_{Ia} - V_{Ib})$ where the suffix a and b refer to direction , we can linearly transform every pixel point (x, y) to a point (x', y') as $y' = s_h * y + t_h$ $x' = s_w * x + t_w$ where $s_w = W_M/W_I$, $t_w = 0$, since all the spectra are aligned with respect to the start of the R-wave. Also, $s_h = \frac{V_I}{V_M} * \frac{H_M}{H_I}$, and $t_h = 0.5 * H_M - y_0$, where y_0 is the baseline for the Doppler spectrum.

4.2   Feature Extraction from Doppler Spectrum

To capture the intensity and shape information from both the velocity envelopes and interior regions, we use the dense SIFT feature descriptor [9]. However, we only apply the descriptor in the region between upper and lower Doppler envelopes to capture the essential clinical information. To reduce the high dimensionality of SIFT features further, we cluster them to form code books similar to the bag of words model. Using these enhancements, the steps in the derivation of visual features are illustrated in Figure 2. Note that even though the SIFT descriptor itself is uninterpretable clinically, its selective application in the clinically relevant Doppler regions produces discriminable features useful for correlating with disease.

5   Ambiguity Reduction Using Machine Learning

Given a set of feature vectors $X = \{x_i\}, i = 1...N$ corresponding to all training images, where each sample x_i is associated with a set of ambiguous labels $Y_i = \{a_{ij}\}, j = 1...M_i$, the problem is to train a classifier that could reduce the ambiguity and obtain at least one label for sample from X. Let the set of possible labels be $\{1, 2..., L\}$. Using the convex optimization formulation proposed in [5], for each class label a, we define a linear classifier as $g^a(x) = w^a \cdot x$. Given scores from all the classifiers $\{g^a(x)\}$ for a sample x, one could obtain the best label as $\arg\max_a g^a(x)$. We denote the overall classifier as $g(x)$, which is parameterized by $\{g^a(x)\}$ or $d \times L$ parameters. Following [5], we learn the parameters of g, by minimizing the following objective function

$$min_w \frac{1}{2}||w||_2^2 + C||\xi||_2^2 \qquad (1)$$

such that $s.t. \frac{1}{|Y_i|} \sum_{a \in Y_i} w^a \cdot x_i \geq 1 - \xi_i, -w^a \cdot x_i \geq 1 - \xi_{ia} \forall a \notin Y_i$. Here w is a concatenation of $\{w^a\}$. This formulation encodes the idea that on an average, over the set of associated ambiguous labels, the classifier should maximize the margin with respect to each incorrect label. Once this classifier has been trained, given a new sample x, we can obtain its classification score with respect to each of the labels, since all w^a are now known. Note that this approach is different

Table 4. Illustration of Doppler envelope detection accuracy in Doppler imaging.

Images tested	ROI accuracy	EKG accuracy	Period accuracy	% Normalization accuracy
7332	99.3%	88.1%	82.2%	97.8%

from training a single SVM for each label or a multi-class SVM, since the best learner is chosen based on minimizing the empirical risk from the ambiguous 0/1 loss defined over the ambiguous label set as shown by the summation term in Equation 1.

6   Results

To validate our methodology, we assembled a large collection of over 7148 cardiac ultrasound studies from about 2059 patients from the electronic health records of a nearby collaborating hospital. Isolating the CW Doppler images within those studies that had associated cardiology reports, we obtained 7332 CW Doppler images that needed ground truth labeling.

6.1   Accuracy of Disease Label Extraction

To evaluate the accuracy of disease label detection in reports, a subset of 800 reports were divided among 5 experts who noted the disease labels and the sentences in which they occurred. The resulting performance is indicated in Table 3 indicating 89% precision and over 83% recall in the label extraction from reports. These numbers outperformed the commercial LanguageWare software that uses an exact string matching algorithm with proprietary negation finding, and the cTakes algorithm[12] as shown in that table. Our method has a better recall due to its ability to tolerate word variations using the LCF algorithm.

Table 5. Illustration of agreement of labels learned with manual verification.

Images	Ambiguity	Maximum	Avg Labels		Manually
tried	set size	Labels	before	after	verified
5641	36	13	3.58	1.03	92.3%

6.2   Accuracy of Doppler Spectrum Extraction

Next, we evaluated the accuracy of Doppler spectrum extraction by manually noting the number of errors for each of the image processing steps of ROI detection, EKG extraction, periodicity estimation, and velocity unit estimation. The results of testing over the 7332 image collection is shown in Table 4 for each stage of the image processing in terms of percentage found correct.

6.3   Ambiguity Reduction Using Machine Learning

By limiting the detected disease labels to be within the most frequent labels (there were 36 diseases that were frequently occurring), we obtained an average of 3.58 labels per image with a maximum of 13 labels for some of the images as shown in Table 5. By applying the ambiguous label learning algorithm, we were able to reduce the ambiguity to an average of 1.03 labels. To evaluate the quality of the labels produced by the learning, we randomly selected a set of 650 images from the labeled collection. We then had experts produce independent labels for the images by observing them within the corresponding ultrasound study and reading the associated echocardiogram report. There was 92% agreement

Table 6. Illustration of classification accuracy improvement using reduced ambiguity labels.

Training images from ground truth	Testing images from ground truth	Ambiguity size	Error with ambiguous labels	Error with reduced labels
4513	1128	36	34.3%	8.2%

in the labels produced by these evaluations with the manual labeling indicating the validity of our method. Interestingly, when the visual features were changed from SIFT code books on and within Doppler envelopes to features only on the Doppler envelope as described in [14], the manual validation accuracy with the resulting labels went down to 64.7%. This indicated that the features within interior regions of the envelopes were relevant for learning the visual-text label associations.

Lastly, to show that label reduction during training helps subsequent classification accuracy, we set aside 20% of the original training data for testing. We used the learning from ambiguous labels framework first with the larger set of labels for each training image (Column 4, Table 6), and then with the smaller set of ambiguous labels (Column 5). As can be seen from Table 6, the overall classification accuracy is higher with smaller set of ambiguous labels than the original labels, thus justifying the ambiguity reduction step in the training stage prior to classification.

7   Conclusions

In this paper, we address for the first time, the problem of candidate ground truth label generation of large medical image collections by combining textual and visual features within an ambiguous label learning framework. While manual verification of the selected labels may still be desirable, the automatic ground truth labeling process is expected to significantly reduce the visual examination burden for clinical experts.

References

1. Babenko, B.: Multiple Instance Learning: Algorithms and Applications. Springer (2009)
2. Barnard, K., et al.: Matching words and pictures. Journal of Machine Learning Research 3, 1107–1135 (2003)
3. Bordes, A., et al.: Label ranking under ambiguous supervision for learning semantic correspondences. In: Proc. 27th Intl. Conf. on Machine Learning, ICML (2010)
4. Chen, T., et al.: Psar: Predictive space aggregated regression and its application in valvular heart disease classification. In: Proc. ISBI (2013)
5. Cour, T., Sapp, B., Ben Taskar, C.J.: Learning from ambiguously labeled images. In: Proceedings CVPR 2009 (2009)
6. Goldstein, I., et al.: Three approaches to automatic assignment of icd9-cm codes to radiology reports. In: Proc. Annual Symposium on American Medical Informatics Association (AMIA), pp. 279–283 (2007)

7. Jin, R., Ghahramani, Z.: Learning with multiple labels. In: Proceedings NIPS, pp. 897–904 (2002)
8. Long, W.: Extracting diagnosis from discharge summaries. In: Proc. Annual Symposium on American Medical Informatics Association (AMIA), pp. 470–474 (2005)
9. Lowe, D.G.: Object recognition from local scale-invariant features. In: Proceedings of the International Conference on Computer Vision, ICCV 1999, vol. 2 (1999)
10. Patrick, J., et al.: Identifying clinical concepts in unstructured clinical notes using existing knowledge within the corpus. In: IEEE International Conference on Computer-based Medical Systems, pp. 66–71 (2010)
11. Rodríguez, A.F., Muller, H.: Ground truth generation in medical imaging: a crowdsourcing-based iterative approach. In: CrowdMM 2012 Proceedings of the ACM Multimedia 2012 Workshop on Crowdsourcing for Multimedia, pp. 9–14 (2012)
12. Savova, G.K.: Mayo clinical text analysis and knowledge extraction system (ctakes): Architecture, component evaluation, and applications. Journal of AMIA 17, 507–513 (2010)
13. Shechner, O., Sheinovitz, M., Feinberg, M., Greenspan, H.: Image analysis of doppler echocardiography for patients with atrial fibrillation. In: Proc. ISBI (2004)
14. Syeda-Mahmood, T., Turaga, P., Beymer, D., Wang, F., Amir, A., Greenspan, H., Pohl, K.: Shape-based similarity retrieval of doppler images for clinical decision support. In: IEEE CVPR, pp. 855–862 (2010)
15. Tschirren, J., Lauer, R.M., Sonka, M.: Automated analysis of doppler ultrasound velocity flow diagrams. IEEE Trans. on Medical Imaging 20, 1422–1425 (2001)

Longitudinal Analysis of Brain Recovery after Mild Traumatic Brain Injury Based on Groupwise Consistent Brain Network Clusters

Hanbo Chen[1,*], Armin Iraji[2,*], Xi Jiang[1], Jinglei Lv[1], Zhifeng Kou[2,**], and Tianming Liu[1,**]

[1] Cortical Architecture Imaging and Discovery Laboratory, Department of Computer Science and Bioimaging Research Center, The University of Georgia, Athens, GA, USA
[2] Biomedical Engineering and Radiology, Wayne State University, Detroit, Michigan, USA

Abstract. Traumatic brain injury (TBI) affects over 1.5 million Americans each year, and more than 75% of TBI cases are classified as mild (mTBI). Several functional network alternations have been reported after mTBI; however, the network alterations on a large scale, particularly on connectome scale, are still unknown. To analyze brain network, in a previous work, 358 landmarks named dense individualized common connectivity based cortical landmarks (DICCCOL) were identified on cortical surface. These landmarks preserve structural connection consistency and maintain functional correspondence across subjects. Hence DICCCOLs have been shown powerful in identifying connectivity signatures in affected brains. However, on such fine scales, the longitudinal changes in brain network of mTBI patients were complicated by the noise embedded in the systems as well as the normal variability of individuals at different times. Faced with such problems, we proposed a novel framework to analyze longitudinal changes from the perspective of network clusters. Specifically, multiview spectral clustering algorithm was applied to cluster brain networks based on DICCCOLs. And both structural and functional networks were analyzed. Our results showed that significant longitudinal changes were identified from mTBI patients that can be related to the neurocognitive recovery and the brain's effort to compensate the effect of injury.

Keywords: traumatic brain injury, brain network clustering, DTI, fMRI, longitudinal analysis, t-test.

1 Introduction

Mild traumatic brain injury (mTBI) accounts for over one million emergency visits each year in the United States [1]. Most mTBI patients have normal findings in clinical neuroimaging. Advanced magnetic resonance imaging (MRI) has detected microstructural damage in major white matter tracts by diffusion tensor imaging (DTI), and

---

* Co-first authors.
** Co-corresponding authors.

© Springer International Publishing Switzerland 2015
N. Navab et al. (Eds.): MICCAI 2015, Part II, LNCS 9350, pp. 194–201, 2015.
DOI: 10.1007/978-3-319-24571-3_24

functional network alternations by functional MRI (fMRI) [2, 3]. However, the field is still short of investigations on the overall extent of structural and functional network disruptions after mTBI and its recovery process. Moreover, there is lack of investigation in the alteration of connectivity on large-scale brain networks after mTBI and their recovery process. We hypothesize that mTBI results in network connectivity changes, and brain structural and functional recovery occurs over time.

In a literature work, Zhu et al. identified 358 landmarks on cortical surface that preserve structural connection consistency across subjects named dense individualized common connectivity-based cortical landmarks (DICCCOL). The previous studies have shown that DICCCOLs are highly reproducible across individuals [4, 5] and they also preserves structural and functional correspondence across individuals [6]. Moreover, in recent studies, Zhu et al. have shown that, by taking these DICCCOLs as network nodes, the connections between them could be taken as connectome signature of mental diseases such as mild cognitive impairment [7] or prenatal cocaine exposure [8]. With DICCCOL framework, the brain network alternations after injury and its recovery process of mTBI patients could be analyzed.

Intuitively, the changes in network connections during brain recovery can be derived by comparing the MRI scans of healthy subjects and the mTBI patients using t-test. Yet a considerable amount of changes in brain network connections were also seen in the two scans of the same group of healthy control (HC) subjects (E.g. the functional connection changes shown in Fig. 1). This result suggested that pairwise network connections comparison is sensitive to individual variability as well as system noise on a fine scale and thus cannot serve our purpose.

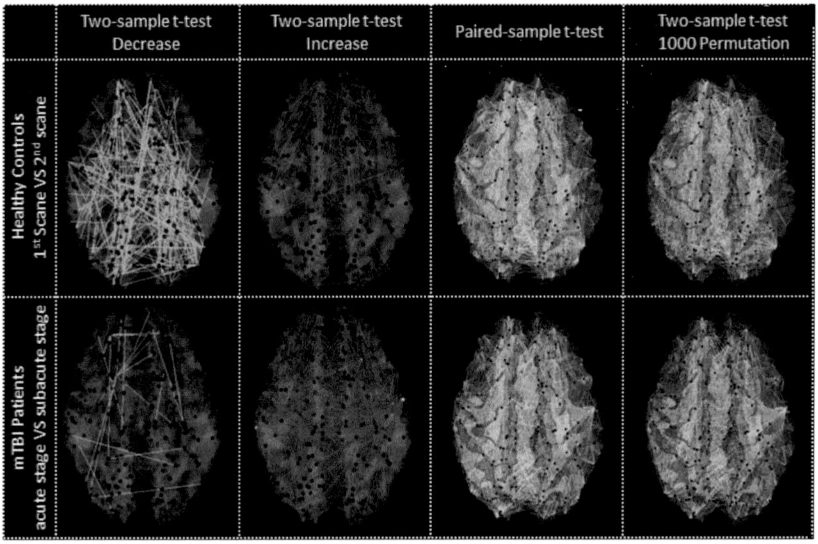

Fig. 1. Significantly different (P<0.05) pairwise functional connections among DICCCOLs between two scans of each population identified by different types of t-test.

Faced with such problem, we addressed the issue from the level of connectivity changes of brain network clusters. Whole brain networks were clustered into group-wisely common sub-networks based on the multiview spectral clustering algorithm. Each network cluster is a subset of nodes that are more densely connected within the cluster than between clusters. By comparing the connection changes within and between the clusters, the noises due to individual variability were greatly diminished and we have observed consistent pattern of disruption in structural and functional networks after mTBI. Interestingly, over time the decrease in structural connectivity is accompanied by the increase in functional connectivity. This finding is in agreement with the temporally evolving and deteriorating nature of brain injury. On the other hand, the increase in functional connectivity suggested that brain is highly plastic as it tries to recruit more regions and remodel the functional connectivity to compensate the alteration in structural connectivity. Together, these results may shed light to the network alteration mechanism of brain recovery and plasticity.

2   Data Acquisition

This study was approved by the local Human Investigation Committee. Written informed consent was obtained from each subject before enrollment. In this study, the DTI and rsfMRI data were acquired from 24 healthy subjects twice in two independent scans and from 16 mTBI patients at both acute and subacute stages after injure. In acute stage, patients were scanned 82.64/17 (average/median) hours after injury. For subacute stage, patients returned 4-6 weeks after injury to take the second scan.

Data were collected on a 3-Tesla Siemens Verio scanner with a 32-channel radiofrequency head-only coil. Diffusion imaging was acquired using a gradient echo EPI sequence in 30 diffusion gradients directions with the following parameters: b = 1000, TR = 13300 ms, TE = 124 ms, slice thickness = 2 mm, pixel resolution =1.333 x 1.333 mm, matrix size = 192 x 192, flip angle = 90°, and number of averages (NEX) =2. Resting state functional imaging was performed by a gradient echo EPI sequence with the following imaging parameters: TR/TE = 2000/30 ms, slice thickness = 3.5 mm, slice gap = 0.595 mm, pixel spacing size = 3.125 x 3.125 mm, matrix size = 64 x 64, flip angle = 90°, 240 volumes for whole-brain coverage, NEX = 1. During resting state scans, subjects were instructed to keep their eyes closed.

3   Method

Each DICCCOL node is a region of interest (ROI) [4]. The connectivity between DICCCOLs was obtained based on DTI/rsfMRI data to construct structural/functional networks. The group-wise common clusters were calculated based on multi-view spectral clustering algorithm [5] for structural or functional networks separately by taking the brain network of each subject as a 'view'. Based on those clusters, we further analyzed the connection changes of mTBI patients over the recovery period.

3.1   Preprocessing

Preprocessing of DTI data was performed using FSL toolbox [9] which includes eddy current correction, skull and background removal, fractional anisotropic (FA) estimation. The white matter (WM)/grey matter (GM) was segmented based on FA image and WM surface was then reconstructed [10, 11]. DTI tractography was performed based on MedINRIA [12] to reconstruct fiber streamlines. For rsfMRI data, the first 5 volumes were removed before preprocessing. Then, brain extraction, motion correction, slice-time correction, spatially smoothing (FWHM=5mm), temporal prewhitening, grand mean removal, and temporally high-pass filter were applied on rsfMRI data accordingly in FSL [9].

3.2   Predict DICCCOLs and Construct Brain Networks

DICCCOLs were predicted based on the DTI derived fiber streamlines and the reconstructed cortical surface by using the tool downloaded from http://dicccol.cs.uga.edu/. In brief, DICCCOL is composed by 358 cortical landmarks obtained based on groupwise training process described in [4]. These landmarks were defined as a patch on cortical surface and the DTI derived fiber connection profile of each patch is consistent across individuals. To predict DICCCOLs on a new subject, the subject's brain will be aligned to the template space. Then for each ROI, the closest point to the template center will be identified on the subject's reconstructed cortical surface as initial location. By searching around the neighborhood of this initial location, the patch with similar structural connection profile to the template will be identified as the location of this ROI on the new subject.

Based on obtained 358 ROIs, brain networks were reconstructed by similar approaches in [5, 7]. The average fractional anisotrophy (FA) value along the fiber streamlines connecting each pair of DICCCOLs was taken as the structural connection strength. And if there is no fiber streamline connecting two DICCCOLs, the connection strength between them will be set 0. The functional connection strength between each pair of DICCCOLs was defined by the Pearson correlation between preprocessed rsfMRI signals derived from GM area of DICCCOLs. The obtained structural and functional connection matrices were represented by symmetric affinity matrices.

3.3   Multi-view Spectral Clustering

To analyze brain network alternations of mTBI patients as well as the network longitudinal changes during recovery, common network clusters were needed for comparison between different populations and different stages. Thus, we applied multi-view spectral clustering which has been shown to be reliable in obtaining group-wisely consistent brain network clusters [5]. Specifically, the brain network of each subjects were taken as a view. Its affinity matrix W will be projected to the eigenspace of the graph Laplacian of other views and then projected back such that:

$$proj(W,U) = (UU^T W + (UU^T W)^T)/2 \qquad (1)$$

where $U = \Re^{n \times k}$ is the first k eigenvectors corresponding to the top k smallest eigenvalues of graph Laplacian of other affinity matrices and $n = 358$. The idea is similar to principal component analysis. Since the space represented by the top eigenvectors of graph Laplacian of affinity matrices can be viewed as the principal direction of corresponding graphs in which the graph expands most, by projecting other graphs to this space, the common part (the connections within clusters) will be retained and the disagreed part (the connections between clusters) will be eliminated. Then by doing so iteratively, the networks will converge to common connections and the common clusters across individuals will be retained. For the detailed mathematical derivation, algorithm description, and experimental validations, one can refer to [5].

4   Results

By performing multi-view spectral clustering on all the 80 affinity matrices derived from the data obtained from the two scans of 24 healthy controls and 16 mTBI patients, the clustering algorithm has converged to 13 common structural network clusters and 8 common functional network clusters (Fig. 2). The network clusters largely agree with the ones obtained from young healthy subjects in previous works [5]. The average within and between clusters connectivity are shown in Fig. 3(a) for structural networks and Fig. 3(c) for functional networks, respectively. It is obvious that within cluster connections is stronger than between cluster connections.

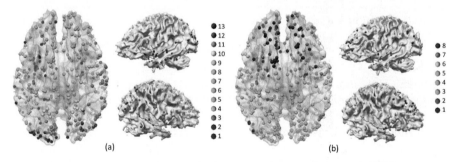

Fig. 2. Visualization of brain network clusters. Each DICCCOL is represented by a bubble color-coded by clusters (color legend on right). (a) 13 group-wise consistent structural network clusters. (b) 8 group-wise consistent functional network clusters.

For structural connections, the connectivity pattern is relatively similar between patient and control populations. Comparing the differences between the two scans of the same group (Fig. 3(b)), the brain network of normal controls is relatively consistent between two scans while those of mTBI patients from the acute stage to the subacute stage presented significant changes in brain networks. However, it is intriguing that the majority of the changes are the decreased connection strength during recovery such as those highlighted by green and red arrows in Fig. 3(b). Another intriguing observation is that, some of these changes were not detected by paired-sample t-test (as highlighted by red arrows in Fig. 3(b)). Meanwhile, with paired-sample t-test, the connections that do not change significantly could be selected (magenta arrows in Fig. 3(b)). This is partially because though the connections strength is extremely small, the t-test will still pick up the connections when there is relative significant difference between groups (E.g. average connection is 0.01 for one set of data and 0.005 for another set). However, we are not interested in such connection in our analysis. And we would like to call attention on the usage of t-test in such applications.

Similar observation has also been obtained in functional connection between clusters. The network connection between and within clusters remained similar between two scans of healthy subjects while significant changes in cluster connections were observed between two stages of mTBI patients Fig. 3(d)).

In our analysis, we noticed that the connection within and between structural cluster 5 and cluster 12 both decreased in subacute stage. By comparing the structural network of mTBI patients and healthy controls, the connections related to these two clusters is also weaker than normal controls for patients (Fig. 4). These two clusters locate at the occipital lobe and temporal lobe of right hemisphere Fig. 5(a). Since the major fiber pathway in this area is inferior longitudinal fasciculus (ILF) and uncinate fasciculus (UF), it may suggest longitudinal degradation of these tracts over time. Interestingly, the functional connection between cluster 2 (temporal lobe, Fig. 5(b)) and other clusters increased significantly during brain recovery, which is in consistency with the observation based on structural networks.

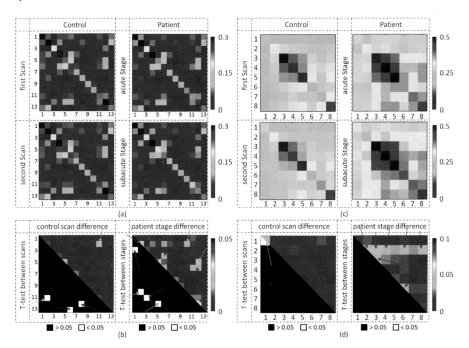

Fig. 3. Average (a) structural connection density or (c) functional connection strength within and between clusters for each group of scans. Comparison between two scans for each population for (b) structural or (d) functional connection were shown on the bottom accordingly. In the matrix shown in (b) and (d), top right part is the absolute difference between the average connection densities of two scans/stages; and bottom left part is the significantly changed connections (P<0.05) tested by paired-sample t-test.

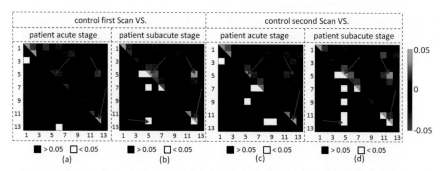

Fig. 4. Comparison of average structural connection densities between healthy controls and mTBI patients. In each subfigure, top right part of the matrix is the difference (control minus patient) and bottom left part is the significant different connections tested by two-sample t-test with 1000 permutations.

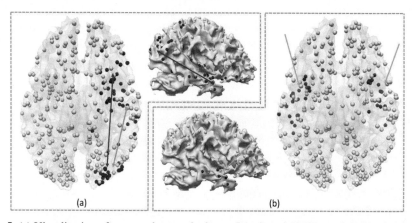

Fig. 5. (a) Visualization of structural network cluster 5 (red) and 12 (blue). (b) Visualization of functional network cluster 2 (red). Each cluster is highlighted by arrows of different colors.

5   Discussion and Conclusion

Mounting evidence in histopathology demonstrates that TBI has a progressive nature. After initial traumatic insult, the axons will undergo a temporal progression of degradation to final disruption. Recent evidence demonstrates that a prior history of brain injury, even a concussion, will make the patient more vulnerable to poor outcome after the second insult. Our structural network finding also demonstrates the progressive degradation nature in large-scale networks in mTBI. Furthermore, despite brain concussion, most mTBI patients enjoy a full recovery within several months from neurocognitive assessment perspective. This leads to the hypothesis that brain is highly plastic. Our data further support this hypothesis. In spite of structurally reduced connectivity in temporal white matter, this area tends to increase functional connectivity with other regions of the brain to compensate. Putting together, our work represents the first finding on progressive pathology of brain injury and functional compensation after mTBI from large scale network perspective. Particularly the identification of brain networks undergoing structural degradation and functional plasticity would help clinicians to make proper neurorehabilitation plan to proactively treat the patient for a speedy recovery.

Acknowledgements. This research was supported in part by the National Institutes of Health (R01DA033393, R01AG042599), by the National Science Foundation Graduate Research Fellowship (NSF CAREER Award IIS-1149260, CBET-1302089, BCS-1439051), by the Department of Defense (award number W81XWH-11-1-0493), and by International Society for Magnetic Resonance in Medicine (ISMRM) Seed Grant award (PI: Zhifeng Kou).

References

1. McCrea, M., Iverson, G.L., McAllister, T.W., Hammeke, T.A., Powell, M.R., Barr, W.B., Kelly, J.P.: An integrated review of recovery after mild traumatic brain injury (MTBI): implications for clinical management. Clin. Neuropsychol. 23, 1368–1390 (2009)
2. Eierud, C., Craddock, R.C., Fletcher, S., Aulakh, M., King-Casas, B., Kuehl, D., LaConte, S.M.: Neuroimaging after mild traumatic brain injury: Review and meta-analysis. NeuroImage. Clin. 4, 283–294 (2014)
3. Iraji, A., Benson, R.R., Welch, R.D., O'Neil, B.J., Woodard, J.L., Ayaz, S.I., Kulek, A., Mika, V., Medado, P., Soltanian-Zadeh, H., Liu, T., Haacke, E.M., Kou, Z.: Resting State Functional Connectivity in Mild Traumatic Brain Injury at the Acute Stage: Independent Component and Seed-Based Analyses. J. Neurotrauma (2015)
4. Zhu, D., Li, K., Guo, L., Jiang, X., Zhang, T., Zhang, D., Chen, H., Deng, F., Faraco, C., Jin, C., Wee, C.-Y., Yuan, Y., Lv, P., Yin, Y., Hu, X.X., Duan, L., Hu, X.X., Han, J., Wang, L., Shen, D., Miller, L.S., Li, L., Liu, T.: DICCCOL: dense individualized and common connectivity-based cortical landmarks. Cereb. Cortex. 23, 786–800 (2013)
5. Chen, H., Li, K., Zhu, D., Jiang, X., Yuan, Y., Lv, P., Zhang, T., Guo, L., Shen, D., Liu, T.: Inferring group-wise consistent multimodal brain networks via multi-view spectral clustering. IEEE Trans. Med. Imaging 32, 1576–1586 (2013)
6. Yixuan, Y., Xi, J., Dajiang, Z., Hanbo, C., Kaiming, L., Peili, L., Xiang, Y., Xiaojin, L., Shu, Z., Tuo, Z., Xintao, H., Junwei, H., Lei, G., Tianming, L.: Meta-analysis of Functional Roles of DICCCOLs. Neuroinformatics (2012)
7. Zhu, D., Li, K., Terry, D.P., Puente, A.N., Wang, L., Shen, D., Miller, L.S., Liu, T.: Connectome-scale assessments of structural and functional connectivity in MCI. Hum. Brain Mapp. (2013)
8. Li, K., Zhu, D., Guo, L., Li, Z., Lynch, M.E., Coles, C., Hu, X., Liu, T.: Connectomics signatures of prenatal cocaine exposure affected adolescent brains. Hum. Brain Mapp. 34, 2494–2510 (2013)
9. Jenkinson, M., Beckmann, C.F., Behrens, T.E., Woolrich, M.W., Smith, S.M.: FSL. Neuroimage 62, 782–790 (2012)
10. Liu, T., Li, H., Wong, K., Tarokh, A., Guo, L., Wong, S.T.C.: Brain tissue segmentation based on DTI data. Neuroimage 38, 114–123 (2007)
11. Liu, T., Nie, J., Tarokh, A., Guo, L., Wong, S.T.C.: Reconstruction of central cortical surface from brain MRI images: method and application. Neuroimage 40, 991–1002 (2008)
12. Toussaint, N., Souplet, J., Fillard, P.: MedINRIA: Medical image navigation and research tool by INRIA. In: MICCAI 2007, pp. 1–8 (2007)

Registration: Method and Advanced Applications

Dictionary Learning Based Image Descriptor for Myocardial Registration of CP-BOLD MR

Ilkay Oksuz[1], Anirban Mukhopadhyay[1], Marco Bevilacqua[1],
Rohan Dharmakumar[2], and Sotirios A. Tsaftaris[1,3]

[1] IMT Institute for Advanced Studies Lucca, Italy
[2] Biomedical Imaging Research Institute, Cedars-Sinai Medical, Los Angeles, USA
[3] Department of Electrical Engineering and Computer Science,
Northwestern University, Evanston, IL, USA

Abstract. Cardiac Phase-resolved Blood Oxygen-Level-Dependent (CP-BOLD) MRI is a new contrast agent- and stress-free imaging technique for the assessment of myocardial ischemia at rest. The precise registration among the cardiac phases in this cine type acquisition is essential for automating the analysis of images of this technique, since it can potentially lead to better specificity of ischemia detection. However, inconsistency in myocardial intensity patterns and the changes in myocardial shape due to the heart's motion lead to low registration performance for state-of-the-art methods. This low accuracy can be explained by the lack of distinguishable features in CP-BOLD and inappropriate metric definitions in current intensity-based registration frameworks. In this paper, the sparse representations, which are defined by a discriminative dictionary learning approach for source and target images, are used to improve myocardial registration. This method combines appearance with Gabor and HOG features in a dictionary learning framework to sparsely represent features in a low dimensional space. The sum of absolute differences of these distinctive sparse representations are used to define a similarity term in the registration framework. The proposed approach is validated on a dataset of CP-BOLD MR and standard CINE MR acquired in baseline and ischemic condition across 10 canines.

Keywords: Registration, Dictionary Learning, Similarity Metric, CP-BOLD MR, CINE MR.

1 Introduction

Nonrigid image registration is an essential step in medical imaging, including automatic segmentation, motion tracking and morphometric analysis [13]. However, since most of the proposed algorithms rely on a (dis)similarity metric build based on the assumptions of consistent intensity and local shape, images with pathologies and locally varying intensity may not be accurately aligned. One example of that is the registration of image sequences of Cardiac Phase-resolved

© Springer International Publishing Switzerland 2015
N. Navab et al. (Eds.): MICCAI 2015, Part II, LNCS 9350, pp. 205–213, 2015.
DOI: 10.1007/978-3-319-24571-3_25

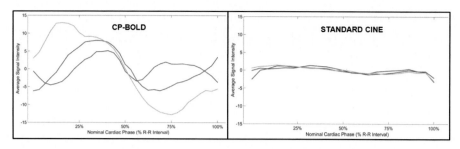

Fig. 1. Exemplary plots of time series extracted from the same corresponding regions in the same subject under baseline (absence of disease) conditions using CP-BOLD MR and standard Cine. Observe how in CP-BOLD, intensity varies with cardiac phase, but in standard CINE MR this variation is minimal.

Blood Oxygen-Level-Dependent (CP-BOLD) MR. CP-BOLD MR is a truly non-invasive method for early diagnosis of an ongoing ischemia, observing changes in myocardial signal intensity patterns as a function of cardiac phase [17]. As Figure 1 illustrates, time series of intensity vary as a function of cardiac phase when BOLD effect is present –it appears maximal in systole and minimal in di-astole. In disease this effect is not present. However, visualizing and quantifying such patterns requires significant post-processing, including myocardial regis-tration to establish pixel-precise time series for identifying such patterns [12]. Such spatio-temporal intensity variations of the myocardial BOLD effect cause the methods developed for standard CINE MR registration to under-perform. Thus, in CP-BOLD in addition to violations of shape invariance (as with stan-dard CINE MR) the principal assumption of appearance invariance (consistent intensity) is violated as well.

As a result, no CP-BOLD MR myocardial registration algorithms exist and due to this absence either segmental information [11] or synthetic data sets are used [12], to obtain pixel-wise time series. We assume that it is due to lack of proper similarity criteria. Rather than relying on low-level features used often for myocardial registration of standard CINE MR, a more distinguishing descriptor should be developed to accommodate the BOLD effect.

In this paper, we propose a feature-based descriptor as a similarity measure of the alignment to register the myocardium in the entire cardiac sequence of CP-BOLD. We adopt a patch-based discriminative dictionary learning technique [4] to learn features from data. Our motivation is to employ a compact and high-fidelity low-dimensional subspace representation, which is able to extract semantic information of the myocardial pixels [5]. We observe that although the patch intensity level varies significantly across the cardiac cycle, sparse represen-tations based on learnt dictionaries are invariant, as well as unique and robust. The discriminative dictionary learning strategy is designed to facilitate this key observation regarding CP-BOLD.

During training, two dictionaries of patches for myocardium and background are learnt offline. To register two images with unknown myocardium masks, the sparse representations that are obtained on the basis of previously trained dictionaries for background and myocardium, are concatenated and considered as the feature for that particular pixel. The similarity term evaluates the match of the sparse features at every iteration on a pixel level. The sum of squared differences of the sparse representations between the target image and warped source image are utilized as similarity criteria.

There are three major contributions of the paper. First of all, we propose a sparse representation-based image descriptor in a registration framework, for the first time to the best of our knowledge. Second, we experimentally validate the fact that BOLD contrast significantly affects the accuracy of registration algorithms (including intensity-based and feature-based methods), which instead perform well in standard CINE MR. Finally, we address the fundamental problem in handling BOLD contrast by designing a set of compact features using discriminative dictionary learning, which can effectively represent the myocardium in CP-BOLD MR.

The remainder of the paper is organized as follows: Section 2 discusses the background and Section 3 presents the method. Based on our experimental results (Section 4), we draw conclusions in Section 5.

2   Background

Automated myocardial registration for standard CINE MR is a well studied problem [15]. Most of these algorithms can be classified into two groups according to similarity criteria used: intensity-based or feature-based. General intensity-based registration algorithms can be summarized as an energy minimization procedure, where the energy functional is [13]:

$$E = \sum_{p \in \Omega} DS(I_s(p), I_t(p + u)) + \lambda E_R, \tag{1}$$

where Ω represents the entire image domain, and p denotes a pixel in the domain. Non-rigid registration consists of minimizing a dissimilarity measure DS between a source image I_s and a target image I_t, u denotes the displacements and E_R denotes the regularization term. In this work, we are particularly interested in the definition of the similarity measure. Sum of squared differences (SSD) and cross correlation (CC), are the earlier metrics utilized in registration. Recently, information theory-based approaches gained attention, e.g., derivatives of Mutual Information (MI), which is based on individual and joint gray level distributions [8].

When registration under inhomogeneity conditions is required, some have proposed modifications on regional intensity distortions (for brain MRI) [14] or spatially intensity variations [19]. Alternatively, feature-based approaches can be used. A recent example is DRAMMS [6], where the similarity is based on optimal Gabor attributes. Another approach, MIND [3], relies on regional information following the footsteps of self-similarity (a method utilized for image denoising) for multi-modality registration.

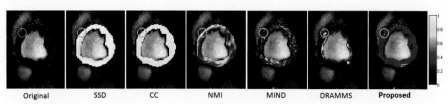

| Original | SSD | CC | NMI | MIND | DRAMMS | Proposed |

Fig. 2. Similarity of patches in two consecutive images. First image shows the test patch (green circle) and the remainder shows responses of each similarity metric inside the myocardium. All metrics are normalized and dissimilarity metrics are inverted.

In this paper, we concentrate on developing a feature-based metric but also learning features instead of using fixed ones. We use sparse representation coefficients of patches, generated by a dictionary trained offline, to define a similarity measure of alignment. In this study, we compare our method with SSD and MI based Free Form Deformations (FFD) [10], optical flow based diffeomorphic demons (ddemons) [18] and symmetric diffeomorphic transformation with CC metric implemented in Advanced Normalization Toolkit (ANTs) [2]. To demonstrate that our proposed approach provides better localized matches, Figure 2 shows the values of matches using several criteria when taking a patch from one image and matching it to myocardial locations in another image.

3   Method

We leverage dictionary learning techniques to learn better representative features. Accordingly, we integrate a Dictionary Learning-based Image Descriptor (DLID) derived from training patches into a similarity term of our proposed registration framework. Features learnt via dictionary learning are used in an image registration framework to evaluate the performance of the proposed descriptor.

3.1   Using Learnt Features in a Registration Framework

When registering a cardiac sequence $I_1, \ldots, I_t$, we aim to find a deformation that can register each image in the sequence to the first one. Here following the formulation of equation 1, we adopt a regularization in the form of

$$\underset{u}{\operatorname{argmin}} \sum_{p \in \Omega} S(I_1(p), I_t(p+u))^2 + \lambda \operatorname{tr}(\nabla u(p)^T \nabla u(p))^2, \qquad (2)$$

where ∇u denotes the gradient of the displacement field. This function is minimized over u with Gauss-Newton optimization as described in [3].

We propose an appropriate similarity term S based on the sparse feature representation of image patches. Assuming two input images, considering I_1 as fixed and I_t as moving, we extract for each pixel location in both, patches, which we represent with appearance and texture features (HoG, Gabor).

Algorithm 1. Dictionary Learning

Input: Training patches for background and myocardium: Y^B and Y^M
Output: Dictionaries for background and myocardium: D^B and D^M

1: **for** C={B,M} **do**
2:    Find intra-class Gram matrix G^C and discard atoms with high values
3:    Learn dictionary and sparse feature matrix with the K-SVD algorithm

$$\underset{D^C, X^C}{\text{minimize}} \|Y^C - D^C X^C\|_2^2, \text{ subject to } \|x_i^C\|_0 \le s$$

4: **end for**
5: Compute inter-class Gram matrix G^{BM}
6: Discard from D^B and D^M atoms with high values in G^{BM}

We create a sparse representation $\hat{X}_p$ for each pixel location for the two images to be registered. The Orthogonal Matching Pursuit (OMP) algorithm [16] is used to compute, two sparse feature matrices $\hat{X}^B$ and $\hat{X}^M$, both with n dimensions, based on previously computed dictionaries D^B and D^M (detailed below). At a certain pixel p of the image, a concatenation of these sparse representation vectors $\hat{X}_p = [\hat{X}^B; \hat{X}^M]$ are used to represent the image instead of the pixel level definitions. The proposed similarity term S at pixel p is defined as the ℓ^1 norm of the difference vector between the sparse representations of the warped source image and the target image as shown in equation 3.

$$S(I_1(p), I_t(p + u)) = \| \hat{X}_p^1 - \hat{X}_{p+u}^t \|_1 \tag{3}$$

3.2 Feature Generation with Discriminative Dictionary Learning

Given some training images (e.g., sequences in the context of cine (BOLD) MRI) and corresponding ground truth labels (i.e., myocardial masks), we obtain two sets of matrices, Y^B and Y^M, where the matrix Y^B contains background information, and Y^M contains information of patches within the myocardium. Information is collected from image patches: $K \times K$ squared patches are sampled around each pixel in the training images. More precisely, the i-th column of the matrix Y^B (and similarly for the matrix Y^M) is obtained by concatenating the normalized patch vector of pixel intensities, taken around the i-th pixel in the background (or myocardium), along with Gabor and HOG features of the same patch. The dictionary learning method takes as input these two sets of training matrices, to learn, two dictionaries, D^B and D^M, with n number of atoms, and two sparse feature matrices, X^B and X^M, with sparsity s. The i-th column of the matrix X^B, x_i^B, is considered as the discriminative feature vector for the particular pixel corresponding to the i-th column in Y_j^B.

Dictionaries and sparse features are trained via the well-known K-SVD algorithm [1], in an optimization problem shown in Algorithm 1. During initialization we first find the "intra-class Gram matrix" to promote diversity. The idea is to have a subset of patches as much diverse as possible to train dictionaries and sparse features. For a given class considered (let us say background) we can define the intra-class Gram matrix as $G^B = (Y^B)^T Y^B$. To ensure a proper discriminative initialization, patches that correspond to high values in the Gram matrix are discarded from the training before performing K-SVD, and K-SVD is initialized obtaining a random set of patches as initial atoms.

We also use pruning, inspired as a greedy approach of [9], which is performed after K-SVD to remove undesired (similar to other) atoms from each dictionary trained. In this case, an "inter-class Gram matrix" between dictionaries is computed $(G^{BM} = (D^B)^T D^M)$, the atoms of each dictionary are sorted according to their cumulative coefficients in G^{BM}, and a chosen percentage of them is discarded to ensure mutual exclusiveness (and better discrimination) between the different dictionaries. These modifications ensure that patches of different origin will have different support and that similar atoms are excluded.

4 Results

This section describes qualitatively and compares quantitatively our proposed dictionary learning-based descriptor with state-of-the-art approaches.

Data Preparation and Parameter Settings: 2D short-axis images of the whole cardiac cycle (2D+time, cine) were acquired at baseline and severe ischemia (inflicted as stenosis of the left-anterior descending coronary artery (LAD)) on a 1.5T Espree (Siemens Healthcare) in the same 10 canines along the mid ventricle using both standard CINE and a flow and motion compensated CP-BOLD acquisition within few minutes of each other [17]. All quantitative experiments are performed in a strict leave-one-subject-out cross-validation. Parameters and settings were optimized for each method used in comparison. For DLID, in this paper we have empirically chosen a dictionary of $n = 1000$ atoms for foreground and background respectively, a sparsity of $s = 4$, and as patch size $K=9$. The regularization weight (λ) is set to 0.8 to ensure smooth deformations.

Visual Evaluation: In an example sequence, we register each image in the sequence throughout the cardiac cycle to the first image using our approach. We take two orthogonal short axis profiles that intersect approximately at the center of the Left Ventricle, and in Figure 3 we show the temporal evolution of the profiles with and without registration (left-most and right-most horizontal and vertical profile, respectively). Our method shows clearly defined structure and the ability to correct for cardiac motion. Notice that BOLD intensity variation is subtle and not perceptible in these images (ie., is not a global change).

Quantitative Comparison: Using again the same process, in a strict-leave-one-out fashion we want to investigate the effect of different similarity metrics in recovering cardiac motion. To evaluate performance, we use again manual delineations of the myocardium provided by experts, and train dictionaries on a set of images and test on one subject. For validation, via segmentation, the myocardial mask from the source image was propagated to the target using the deformation field found with the algorithms, and its overlap with the ground

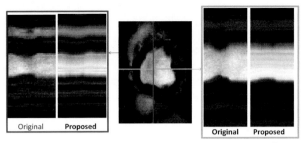

Fig. 3. Temporal evolution of two orthogonal short axis profiles (red and green line) intersecting approximately at the center of the left ventricle, without registration (original) and with registering every image in the sequence with the first image (proposed).

Table 1. Dice overlap comparison for different similarity metrics

Methods	Baseline		Ischemia	
	Standard Cine	CP-BOLD	Standard Cine	CP-BOLD
ANTs (CC metric) [2]	0.60 ∓ 0.11	0.55 ∓ 0.10	0.55 ∓ 0.15	0.51 ∓ 0.12
dDemons [18]	0.59 ∓ 0.11	0.51 ∓ 0.16	0.58 ∓ 0.13	0.45 ∓ 0.13
DRAMMS [6]	0.67 ∓ 0.09	0.61 ∓ 0.07	0.59 ∓ 0.10	0.54 ∓ 0.06
FFD-SSD [10]	0.49 ∓ 0.07	0.45 ∓ 0.16	0.48 ∓ 0.14	0.39 ∓ 0.13
FFD-MI [10]	0.54 ∓ 0.12	0.48 ∓ 0.08	0.53 ∓ 0.06	0.38 ∓ 0.07
MIND [3]	0.62 ∓ 0.07	0.62 ∓ 0.12	0.61 ∓ 0.15	0.53 ∓ 0.09
Proposed without sparsity	0.55 ∓ 0.08	0.52 ∓ 0.11	0.45 ∓ 0.09	0.42 ∓ 0.12
Proposed	0.63 ∓ 0.07	0.66 ∓ 0.09	0.58 ∓ 0.07	0.60 ∓ 0.13

truth mask of the fixed is measured using the Dice overlap metric [7]. Note that these masks are unknown to the algorithms and are used only for comparison.

Our findings in Table 1, show that using discriminative features and our similarity term significantly improve the performance for CP-BOLD cardiac sequence registration either under baseline or ischemia conditions w.r.t. other approaches. To highlight the unique challenge of BOLD, we also include results based on standard CINE. Our proposed method, although not its main focus, performs as good as other algorithms even in this case. To emphasize the importance of sparsity and learning we also use directly the ℓ^2 norm between input patches, instead of spare representations. Lower performance in ischemia for all algorithms could be attributed to changes in myocardial contractility.

5   Discussions and Conclusion

We propose a new dictionary learning-based image descriptor (DLID) for myocardial registration. The experiments clearly underline the need for a new representation in image registration. Their integration into analytical tools are necessary to meet new challenges posed by myocardial CP-BOLD MR. In particular, this study pin-pointed the challenges the BOLD effect poses on common assumptions made when registering the myocardium and quantitatively analyzed the performance of the descriptor both under baseline and ischemia conditions. Moreover, in this study we showed that by learning appropriate features to best represent texture and appearance in CP-BOLD, it is possible to obtain better correspondences for the entire cardiac sequence. The proposed method can be utilized for other challenges, where spatio-temporal intensity is a biomarker of disease, especially in the presence of motion. One limitation is computational time, since calculating sparse representations is the bottleneck of the problem. The successful application of this post-processing tools are foreseen to be critical in the clinical translation of cardiac CP-BOLD MR.

References

1. Aharon, M., et al.: K-SVD: An Algorithm for Designing Overcomplete Dictionaries for Sparse Representation. IEEE TSP 54(11), 4311–4322 (2006)
2. Avants, B.B., et al.: Symmetric diffeomorphic image registration with cross-correlation: evaluating automated labeling of elderly and neurodegenerative brain. MIA 12(1), 26–41 (2008)
3. Heinrich, M.P., et al.: MIND: Modality independent neighbourhood descriptor for multi-modal deformable registration. MIA 16(7), 1423–1435 (2012)
4. Huang, X., et al.: Contour tracking in echocardiographic sequences via sparse representation and dictionary learning. MIA 18, 253–271 (2014)
5. Mukhopadhyay, A., Oksuz, I., Bevilacqua, M., Dharmakumar, R., Tsaftaris, S.A.: Data-driven feature learning for myocardial segmentation of CP-BOLD MRI. In: van Assen, H., Bovendeerd, P., Delhaas, T. (eds.) FIMH 2015. LNCS, vol. 9126, pp. 189–197. Springer, Heidelberg (2015)
6. Ou, Y., et al.: DRAMMS: Deformable registration via attribute matching and mutual-saliency weighting. MIA 15(4), 622–639 (2011)
7. Ou, Y., Ye, D.H., Pohl, K.M., Davatzikos, C.: Validation of DRAMMS among 12 popular methods in cross-subject cardiac MRI registration. In: Dawant, B.M., Christensen, G.E., Fitzpatrick, J.M., Rueckert, D. (eds.) WBIR 2012. LNCS, vol. 7359, pp. 209–219. Springer, Heidelberg (2012)
8. Pluim, J.P.W., et al.: Mutual-information-based registration of medical images: a survey. TMI 22(8), 986–1004 (2003)
9. Ramirez, I., et al.: Classification and clustering via dictionary learning with structured incoherence and shared features. In: IEEE CVPR, pp. 3501–3508 (2010)
10. Rueckert, D., et al.: Nonrigid registration using free-form deformations: application to breast MR images. TMI 18(8), 712–721 (1999)
11. Rusu, C., Tsaftaris, S.A.: Structured dictionaries for ischemia estimation in cardiac BOLD MRI at rest. In: Golland, P., Hata, N., Barillot, C., Hornegger, J., Howe, R. (eds.) MICCAI 2014, Part II. LNCS, vol. 8674, pp. 562–569. Springer, Heidelberg (2014)
12. Rusu, C., et al.: Synthetic generation of myocardial blood-oxygen-level-dependent MRI time series via structural sparse decomposition modeling. IEEE TMI 7(33), 1422–1433 (2014)
13. Sotiras, A., et al.: Deformable Medical Image Registration: A Survey Medical Imaging. IEEE TMI 7(32), 1153–1190 (2013)

14. Studholme, C., et al.: Deformation-based mapping of volume change from serial brain MRI in the presence of local tissue contrast change. IEEE TMI 5(25), 626–639 (2006)
15. Tavakoli, V., et al.: A Survey of shape-based registration and segmentation techniques for cardiac images. CVIU 117, 966–989 (2013)
16. Tropp, J., et al.: Signal recovery from random measurements via orthogonal matching pursuit. IEEE T. Information Theory 53(12), 4655–4666 (2007)
17. Tsaftaris, S.A., et al.: Detecting myocardial ischemia at rest with cardiac phase–resolved blood oxygen level–dependent cardiovascular magnetic resonance. Circulation: Cardiovascular Imaging 6(2), 311–319 (2013)
18. Vercauteren, T., Pennec, X., Perchant, A., Ayache, N.: Non-parametric diffeomorphic image registration with the demons algorithm. In: Ayache, N., Ourselin, S., Maeder, A. (eds.) MICCAI 2007, Part II. LNCS, vol. 4792, pp. 319–326. Springer, Heidelberg (2007)
19. Zhuang, X., et al.: A nonrigid registration framework using spatially encoded mutual information and free-form deformations. IEEE TMI 10(30), 1819–1828 (2011)

Registration of Color and OCT Fundus Images Using Low-dimensional Step Pattern Analysis

Jimmy Addison Lee, Jun Cheng, Guozhen Xu, Ee Ping Ong, Beng Hai Lee,
Damon Wing Kee Wong, and Jiang Liu

Institute for Infocomm Research, Agency for Science,
Technology and Research (A*STAR), Singapore
{jalee,jcheng,xug,epong,benghai,wkwong,jliu}@i2r.a-star.edu.sg

Abstract. Existing feature descriptor-based methods on retinal image registration are mainly based on scale-invariant feature transform (SIFT) or partial intensity invariant feature descriptor (PIIFD). While these descriptors are many times being exploited, they have not been applied to color fundus and optical coherence tomography (OCT) fundus image pairs. OCT fundus images are challenging to register as they are often degraded by speckle noise. The descriptors also demand high dimensionality to adequately represent the features of interest. To this end, this paper presents a registration algorithm coined low-dimensional step pattern analysis (LoSPA), tailored to achieve low dimensionality while providing sufficient distinctiveness to effectively register OCT fundus images with color fundus photographs. The algorithm locates hypotheses of robust corner features based on connecting edges from the edge maps, mainly formed by vascular junctions. It continues with describing the corner features in a rotation invariant manner using step patterns. These customized step patterns are insensitive to intensity changes. We conduct comparative evaluation and LoSPA achieves a higher success rate in registration when compared to the state-of-the-art algorithms.

Keywords: Registration, optical coherence tomography, feature descriptor, LoSPA.

1 Introduction

Optical coherence tomography (OCT) is a micrometer-scale, cross-sectional imaging modality for biological tissue. An OCT fundus image constructed by integration of the 3D tomogram along depth provides a view similar to traditional en-face imaging modalities, such as color fundus photographs. Examples of color fundus and OCT fundus image pairs are shown in Fig. 1. Registration of the color fundus and OCT fundus images allows ophthalmologists to obtain a more complete detail of the subject by correlating the cross-sectional scattering properties of the retina with the familiar information of the color fundus photographs. The main challenges in this registration are the intensity differences between the two modalities and the poor quality of the OCT fundus images which are adversely affected by speckle noise or pathologies.

The literature on retinal image registration is extensive, with many existing work on same modality [1,2,3,4,5] and few on multimodality [6,7,8,9,10]. Among multimodality, work on registration between color fundus and OCT fundus images is very limited

© Springer International Publishing Switzerland 2015
N. Navab et al. (Eds.): MICCAI 2015, Part II, LNCS 9350, pp. 214–221, 2015.
DOI: 10.1007/978-3-319-24571-3_26

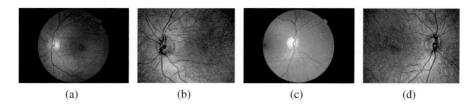

Fig. 1. Two pairs of color fundus and OCT fundus images. (a) and (b) is one pair and (c) and (d) is another pair. Color fundus is on the left and OCT fundus is on the right of each pair.

and is mainly based on vasculature [8,10]. For example, curvelet transform [10] is used to extract vessels in both modalities. The extracted vessels from the two modalities are registered together. There are several other work [1,2,4,8] that utilize vessels for image registration. Although vessels are invariant to intensity variations, their localizations are often inaccurate [11]. In addition, vessel-based approaches rely heavily on vascular structures and usually involve extensive preprocessing such as segmentation and skeletonization. Extracting of vessels is difficult in poor quality images [7].

Recently, feature descriptor-based registration approaches that do not rely on vasculature are becoming more popular. SIFT algorithm [12] detects feature points as the extrema in the difference of Gaussian (DoG) scale space. For each feature point, the intensity gradient vectors within its neighbors are collected in histograms to form a descriptor of 128 dimensions. However, the algorithm fails to identify stable and uniformly distributed feature points in multimodal retinal images [6,13,14], and it is more suitable for monomodal image registration [6]. Therefore, enhancement methods are proposed. A generalized dual-bootstrap iterative closest point (GDB-ICP) [5] uses SIFT with the alignment process driven by two types of feature points: corner points and face points. To better deal with the multimodal registration problem, an edge-driven DB-ICP (ED-DB-ICP) [9] algorithm is developed by enriching SIFT with shape context using edge points, summing up to a 188-dimensional vector descriptor. The resulting descriptor is not robust to scale changes and images affected by pathologies or noise [6,7]. The partial intensity invariant feature descriptor (PIIFD) [15] is later introduced. Similar to SIFT constituting of a 128-dimensional vector, PIIFD combines constrained gradient orientations between 0 to π linearly, and performs a rotation to address the multimodal problem of gradient orientations of corresponding points in opposite directions. A Harris-PIIFD [6] framework is later proposed where PIIFD is used to describe surrounding fixed size regions of Harris corners [16]. However, the Harris corners are not uniformly distributed [7,13] and the repeatability rate is poor when the scale changes between images go beyond 1.5 or in the presence of pathologies or noise in the retina [7]. To circumvent the problems, Harris method is replaced with an uniform robust SIFT (UR-SIFT) [7] method. The improvement is the more stable UR-SIFT features of higher contrast in the uniform distribution of both the scale and image spaces to compute the PIIFD descriptor. However, the algorithm has not been applied to register color fundus and OCT fundus image pairs.

In this paper, we propose a registration algorithm which comes with a low-dimensional feature descriptor that is insensitive to intensity changes, and provides sufficient distinctiveness to register color fundus and OCT fundus images. In addition, to the best of our knowledge, this is the first work to conduct comparative evaluation between existing feature descriptor-based registration methods on color and OCT fundus image pairs.

The rest of the paper is organized as follows. Section 2 presents our methodology. Experimental results follow in section 3 and section 4 concludes the paper.

2   Methodology

2.1   Geometric Corner Extraction

We exploit the geometric corner extraction method [13] to locate hypotheses of robust corner features. Extracted edges from the edge maps may be fractured due to missing edge pixels. To circumvent this problem, a post-processing step [13] is applied to identify and fix broken edges with end-points and angles of close proximity. The purpose is to eventually remove edges that are isolated or insignificant, e.g. edges < 5 pixels which are mainly noise. The subsequent step is to locate intersecting points from connecting edges which are called geometric corners [13]. Geometric corners are always true corners where each geometric corner g_i comes from an intersecting point of two edges $\ell_1^{g_i}$ and $\ell_2^{g_i}$. For robustness, we exclude two edges of similar angles as a candidate for g_i. The smaller internal angle between $\ell_1^{g_i}$ and $\ell_2^{g_i}$ must be between $25°$ and $155°$.

2.2   LoSPA Description

Due to non-linear intensity changes, corresponding images of different modalities often do not correlate well. Therefore, we have to focus on the intensity change patterns instead of the intensity change values. We first rotate the input image relative to a mutual orientation derived from $\ell_1^{g_i}$ and $\ell_2^{g_i}$ to achieve rotation invariance. The center of rotation is at g_i, and the angle-to-rotate $\theta_{rot}^{g_i}$ is derived as follows:

$$\theta_{rot}^{g_i} = \theta_{min}^{g_i} + [\delta]\,(\theta_{max}^{g_i} - \theta_{min}^{g_i}), \tag{1}$$

where $\theta_{max}^{g_i}$ and $\theta_{min}^{g_i}$ denote the maximum and minimum angles from $\ell_j^{g_i}$ to the positive x-axis respectively, with $\forall j \in \{1,2\}$. [.] is a binary indicator function, and δ is the inequality formalized as:

$$\theta_{max}^{g_i} - \theta_{min}^{g_i} > 180°. \tag{2}$$

After rotation, we extract a local window $\mathbf{W}_{rot}^{g_i}$ (e.g. 15×15) centered at g_i from the rotated image. In this paper, we propose to divide $\mathbf{W}_{rot}^{g_i}$ into equal-sized subregions using two straight lines and a set of rules. For example, the first step pattern in Fig. 2(a) is formed by two parallel lines dividing a square into three equal-sized subregions. By rotating the two parallel lines by $45°$, $90°$ and $135°$, we form three other step patterns as shown in Fig. (2(b)-2(d)). Fig. 2(e) is formed by drawing two lines starting from the center of one edge of the square to separate the square into three equal-sized subregions. Fig. (2(f)-2(h)) are also formed similarly with the two lines starting at different edges. The rest of the step patterns are formulated by similar rules. We then compare the average intensities between the subregions, which will be computed as a feature representation for $\mathbf{W}_{rot}^{g_i}$. 28 different patterns are empirically proposed, which represent

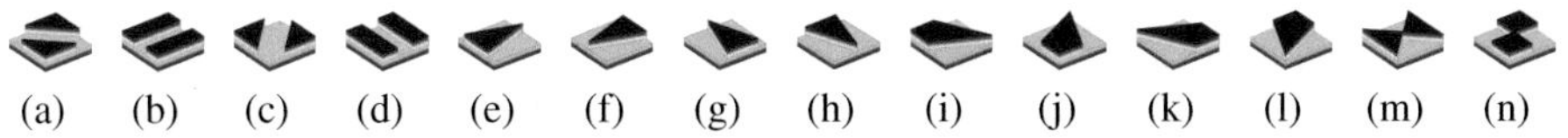

(a)   (b)   (c)   (d)   (e)   (f)   (g)   (h)   (i)   (j)   (k)   (l)   (m)   (n)

Fig. 2. Two-level step patterns.

(a)   (b)   (c)   (d)   (e)   (f)   (g)   (h)   (i)   (j)   (k)   (l)   (m)   (n)

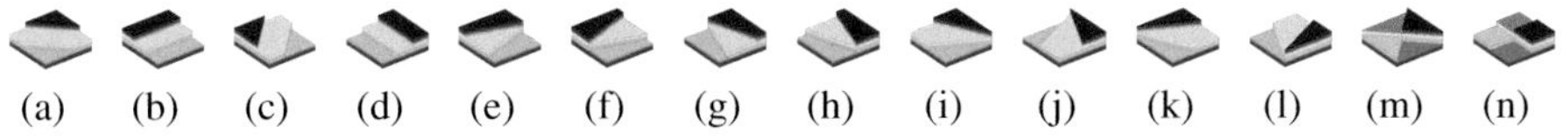

Fig. 3. Three- and four-level step patterns.

most of the possible patterns with equal-sized subregions as shown in Fig. 2 and 3. The patterns are called step patterns. As the name implies, these patterns come in step forms of two to four height levels where the higher level steps indicate subregions of higher average intensity values. Taking Fig. 2(b) as an exemplar to be depicted in Fig. 4(a), the number of pixels in the subregions $\mathbf{R_1}$, $\mathbf{R_2}$ and $\mathbf{R_3}$ are equal. For average intensity value $I_{avg}^{\mathbf{R_k}}$ in $\mathbf{R_k}$ where $\forall \mathbf{k} \in \{1,2,3\}$, we formulate as follows:

$$I_{avg}^{\mathbf{R_k}} = \frac{1}{N} \sum_{(x,y) \in \mathbf{R_k}} \mathbf{W}_{rot}^{g_i}(x,y), \tag{3}$$

where N is the number of pixels in $\mathbf{R_k}$. Each $\mathbf{W}_{rot}^{g_i}$, in relation with its respective g_i, can be described using the equation:

$$d_1 = \left[I_{avg}^{\mathbf{R_1}} - I_{avg}^{\mathbf{R_2}} > \tau \right] \cdot \left[I_{avg}^{\mathbf{R_3}} - I_{avg}^{\mathbf{R_2}} > \tau \right], \tag{4}$$

where d_1 is a binary result to indicate the existence of the step pattern in Fig. 4(a), and τ denotes a position integer value. In this paper, we set $\tau = 1$ to avoid noise. To deal with contrast reversal problem such as the change in intensities between the local neighborhood of two image modalities (for instance, the optic discs become dark in the OCT fundus images), the step pattern is reversible as illustrated in Fig. 4(b). Hence, the equation for the reversed step pattern in Fig. 4(b) can be rearranged as:

$$d_2 = \left[I_{avg}^{\mathbf{R_2}} - I_{avg}^{\mathbf{R_1}} > \tau \right] \cdot \left[I_{avg}^{\mathbf{R_2}} - I_{avg}^{\mathbf{R_3}} > \tau \right]. \tag{5}$$

The final equation to describe $\mathbf{W}_{rot}^{g_i}$ is given by:

$$d_3 = d_1 + d_2, \tag{6}$$

and d_3 is still a binary result. For the rest of the patterns in Fig. 2 and 3, $I_{avg}^{\mathbf{R_k}}$ can be computed similarly by applying Eq. (3). d_1 to d_3 in Eq. (4-6) are also computed similarly for the two-level step patterns in Fig. 2. For the three- and four-level step patterns in Fig. 3, d_1 and d_2 are expressed in an increasing or decreasing step manner instead. Hence, the equations can be mathematically revised as:

$$d_1 = \prod_{i=1}^{p-1} \left[I_{avg}^{\mathbf{R_{i+1}}} - I_{avg}^{\mathbf{R_i}} > \tau \right] \quad and \quad d_2 = \prod_{i=1}^{p-1} \left[I_{avg}^{\mathbf{R_i}} - I_{avg}^{\mathbf{R_{i+1}}} > \tau \right], \tag{7}$$

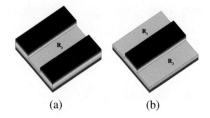

(a)   (b)

Fig. 4. A two-level step pattern is shown in (a), and its reversed step pattern for invariant to contrast reversal is shown in (b).

where $p \in \{3, 4\}$ is the number of steps in the pattern. d_3 remains the same as in Eq. (6).

In order to describe the inner and outer regions of the local neighborhood surrounding g_i, two $\mathbf{W}_{rot}^{g_i}$ of different scales are deployed. We also include the angle between $\ell_1^{g_i}$ and $\ell_2^{g_i}$, and the angle-to-rotate $\theta_{rot}^{g_i}$, which are two important attributes for robust matching and verification. We set the window scales of $\mathbf{W}_{rot}^{g_i}$ to fixed 15×15 and 21×21 pixels for the reason that the scale difference in retinal images is usually slight. For improved robustness to scale changes, we include an additional window scale of 27×27, resulting in a 86-dimensional ($28 \times 3 + 2$) LoSPA feature vector.

2.3 Feature Matching, Outlier Rejection and Transformation Function

We find matches by Euclidean distance, using the k-dimensional data structure and search algorithm [17] with $k = 3$. Each match comprises two window scales, thus we have four match combinations resulting from an additional window scale to switch with. Among the four, the one which returns the highest number of matches is considered as the best fit. Each match takes only 29.4 milliseconds (in MATLAB) so we can afford to perform matching more than once. $\theta_{rot}^{g_i}$ is not included in for matching, it is used for rejecting incorrect matches instead. It is obvious that the differences between $\theta_{rot}^{g_i}$ for all matched feature pairs are similar. Suppose that the sets of matched gi between two images are $\mathbf{G_{1m}} = \{g_{1mi}\}$ and $\mathbf{G_{2m}} = \{(g'_{2mi}, g''_{2mi}, g'''_{2mi})\}$ where i is the corresponding number index, and $(g'_{2mi}, g''_{2mi}, g'''_{2mi})$ correspond to g_{1mi}'s three closest neighbors respectively, we compute the difference between $\theta_{rot}^{g_i}$ of every single pair as:

$$(\|\theta_{rot}^{g_{1mi}} - \theta_{rot}^{g_{2mi}^j}\|) \bmod 180°, \qquad (8)$$

and put them into their respective bins of 12, each of $30°$ range with half overlapping in between each pair. The bin with the highest number of votes is denoted as bin'_{hi}. bin''_{hi} only exists if it is the closest neighbor (direct left or right) of bin'_{hi} and its number of votes is above 60% of bin'_{hi}. The matched feature pairs in $\mathbf{G_{1m}}$ and $\mathbf{G_{2m}}$ that do not fall within bin'_{hi} and bin''_{hi} are rejected. Most incorrect matches are actually rejected according to this criterion. Next, we validate the remaining pairs in a global transformation function between the two images. Random sample consensus (RANSAC) [18] with affine transformation setting is applied to all remaining matched pairs. We can exclude the remaining incorrect matches with this method.

We exploit affine model [19] as the transformation function in our framework. When it has been applied on the floating retinal image, we simply superpose the transformed

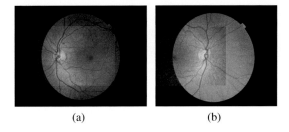

(a)   (b)

Fig. 5. Mosaic results of the proposed algorithm (LoSPA) for the color fundus and OCT fundus image pairs shown in Fig. 1(a) and 1(b), and Fig. 1(c) and 1(d).

retinal image on the fixed retinal image to produce a retinal mosaic. Some mosaic results of image pairs in Fig. 1 are shown in Fig. 5.

3 Experimental Results

We conduct robustness and comparative experiments on a dataset comprising 52 pairs of color fundus and corresponding OCT fundus images. The color fundus photographs were acquired with a TRC-NW8 non-mydriatic fundus camera and the 3D OCT data were obtained from a Topcon DRI OCT-1 machine with a size of $992 \times 512 \times 256$ voxels. The OCT fundus images were formed by intensity averaging along A-scans. The resized color fundus and OCT fundus images are 1016×675 and 513×385 respectively. We select 8 pairs of corresponding points in each image pair manually to generate ground truth. The points have to be distributed uniformly with an accurate localization. The main advantage of this method is that it can handle poor quality OCT fundus images which are degraded by speckle noise or pathologies. We compute the root-mean-square-error (RMSE) between the corresponding points in each registered image pair [7,14,20]. For successful registration, we consider the RMSE < 5 pixels in proportion to the image resolution in [7]. In addition, a significant error such as the maximal error (MAE) > 10 pixels [6] also results in a registration failure.

3.1 Robustness Test Results

This part evaluates the robustness of LoSPA to rotation invariance and scale insensitivity. We select 10 image pairs from the dataset to perform rotation and rescaling.

Rotation Invariance Test. We rotate the floating images in the selected image pairs from $0°$ to $180°$ with a $20°$ step. It should be noted that the reference images are held fixed. We apply the LoSPA algorithm on the reference images and the rotated floating images. The result of this test shows that LoSPA successfully registered all image pairs regardless of the rotation angle, demonstrating that LoSPA is rotation invariant.

Scale Change Test. We rescale the floating images with a scaling factor from 1 to 2.8, and apply the LoSPA algorithm on all the images. The registration rates across a range of scale changes are shown in Table 1. The experiment indicates that LoSPA can provide robust registration when the scale factor is 1.8 and below. However, LoSPA usually fails when the scale factor is above 1.8. This is still acceptable as most of these clinical images are of very small scale differences and are usually less than 1.5 [6].

Table 1. Successful registration relative to scale factor.

Scale factor	1	1.2	1.4	1.6	1.8	2	2.2	2.4	2.6	2.8
Success rate (%)	100	100	100	100	80	40	10	0	0	0

3.2   Comparative Evaluation Results

We run comparative evaluation between the 7 algorithms discussed earlier: SIFT [12], UR-SIFT-PIIFD [7], Harris-PIIFD [6], Curvelet transform (CT) [10], GDB-ICP [5], ED-DB-ICP [9], and LoSPA. It should be noted that CT is a vessel-based approach, however we include it for comparison purpose. Table 2 shows the comparison results. For SIFT, it registers only 3 image pairs. UR-SIFT-PIIFD, Harris-PIIFD, and CT perform better but still do not make it beyond the 50% success rate. For CT, many of the vessels are not being extracted and therefore induced failure during registration. The rest of the algorithms pass the 50% success rate mark, with LoSPA dominating in the scores. Some registration image results of LoSPA are shown in Fig. 5. The comparison shows that the deployment of LoSPA to color fundus and OCT fundus image registration translates into lower dimensionality and higher registration success rate.

Running LoSPA in MATLAB on a 3.5GHz Intel Core i7 desktop with 32GB memory, the average execution time is 4.48 seconds (s) for feature extraction, 3.31s for LoSPA feature description, 29.4ms for feature matching, and 0.2s for outlier rejection.

Table 2. Registration results of 7 algorithms on a dataset of 52 color fundus and OCT fundus image pairs. Number of successfully registered pairs and success rate of registration are shown.

	SIFT	UR-SIFT-PIIFD	Harris-PIIFD	CT	GDB-ICP	ED-DB-ICP	LoSPA
Registered pairs	3	11	12	15	26	26	**41**
Success rate (%)	5.77	21.15	23.08	28.85	50	50	**78.85**

4   Conclusion

We have presented a low-dimensional feature descriptor-based algorithm LoSPA, which shows high potential in multimodal image registration application. The algorithm is not only low in dimensionality, but more crucially without compromising on its distinctiveness and effectiveness, it is able to robustly register color and OCT fundus image pairs. LoSPA is invariant to non-linear intensity changes which is an important requisite for multimodal registration. We have conducted a comparative evaluation of algorithms on a color and OCT fundus image dataset. Results indicated that LoSPA achieves significantly higher registration success rate which easily frustrates the other algorithms.

References

1. Can, A., Stewart, C., Roysam, B., Tanenbaum, H.: A feature-based, robust, hierarchical algorithm for registering pairs of images of the curved human retina. TPAMI 24(3), 347–364 (2002)
2. Laliberté, F., Gagnon, L., Sheng, Y.: Registration and fusion of retinal images - an evaluation study. T-MI 22(5), 661–673 (2003)
3. Ritter, N., Owens, R., Cooper, J., Eikelboom, R.H., Saarloos, P.P.V.: Registration of stereo and temporal images of the retina. T-MI 18(5), 404–418 (1999)
4. Stewart, C., Tsai, C.L., Roysam, B.: The dual-bootstrap iterative closest point algorithm with application to retinal image registration. T-MI 22(11), 1379–1394 (2003)
5. Yang, G., Stewart, C.V., Sofka, M., Tsai, C.L.: Alignment of challenging image pairs: Refinement and region growing starting from a single keypoint correspondence. TPAMI 23(11), 1973–1989 (2007)
6. Chen, J., Tian, J., Lee, N., Zheng, J., Smith, R.T., Laine, A.F.: A partial intensity invariant feature descriptor for multimodal retinal image registration. TBME 57(7), 1707–1718 (2010)
7. Ghassabi, Z., Sedaghat, A., Shanbehzadeh, J., Fatemizadeh, E.: An efficient approach for robust multimodal retinal image registration based on UR-SIFT features and PIIFD descriptors. IJIVP 2013(25) (2013)
8. Li, Y., Gregori, G., Knighton, R.W., Lujan, B.J., Rosenfeld, P.J.: Registration of OCT fundus images with color fundus photographs based on blood vessel ridge. Opt. Express 19(1), 7–16 (2011)
9. Tsai, C.L., Li, C.Y., Yang, G., Lin, K.S.: The edge-driven dual-bootstrap iterative closest point algorithm for registration of multimodal fluorescein angiogram sequence. T-MI 29(3), 636–649 (2010)
10. Golabbakhsh, M., Rabbani, H.: Vessel-based registration of fundus and optical coherence tomography projection images of retina using a quadratic registration model. IET Image Processing 7(8), 768–776 (2013)
11. Tsai, C.L., Stewart, C.V., Tanenbaum, H.L., Roysam, B.: Model-based method for improving the accuracy and repeatability of estimating vascular bifurcations and crossovers from retinal fundus images. Trans. Info. Tech. Biomed. 8(2), 122–130 (2004)
12. Lowe, D.G.: Distinctive image features from scale-invariant keypoints. IJCV 60(2), 91–110 (2004)
13. Lee, J.A., Lee, B.H., Xu, G., Ong, E.P., Wong, D.W.K., Liu, J., Lim, T.H.: Geometric corner extraction in retinal fundus images. In: Proc. EMBC (2014)
14. Li, J., Chen, H., Chang, Y., Zhang, X.: A robust feature-based method for mosaic of the curved human color retinal images. In: Proc. BMEI, pp. 845–849 (2008)
15. Chen, J., Smith, R.T., Tian, J., Laine, A.F.: A novel registration method for retinal images based on local features. In: Proc. EMBC, pp. 2242–2245 (2004)
16. Harris, C., Stephens, M.: A combined corner and edge detector. In: Proc. AVC, pp. 147–151 (1988)
17. Bentley, J.L.: Multidimensional binary search trees used for associative searching. Comm. ACM 18(9), 509–517 (1975)
18. Fischler, M.A., Bolles, R.C.: Random sample consensus: a paradigm for model fitting with applications to image analysis and automated cartography. Comm. ACM 24(6), 381–395 (1981)
19. Jagoe, R., Blauth, C.I., Smith, P.L., Smith, J.V., Arnold, J.V., Taylor, K., Wootton, R.: Automatic geometrical registration of fluorescein retinal angiograms. Comp. and Biomed. Research 23(5), 403–409 (1990)
20. Matsopoulos, G.K., Asvestas, P.A., Mouravliansky, N.A., Delibasis, K.K.: Multimodal registration of retinal images using self organizing maps. T-MI 23(12), 1557–1563 (2004)

Estimating Patient Specific Templates for Pre-operative and Follow-Up Brain Tumor Registration

Dongjin Kwon, Ke Zeng, Michel Bilello, and Christos Davatzikos

Center for Biomedical Image Computing and Analytics,
University of Pennsylvania, Philadelphia, PA, USA

Abstract. Deformable registration between pre-operative and follow-up scans of glioma patients is important since it allows us to map post-operative longitudinal progression of the tumor onto baseline scans, thus, to develop predictive models of tumor infiltration and recurrence. This task is very challenging due to large deformations, missing correspondences, and inconsistent intensity profiles between the scans. Here, we propose a new method that combines registration with estimation of patient specific templates. These templates, built from pre-operative and follow-up scans along with a set of healthy brain scans, approximate the patient's brain anatomy before tumor development. Such estimation provides additional cues for missing correspondences as well as inconsistent intensity profiles, and therefore guides better registration on pathological regions. Together with our symmetric registration framework initialized by joint segmentation-registration using a tumor growth model, we are also able to estimate large deformations between the scans effectively. We apply our method to the scans of 24 glioma patients, achieving the best performance among compared registration methods.

1 Introduction

Glioblastoma is a very aggressive brain tumor, which infiltrates well beyond visible tumor boundaries. Finding imaging signatures that can predict tumor infiltration and subsequent tumor recurrence is very important in treatment of brain gliomas, as it could potentially affect treatment decisions at baseline patient evaluations [1]. This necessitates the development of accurate deformable registration methods that establish spatial correspondences between the pre-operative and follow-up brain scans, which allow follow-up information to be mapped onto baseline scans and elucidate imaging signatures for more aggressively infiltrated tissue, and accordingly inform pre-surgical planning procedures. This process must account for large deformations present in the pre-operative scan due to mass effect by tumor, as well as in the follow-up scan after tumor resection and tissue relaxation. Moreover, edema and tumor infiltration further confound the anatomy around the tumor. Even though the scans come from the same patient, this intra-subject registration task is very challenging due to these large deformations, missing correspondences, and inconsistent intensity profiles between the scans.

© Springer International Publishing Switzerland 2015
N. Navab et al. (Eds.): MICCAI 2015, Part II, LNCS 9350, pp. 222–229, 2015.
DOI: 10.1007/978-3-319-24571-3_27

Most existing registration methods exclude the pathological regions to deal with missing correspondences [9,3,7]. The concept of guiding registration via segmentation is used by methods performing intra-subject registration of scans capturing an evolving tumor [7] or inter-subject registration of scans for healthy brains and the one with pathology [9,3]. However, it is difficult to estimate large deformations on brain tumors by simply excluding the pathology. To take account of pathological regions, there exist different approaches performing inter-subject registrations by inpainting pathological regions [11] or estimating low-rank images iteratively [6]. For intra-subject registrations, Kwon et al. [4], design a registration framework specific to the pre-operative and post-recurrence scans. This method estimates a patient specific probabilistic prior aligned with the follow-up scan and jointly segments and registers with the pre-operative scan by growing a tumor from the location of resection. However, pathological regions, such as edema, are excluded in the matching cost, as one could not establish correspondences for these regions. As a result, the deformation field is solely determined through associated displacements of surrounding tissues via regularization, a procedure that could potentially compromise registration accuracy.

In this paper, we propose a new method combining registration and estimation of patient specific templates for pre-operative and follow-up brain tumor scans. As the follow-up scan is freed from an often huge mass effect and intense peritumoral edema by surgical resection of the glioma, we assume that the follow-up scans contain enough information for us to estimate the patient's brain anatomy before tumor development, using informative prior knowledge of brain structure provided by a set of healthy brain scans. Such estimation could be propagated to the pre-operative space, given the reasonable mapping between scans. Our method estimates this mapping by registering pre-operative and follow-up scans by excluding pathological regions estimated by [4] in calculating matching cost. After estimating patient specific templates on both scans, pathological regions that have been confidently estimated no longer need to be masked out in the matching cost, providing extra information to the registration process in order to identify correspondences. Note that we use the term "inpainting" for our estimation of patient specific templates, considering the similarities of the task that fills missing areas using prior knowledge.

In the rest of this paper, we describe the segmentation methods for pre-operative and follow-up brain tumor scans in Sec. 2 and our combined registration and inpainting framework in Sec. 3. In Sec. 4, we present our quantitative and qualitative evaluations and conclude the paper in Sec. 5.

2   Segmentation of Pre-operative and Follow-Up Scans

In this section, we estimate posterior probabilities of the pre-operative (baseline) scan B and follow-up scan F and the initial mapping between B and F based on [4]. As F is usually closer to the normal anatomy by the surgical resection of the glioma, we firstly segment F by aligning an atlas of the healthy population to F. Then we segment B and simultaneously register B and F by simulating

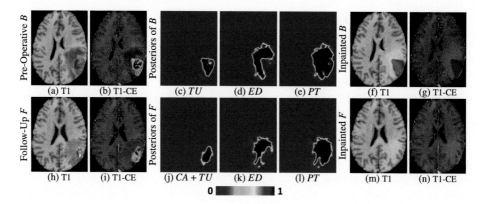

Fig. 1. An example of posteriors and estimated patient specific templates by inpainting pathological regions. For the pre-operative scan B, we show subject scans in (a)-(b), posteriors for tumor (TU), edema (ED), and pathological regions (PT) in (c)-(e), patient specific templates in (f)-(g). In (f)-(g), tumor regions are masked as they don't belong to the normal anatomy. For the follow-up scan F, we show subject scans in (h)-(i), posteriors of cavity (CA) with tumor, edema, and pathological regions in (j)-(l), patient specific templates in (m)-(n).

tumor growths on this aligned atlas. We denote by '$\mathcal{T}_t|\mathbf{x}$' the tissue type being t at voxel $\mathbf{x}$, namely '$\mathcal{T} = t|\mathbf{x}$'. The atlas p_A is defined as a set of probability maps $p_A(\mathcal{T}_t|\mathbf{x})$ for white matter (WM), gray matter (GM), and cerebrospinal fluid (CSF), i.e. $t \in \{WM, GM, CSF\}$.

For segmenting F, we define spatial probabilities $p_F(\mathcal{T}_t|\mathbf{x})$ of F for each tissue type t by combining p_A with a simple model for pathology described in [4]. This model generates a spatial probability for pathological regions, such as cavity $(t=CA)$, tumor recurrences $(t=TR)$ and edema $(t=ED)$, using the generalized logistic function given the approximated center point and radius for each region of the cavity or tumor recurrence. We then estimate the mapping h_F^* and the posterior probabilities $p_F(\mathcal{T}_t|F,\mathbf{x})$ by registering $p_F(\mathcal{T}_t|\mathbf{x})$ with F via the expectation-maximization (EM) algorithm. We show an example of posteriors for pathological regions in Fig. 1 (j)-(l).

To segment B and estimate the initial mapping between B and F, we apply a joint segmentation-registration method [5] on the atlas aligned with F, defined as $p_S(\mathcal{T}_t|\mathbf{x}) \triangleq p_A(\mathcal{T}_t|h_F^*(\mathbf{x}))$. This method generates the spatial probabilities of tumor $(t=TU)$ and edema $(t=ED)$ by applying a tumor growth model on the space of F and combine them with p_S to define spatial probabilities $p_B(\mathcal{T}_t|\mathbf{x})$ of B. Similar to the method for F, it estimates the mapping h_B^* and the posterior probabilities $p_B(\mathcal{T}_t|B,\mathbf{x})$ by registering $p_B(\mathcal{T}_t|\mathbf{x})$ with B via the EM algorithm. Then the initial mapping between B and F, denoted by f_{BF}^0, is obtained by concatenating h_B^* and the mapping $\mathbf{u}^*$ representing the mass effect from the tumor growth model. The mapping f_{BF}^0 approximates the mapping between B and F as the spatial probabilities p_S having smoothed anatomical information is used for the alignment instead of F. We show an example of posteriors for pathological regions in Fig. 1 (c)-(e).

3   Combined Registration and Inpainting Framework

Having defined the posterior probabilities p_B and p_F and the initial mapping $\boldsymbol{f}_{BF}^0$, we now describe our combined registration and inpainting framework to obtain final mapping $\boldsymbol{f}_{BF}$. To determine the large deformation reliably, we apply a symmetric registration scheme to match both scans to a center coordinate system Ω_C. Then we split the mapping $\boldsymbol{f}_{BF}$ into a mapping from Ω_C to Ω_B, $\boldsymbol{f}_{CB}$ and a mapping from Ω_C to Ω_F, $\boldsymbol{f}_{CF}$ as follows:

$$\boldsymbol{f}_{BF} \triangleq \boldsymbol{f}_{CF} \circ (\boldsymbol{f}_{CB})^{-1}, \tag{1}$$

where "$\circ$" concatenates two mappings. For registration, we model an energy function $E(\cdot)$ composed of a correspondence term E_C, a pathology term E_P, and a smoothness term E_S and estimate optimal mappings $\{\boldsymbol{f}_{CB}^*, \boldsymbol{f}_{CF}^*\}$ by minimizing $E(\cdot)$:

$$\{\boldsymbol{f}_{CB}^*, \boldsymbol{f}_{CF}^*\} = \arg \min_{\boldsymbol{f}_{CB}, \boldsymbol{f}_{CF}} E(\boldsymbol{f}_{CB}, \boldsymbol{f}_{CF}; B, F, p_B, p_F) . \tag{2}$$

Then we calculate optimal mappings $\boldsymbol{f}_{BF}^*$ and $\boldsymbol{f}_{FB}^* \triangleq (\boldsymbol{f}_{BF}^*)^{-1}$ using (1). Our framework firstly estimates the optimal mappings while masking out correspondences on the pathological regions using p_B and p_F, then we estimate patient specific templates by inpainting pathological regions of B and F using aligned healthy brain sets. After estimating patient specific templates, we update the optimal mappings by including correspondences on the pathological regions. The remainder of this section describes our inpainting method and then our energy function in detail.

To inpaint pathological regions of F, let $\mathcal{I}_F = \{I_n\}_{n=1}^N$ be a set of N healthy brain templates aligned with F by applying a nonrigid registration method [2] (with the histogram matching) to each pair of I_n and F with the foreground mask computed using p_F. Based on our observation that F is closer to the normal anatomy compared with B, we register healthy brain templates on F rather than B. We also provide the foreground mask computed using p_F. For each voxel $\mathbf{x} \in \Omega_F$ having non-zero posteriors of pathological regions ($t \in \{CA, TR, ED\}$), we find the index of the best matching template $n_F^*(\mathbf{x})$ by minimizing patch-based distances between I_n and F and between I_n and $B \circ \boldsymbol{f}_{FB}^*$ (aligning B into F).

$$n_F^*(\mathbf{x}) = \arg \min_n D_{SSD}(F, I_n, \mathbf{x}) + \alpha \cdot D_{SSD}(B \circ \boldsymbol{f}_{FB}^*, I_n, \mathbf{x}) , \tag{3}$$

where $D_{SSD}(\cdot, \cdot, \mathbf{x})$ is the sum of squared distance (SSD) between patches of two input scans centered on $\mathbf{x}$. After estimating $n_F^*(\mathbf{x})$ for pathological regions, we synthesize these regions of F by simply averaging the best matching patches while other advanced methods could also be applied [10]. To inpaint B, we align the set of healthy brain templates into B by applying $\boldsymbol{f}_{BF}^*$ to each template, i.e. $\mathcal{I}_B = \{I_n \circ \boldsymbol{f}_{BF}^*\}_{n=1}^N$. Similar to the case of F, the index of the best matching template $n_B^*(\mathbf{x})$ is estimated for each voxel having non-zero posteriors of pathological regions ($t \in \{TU, ED\}$) by

$$n_B^*(\mathbf{x}) = \arg \min_n D_{SSD}(B, I_n \circ \boldsymbol{f}_{BF}^*, \mathbf{x}) + \alpha \cdot D_{SSD}(F \circ \boldsymbol{f}_{BF}^*, I_n \circ \boldsymbol{f}_{BF}^*, \mathbf{x}) . \tag{4}$$

In (3) and (4), the best matching patch would be consistent with both scans when $\alpha > 0$. We iterate the estimation of the index $\{n_F^*, n_B^*\}$ by applying synthesized scans F and B on the previous iteration in (3) and (4). On the first iteration, we set $\alpha = 0$ and compute D_{SSD} only on the healthy regions (when posteriors of pathological regions are zero). If there exists limited healthy brain regions in the patch, we adaptively double the size of the patch until including enough healthy regions. For the following iterations, we set $\alpha = 1$ and compute D_{SSD} on entire brain regions. This approach improves the coherence of the synthesis as shown in [12]. In Fig. 1 (f)-(g) and (m)-(n), we show inpainted scans for B (a)-(b) and F (h)-(i), respectively.

Now we describe each energy term of $E(\cdot)$ in (2) and then how to optimize it. For the correspondence term E_C, we apply the normalized cross correlation (NCC) distance D_{NCC} between B and F aligned on Ω_C and the cost function masking using posterior probabilities on the pathological regions (PT):

$$E_C(\boldsymbol{f}_{CB}, \boldsymbol{f}_{CF}; B, F, p_B, p_F) \triangleq \int_{\mathbf{x} \in \Omega_C} \{1 - p_{B,PT}(\boldsymbol{f}_{CB}(\mathbf{x}))\}$$
$$\cdot \{1 - p_{F,PT}(\boldsymbol{f}_{CF}(\mathbf{x}))\} \cdot D_{NCC}(B \circ \boldsymbol{f}_{CB}, F \circ \boldsymbol{f}_{CF}, \mathbf{x}) \, d\mathbf{x} \,, \quad (5)$$

where $p_{\cdot,PT}$ is a summation of posteriors for tissue types to be excluded in calculating E_C. Before the inpainting stage, we include whole pathological regions in $p_{B,PT}$ and $p_{F,PT}$ to exclude those regions from calculating correspondences. After the inpainting stage, we only include the tumor region ($t=TU$) in $p_{B,PT}$ and the cavity region ($t=CA$) in $p_{F,PT}$, so the inpainted regions are used for computing E_C. The pathological term E_P penalizes mismatched regions between posteriors of tumor in B ($p_{B,TU}$) and cavity in F ($p_{F,CA}$):

$$E_P(\boldsymbol{f}_{CB}, \boldsymbol{f}_{CF}; p_B, p_F) \triangleq \int_{\mathbf{x} \in \Omega_C} \{p_{B,TU}(\boldsymbol{f}_{CB}(\mathbf{x})) - p_{F,CA}(\boldsymbol{f}_{CF}(\mathbf{x}))\}^2 \, d\mathbf{x} \,. \quad (6)$$

The smoothness term $E_S(\boldsymbol{f}_{CB}, \boldsymbol{f}_{CF})$ is a regularizer based on Tikhonov operator which measures the smoothness of the mappings $\boldsymbol{f}_{CB}$ and $\boldsymbol{f}_{CF}$. To minimize $E(\cdot)$ in (2), we use the discrete-continuous optimization method proposed in [4]. This method updates the initial mapping $\boldsymbol{f}_{BF}^0$ by finding a global solution on the coarse search space through discrete optimization and then refining the solution using continuous optimization.

4   Experiments

We tested our method on a set composed of pre-operative and follow-up MR brain scans of 24 glioma patients. For preprocessing, we co-registered all four modalities (T1, T1-CE, T2, and FLAIR), corrected MR field inhomogeneity, and scaled intensities to fit $[0, 255]$. For all 24 subjects, an expert manually segmented tumor on the pre-operative scan and cavity on the follow-up scan. We computed the Dice score between the tumor region and the cavity region aligned to the pre-operative scan by the method. Also, two experts placed landmarks on the

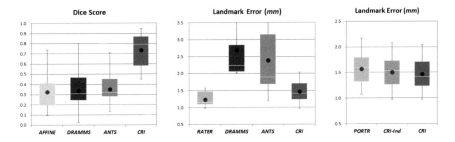

Fig. 2. Box-and-whisker plots of Dice scores on segmentation of pathology (left) and average landmark errors (middle and right). Bars start at the lower quartile and end at the upper quartile with the white line representing the median. Black dots represent the mean errors. *AFFINE* shows the errors of the affine registration and *RATER* denotes the landmark errors of the second rater.

scans of 10 randomly selected subjects. One expert defined 20 landmarks inside 30 mm distance to the tumor boundary on the pre-operative scan. Then both experts independently found corresponding landmarks in the follow-up scan. The landmark error is defined as the mean distance between the landmarks aligned by the method and the corresponding ones set by the expert.

Our method, denoted as *CRI*, requires minimal user inputs including seed point and radius for each tumor and initial mean values for each tissue type for segmenters described in Sec. 2. The correspondence term (5) is only based on T1 and T1-CE as the other two modalities (T2 and FLAIR) decrease the accuracy due to their lower resolutions. We thus applied inpainting on T1 and T1-CE only. For inpainting, we used $N = 64$ T1 healthy brain templates, and applied 10 iterations which is sufficient to create coherent synthesis. We represent *PORTR* as the method runs without inpainting, which corresponds to [4], and *CRI-Ind* as applying independent inpainting by always setting $\alpha = 0$ in (3) and (4). We also applied state-of-the-art registration methods including *DRAMMS* [8] and *ANTS* [2] on our test set. For both methods, we provide the foreground mask to be used for masking out pathological regions.

Fig. 2 (left) shows results on Dice scores for the pathological regions. The average Dice score of *CRI* shows 56%, 54%, and 52% higher than *AFFINE*, *DRAMMS*, and *ANTS*, respectively. *CRI* performed significantly better than the other comparing methods ($p < 0.0001$). Fig. 2 (middle and right) shows results on landmark errors. In the middle figure, *CRI* has the lowest mean error, closest to that of *RATER* and its mean error is 46% lower than *DRAMMS* and 39% lower than *ANTS*. In the right figure, the method using inpainting, *CRI* and *CRI-Ind* performed better than *PORTR* the one without inpainting. The mean error of *CRI* is 7% lower than *PORTR* and 2% lower than *CRI-Ind*. *CRI* performed significantly better than *PORTR* ($p < 0.01$). In Fig. 3, we visually compare the registration results of selected subjects. The aligned follow-up of *CRI* (e) matches better with the pre-operative scan (a) than those of other methods (c)-(d). Also, estimated patient specific templates shown in (f)-(g) shows reasonable restorations of the normal anatomy specific to the scan.

228   D. Kwon et al.

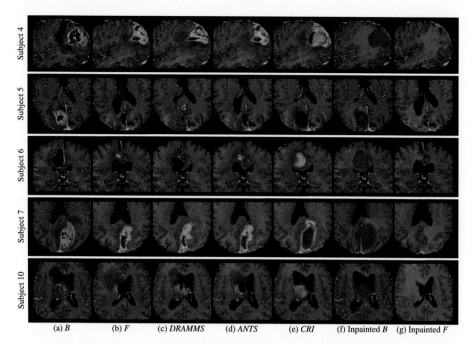

(a) B   (b) F   (c) DRAMMS   (d) ANTS   (e) CRI   (f) Inpainted B   (g) Inpainted F

Fig. 3. Registration results for each method. In each row, we show T1-CE images of the
pre-operative scan B in (a) and the follow-up scan F in (b). (c)-(e) show the registered
F using *DRAMMS*, *ANTS*, and *CRI*, respectively. For B and registered F, boundaries
of segmented tumor is overlaid. (f)-(g) show B and F inpainted by *CRI*. In (f), tumor
regions are masked as they don't belong to the normal anatomy.

5   Conclusion

In this paper, we proposed a new method combining registration and estimation
of patient specific templates for pre-operative and follow-up brain tumor scans.
We estimated large deformations on the pre-operative scan using the symmetric
registration framework initialized by the joint segmentation-registration which
grows a tumor on the atlas aligned on the follow-up scan. The registration on
tumor regions of the pre-operative scan was guided to match with cavity on
the follow-up scan by the pathological term E_P. To estimate the registration
on the entire pathological regions reliably, we estimated patient specific templates by inpainting pathological regions using the patch-based synthesis based
on the healthy brain population. Therefore, we were able to explicitly address
missing correspondences and inconsistent intensity profile problems. Our method
was evaluated on the scans of 24 glioma patients and performed the best among
compared registration methods.

Acknowledgement. This work was supported by the National Institutes of
Health (NIH) under Grant R01 NS042645.

References

1. Akbari, H., Macyszyn, L., Da, X., Wolf, R.L., Bilello, M., Verma, R., O'Rourke, D.M., Davatzikos, C.: Pattern Analysis of Dynamic Susceptibility Contrast-enhanced MR Imaging Demonstrates Peritumoral Tissue Heterogeneity. Radiology 273(2), 502–510 (2014)
2. Avants, B.B., Epstein, C.L., Grossman, M., Gee, J.C.: Symmetric diffeomorphic image registration with cross-correlation: Evaluating automated labeling of elderly and neurodegenerative brain. Med. Image Anal. 12(1), 26–41 (2008)
3. Chitphakdithai, N., Duncan, J.S.: Non-rigid registration with missing correspondences in preoperative and postresection brain images. In: Jiang, T., Navab, N., Pluim, J.P.W., Viergever, M.A. (eds.) MICCAI 2010, Part I. LNCS, vol. 6361, pp. 367–374. Springer, Heidelberg (2010)
4. Kwon, D., Niethammer, M., Akbari, H., Bilello, M., Davatzikos, C., Pohl, K.M.: PORTR: Pre-Operative and Post-Recurrence Brain Tumor Registration. IEEE Trans. Med. Imaging 33(3), 651–667 (2014)
5. Kwon, D., Shinohara, R.T., Akbari, H., Davatzikos, C.: Combining generative models for multifocal glioma segmentation and registration. In: Golland, P., Hata, N., Barillot, C., Hornegger, J., Howe, R. (eds.) MICCAI 2014, Part I. LNCS, vol. 8673, pp. 763–770. Springer, Heidelberg (2014)
6. Liu, X., Niethammer, M., Kwitt, R., McCormick, M., Aylward, S.R.: Low-rank to the rescue – atlas-based analyses in the presence of pathologies. In: Golland, P., Hata, N., Barillot, C., Hornegger, J., Howe, R. (eds.) MICCAI 2014, Part III. LNCS, vol. 8675, pp. 97–104. Springer, Heidelberg (2014)
7. Niethammer, M., Hart, G.L., Pace, D.F., Vespa, P.M., Irimia, A., Van Horn, J.D., Aylward, S.R.: Geometric metamorphosis. In: Fichtinger, G., Martel, A., Peters, T. (eds.) MICCAI 2011, Part II. LNCS, vol. 6892, pp. 639–646. Springer, Heidelberg (2011)
8. Ou, Y., Sotiras, A., Paragios, N., Davatzikos, C.: DRAMMS: Deformable registration via attribute matching and mutual-saliency weighting. Med. Image Anal. 15(4), 622–639 (2011)
9. Periaswamy, S., Farid, H.: Medical image registration with partial data. Med. Image Anal. 10(3), 452–464 (2006)
10. Roy, S., Carass, A., Prince, J.L.: Magnetic Resonance Image Example-Based Contrast Synthesis. IEEE Trans. Med. Imaging 32(12), 2348–2363 (2013)
11. Sdika, M., Pelletier, D.: Nonrigid registration of multiple sclerosis brain images using lesion inpainting for morphometry or lesion mapping. Hum. Brain Mapp. 30(4), 1060–1067 (2009)
12. Ye, D.H., Zikic, D., Glocker, B., Criminisi, A., Konukoglu, E.: Modality propagation: coherent synthesis of subject-specific scans with data-driven regularization. In: Mori, K., Sakuma, I., Sato, Y., Barillot, C., Navab, N. (eds.) MICCAI 2013, Part I. LNCS, vol. 8149, pp. 606–613. Springer, Heidelberg (2013)

Topography-Based Registration of Developing Cortical Surfaces in Infants Using Multidirectional Varifold Representation

Islem Rekik, Gang Li, Weili Lin, and Dinggang Shen*

Department of Radiology and BRIC,
University of North Carolina at Chapel Hill, NC, USA
dgshen@med.unc.edu

Abstract. Cortical surface registration or matching facilitates atlasing, cortical morphology-function comparison and statistical analysis. Methods that geodesically shoot surfaces into one another, as currents or varifolds, provide an elegant mathematical framework for generic surface matching and dynamic local features estimation, such as deformation momenta. However, conventional current and varifold matching methods only use the normals of the surface to measure its geometry and guide the warping process, which overlooks the importance of the direction in the convoluted cortical sulcal and gyral folds. To cope with the stated limitation, we decompose each cortical surface into its normal and tangent varifold representations, by integrating principal curvature direction field into the varifold matching framework, thus providing rich information for the direction of cortical folding and better characterization of the cortical geometry. To include more informative cortical geometric features in the matching process, we *adaptively* place control points based on the surface topography, hence the deformation is controlled by points lying on gyral crests (or "hills") and sulcal fundi (or "valleys") of the cortical surface, which are the most reliable and important topographic and anatomical landmarks on the cortex. We applied our method for registering the developing cortical surfaces in 12 infants from 0 to 6 months of age. Both of these variants *significantly* improved the matching accuracy in terms of closeness to the target surface and the precision of alignment with regional anatomical boundaries, when compared with several state-of-the-art methods: (1) diffeomorphic spectral matching, (2) current-based surface matching and (3) original varifold-based surface matching.

1 Introduction

Advancing our understanding of the cerebral cortex development, neuroplasticity, aging and disorders is of tremendous value in modern neuroscience and psychology. The ever-growing acquisition of neuroimaging datasets mined for morphometric and functional brain studies continues to churn out wide spectrums of computational neuroanatomy methods. In particular, registration methods have been exhaustively developed in order to better align the imaging data

---

* Corresponding author.

© Springer International Publishing Switzerland 2015
N. Navab et al. (Eds.): MICCAI 2015, Part II, LNCS 9350, pp. 230–237, 2015.
DOI: 10.1007/978-3-319-24571-3_28

to a common space, where statistical analyses can be performed. Due to the remarkable convolution and inter-subject variability of cortical foldings, volume-based warping typically produced poorly aligned sulcal and gyral folds [1]. In contrast, cortical surface-based registration can better align the convoluted and variable cortical folding, owing to respecting the inherent topological property of the cortex during registration. Recently, Lombaert *et al.* incorporated more local geometric features in an *exact* surface matching framework, which estimated a diffeomorphic correspondence map *via* a simple closest neighbor search in the surface spectral domain [2]. Its accuracy measured up to the performance of Freesurfer [3] and Spherical Demons [4]. However, both of these methods [3,4] do not directly operate on the cortical surface, as they inflate each cortical hemisphere into a sphere and then register them in the spherical space, which inevitably introduces distortion to surface metrics.

On the other hand, *inexact* surface matching methods, based on geodesically shooting one surface into another, present a spatially consistent method for establishing diffeomorphic correspondences between shapes and measuring their dissimilarity. In [5], the *current metric* provided groundwork for developing a generic diffeomorphic surface registration and regression model without having to establish the point-to-point surface landmark correspondence on the longitudinal shapes. One key strength of this mathematical model is that it measures dissimilarities between complex shapes of different dimensions such as distributions of unlabelled points (e.g. anatomical landmarks), curves (e.g. fiber tracts) and surfaces (e.g. cortices); thereby, *simultaneously and consistently* tracking local deformations in a set of *multi-dimensional shapes* within a large deformation morphometric mapping (LDDMM) framework. One drawback of this method is that it annihilates the sum of two shapes with opposing normals. Recently, Charon *et al.* in [6] solved this problem by proposing the use of the *varifold metric* –a variant of the current metric– for matching shapes with inconsistent orientations. Surfaces are encoded as a set of non-oriented normals, which are embedded into a space endowed with the varifold dissimilarity metric.

However, the conventional varifold matching framework developed in [6,7] does not consider the principal curvature direction of the deforming surface, whereas this represents a key feature of the convoluted cortical surface by encoding the local direction of sulcal and gyral folds that marked previous work on the cortex [8]. In this paper, we propose a novel surface matching method by extending the previous work of [6] and [7] for integrating topography-based surface features to achieve a more anatomically consistent and accurate matching of cortical surfaces in infants with dynamic cortex growth. First, we automatically and adaptively lay the control points on the cortex high hills (gyral crests) and deep valleys (sulcal fundi) through a supervertex surface partition for guiding the shape deformation from a source surface to a target surface. Second, we add a novel varifold surface representation encoded by its principal curvature direction, which will be combined to its normal varifold representation to solve a variational problem leading to a gradient shape matching. Finally, we compare the accuracy of our method with: (1) diffeomorphic spectral cortical matching [2], (2) current-based surface matching [5], and (3) original varifold-based surface matching methods [6,7] in terms of geometric concordance between target and warped shapes and alignment with the boundaries of anatomical cortical regions.

2   Varifold-Based Surface Matching

The concept of varifold in geometric measure theory was recently used to solve shape matching problems in [6,7]. We begin by reviewing the basic concepts for matching two shapes using the varifold metric as exposed by [6,7].

Surface Representation as a Varifold. In the varifold framework, a surface S is embedded in a vector space E (here $\mathbb{R}^3$) and encoded by a set of its *nonoriented* normals $n(x)$ attached at each of its vertices x (Fig. 1). These nonoriented vectors belong to the Grassman manifold $G_d(E)$ (the space of non-oriented tangent spaces), which in the case of surfaces, is defined as the quotient of the unit sphere $\mathbb{S}$ in $\mathbb{R}^3$ by two group elements $\{\pm Id_{\mathbb{R}^3}\}$. This quotient space $G_d(E)$ contains elements u that are equivalent to $u/|u|$ and $-u/|u|$, denoted as $\overleftrightarrow{u}$. Any surface is thereby represented as a distribution of non-oriented spaces tangent to each of its vertices and spread in the embedding space E.

In a similar construction of currents, a varifold surface is defined as a continuous linear form that integrates a vector field $\omega \in W$: $S(\omega) = \int_{\Omega_S} \omega(x, \overleftrightarrow{n(x)}) |n(x)| dx$. The vector space W is defined as a Reproducing Kernel Hilbert Space (RKHS) on the square-integrable space $C_0(E \times G_d(E))$. The reproducing kernel k on the space of varifolds is the tensor product of kernels on E and on $G_d(E)$: $k = k_e \otimes k_t$, where k_e denotes a positive continuous kernel on the space E (same as currents) and k_t denotes an additional linear continuous kernel of non-oriented vectors on the manifold $G_d(E)$. In particular, for $x, y \in E$ and $\overleftrightarrow{u}, \overleftrightarrow{v} \in G_d(E)$, the varifold kernel is defined as $k((x, \overleftrightarrow{u}), (y, \overleftrightarrow{v})) = k_e(x, y) \left(\frac{u^T v}{|u||v|} \right)^2$, where $k_e(x, y) = exp(-|x-y|^2/\sigma_e^2)$ is a Gaussian scalar kernel that decays with a rate σ_e. This kernel parameter controls the scale under which geometric details are ignored when measuring the surface using the varifold metric. The space of varifold is then defined as the *dual* space W^* (*i.e.* the space of linear mappings from W into $\mathbb{R}$). By the reproducing property, any varifold in W^* is defined as: $\omega(x, \overleftrightarrow{u}) = \delta_{(x, \overleftrightarrow{u})}(\omega) = < k((x, \overleftrightarrow{u}), \cdot), \omega >_W$, where $\delta_{(x, \overleftrightarrow{u})}$ defines a Dirac varifold that acts on ω. A surface S with N meshes (triangles) is then approximated by the sum of Dirac varifolds parameterized by the positions x_i of the centers of its meshes and their corresponding normals: $S = \sum_{i=1}^{N} \delta_{(x_i, \overleftrightarrow{n_i})}$. The Dirac varifold does not depend on the orientation given to each triangle. More importantly, the varifold space is endowed with a dot-product that induces a norm used for measuring the difference between pairs of shapes $S = \sum_i \delta_{(x_i, \overleftrightarrow{n_i})}$ and $S' = \sum_j \delta_{(x'_j, \overleftrightarrow{n'_j})}$:

$$< S, S' >_{W^*} = \sum_i \sum_j k_e(x_i, x'_j) \frac{(n_i^T n'_j)^2}{|n_i||n'_j|} \tag{1}$$

Varifold Registration Using LDDMM. Geodesically shooting a source varifold S_0 onto a target varifold S_1 is fully defined by the initial momenta of

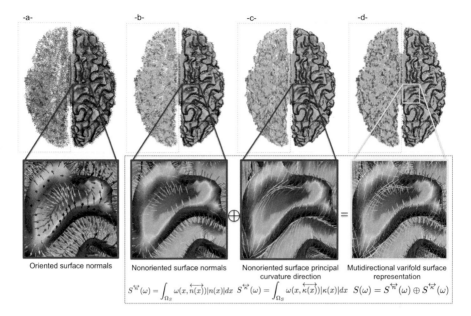

Fig. 1. *Cortical surface representations.* (a) The surface is represented using its oriented normals located at the centers of its meshes (*i.e.* a current) or (b) using its nonoriented normals (*i.e.* a varifold). (d) We propose to represent the surface S as a sum of two directional varifolds ($S^{\overleftrightarrow{n}}$ and $S^{\overleftrightarrow{\kappa}}$): one generated by its nonoriented normals (b) and the other by the nonoriented principal curvature direction (c).

deformation p_0. Geodesics (optimal deformation trajectories) are the solution of the flow equation: $\frac{d\phi_t(x)}{dt} = v_t \circ \phi_t(x)$, $t \in [0,1]$ with $\phi_0 = Id_{\mathbb{R}^3}$. ϕ_t is the diffeomorphism which acts on each mesh center x of S_0 to deform into $S_1 = \phi_1 \cdot S_0$. The time-varying deformation velocity v_t belongs to the RKHS V, densely spanned by a reproducing Gaussian kernel k_V which decays at a rate σ_V (the scale under which there is no deformation). In [7], the dense deformation was guided by a set of *control points* $\{c_k\}_{k=1,\ldots,N_c}$ that are estimated along with the initial momenta of deformation and the positions of the vertices in the warped surface. The velocity at any point $x \in E$ is defined as the sum of the scalar functions k_V (located at a set of control points $\{c_k\}_{1,\ldots,Nc}$) convoluted with their deformation momenta $\{p_k\}$: $v(x) = \sum_{k=1}^{N_c} k_V(x, c_k)p_k$.

Objective Functional. The estimation of the optimal initial deformation momenta, optimal control points and optimal warped vertices' positions is achieved through minimizing the following energy functional:

$J = \frac{1}{2} \int_0^1 |v_t|_V^2 dt + \gamma ||\phi_1^v \cdot S_0 - S_1||_{W^*}^2$

The first energy term forces the warping trajectory to be smooth and the second makes the trajectory end close enough to the target surface. The parameter γ defines the trade-off between both of these terms. The objective functional J is minimized through a gradient descent algorithm as in [7].

3   Topography-Based Cortical Surface Matching Using Varifold Metric

Surface Multidirectional Varifold Representation. To better guide the geometric varifold warping, we propose a novel formula for surface varifold representation by adding the principal curvature direction κ: $S(\omega) = S^{\overleftrightarrow{n}}(\omega) \oplus S^{\overleftrightarrow{\kappa}}(\omega)$, where $S^{\overleftrightarrow{n}}(\omega) = \int_{\Omega_S} \omega(x, \overleftrightarrow{n(x)})|n(x)|dx$ and $S^{\overleftrightarrow{\kappa}}(\omega) = \int_{\Omega_S} \omega(x, \overleftrightarrow{\kappa(x)})|\kappa(x)|dx$.

Decomposing the surface into both of these 'orthogonal' components means that, instead of *reading* the shape of a surface in one direction using only the set of normals associated with its meshes, we perform an additional tangential reading in the principal curvature direction; thereby, collecting more geometric features that help register cortical surfaces through capturing important orientation information of cortical folding (Fig. **1**). However, unlike the computation of surface normals, the estimation of the principal direction is challenging as it may be noisy and ambiguous at flat cortical areas where both minimum and maximum principal curvatures are very small (Fig. **2**). To solve this problem, we first compute the principal directions and curvature derivatives using an efficient finite difference method. Second, we adopt a robust method developed in [9] to estimate smooth principal curvature directions that uniformly point towards the direction parallel to its folds –without diverting them from the original principal direction field. These are estimated through solving the variational diffusion equation: $E_d = \int_{\Omega_S} |\nabla \kappa(x)|^2 + f(x)|\kappa(x) - \eta(x)|^2 dx$ with respect to $\kappa(x) \cdot n(x) = 0$; where η denotes the original principal curvature direction, κ represents the diffused principal curvature direction, and $f(x)$ is set to the absolute value of the principal curvature at each vertex x. This propagates reliable and informative principal directions at sulcal bottoms and gyral crests to flat regions with unreliable principal directions, thereby generating a smooth tangential varifold which provides rich information of cortical folding. Subsequently, the varifold dot-product between two surfaces S and S' becomes:

$$< S, S' >_{W^*} = \frac{1}{2}\sum_i \sum_j k_e(c_i, c'_j)\frac{(n_i^T n'_j)^2}{|n_i||n'_j|} + \frac{1}{2}\sum_i \sum_j k_e(c_i, c'_j)\frac{(\kappa_i^T \kappa'_j)^2}{|\kappa_i||\kappa'_j|}$$

Topography-Based Control Points Selection. Instead of estimating the optimal control points near the most variable parts of the mean shape for both source and target shapes during energy minimization as in [7], we explore the highly variable topography of the cortical surface and adaptively place them on high gyral crests and low sulcal fundi. This allows for better exploration of the topography in the deforming cortical surface. We then feed them as inputs to the objective functional J. For this purpose, we adopt the supervertex cortical surface partition method developed by [10]. Supervertices seeds are uniformly placed on cortical surface and then a partition, that aligns the supervertices boundaries with gyral crests and sulcal fundi, is generated via minimizing an energy function using graph cuts. For our application, we choose to place the control points in cortical areas that will guide the deformation of the multidirectional surface varifold around each supervertex edge located at gyral crests and sulcal bottoms of the cortical surface by automatically checking the maximum principal curvature value (Fig. **2**).

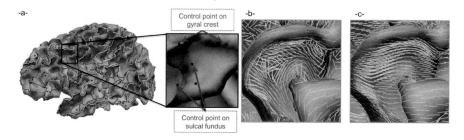

Fig. 2. *Key elements of the proposed method.* (a) Surface partition into supervertices and the control point placement on gyral crests and sucal fundi. Noisy principal direction (b) transformed into a smooth principal direction field (c).

Objective Functional. To estimate the initial momenta of deformation attached to each topographic control point placed on the target surface, we now minimize the following new energy using the numerical scheme proposed in [7]:

$$J_{new} = \tfrac{1}{2}\int_0^1 |v_t|_V^2 \, dt + \gamma_n ||\phi_1^v \cdot S_0^{\overleftrightarrow{n}} - S_1^{\overleftrightarrow{n}}||_{W^*}^2 + \gamma_\kappa ||\phi_1^v \cdot S_0^{\overleftrightarrow{\kappa}} - S_1^{\overleftrightarrow{\kappa}}||_{W^*}^2$$

4   Results

Data and Parameters Setting. We evaluated the proposed framework on inner cortical surfaces of 12 infants, each with MRI scans acquired at around birth and 6 months of age. We empirically fixed the current and varifold parameters at the same values for all infants: $\sigma_e = 5$, $\sigma_V = 20$ and $\gamma = 0.1$. For the novel varifold matching framework, we set $\gamma_n = 0.1$ and $\gamma_\kappa = 0.2$ to assign more weight to the fidelity-to-data term, depending on the surface principal curvature direction. In our experiments, we only used the minimum principal curvature direction which traces the gyral folding as a line.

Table 1. *Matching accuracy for twelve 0-to-6 month cortical surfaces.*

12 infants	Vertex-wise distance error (mm)	Average Dice over 36 ROIs
Spectral diffeomorphic exact matching	–	0.86 ± 0.004 ($p = 0.001$)
Current-based surface matching	1.15 ± 3.14	0.86 ± 0.03 ($p = 0.0002$)
Original varifold-based surface matching	0.64 ± 0.73	0.87 ± 0.015 ($p = 0.002$)
Proposed varifold-based surface matching	$\mathbf{0.60 \pm 0.65}$	$\mathbf{0.88 \pm 0.006}$

Benchmark with Three State-of-the Art Methods. We compared the results of the proposed method with: (1) diffeomorphic spectral cortical matching[1] where we used the mean curvature as a feature to refine the registration as pinpointed in [2], (2) current-based surface matching [5], and (3) original varifold-based surface matching methods[2] [6,7]. To evaluate the matching performance, we used two different criteria: (i) Euclidean distance (in mm) between the warped and the target

---

[1] The source code was kindly shared by first author in [2]

[2] We thank deformetrica research team for sharing the current-based and varifold-based matching code at http://www.deformetrica.org/

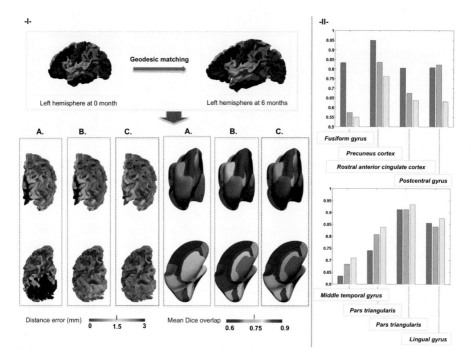

Fig. 3. *Euclidean distance error between the warped and the target hemispheres (left) and mean Dice overlap between warped and target parcellated hemispheres into 36 anatomical regions (right), both averaged across all subjects.* We overlay the average distance and mean Dice maps on a template for the current-based matching method (I-A), the original varifold matching method (I-B), and the proposed method (I-C). Bar plots represent the mean distance error (II-top) and mean Dice index (II-bottom) averaged across subjects in multiple highly folded and variable cortical areas for current (dark green), original varifold (light green) and proposed method (yellow). Our proposed method shows the best performance for (I-left) and performs at least as good as methods (A) and (B) and better in the majority of cortical areas for (I-right).

surfaces; and (ii) the accuracy of alignment with target anatomical region boundaries measured using the mean Dice area overlap index $d(S, S') = \frac{2|S \cap S'|}{|S|+|S'|}$ over 36 anatomical cortical regions. Table **1** shows that the proposed method achieves the best performance *w.r.t* both criteria. Our performance has improved with a rate similar to the Dice overlap ratios reported in [2] when compared to FreeSurfer and Spherical Demons. This improvement is notably visible in Fig. **3**, which displays the distance error map between the warped and the target surfaces and the mean Dice ratio between warped and target 36 boundaries of anatomical regions averaged across all subjects. The matching performance gradually ameliorates from the current-based method (Fig. **3**–I-A) to the original varifold method (Fig. **3**–I-B) and reaches its apex for the proposed method (Fig. **3**–I-C). The proposed method also outperforms other methods significantly in some highly variable and folded cortical regions (e.g. precuneus cortex and rostral anterior cingulate cortex) (Fig. **3**–II).

5   Discussion and Conclusion

We presented the first cortical surface registration method involving multiple directions for surface representation using the varifold metric and guided by topographic control points lying on the highs and the dips of the surface. Notably, the proposed framework capitalizes on a rich topographic and orthogonal reading of the deforming surface, applied for the first time to developing infant brains. Through surpassing the performance of several other state-of-the art surface registration methods, our proposed method can be used for building cortical surface atlases and better examining subjects with abnormal cortical development.

References

1. Thompson, P., Toga, A.: A surface-based technique for warping three-dimensional images of the brain. IEEE Trans. Med. Imaging 15, 402–417 (1996)
2. Lombaert, H., Sporring, J., Siddiqi, K.: Diffeomorphic spectral matching of cortical surfaces. Inf. Process. Med. Imaging 23, 376–389 (2013)
3. Fischl, B., Sereno, M., Tootell, R., Dale, A.: High-resolution intersubject averaging and a coordinate system for the cortical surface. Hum. Brain Mapp. 8, 272–284 (1999)
4. Yeo, B., Sabuncu, M., Vercauteren, T., Ayache, N., Fischl, B., Golland, P.: Spherical demons: fast diffeomorphic landmark-free surface registration. IEEE Trans. Med. Imaging 29, 650–668 (2010)
5. Durrleman, S., Pennec, X., Trouvé, A., Ayache, N.: Statistical models of sets of curves and surfaces based on currents. Medical Image Analysis 13, 793–808 (2009)
6. Charon, N., Trouvé, A.: The varifold representation of non-oriented shapes for diffeomorphic registration. SIAM Journal on Imaging Sciences 6, 2547–2580 (2013)
7. Durrleman, S., Prastawa, M., Charon, N., Korenberg, J., Joshi, S., Gerig, G., Trouvé, A.: Morphometry of anatomical shape complexes with dense deformations and sparse parameters. Neuroimage 101, 35–49 (2014)
8. Boucher, M., Evans, A., Siddiqi, K.: Oriented morphometry of folds on surfaces. Inf. Process. Med. Imaging 21, 614–625 (2009)
9. Li, G., Guo, L., Nie, J., Liu, T.: Automatic cortical sulcal parcellation based on surface principal direction flow field tracking. NeuroImage 46, 923–937 (2009)
10. Li, G., Nie, J., Shen, D.: Partition cortical surfaces into supervertices: Method and application. In: Levine, J.A., Paulsen, R.R., Zhang, Y. (eds.) MeshMed 2012. LNCS, vol. 7599, pp. 112–121. Springer, Heidelberg (2012)

A Liver Atlas Using the Special Euclidean Group

Mohamed S. Hefny[1,*], Toshiyuki Okada[2], Masatoshi Hori[3], Yoshinobu Sato[4],
and Randy E. Ellis[1]

[1] Queen's University, Kingston, Ontario, Canada
{hefny,ellis}@cs.queensu.ca
[2] Tsukuba University, Tsukuba, Japan
okada.t@md.tsukuba.ac.jp
[3] Osaka University, Osaka, Japan
mhori@radiol.med.osaka-u.ac.jp
[4] Nara Institute of Science and Technology, Nara, Japan
yoshi@is.naist.jp

Abstract. An atlas is a shape model derived using statistics of a population. Standard models treat local deformations as pure translations and apply linear statistics. They are often inadequate for highly variable anatomical shapes. Non-linear methods has been developed but are generally difficult to implement.

This paper proposes encoding shapes using the special Euclidean group $\mathbb{SE}(3)$ for model construction. $\mathbb{SE}(3)$ is a Lie group, so basic linear algebra can be used to analyze data in non-linear higher-dimensional spaces. This group represents non-linear shape variations by decomposing piecewise-local deformations into rotational and translational components.

The method was applied to 49 human liver models that were derived from CT scans. The atlas covered 99% of the population using only three components. Also, the method outperformed the standard method in reconstruction. Encoding shapes as ensembles of elements in the $\mathbb{SE}(3)$ group is a simple way of constructing compact shape models.

Keywords: Statistical Shape Model · Special Euclidean Group · Lie Groups · Lie Algebras · Anatomical Atlas

1 Introduction

Statistical shape models, or atlases, are shape descriptors, derived using statistical analysis on a population, that was introduced by Cootes *et al.* [2]. Atlases have been widely used in medical applications such as shape analysis, segmentation, and treatment planning. The concept is to reduce the dimensionality of a large dataset by capturing variations and removing redundancies. This is often performed using classical principal component analysis (PCA) [12], which assumes the shape space to be Euclidean so that pure translations will describe point-wise deformations. Although this might be a legitimate assumption in some datasets, it is not useful for highly variable human anatomy such as the liver.

---

* Corresponding author.

© Springer International Publishing Switzerland 2015
N. Navab et al. (Eds.): MICCAI 2015, Part II, LNCS 9350, pp. 238–245, 2015.
DOI: 10.1007/978-3-319-24571-3_29

Many attempts have been made to construct compact and accurate shape models of the human liver. Lamecker *et al.* [13] divided the liver into four patches and encoded local distortions by mapping each patch to a disk. Davatzikos *et al.* [3] used wavelet transforms to construct hierarchical shape models. Feng *et al.* [5] used a multi-resolution method for model construction. Okada *et al.* [14] considered inter-organ relationships to handle large variations of shapes. Foruzan *et al.* [7] employed classification of samples to construct population-based models. These models adapted the original PCA formulation, with limited success.

There has been some previous work on applying non-linear statistical analysis for shape model construction. Heap and Hogg [8] extended the PDM using polar coordinates. Fletcher *et al.* [6] presented principal geodesic (PGA) as a generalization of PCA to non-linear spaces; the method approximated geodesics by performing the analysis on the tangent space of the data manifold. The method was applied to medial representations and diffusion tensor images. Sommer *et al.* [16] introduced exact-PGA that performed intrinsic computations on the manifold; this was more accurate, but less efficient than, PGA. Hefny *et al.* [9,11,10] introduced constructing shape models by encoding shapes as elements of a matrix Lie group to enable accurate and efficient non-linear analysis, applying the method to quadrilateral meshes extracted from CT images.

This work proposes modeling a triangulated shape as triples of homogeneous four-vectors and encoding them as rigid transformation matrices. These transformation matrices are members of the special Euclidean Lie group $\mathbb{SE}(3)$. This encoding captures deformations caused by translating or rotating the triples in 3D. A Lie group has an associated Lie algebra, with an exact mapping that maps simple computations on the algebra back to the non-linear group.

The rest of the paper has the following structure. The special Euclidean group $\mathbb{SE}(3)$ is introduced in Section 2. Shape encoding and model construction are developed in Section 3. Experiments and results are presented in Section 4. Discussions and conclusions are drawn in Section 5.

2   The Special Euclidean Group $\mathbb{SE}(3)$

The special Euclidean group $\mathbb{SE}(3)$ is the Lie group of rigid transformations in $\mathbb{R}^3$. $\mathbb{SE}(3)$ is defined as the semi-direct product of the special orthogonal group $\mathbb{SO}(3)$ and the real-valued three-vector group $\mathbb{R}^3$. A transformation $T \in \mathbb{SE}(3)$ has the structure

$$T = \begin{bmatrix} R & t \\ 0\,0\,0 & 1 \end{bmatrix}$$

where $R \in \mathbb{SO}(3)$ is a rotation matrix, and $t \in \mathbb{R}^3$ is a translation vector.

The group $\mathbb{SE}(3)$ is isomorphic to a subset of the general linear group $\mathbb{GL}(4,\mathbb{R})$ because it is a real-valued 4×4 matrix. The group identity is the identity matrix I. The group operation $\circ$ is defined as the standard matrix multiplication, so

$$T_i \circ T_j = T_i T_j = \begin{bmatrix} R_i & t_i \\ 0\,0\,0 & 1 \end{bmatrix} \begin{bmatrix} R_j & t_j \\ 0\,0\,0 & 1 \end{bmatrix} = \begin{bmatrix} (R_i R_j) & (R_i t_j + t_i) \\ 0\,0\,0 & 1 \end{bmatrix}$$

Each transformation $T \in \mathbb{SE}(3)$ has an inverse transformation $T^{-1} \in \mathbb{SE}(3)$ that is the matrix inverse.

The group $\mathbb{SE}(3)$ has the Lie algebra $\mathfrak{se}(3)$ with 6 generators that are 4×4 matrices corresponding to the 6 degrees of freedom of each group element. Three infinitesimal translations are represented by the three matrices G_{t_x}, G_{t_y} and G_{t_z}:

$$
G_{t_x} = \begin{bmatrix} 0 & 0 & 0 & 1 \\ 0 & 0 & 0 & 0 \\ 0 & 0 & 0 & 0 \\ 0 & 0 & 0 & 0 \end{bmatrix} \quad
G_{t_y} = \begin{bmatrix} 0 & 0 & 0 & 0 \\ 0 & 0 & 0 & 1 \\ 0 & 0 & 0 & 0 \\ 0 & 0 & 0 & 0 \end{bmatrix} \quad
G_{t_z} = \begin{bmatrix} 0 & 0 & 0 & 0 \\ 0 & 0 & 0 & 0 \\ 0 & 0 & 0 & 1 \\ 0 & 0 & 0 & 0 \end{bmatrix}
$$

Three infinitesimal rotations are represented by the three skew-symmetric matrices G_{η_x}, G_{η_y} and G_{η_z}:

$$
G_{\eta_x} = \begin{bmatrix} 0 & 0 & 0 & 0 \\ 0 & 0 & -1 & 0 \\ 0 & 1 & 0 & 0 \\ 0 & 0 & 0 & 0 \end{bmatrix} \quad
G_{\eta_y} = \begin{bmatrix} 0 & 0 & 1 & 0 \\ 0 & 0 & 0 & 0 \\ -1 & 0 & 0 & 0 \\ 0 & 0 & 0 & 0 \end{bmatrix} \quad
G_{\eta_z} = \begin{bmatrix} 0 & -1 & 0 & 0 \\ 1 & 0 & 0 & 0 \\ 0 & 0 & 0 & 0 \\ 0 & 0 & 0 & 0 \end{bmatrix}
$$

The algebra $\mathfrak{se}(3)$ is a linearization of the manifold $\mathbb{SE}(3)$, so it can be represented by a coordinate vector $\vec{k} \in \mathbb{R}^6$ as

$$
\vec{k} = [t_x, t_y, t_z, \eta_x, \eta_y, \eta_z]^T
$$

An arbitrary element $K \in \mathfrak{se}(3)$ is described by multiplying its linear coordinate with the generators such that

$$
K = t_x G_{t_x} + t_y G_{t_y} + t_z G_{t_z} + \eta_x G_{\eta_x} + \eta_y G_{\eta_y} + \eta_z G_{\eta_z}
$$

The exponential mapping $exp : \mathfrak{se}(3) \to \mathbb{SE}(3)$ produces a matrix that corresponds with the element K. This mapping is well-defined and surjective. It is commonly represented as a Taylor series expansion

$$
\exp(K) = e^{[K]} = \sum_{i=0}^{\infty} \frac{K^i}{i!} = I + K + \frac{K^2}{2!} + \frac{K^3}{3!} + \cdots
$$

Because the generator matrices G_α are nilpotent, the Taylor expansion can be easily computed as a rotation sub-matrix and a translation sub-vector [11]. The exponential map takes any element of the Lie algebra $\mathfrak{se}(3)$ to the transformation in the Lie group $\mathbb{SE}(3)$. The logarithmic mapping $log : \mathbb{SE}(3) \to \mathfrak{se}(3)$ is the inverse process, or the natural logarithm of a matrix, which is well defined because for a 4×4 homogeneous transform T we always have $\det(T) = 1$.

Both mappings can be used to compute the mean and covariance of samples in the Lie group $\mathbb{SE}(3)$ using known methods [15]. For a dataset of n samples $\{s_0, ..., s_{n-1}\} \in \mathbb{SE}(3)$, both moments can be computed iteratively. An initial mean μ_0 is arbitrarily selected from the dataset. The deviation of the mean is computed in the tangent space as

$$k_{i,j} \equiv log\left(s_i \cdot \mu_j^{-1}\right)$$

where i indexes the samples and j is an iteration index. The mean can be iteratively computed as

$$\mu_{j+1} = exp\left(\frac{1}{n}\sum_i k_{i,j}\right) \cdot \mu_j \tag{1}$$

At each iteration j, the covariance can be computed iteratively as

$$\Sigma_j = \frac{1}{n}\sum_i \left(k_{i,j} \cdot k_{i,j}^T\right) \tag{2}$$

These means and covariances will be used to statistically analyze the data after encoding the shapes as $\mathbb{SE}(3)$ transformation.

3   Shape Encoding and Model Construction

A dataset consists of a population of shape samples with a previously established point correspondence. Shapes must be aligned to remove global rigid transformations and scaling. An important assumption in our work is that the data are a triangulated mesh, so each sample can be handled as an ensemble of point triples or triangles. A non-degenerate triangle $\triangle P_i$ can be represented, in homogeneous coordinates, by the matrix

$$P_i = \begin{bmatrix} p_{i,0}^x & p_{i,1}^x & p_{i,2}^x \\ p_{i,0}^y & p_{i,1}^y & p_{i,2}^y \\ p_{i,0}^z & p_{i,1}^z & p_{i,2}^z \\ 1 & 1 & 1 \end{bmatrix} \tag{3}$$

where the order of the points $p_{i,0}$, $p_{i,1}$, and $p_{i,2}$ is arbitrary but must be consistent across the point correspondence of all samples. We will refer to point $p_{i,0}$ as the *base vertex* of triangle #i.

Any triangle $\triangle P_i$ that is represented by Equation 3 can also be written as a transformation of a canonical matrix. Consider a canonical triangle in the **XY** plane that has one vertex at the origin and one on the **X** axis; its form is

$$P_i^* = \begin{bmatrix} 0 & p_{i,1}^{x*} & p_{i,2}^{x*} \\ 0 & 0 & p_{i,2}^{y*} \\ 0 & 0 & 0 \\ 1 & 1 & 1 \end{bmatrix} \tag{4}$$

This can be mapped to the general triangle $\triangle P_i$ as

$$\triangle P_i = T_i P_i^* \tag{5}$$

where the origin of the canonical triangle is mapped to the base vertex of the general triangle. An important class of triangulated meshes are simple closed meshes. Topologically, these are diffeomorphic to a closed shape (such as a sphere or a torus) and have a key constraint:

Every non-base vertex is in the plane of some other general triangle

With this constraint in mind, for the purposes of constructing an atlas, we can neglect the canonical triangle because the positions of its non-base vertices will be completely described as the base vertex of some other general triangle. (This is not strictly true for other topologies but works for completely closed surfaces.)

We can therefore perform computation just on the transformation matrices T_i that describe each triangulated sample shape. A shape can be encoded as a list of elements in $\mathbb{SE}(3)$. This has the distinct advantage over point-based PCA by handling both rotations and translations, instead of handling only translations. Since translations and rotations are in difference units, the translational components were scaled to be in comparable units with the rotational components.

To construct a statistical atlas, every shape is converted from an ensemble of triangles to an ensemble of rigid transformation matrices. The mean of corresponding matrices is computed using Equation 1 and the covariance is computed using Equation 2. Finally, an eigenvalue decomposition is applied to the covariance matrix. The statistical atlas consists of the mean shape and the eigenvectors as modes of variation.

4   Experiments and Results

Our dataset consists of 49 liver triangular meshes extracted from computed tomography (CT) scans obtained using GE Lightspeed Ultra scanner (General Electric, Milwaukee, USA). The data collection was approved by the relevant Institutional Review Board. The images were manually segmented by a specialized physician and automatically triangulated. Point correspondence between meshes was established using the minimum description length algorithm [4]. Both standard PCA and the proposed method were implemented using MAT-LAB Parallel Computing Toolbox (Mathworks, Natick, USA) and executed on an NVIDIA Tesla K40 GPU (Nvidia, Santa Clara, USA).

One interesting comparison criteria is the parsimony of the model description. For dimensionality reduction, it is desirable to minimize the number of deduced descriptive features that capture most of the variability. The first component of the standard PCA covered 47% of the population variability; it required 11 components to cover 95% and 27 components to cover 99%. The first component of the $\mathbb{SE}(3)$ atlas covered 66%; it required 2 components to cover 95% and 3 components to cover 99% of the population. It is clear that the $\mathbb{SE}(3)$ implementation outperformed the standard implementation of PCA. Figure 1 shows the plots of the accumulated eigenvalues of both methods.

The volumes were reconstructed using both the $\mathbb{SE}(3)$ and PDM methods with just two components. Three evaluation methods were implemented, namely relative volume reconstruction error, average point distance error, and Dices's

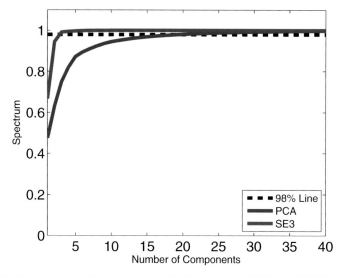

Fig. 1. Accumulated Eigenvalues for both standard PCA and $\mathbb{SE}(3)$ encoding.

Table 1. Summary of Results

Method	Relative volume error	Average point distance error	Dice's coefficient
$\mathbb{SE}(3)$	7.97% ($\pm$ 4.51%)	4.13 mm ($\pm$ 1.61 mm)	92% ($\pm$ 7.13%)
PDM	17.01% ($\pm$ 6.82%)	17.06 mm ($\pm$ 2.25 mm)	76% ($\pm$ 5.60%)

coefficient of overlapping volumes as explained in [1]. The three evaluation methods were applied to each sample, and both mean and standard deviation were computed for the population.

The volumes enclosed within the triangulated surfaces were computed for the original meshes and the reconstructions, as was the relative error in volume reconstruction. The mean relative volume error was 7.28% with a standard deviation of 4.5% for the proposed method, while it was 17.01% with a standard deviation of 6.82% for the standard PDM method. The mean average point distance error was 4.13 mm with a standard deviation of 1.61 mm for the proposed method, while it was 17.06 mm with a standard deviation of 2.25 mm for the standard PDM method. The mean Dice's coefficient was 92% with a standard deviation of 7.13% for the proposed method, while it was 76% with a standard deviation of 5.60% for the standard PDM method. All these errors are statistically significantly different, with $p < 0.001$. Table 1 summarizes the results.

5   Discussion and Conclusions

This work proposed using the special Euclidean group $\mathbb{SE}(3)$ of rigid transformations to encode anatomical shapes for statistical analysis and shape model construction. The shapes were processed as triples of points, instead of independent points as in the standard method. Processing shapes as triples enabled a decomposition of local patch transformations into rotations and translations, rather than using only points that accounts for only translations. The shape can be easily retrieved using those transformations.

The significance of this encoding that it takes the form of a Lie group. A Lie group is a powerful mathematical structure that is simultaneously an algebraic group and a smooth manifold, so complicated geometric data can be processed using simple tools of algebra. Here, we began with the oriented plane of a triangle in a mesh; this geometric element can be represented as an algebraic element in the form of a 4×4 homogeneous rigid transformation which is in the $\mathbb{SE}(3)$ Lie group. The rigid transformation between two planes can be parameterized as a geodesic curve, which is also a 1-parameter 4×4 transformation that can be exactly computed using ordinary matrix algebra. The tangent spaces of the $\mathbb{SE}(3)$ group are linear vector spaces that can be found by taking the matrix logarithm and extracting the 6 infinitesimal transformation parameters; in a tangent space, linear algebra such as PCA can be used to compute statistics such as deformations. These linear differences in the tangent space can be mapped back to the manifold to find the rigid transformations that they describe.

We applied this method to a highly variable human liver dataset. The method outperformed the standard PCA in parsimony of representation. The Lie group formulation required only 2 components to cover 95% of the data, whereas the standard method required 11 components to cover the same percentage. The method was able to reconstruct the data, using only these two components, with a relative mean enclosed volume error of 7.28% that had a standard deviation of 4.5%, mean average point distance error 4.13 mm with a standard deviation of 1.61 mm, and mean Dice's coefficient of overlapping volumes of 92% with a standard deviation of 7.13%.

In conclusion, encoding anatomical shapes using the special linear group $\mathbb{SE}(3)$ is a promising method for construction of statistical shape models. The method represents both local rotations and translations between samples. It outperformed the standard PCA that is in common use. Moreover, the Lie group method is easy to implement. Future work might extend to use of other easily computed matrix Lie groups to large sets of data that are not simple vectors.

Acknowledgments. This work was supported in part by the Natural Sciences and Engineering Research Council of Canada grant #43515, the Collaborative Health Research Program grant #385914, and the MEXT KAKENHI #26108004. The Tesla K40 used for this research was donated by the NVIDIA Corporation.

References

1. Babalola, K.O., Patenaude, B., Aljabar, P., Schnabel, J.A., Kennedy, D., Crum, W.R., Smith, S., Cootes, T.F., Jenkinson, M., Rueckert, D.: Comparison and evaluation of segmentation techniques for subcortical structures in brain MRI. In: Metaxas, D., Axel, L., Fichtinger, G., Székely, G. (eds.) MICCAI 2008, Part I. LNCS, vol. 5241, pp. 409–416. Springer, Heidelberg (2008)

2. Cootes, T.F., Taylor, C.J., Cooper, D.H., Graham, J.: Active shape models - their training and application. Comput. Vis. Image Underst. 61(1), 38–59 (1995)
3. Davatzikos, C., Tao, X., Shen, D.: Hierarchical active shape models, using the wavelet transform. IEEE Trans. Med. Imaging (USA) 22(3), 414–423 (2003)
4. Davies, R.H., Twining, C.J., Cootes, T.F., Waterton, J.C., Taylor, C.J.: A minimum description length approach to statistical shape modeling. IEEE Trans. Med. Imaging 21(5), 525–537 (2002)
5. Feng, J., Ip, H.H.S.: A muti-resolution statistical deformable model (MISTO) for soft-tissue organ reconstruction. Pattern Recognit. 42(7), 1543–1558 (2009)
6. Fletcher, P.T., Lu, C., Pizer, S.M., Joshi, S.: Principal geodesic analysis for the study of nonlinear statistics of shape. IEEE Trans. Med. Imaging 23(8), 995–1005 (2004)
7. Foruzan, A.H., Chen, Y.W., Hori, M., Sato, Y., Tomiyama, N.: Capturing large shape variations of liver using population-based statistical shape models. Int. J. Comp. Assist. Radiol. Surg. 9, 967–977 (2014)
8. Heap, T., Hogg, D.: Extending the point distribution model using polar coordinates. In: Hlaváč, V., Šára, R. (eds.) CAIP 1995. LNCS, vol. 970, pp. 130–137. Springer, Heidelberg (1995)
9. Hefny, M.S.: Analysis of Discrete Shapes Using Lie Groups. Ph.D. thesis, Queen's University (2014)
10. Hefny, M.S., Pichora, D.R., Rudan, J.F., Ellis, R.E.: Manifold statistical shape analysis of the distal radius. Int. J. Comp. Assist. Radiol. Surg. 9(supp. 1), S35–S42 (2014)
11. Hefny, M.S., Rudan, J.F., Ellis, R.E.: A matrix lie group approach to statistical shape analysis of bones. Stud. Health Technol. Inform. 196, 163–169 (2014)
12. Hotelling, H.: Analysis of a complex of statistical variables into principal components. J. Educ. Psychol. 24, 417–441 (1933)
13. Lamecker, H., Lange, T., Seebass, M.: A statistical shape model for the liver. In: Dohi, T., Kikinis, R. (eds.) MICCAI 2002, Part II. LNCS, vol. 2489, pp. 421–427. Springer, Heidelberg (2002)
14. Okada, T., Linguraru, M.G., Yoshida, Y., Hori, M., Summers, R.M., Chen, Y.-W., Tomiyama, N., Sato, Y.: Abdominal multi-organ segmentation of CT images based on hierarchical spatial modeling of organ interrelations. In: Yoshida, H., Sakas, G., Linguraru, M.G. (eds.) Abdominal Imaging. LNCS, vol. 7029, pp. 173–180. Springer, Heidelberg (2012)
15. Pennec, X.: Intrinsic statistics on Riemannian nanifolds: basic tools for geometric measurements. J. Math. Imag. Vis. 25, 127–154 (2006)
16. Sommer, S., Lauze, F., Hauberg, S., Nielsen, M.: Manifold valued statistics, exact principal geodesic analysis and the effect of linear approximations. In: Daniilidis, K., Maragos, P., Paragios, N. (eds.) ECCV 2010, Part VI. LNCS, vol. 6316, pp. 43–56. Springer, Heidelberg (2010)

Multi-scale and Multimodal Fusion of Tract-Tracing, Myelin Stain and DTI-derived Fibers in Macaque Brains

Tuo Zhang[1,2], Jun Kong[3], Ke Jing[4], Hanbo Chen[2], Xi Jiang[2], Longchuan Li[3], Lei Guo[1], Jianfeng Lu[4], Xiaoping Hu[3], and Tianming Liu[2]

[1]Northwestern Polytechnical University, Xi'an, Shaanxi, China
[2]Cortical Architecture Imaging and Discovery Lab, The University of Georgia, Athens, Georgia, USA
[3]Emory University, Atlanta, GA, USA
[4]Nanjing University of Science and Technology, Nanjing, Jiangsu, China

Abstract. Assessment of structural connectivity patterns of brains can be an important avenue for better understanding mechanisms of structural and functional brain architectures. Therefore, many efforts have been made to estimate and validate axonal pathways via a number of techniques, such as myelin stain, tract-tracing and diffusion MRI (dMRI). The three modalities have their own advantages and are complimentary to each other. From myelin stain data, we can infer rich in-plane information of axonal orientation at micro-scale. Tract-tracing data is considered as 'gold standard' to estimate trustworthy meso-scale pathways. dMRI currently is the only way to estimate global macro-scale pathways given further validation. We propose a framework to take advantage of these three modalities. Information of the three modalities is integrated to determine the optimal tractography parameters for dMRI fibers and identify cross-validated fiber bundles that are finally used to construct atlas. We demonstrate the effectiveness of the framework by a collection of experimental results.

Keywords: Tract-tracing, myelin stain, DTI, multi-scale and multimodal fusion, atlas.

1 Introduction

Accurate assessment of structural connectivity patterns on primate brains provides an effective vehicle to understand structural architectures, mechanisms of cortical convolution and brain function [1]. Many advanced techniques have been developed for and applied to structural pathway investigations [2-4]. Among them, diffusion MRI (dMRI) and tractography approaches have been widely applied to estimate major macro-scale white matter pathways in primate brains *in vivo* [2]. A large number of reports on dMRI performance evaluation can be found where it is compared to other data modalities (e.g., [5,7]), such as tract-tracing [7] and myelin stain [5] which are deemed as trustworthy proof for either the existence of 3D inter-regional connections [6] or local in-plane axonal orientations [5]. As for tract-tracing approaches, it is

© Springer International Publishing Switzerland 2015
N. Navab et al. (Eds.): MICCAI 2015, Part II, LNCS 9350, pp. 246–254, 2015
DOI: 10.1007/978-3-319-24571-3_30

difficult to conduct this method on primate brains due to ethical concerns [8]. Also, available reports are based on a variety of partition schemes [11]. Thanks to the "Collation of Connectivity Data for the Macaque" (CoCoMac) database [9], researchers can now estimate and quantify a meso-scale whole-brain connectivity diagram on a user-selected brain map based on hundreds of reports. However, the absence of inter-plane information in myelin stain data and absence of pathways in CoCoMac data make it impossible to construct a whole brain wiring diagram in 3D space.

In this paper, we take the complementary advantages of the abovementioned three modalities. Multi-scale information from them is integrated to determine the optimal tractography parameters for dMRI fibers (step 1 & 2 in Fig. 1) and identify cross-validated fiber bundles that are finally used to construct a 'hybrid' fiber atlas (step 3), which provides trustworthy pathways rarely found in available macaque tract-tracing databases and integrates the myelin-validated coherent score to them. Several evaluation experiments demonstrate the effectiveness of this framework and the derived atlases.

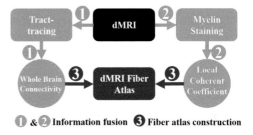

Fig. 1. Flowchart of the framework.

2 Materials and Preprocessing

dMRI Dataset: MRI scans were conducted on twenty macaques under IACUC approval. T1-weighted MRI: repetition time/inversion time/echo time of 2500/950/3. 49 msec, a matrix of 256×256×192, resolution of 0.5×0.5×0.5 mm^3. DTI: diffusion-weighting gradients applied in 60 directions with a b value of 1000 sec/mm^2, repetition time/echo time of 7000/108 msec, matrix size of 128×120×43, resolution of 1.1×1.1×1.1 mm^3. **Caret dataset:** It includes the macaque 'F99' atlas with both surface and volume (T1-weighted, 0.5 mm resolution) templates, to which *LVE00* brain map have been mapped [10]. **CoCoMac database:** It includes 40,000 reports on macaque anatomical connections [9]. We can retrieve wiring information from those collated reports and construct meso-scale tract-tracing connectivity matrix based on the *LVE00* brain map. **Myelin stain database:** 36 coronal Weil's stain slices covering whole brain of one adult macaque brain are available in http://brainmaps.org. The myelin structures are stained dark blue and red cells are stained brown. The in-plane resolution is 0.46 mircon/pixel. The slice thickness is 40 microns.

Preprocessing: dMRI Data: We conduct skull removal and eddy current correction in FSL-FDT with DTI data. We adopt deterministic tractography via DTI Studio to reconstruct streamline fibers. T1-weighted MRI is used as the intra-subject standard space. We perform co-registration by aligning FA map to T1-weighted MRI via FSL-FLIRT. **Myelin stain data**: To align myelin staining to the same space, we use the 8-fold down sampled images (sampling factor is 2) and conduct rigid body 2D image co-registration with maximization of mutual information [12]. By selecting slice #22 as a reference, the slices after it are consecutively registered onto the previous one. Those slices before it are consecutively registered onto the latter one. Original images are aligned accordingly. **Caret data:** The 'F99' atlas is used as the cross-subject and cross modality common space. Individual T1-weighted MRI is registered to the atlas via FSL-FLIRT. All data in individual space is linearly transformed accordingly. The reconstructed 3D myelin staining images are linearly aligned to 'F99' atlas via FSL-FLIRT. As *LVE00* brain map has been mapped to the atlas surface [10], connectivity derived from CoCoMac database is in the common space. It should be noted that macaque brains are less convoluted, making it feasible to register all four aforementioned datasets into the same macaque atlas space with acceptable misalignment error. It is noted that linear registration was used across subjects and modalities because nonlinear registration method may impose interpolation on myelin stain data and tensors derived from dMRI. The axonal orientations and pathways estimated may not be trustworthy.

3   Methods

3.1   Micro-scale Myelin Stain Pathway Orientations

Micro-scale myelin stain pathway orientations were estimated on 256×256 size image blocks. On each block, we estimated one myelin direction.

Step 1: The blood cells, myelin structures and others have different colors (brown, dark blue and white). We used support vector machine (SVM) method [13] to decompose each image block into three probabilistic color maps. We randomly selected 500 training voxels and manually labeled the three tissues. RGB colors were used as features to train the classification model. The training model was applied to all image blocks. Fig. 2(b) illustrates the 'myelin' probabilistic color maps. We use $m(x)$ to denote the myelin probability at pixel x in image $I(x)$.

Step 2: We analyzed the texture to estimate the probability of myelin after converting the color image to the gray-scale. We applied Hessian matrix to filter the image:

$$H(x) = \begin{bmatrix} L_{xx}(x) & L_{xy}(x) \\ L_{xy}(x) & L_{yy}(x) \end{bmatrix} \tag{1}$$

The Hessian matrices were computed with a series of smoothed images. The derivatives $L_i(x)$ in Eq. (1) associated with the ith smoothing scale were obtained by convolving image with a Gaussian kernel of scale σ_i. On $H(x)$, we computed the eigen values $l_1(x)$ and $l_2(x)$ ($|l_1(x)| > |l_2(x)|$). Line shape descriptor is defined as follows:

$$f(x) = e^{-(l_2(x)/l_1(x))^2/\sigma_r} \cdot \left(1 - e^{-\left(l_1^2(x)+l_2^2(x)\right)/\sigma_s}\right) \tag{2}$$

Because each pixel x has a series of $f_i(x)$ values at different smoothing scales, the extrema $f_{max}(x)$ was used to represent the line shape probability (Fig. 2(c)).

Step 3: Final probabilistic map $p(x)$ is the product of $f_{max}(x)$ and $m(x)$.

Step 4: we estimated the myelin orientations in a binary image resulting from thresholding the map $p(x)$ by 0.05(Fig. 2(d)). Connected components were extracted from the binary image. The orientation α measures the angle (in degrees ranging from -90° to 90°) between the x-axis and the major axis of the ellipse that has the same second-moments as the connected component. The connected components less than 20 pixels were eliminated. We used unimodal Gaussian model to fit the distribution of connected component orientation in Fig. 2(e). The expectation (i.e., 50 degrees in Fig. 2(e)) was used as myelin orientation feature for the image block in Fig. 2(a). One direction was estimated because we jointly analyzed the data with DTI fibers, on which only one direction was estimated from diffusion tensors. The orientation distribution is found to be robust to errors introduced by myelin identification.

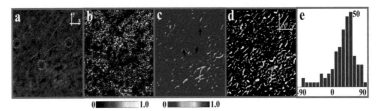

Fig. 2. Myelin orientation estimation method. Circled numbers represent processing steps (see text for details). (a) Original 256×256 myelin stain image block. Black arrows highlight sample stained myelin represented by white dashed curves; white circles highlight sample red cells; (b) The probabilistic map of dark blue color channel; (c) The probabilistic map of myelin texture shape; (d) Binary joint probabilistic map of myelin based on (b) and (c); (e) Orientations distribution of disconnected components in (d). Probabilistic color bars are shown beneath (b)&(c).

3.2   Meso-scale Tract-Tracing and Macro-scale DTI Connectivity Matrices

We used E to denote the tract-tracing connectivity matrix, and A to denote the DTI connectivity matrix. 91 *BrainSites* on each hemisphere under *LEV00* parcellation scheme were used as nodes for the matrices. e_{ij} of E was set to be '1' if *BrainSite i* is an injected *BrainSite* and *BrainSite j* is a labeled region in the CoCoMac database. The matrix is not guaranteed to be symmetric. More technical details can be found in [14]. As for A, Element a_{ij} is the number of fibers which pass through *BrainSite i* and j simultaneously. Within each subject, A was divided by the total fiber number for normalization, so that we obtained an average matrix $\overline{A}$ of all subjects to represent group-wise information. As the meso-scale connectivity matrix E is binary, threshold α was applied to $\overline{A}$ to binarize it by setting all values below it to zero.

3.3   Data Fusion and Atlas Construction

3.3.1 Macro- and Meso-scale Data Fusion

The fusion of macro-scale and meso-scale data was conducted on connectivity matrix base. $\overline{A}$ is regulated by tractography parameters such as angular value, FA value and the threshold α. An optimal set of parameters is the one that makes the corresponding $\overline{A}$ maximally matched with E. The matrix matching problem is equivalent to evaluation of a binary classifier performance. Using E as ground truth, we adopted receiver operating characteristic (ROC) curves to evaluate the performance of $\bar{A}$s under different sets of parameters (see Fig. 3(a)). For each ROC, we had a Youden's index, denoted as Y. The maximal Y represents the maximal matching between $\bar{A}$ and E, and also determines the optimal parameter set. Details can be found in [14].

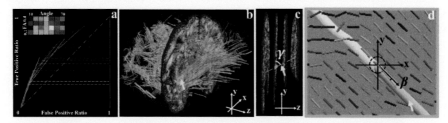

Fig. 3. (a) ROC curves of matching $\bar{A}$ and E; (b) DTI fibers (white curves) and myelin stain slices; (c) and (d): How to measure the similarity between fiber local orientation and myelin orientation. Green boxes highlight the local region where the fiber tract penetrates the slice at dashed black circle location. Short lines in (d) represent myelin orientations, black arrow illustrates the local orientation of the fiber tract and the blue arrow illustrates the myelin orientation.

3.3.2 Macro- and Micro-scale Data Fusion
We attempted to score the points on a DTI fiber tract by measuring if their local orientations are coherent with counterparts on myelin data. We used $t(x)$ to denote a fiber tract, where x is the point on it. In Fig. 3(b)&(c), we illustrate a fiber tract highlighted by yellow arrow, which penetrate four myelin slices. At a penetrating location, as illustrated in Fig. 3(d), we used the angle β ($0° \leq \beta \leq 90°$) between myelin orientation (blue arrow) and fiber orientation (black arrow) to measure if they are coherent.

For each x on $t(x)$, we found the nearest voxel on orientation slices to compute β. If the nearest distance is greater than $1mm$, we marked the point as 'unlabeled'. Also, as the myelin stain slices only contain in-plane information (x-y plane in Fig. 3(b)-(d)), we also measured the angle between local fiber orientation and the myelin plane for each point x, denoted by γ ($0° \leq \gamma \leq 90°$) in Fig 3.(c). If $\gamma = 90°$, no accurate information can be projected onto the slice. Finally, an overall coherent coefficient C for all fiber tracts on a subject can be obtained by:

$$C = \sum_{m=1}^{M} \sum_{n}^{N_m} \frac{(90-\beta_m(x_n))}{90} \times \frac{(90-\gamma_m(x_n))}{90} \ if \ x_n \ is \ not \ 'unlabeled' \qquad (3)$$

where M is the number of fiber tracts and N_m is point number on fiber tract #m. The product term is local coherent coefficient. Similar to Y in section 3.3.1, we measured the average C across subjects for every combination of FA and angular values.

3.3.3 Three Modality Data Fusion and DTI Fiber Atlas Construction
We fused the three data modalities using the following equation:

$$arg\ max_{fa,angle}(\lambda Y(fa, angle) + (1 - \lambda)C(fa, angle)) \qquad (4)$$

Based on Eq. (4), we identified a set of parameters so that the linear combination of Y and C can reach the maximal value. That is, with this set of tractography parameters, the DTI fibers derived macro-scale global connectivity matrix can maximally match the tract-tracing derived meso-scale connectivity matrix, while the DTI fibers can be locally coherent to myelin derived micro-scale orientations.

Finally, a fiber atlas was constructed on the optimal set of parameters. We obtained the corresponding binary DTI connectivity matrix and overlaid it with the tract-tracing one (Fig. 4(b)). 'Both' connections (detected by both DTI and tract-tracing) were identified and the DTI fiber bundles are extracted from individuals. The points on those atlas fiber bundles also have coherent coefficients validated by myelin data.

4   Experimental Results

The framework was conducted on ten DTI training subjects. The parameters used for myelin orientation estimation are experimentally determined (σ_r=0.5, σ_s=450). 11 σ_i are sampled from [1, 3] with equal spacing. Ys and Cs based on different FA and angular values are shown in Fig. 4(a). Values in the two matrices are normalized to [0, 1], respectively. Optimal parameters are determined (white box, FA=0.3 and angular value=70°) where the two measurements equally contribute (λ=0.5). The optimal threshold α is also determined on the ROC curve of FA=0.3 and angular value=70°, by searching for the maximal Y. We use this parameter set in the following analysis.

We overlay the binary DTI connectivity matrix $\overline{A}$ obtained via the optimal parameter set with the E (Fig. 4(b)). We also map the local myelin coherent coefficients onto the DTI fibers (Fig. 4(c)). Finally, for each 'both' connection, we extract myelin coherent coefficients mapped fiber bundles from subjects individually. The average local myelin coherent coefficients are then computed and assigned to 'both' connections. The final matrix in Fig. 4(d) shows the 'both' connections identified by DTI and tract-tracing data as well as the associated myelin coherent coefficients. This matrix integrates group-wise, multi-scale and multi-modal data information.

Fig.4(e) shows the DTI fiber bundles extracted from 'both' connections in Fig.4(b). Six randomly selected training subjects are shown in the left panel. The myelin coherent coefficients are mapped onto those fiber bundles, shown in Fig. 4(f). We also apply the optimal tractography parameters to two new testing subjects and extracted the corresponding fibers as well. Generally, we can observe the consistency of those fiber bundles across subjects within and across groups. Those fiber bundles in Fig. 4(e)&(f) contain rich information and defined as a 'hybrid' atlas.

We take the injected BrainSite VIPm (ventral intraparietal cortex, medial part on the 43rd row of matrix in Fig. 4(b)&(d)) as an example to quantitatively validate the consistency of those atlas fiber bundles across subjects. We extract DTI fiber bundles emanating from VIPm and connecting to other regions via either 'both' or 'DTI-only' connections. The results from four training subjects are shown Fig. 4(g). Missing fiber bundles highlighted by arrows in 'DTI-only' panel suggest worse fiber consistency as compared with those in 'both' panel. Therefore, we define a missing ratio for each connection to describe portions of training subjects with no fibers on such connection.

In the whole connectivity matrix, the missing ratio on 'DTI-only' connections is significantly greater than the one on 'both' connections with $p = 0.02$ via right-tail ('DTI-only' > 'both', $\alpha=0.05$) t-test. Finally, we compute the myelin coherent coefficients on 'DTI-only' connections, similar to those on 'both' connections shown in Fig. 4(d). The average coherent coefficient on 'both' connections is 0.41. It is significantly greater than the one on 'DTI-only' connections (0.36) with $p = 5.72 \times 10^{-5}$ via right-tail ('both' > 'DTI-only', $\alpha=0.05$) t-test. Those results suggest the effectiveness and robustness of atlas constructed on the cross-validated DTI fiber bundles.

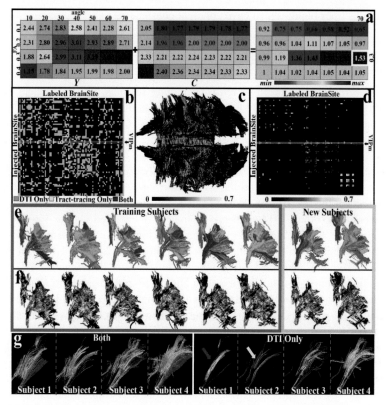

Fig. 4. (a) Y and C measurements based on different parameter combinations and the final fusion result on the right-most matrix; (b) Overlapped matrices E and $\bar{A}$ based on the optimal parameters; (c) The optimal parameters derived DTI fibers, onto which coherent coefficients between myelin and orientations are mapped; (d) The average coherent coefficients of the 'both' connections in (b); (e) DTI fiber bundles extracted from the 'both' connections in (b); (f) 'both' connection DTI fiber bundles, onto which myelin coherent coefficients are mapped; (g) Left panel: 'both' connection DTI fiber bundles on the 43rd row of matrix in Fig. 4(b). Right panel: 'DTI-only' connection fiber bundles. Arrows in indicate missing fiber bundles. Corresponding fiber bundles across subjects are of the same color in (e)&(g).

5   Discussion and Conclusion

This work provides a novel framework to identify cross-validated white matter pathways by fusing multi-scale and multi-modal data. The identified DTI fibers are used to construct atlases. The merits of the framework are summarized as follows: 1) the framework suggests a set of optimal parameters for deterministic streamline tractography; 2) the 'hybrid' fiber atlas is not only cross-validated by multi-scale and multi-modal data, but also contains rich information. The fiber atlases have the potential to be used as trust-worthy 'ground truth' pathways not available in macaque tract-tracing or myelin stain databases. We will take further studies on other dMRI modalities, such as HARDI and tractography models in the future.

Acknowledgement. This work is supported by NIH K25CA181503 and in part by Jiangsu Natural Science Foundation (Project No. BK20131351) by the 111 Project.

References

1. Van Essen, D.: A tension-based theory of morphogenesis and compact wiring in the central nervous system. Nature 385(6614), 313–318 (1997)
2. Chédotal, A., Richards, L.: Wiring the brain: the biology of neuronal guidance. Cold Spring Harb. Perspect. Biol. 2(6), a001917 (1917)
3. Mikula, S., Trotts, I., Stone, J., Jones, E.G.: Internet-Enabled High-Resolution Brain Mapping and Virtual Microscopy. NeuroImage 35(1), 9–15 (2007)
4. Parker, G.J., Stephan, K.E., Barker, G.J., Rowe, J.B., MacManus, D.G., Wheeler-Kingshott, C.A., Ciccarelli, O., Passingham, R.E., Spinks, R.L., Lemon, R.N., Turner, R.: Initial demonstration of in vivo tracing of axonal projections in the macaque brain and comparison with the human brain using diffusion tensor imaging and fast marching tractography. Neuroimage 15(4), 797–809 (2002)
5. Leergaard, T.B., White, N.B., de Crespigny, A., Bolstad, I., D'Arceuil, H., Bjaalie, J.G., Dale, A.: Quantitative histological validation of diffusion MRI fiber orientation distributions in the rat brain. PLoS One 5(1), e8595 (2010)
6. Jbabdi, S., Lehman, J.F., Haber, S.N., Behrens, T.: Human and monkey ventral prefrontal fibers use the same organizational principles to reach their targets: tracing versus tractography. J. Neurosci. 33, 3190–3201 (2013)
7. Sporns, O.: Networks of the Brain. MIT Press, Cambridge (2010)
8. Bakker, R., Wachtler, T., Diesmann, M.: CoCoMac 2.0 and the future of tract-tracing databases. Front Neuroinform 6, 30 (2012)
9. Kötter, R.: Online retrieval, processing, and visualization of primate connectivity data from the CoCoMac database. Neuroinformatics 2, 127–144 (2004)
10. Van Essen, D.C.: Surface-based approaches to spatial localization and registration in primate cerebral cortex. Neuroimage 23(suppl. 1), S97–S107 (2004)
11. Markov, N.: A weighted and directed interareal connectivity matrix for macaque cerebral cortex 24(1), 17–36 (2012)

12. Lu, X., Zhang, S., Su, H., Chen, Y.: Mutual information-based multimodal image registration using a novel joint histogram estimation. Comput. Med. Imaging Graph. 32(3), 202-9 (2008)
13. Chang, C., Lin, C.: LIBSVM: a library for support vector machines. ACM Transactions on Intelligent Systems and Technology 2, 27:1–27:27
14. Jing, K., Zhang, T., Lu, J., Chen, H., Guo, L., Li, L., Hu, X., Liu, T.: Multiscale and multimodal fusion of tract-tracing and DTI-derived fibers in macaque brains. In: ISBI (in press, 2015)

Space-Frequency Detail-Preserving Construction of Neonatal Brain Atlases

Yuyao Zhang, Feng Shi, Pew-Thian Yap, and Dinggang Shen

Department of Radiology and BRIC, University of North Carolina at Chapel Hill, NC, USA

Abstract. Brain atlases are an integral component of neuroimaging studies. However, most brain atlases are fuzzy and lack structural details, especially in the cortical regions. In particular, neonatal brain atlases are especially challenging to construct due to the low spatial resolution and low tissue contrast. This is mainly caused by the image averaging process involved in atlas construction, often smoothing out high-frequency contents that indicate fine anatomical details. In this paper, we propose a novel framework for detail-preserving construction of atlases. Our approach combines space and frequency information to better preserve image details. This is achieved by performing reconstruction in the space-frequency domain given by wavelet transform. Sparse patch-based atlas reconstruction is performed in each frequency subband. Combining the results for all these subbands will then result in a refined atlas. Compared with existing atlases, experimental results indicate that our approach has the ability to build an atlas with more structural details, thus leading to better performance when used to normalize a group of testing neonatal images.

1 Introduction

Brain atlases are spatial representations of anatomical structures, allowing integral brain analysis to be performed in a standardized space. They are widely used for neuroscience studies, disease diagnosis, and pedagogical purposes [1,2].

An ideal brain atlas is expected to contain sufficient anatomical details and also to be representative of the images in a population. It serves as a non-bias reference for image analysis. Generally, atlas construction involves registering a population of images to a common space and then fusing them into a final atlas. In this process, structural misalignment often causes the fine structural details to be smoothed out, which results in blurred atlases. The blurred atlases can hardly represent real images, which are normally rich with anatomical details.

To improve the preservation of details in atlases, the focus of most existing approaches [3-7] has been on improving image registration. For instance, Kuklisova-Murgasova *et al.* [3] constructed atlases for preterm infants by affine registration of all images to a reference image, which was further extended in [4] by using group-wise parametric diffeomorphic registration. Oishi *et al.* [5] proposed to combine affine and non-linear registrations for hierarchically building an infant brain atlas. Using adaptive kernel regression and group-wise registration, Serag *et al.* [6] constructed a spatio-temporal atlas of the developing brain. In [7], Luo *et al.* used both intensity

© Springer International Publishing Switzerland 2015
N. Navab et al. (Eds.): MICCAI 2015, Part II, LNCS 9350, pp. 255–262, 2015.
DOI: 10.1007/978-3-319-24571-3_31

and sulci landmark information in the group-wise registration for constructing a tod-dler atlas. However, all these methods perform simple weighted averaging of the reg-istered images and hence have limited ability in preserving details during image fu-sion. For more effective image fusion, Shi *et al.* [8] utilized a sparse representation technique for patch-based fusion of similar brain structures that occur in the local neighborhood of each voxel. The limitation of this approach is that it lacks an explicit attempt to preserve high frequency contents for improving the preservation of ana-tomical details. In [9], Wei *et al.* proposed to use wavelet transform to reveal detailed information from motion-corrupted diffusion-weighted images of the human heart. It is shown that pyramidal decomposition of images encodes coarse and fine image contents in different frequency subbands.

In this paper, we propose a novel image fusion approach for obtaining neonatal brain atlases with rich details. We employ information in both frequency and space domains given by wavelet transform for atlas construction. **Frequency domain:** By decomposing each brain image into multiple scales and orientations using wavelet transform, fine and latent anatomical structures become more apparent in certain fre-quency subbands. It is hence easier to design constraints to preserve these structures.

Space Domain: The neighboring patches are group-constrained for spatial consisten-cy during reconstruction. We apply our method to construct brain atlases for neonatal MR images, which is challenging due to the low spatial resolution and low tissue contrast. Experimental results indicate that the proposed method can generate atlases of much higher quality, compared to the existing state-of-the-art neonatal atlases.

2   Method

2.1   Overview

The overall pipeline of the proposed method is shown in Fig. 1. First, all individual subject images are aligned to a common space using group-wise registration to generate a mean image. Wavelet transform is then used to decompose both the aligned individual images and the mean image into the frequency domain. In each frequency subband, we then construct an atlas using patch-by-patch sparse reconstruction. To avoid inconsistency, the immediate neighbors of each patch are group-constrained to have similar sparse coefficients. Finally, the reconstructed frequency subband atlases are combined together to construct a final atlas.

2.2   Image Preprocessing

All images were preprocessed with a standard pipeline, including resampling, bias correction, skull stripping, and tissue segmentation. We use a publicly available group-wise registration method [10] (http://www.nitrc.org/projects/glirt) to align all images to a common space. We can then obtain a set of N registered images $\{I_n \mid n = 1, \cdots, N\}$, $I_n \in \mathbb{R}^3$. These images are averaged to form a mean image $I_{mean} = \frac{1}{N}\sum_{n=1}^{N} I_n$.

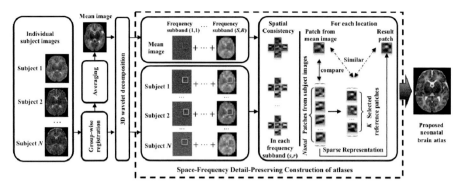

Fig. 1. Flow chart of the proposed atlas construction framework

2.3   Frequency Domain Reconstruction

We combine atlases generated from different frequency subbands of the images to better preserve high-frequency image details. We first perform pyramidal decomposition using 3D wavelet on all images:

$$I = \sum_{s=1}^{S}\sum_{r=1}^{R} I^{(s,r)} = \sum_{s=1}^{S}\sum_{r=1}^{R} D^{(s,r)} \cdot a^{(s,r)} \tag{1}$$

where scale $s = 1, \cdots, S$ denotes that the image has been down-sampled s times. For each scale s, images are further decomposed into orientation subband $r = 1, \cdots, R$. For each scale s, we fixed $R = 8$, and the corresponding orientation subbands in 3D are denoted as '*LLL*', '*HLL*', '*LHL*', '*HHL*', '*LLH*', '*HLH*', '*LHH*', and '*HHH*' filters, where '*L*' indicates low-pass filtering and '*H*' indicates high-pass filtering, i.e., '*HLH*' denotes high-pass filtering in x and z directions and low-pass filtering in y direction. $D^{(s,r)}$ denotes the wavelet basis of subband (s,r), and $a^{(s,r)}$ denotes the wavelet coefficients in subband (s,r). The wavelet coefficients of subband (s,r) of all images $\{I_n | n = 1, \cdots, N\}$ are denoted as $\left\{a_n^{(s,r)} | n = 1, \cdots, N\right\}$.

Atlas construction is performed in a patch-by-patch manner. We consider a local cubic patch $p_{mean}^{(s,r)}$ centered at location (x, y, z) in the mean image I_{mean}. The patch is represented as a vector of length $V = v \times v \times v$, where v is the patch diameter in each dimension. We sparsely refine the mean patch $p_{mean}^{(s,r)}$ using a dictionary, formed by including all patches at the same location in all N training images, i.e., $P^{(s,r)} = \left[p_1^{(s,r)}, p_2^{(s,r)}, \cdots, p_N^{(s,r)}\right]$, thereby generating the reconstructed detail-preserving atlas patch $p_{atlas}^{(s,r)}$. To compensate for possible registration error, we enrich the dictionary by including patches from neighboring locations, i.e., 26 locations immediately adjacent to (x, y, z). Therefore, from all N aligned images, we will have a total of $N_{total} = 27 \times N$ patches in the dictionary, i.e., $P^{(s,r)} = \left[p_1^{(s,r)}, p_2^{(s,r)}, \cdots, p_{N_{total}}^{(s,r)}\right]$. We use this dictionary to reconstruct the refined atlas patch $p_{atlas}^{(s,r)}$ by estimating a sparse coefficient vector $\hat{\beta}^{(s,r)}$, with each element denoting the weight of the contribution of a patch in the dictionary.

To further enhance robustness, we constrain the reconstructed atlas patch $p_{atlas}^{(s,r)}$ to be similar to the appearance of a small set of K ($K \leq N_{total}$) neighboring patches $\{p_k^{(s,r)} | k = 1, \cdots, K\}$ from $P^{(s,r)}$ that are most similar to $p_{mean}^{(s,r)}$. The reconstruction problem can now be formulated as

$$\hat{\beta}^{(s,r)} = \underset{\hat{\beta}^{(s,r)}>0}{\operatorname{argmin}} \sum_{k=1}^{K} \left\| p_k^{(s,r)} - P^{(s,r)} \cdot \beta^{(s,r)} \right\|_2^2 + \lambda \left\| \beta^{(s,r)} \right\|_1 \qquad (2)$$

where λ is a non-negative parameter controlling the influence of the regularization term. Here, the first term measures the discrepancy between observations $p_k^{(s,r)}$ and the reconstructed atlas patch $p_{atlas}^{(s,r)} = P^{(s,r)} \cdot \hat{\beta}^{(s,r)}$, and the second term is for L_1-regularization on the coefficients in $\beta^{(s,r)}$. Considering that the dictionary $P^{(s,r)}$ and the observations $p_k^{(s,r)}$ share the same basis $D^{(s,r)}$, we can combine Eq. (1) and Eq. (2) for a wavelet representation version of the problem:

$$\hat{\beta}^{(s,r)} = \underset{\hat{\beta}^{(s,r)}>0}{\operatorname{argmin}} \sum_{k=1}^{K} \left\| D^{(s,r)} \cdot \left(c_k^{(s,r)} - C^{(s,r)} \cdot \beta^{(s,r)} \right) \right\|_2^2 + \lambda \left\| \beta^{(s,r)} \right\|_1 \qquad (3)$$

where $c_k^{(s,r)}$ is a vector consisting of the wavelet coefficients of $p_k^{(s,r)}$, and $C^{(s,r)} = \left[c_1^{(s,r)}, c_2^{(s,r)}, \cdots, c_{N_{total}}^{(s,r)} \right]$ is a matrix containing the wavelet coefficients of the patches in dictionary $P^{(s,r)}$. Finally, the atlas is constructed as

$$I_{atlas} = \sum_{s=1}^{S} \sum_{r=1}^{R} I_{atlas}^{(s,r)} = \sum_{s=1}^{S} \sum_{r=1}^{R} D^{(s,r)} \cdot C^{(s,r)} \cdot \hat{\beta}^{(s,r)} \qquad (4)$$

2.4   Spatial Consistency

To promote local consistency, multi-task LASSO [11] is used for spatial regularization in the space-frequency domain to simultaneously estimate G neighboring atlas patches, indexed as $g = 1, \cdots, G$.

We denote the dictionary, training patch, and sparse coefficient vector for the g-th neighbor respectively as $P_g^{(s,r)}$, $p_{k,g}^{(s,r)}$ and $\beta_g^{(s,r)}$. For simplicity, we let $B^{(s,r)} = [\beta_1^{(s,r)}, \cdots, \beta_G^{(s,r)}]$, which can also be written in the form of row vectors: $B^{(s,r)} = \begin{bmatrix} \gamma_1^{(s,r)} \\ \vdots \\ \gamma_M^{(s,r)} \end{bmatrix}$, where $\gamma_m^{(s,r)}$ is the m-th row in the matrix $B^{(s,r)}$ (with totally M rows). Then, we reformulate Eq. (2) using multi-task LASSO:

$$\hat{B}^{(s,r)} = \underset{\hat{B}^{(s,r)}>0}{\operatorname{argmin}} \sum_{g=1}^{G} \sum_{k=1}^{K} \left\| p_{g,k}^{(s,r)} - P_g^{(s,r)} \cdot \beta_g^{(s,r)} \right\|_2^2 + \lambda \left\| B^{(s,r)} \right\|_{2,1}$$

$$\qquad (5)$$

$$= \underset{\hat{B}^{(s,r)}>0}{\operatorname{argmin}} \sum_{g=1}^{G} \sum_{k=1}^{K} \left\| D^{(s,r)} \cdot \left(c_{g,k}^{(s,r)} - C_g^{(s,r)} \cdot \beta_g^{(s,r)} \right) \right\|_2^2 + \lambda \left\| B^{(s,r)} \right\|_{2,1}$$

where $\left\|B^{(s,r)}\right\|_{2,1} = \sum_{m=1}^{M}\left\|\gamma_m^{(s,r)}\right\|_2$. The first term is a multi-task sum-of-squares term for all G neighboring atlas patches. The second term is for multi-task regularization using a combination of L_2 and L_1 norms. L_2 norm penalization is imposed on each row of matrix $B^{(s,r)}$ (i.e., $\gamma_m^{(s,r)}$) to enforce similarity of neighboring patches. L_1 norm penalization is to ensure representation sparsity. This combined penalization ensures that the neighboring patches have similar sparse coefficients. The multi-task LASSO in Eq. (5) can be solved efficiently by using the algorithm described in [11].

3   Experiments

Dataset. We use neonatal brain scans to demonstrate the performance of the proposed atlas construction method. Specifically, 73 healthy neonatal subjects (42 males / 31 females) were used in this study. MR images of the subjects were scanned at postnatal age of 24±10 (9-55) days using a Siemens head-only 3T scanner. T2-weighted images were obtained with 70 axial slices using a turbo spin-echo (TSE) sequence for a resolution of 1.25×1.25×1.95mm^3. All 73 images were resampled to have an isotropic resolution of 1×1×1 mm^3, bias-corrected, skull-stripped, and tissue-segmented.

Implementation Details. There are several parameters in the proposed method: the patch size v, the number of nearest patches K, the regularization parameter λ, and the number of wavelet scale levels S. We performed a grid search for parameters that produced the atlas with the highest signal energy. Then we fixed the patch size as $v = 6$ ($V = 6 \times 6 \times 6$) and set the number of closest patches to $K = 10$. We also set the regularization parameter to $\lambda = 10^{-4}$. We used 'symlets 4' as the wavelet basis for image decomposition. The number of scale levels for wavelet decomposition was set to $S = 3$. The low-frequency content of a single subject image was similar to the low-frequency content of the average atlas when using atlas when using 3 or more scales. This suggests that it is sufficient to use 3 scales.

Atlas Construction Performance Using 73 Subjects. Fig. 2 (a-e) show five representative axial slices of the neonatal brain atlas built by the proposed method. Despite the large number of subjects (73) used for atlas construction, the atlas still contains clear structural details especially in the cortical regions.

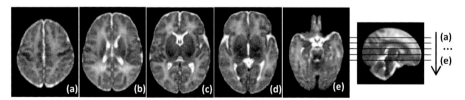

Fig. 2. Neonatal atlas constructed from 73 subjects.

Comparison with State-of-the-Art Neonatal Atlases. Four state-of-the-art neonatal atlases are included for visual inspection. Atlas-A: The 41-th week atlas created by Kuklisova-Murgasova *et al.* [3], longitudinally for each week from week 28.6 to week

47.7 using 142 neonatal subjects. <u>Atlas-B</u>: The atlas constructed by Oishi *et al.* [5] using 25 brain images from neonates of 0-4 days of age. <u>Atlas-C</u>: The 41-th week atlas built by Serag *et al.* [6] involving 204 premature neonates between 26.7 and 44.3 gestational weeks. <u>Atlas-D</u>: The neonatal atlas created by Shi *et al.* [8], involving the same neonatal brain images as used in this work. An atlas created by simply averaging the 73 aligned neonatal images is also included for comparison. One can easily observe from Fig. 3 that the atlas generated by the proposed method provides the clearest structural details. Note that, Atlas-A, Atlas-B and Atlas-C are constructed using datasets different from ours and thus may have different appearances from our atlas. Atlas-D, Averaging atlas, and the Proposed atlas are built from the same dataset.

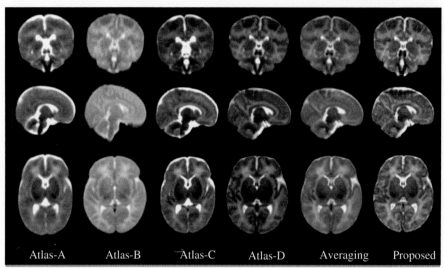

Atlas-A   Atlas-B   Atlas-C   Atlas-D   Averaging   Proposed

Fig. 3. Comparison of neonatal atlases constructed by Kuklisova-Murgasova *et al.* (Atlas-A, 2010), Oishi *et al.* (Atlas-B, 2011), Serag *et al.* (Atlas-C, 2012), Shi *et al.* (Atlas-D, 2014), simple averaging (Averaging), and our proposed method (Proposed) on the 73 aligned images. Similar slices were selected from each of these six atlases for easy comparison.

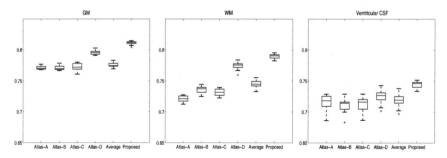

Fig. 4. Box plots for the *Dice Ratio* ($DR = 2|A \cap B| / (|A| + |B|)$, where A and B are the two segmentation maps) values associated with the five state-of-the-art atlases and the proposed atlas. Red lines in the boxes mark the medians. The boxes extend to the lower and upper quartiles (i.e., 25% and 75%). Whiskers extend to the minimum and maximum values in one-and-a-half interquartile range. Outliers beyond this range are marked by red "+" symbols.

Evaluation of Atlas Representativeness. We evaluate the 6 neonatal atlases shown in Fig. 3 in terms of how well they can spatially normalize a **testing** population of neonatal images. MR images of 20 **new** healthy neonatal subjects (10 males/ 10 females) were obtained at 37-41 gestational weeks, using TSE sequences with parameters: TR=6200 ms, TE=116 ms, Flip Angle=150°, and resolution=1.25×1.25×1.95 mm³. Similar image preprocessing was performed, which includes resampling to 1×1×1 mm³, bias correction, skull stripping, and tissue segmentation. All these 20 test images are aligned to each of the 6 atlases by first using affine registration and then nonlinear deformable registration with Diffeomorphic Demons [12], respectively. For each atlas, a mean segmentation image is built by voxel-wise majority voting using all aligned segmentation images. The segmentation images of all individuals, warped to the atlas space, are then compared with this mean segmentation image by means of *Dice Ratio*: $DR = 2|A \cap B| / (|A| + |B|)$, where A and B are the two segmentation maps. DR ranges from 0 (for totally disjoint segmentations) to 1 (for identical segmentations). The structural agreement is calculated in pair of each aligned image and the voted mean segmentation image, which denotes the ability of each atlas for guiding test images into a common space. Statistical analysis (Fig. 4) indicates that the proposed atlas outperforms all other atlases in GM, WM and CSF alignment. Two-sample t-tests based on the *Dice Ratios* demonstrate that the proposed method significantly outperforms all other comparison methods (p<0.001).

Evaluation of Energy Distribution. We assess the image energy variation across all frequency subbands for the 6 neonatal atlases shown in Fig. 3 and then compare with the individual images. For fair comparison, the intensity ranges of all atlases are normalized to interval [0,255]. Low variation of high-frequency components indicates loss of anatomical details. The energy of each frequency subband is defined as the L_2 norm of wavelet coefficients in that subband. The average energy is computed for each of the 24 wavelet subbands (including 3 scales, and 8 orientations for each scale) of the 73 neonatal subject images. Fig. 5 shows the energy distributions for different scale levels and orientations. For the atlases created with simple averaging, the energy loss is significant in the high frequency subbands (e.g., from subband '*HLL*' to '*HHH*' in Scale 1), compared to the atlas created using the proposed method. The energy loss can also be observed in the higher frequency subbands (e.g., subband '*HHH*') of Scale 2 and Scale 3. The proposed atlas mitigates the energy loss problem, illustrating that the proposed atlas preserves more anatomical details from individual images and is hence more representative of the population.

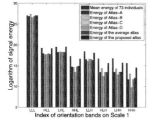 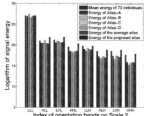 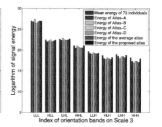

Fig. 5. Image energy distributions across orientations and scales, for the individual images, and the 6 neonatal atlases shown in Fig. 3. Higher energy values in high frequency subbands represent better preservation of anatomical details. It can be seen that the proposed atlas preserves more details from individual images, compared with state-of-the-art atlases.

4   Conclusion

In this paper, we presented a novel space-frequency domain based sparse representation method to better preserve structural details in neonatal brain atlases. Our approach employs a hierarchical strategy in reconstructing the atlas through combining atlases reconstructed from the frequency subbands using wavelet decomposition. Experimental results demonstrated that our approach preserves richer anatomical details (with better performance on neonatal image normalization) than other state-of-the-art neonatal atlases.

References

1. Evans, A., Janke, A., Collins, D., Baillet, S.: Brain templates and atlases. Neuroimage 62, 911–922 (2012)
2. Jin, Y., Shi, Y., Zhan, L., Gutman, B., De Zubicaray, D., McMahon, K., Wright, M., Toga, A., Thompson, P.: Automatic clustering of white matter fibers in brain diffusion MRI with an application to genetics. NeuroImage 100, 75–90 (2014)
3. Kuklisova-Murgasova, M., Aljabar, P., Srinivasan, L., Counsell, S.L., Doria, V., Serag, A., Rueckert, D.: A dynamic 4D probabilistic atlas of the developing brain. NeuroImage 54(4), 2750–2763 (2011)
4. Schuh, A., et al.: Construction of a 4D brain atlas and growth model using diffeomorphic registration. In: Durrleman, S., Fletcher, T., Gerig, G., Niethammer, M., Pennec, X. (eds.) STIA 2014, LNCS 8682. LNCS, vol. 8682, pp. 27–37. Springer, Heidelberg (2015)
5. Oishi, K., Mori, S., Donohue, P., Ernst, T., Anderson, L., Buchthal, S., Chang, L.: Multi-contrast human neonatal brain atlas: application to normal neonate development analysis. NeuroImage 56(1), 8–20 (2011)
6. Serag, A., Aljabar, P., Ball, G., Counsell, S., Boardman, J., Rutherford, M., Rueckert, D.: Construction of a consistent high-definition spatio-temporal atlas of the developing brain using adaptive kernel regression. NeuroImage 59(3), 2255–2265 (2012)
7. Luo, Y., Shi, L., Weng, J., He, H., Chu, W., Chen, F., Wang, D.: Intensity and sulci landmark combined brain atlas construction for Chinese pediatric population. Human Brain Mapping 35(8), 3880–3892 (2014)
8. Shi, F., Wang, L., Wu, G., Li, G., Gilmore, J., Lin, W., Shen, D.: Neonatal atlas construction using sparse representation. Human Brain Mapping 35(9), 4663–4677 (2014)
9. Wei, H., Viallon, M., Delattre, B., Moulin, K., Yang, F., Croisille, P., Zhu, Y.: Free-Breathing Diffusion Tensor Imaging and Tractography of the Human Heart in Healthy Volunteers using Wavelet-Based Image Fusion. IEEE Trans. Med. Imaging 34(1), 306–316 (2015)
10. Wu, G., Wang, Q., Jia, H., Shen, D.: Feature based group-wise registration by hierarchical anatomical correspondence detection. Human Brain Mapping 33(2), 253–271 (2012)
11. Liu, J., Ji, S., Ye, J.: Multi-task feature learning via efficient l 2, 1-norm minimization. In: Proceedings of the Twenty-Fifth Conference on Uncertainty in Artificial Intelligence, pp. 339–348. AUAI Press, June 2009
12. Vercauteren, T., Pennec, X., Perchant, A., Ayache, N.: Diffeomorphic demons: Efficient non-parametric image registration. NeuroImage 45(1), S61–S72 (2009)

Mid-Space-Independent Symmetric Data Term
for Pairwise Deformable Image Registration

Iman Aganj[1], Eugenio Iglesias[2], Martin Reuter[1,3], Mert R. Sabuncu[1,3], and Bruce Fischl[1,3]

[1]Martinos Center, Massachusetts General Hospital, Harvard Medical School, Boston, USA
{iman,mreuter,msabuncu,fischl}@nmr.mgh.harvard.edu
[2]Basque Center on Cognition, Brain and Language (BCBL), San Sebastian, Spain
e.iglesias@bcbl.eu
[3]CSAIL, Massachusetts Institute of Technology, Cambridge, USA

Abstract. Aligning a pair of images in a mid-space is a common approach to ensuring that deformable image registration is symmetric – that it does not depend on the arbitrary ordering of the input images. The results are, however, generally dependent on the choice of the mid-space. In particular, the set of possible solutions is typically affected by the constraints that are enforced on the two transformations (that deform the two images), which are to prevent the mid-space from drifting too far from the native image spaces. The use of an implicit atlas has been proposed to define the mid-space for registration. In this work, by aligning the atlas to each image in the native image space, we make implicit-atlas-based pairwise registration independent of the mid-space, thereby eliminating the need for anti-drift constraints. We derive a new symmetric data term that only depends on a single transformation morphing one image to the other, and validate it through diffeomorphic registration experiments on brain MR images.

1 Introduction

Image registration – i.e., computation of a set of dense spatial correspondences among images – is a central step in most population and longitudinal imaging studies. Since linear transformation is usually not sufficient to account for cross-subject variation and temporal changes in the anatomy, deformable image registration often becomes necessary. In pairwise deformable registration, the choice of the reference space in which the two images are compared affects the registration, making the resulting deformation field dependent on this choice, and leading to registration *asymmetry* [1-11]. Pairwise registration has been proposed to be symmetrized by minimizing the average of two cost functions, each using one input image as the reference space [1-4], yet integrating the mismatch measure non-uniformly in the native space of the interpolated image [11].

In a different approach to achieve symmetry, both images are deformed and compared in a *mid-space*, hence the invariance to the ordering of images [5-10]. Such approaches essentially minimize their cost functions with respect to *two*

© Springer International Publishing Switzerland 2015
N. Navab et al. (Eds.): MICCAI 2015, Part II, LNCS 9350, pp. 263–271, 2015.
DOI: 10.1007/978-3-319-24571-3_32

transformations T_1 and T_2 that take the two input images to the mid-space. However, without additional constraints, this increases the degrees of freedom of the problem twofold, compared to the end result of pairwise registration that is the *one* transformation, $T = T_2 \circ T_1^{-1}$, taking the second input image to the first. Furthermore, if the images are compared in the mid-space (that depends on T_1 and T_2), the optimization algorithm is allowed to update the mid-space so as to decrease the cost function without necessarily changing the final result T. For example, the algorithm can shrink the regions with mismatching image intensities to make the deformed images look more similar in the mid-space, without necessarily making them more similar in the two native spaces. To alleviate these issues, additional constraints are used to keep the mid-space "in between" the native image spaces. These *anti-drift* constraints, which are different from those regularizing the transformations, define the mid-space. They typically either restrict the space of possible T_1 and T_2 (resulting in fewer degrees of freedom), or penalize the values of T_1 and T_2 that move the mid-space away from the native spaces. The most common such constraints, proposed for mid-space registration and atlas construction, are restrictions on T_1 and T_2 to have opposite displacement [7, 8, 12-14] or velocity [9, 10, 15] fields. In large deformation models, geodesic averaging of the deformations has also been proposed [5, 6, 16]. The choice of the anti-drift constraints may bias the algorithm towards favoring a particular set of transformations, thereby affecting the resulting T.

Unbiased *atlas* construction techniques, when applied to a pair of images, can constitute mid-space pairwise registration [10, 16, 17]. Given that the desired output of registration is the deformation field, but not the auxiliary atlas, one can substitute the atlas in the cost function with an analytical expression of the two deformed images, leading to an implicit-atlas cost function. To that end, it was initially proposed to compare the deformed images to the atlas in the abstract mid-space [16]. A better justified generative model, however, progresses from the atlas to the images and compares the deformed atlas to the images (i.e., in the native image spaces) [18, 19]. Taking advantage of this native-space atlas construction resolves the issue of susceptibility to shrinkage-type problems, leading to a proper implicit-atlas cost function for mid-space pairwise registration [10]. Nevertheless, the registration still remains a function of *two* transformations taking the images to a mathematically defined mid-space.

In this work, we point out for the first time the key fact that implicit-atlas pairwise registration is inherently independent of the mid-space. We show that the data term only depends on the overall image-to-image transformation T, implying that the individual image-to-atlas transformations T_1 and T_2 are redundant and unnecessary to keep, and that anti-drift constraints are indeed not needed. We derive a new cost function that, in contrast to the existing mid-space approaches, can be minimized directly with respect to T, with no anti-drift constraints. The proposed cost function is general and can be used with any transformation model, such as the displacement and velocity fields.

2   Methods

2.1   Mid-Space Approach to Registration Symmetry

Let $I_1, I_2 : \Omega \to \mathbb{R}$ be two d-dimensional input images to be registered, where $\Omega \subseteq \mathbb{R}^d$. We want to compute the regular transformation $T : \Omega \to \Omega$ that deforms I_2 so as to make I_1 and $I_2 \circ T$ most similar to each other; a task that is often done by minimizing a cost function with respect to T. The common sum of squared differences (SSD) data term can be formulated, for instance, as $\|I_1 - I_2 \circ T\|_2^2$ or $\|I_1 \circ T^{-1} - I_2\|_2^2$. These two forms are not equivalent though, because the transformed image – which is different in each case – is integrated non-uniformly [1-4, 11], resulting in registration asymmetry.

In a popular approach to derive a symmetric cost function, both images are deformed to a *mid-space* [5-10]. Consequently, these cost functions depend on two transformations, $T_1, T_2 : \Omega \to \Omega$, deforming images I_1 and I_2, respectively. The deformed images are then often compared in the mid-space through a cost function such as $\|I_1 \circ T_1 - I_2 \circ T_2\|_2^2$, and the output is eventually computed as $T = T_2 \circ T_1^{-1}$. The mid-space cost function is by definition invariant with respect to the ordering of the images.

With no additional constraints, the dimension of the mid-space registration problem (solving for T_1 and T_2) is twice as big as the standard asymmetric problem (solving for T). Also, the mid-space can drift arbitrarily far away from the native spaces of the images due to large changes in T_1 and T_2, for instance through combination with a transformation h, as $T_1 \circ h$ and $T_2 \circ h$, which decreases the mid-space cost function without changing the final $T = T_2 \circ h \circ h^{-1} \circ T_1^{-1} = T_2 \circ T_1^{-1}$. To avoid these issues, additional constraints are often employed to keep the mid-space "in between" the native spaces. For instance, the two transformations may be forced to have opposite-sign displacement fields, as $T_1(x) = x + u(x)$ and $T_2(x) = x - u(x)$, resulting in the constraint $T_1(x) + T_2(x) = 2x$ (or similarly $T_1^{-1}(x) + T_2^{-1}(x) = 2x$) [7, 8, 12-14]. This reduces the degrees of freedom and to some extent prevents the mid-space drift, however, at the expense of limiting our ability to model all possible transformations T. An extreme example of this would be the 2D case with the true transformation T being a 180° rotation about the origin, i.e. $T(x) = -x$, where no T_1 and T_2 will simultaneously satisfy both $T_1(x) + T_2(x) = 2x$ and $T_2(x) = T \circ T_1(x)$. For large deformations, opposite-sign velocity fields [9, 10, 15] and geodesic averaging are used to preserve the properties of the transformations [5, 6, 16]. Since there is no unique way to define the mid-space, the registration results can depend on the choice of the constraints imposed on T_1 and T_2.

Mid-space pairwise registration can also be performed by constructing an unbiased atlas from two images [10, 16, 17]. In atlas construction, the observed images are assumed to be instances generated from an atlas image with some geometrical and intensity variation. Therefore, the problem boils down to finding an atlas, $A : \Omega \to \mathbb{R}$, and regular transformations T_1^{-1} and T_2^{-1} that take the atlas from the mid-space to the native spaces of the two images, in such a way that the deformed versions of the atlas resemble the observed images. Using the SSD metric, the data term for such an optimization is the sum of two (asymmetric [18, 19]) subject-atlas distance terms, as in:[1]

$$\hat{T}_1, \hat{T}_2, \hat{A} = \underset{T_1,T_2,A}{\operatorname{argmin}} \left[\int_\Omega \left(I_1(x) - A \circ T_1^{-1}(x) \right)^2 dx + \int_\Omega \left(I_2(z) - A \circ T_2^{-1}(z) \right)^2 dz \right]. \quad (1)$$

Comparing the images to the atlas in the physically meaningful native image spaces complies with the generative model assumption that the image is generated as a deformed version of the atlas (not vice versa), and that the Gaussian noise is added to the deformed atlas [18, 19]. The changes of variables $x = T_1(y)$ and $z = T_2(y)$ leads to:

$$\underset{T_1,T_2,A}{\operatorname{argmin}} \int_\Omega \left[\left(I_1 \circ T_1(y) - A(y) \right)^2 J_1(y) + \left(I_2 \circ T_2(y) - A(y) \right)^2 J_2(y) \right] dy, \quad (2)$$

where $J_1(y) := \det \partial T_1(y)$ and $J_2(y) := \det \partial T_2(y)$ are the Jacobian determinants of the two transformations. The $\hat{A}(y)$ minimizing the cost function is derived as [18]:

$$\hat{A}(y) = \frac{J_1(y)I_1 \circ T_1(y) + J_2(y)I_2 \circ T_2(y)}{J_1(y) + J_2(y)}. \quad (3)$$

In an explicit-atlas scheme, the transformations and the atlas can be iteratively computed from Eq. (1) and Eq. (3) [17]. However, the atlas can indeed be eliminated in Eq. (2) by substituting $A(y)$ with $\hat{A}(y)$, leading to an implicit-atlas data term [10]:

$$\hat{T}_1, \hat{T}_2 = \underset{T_1,T_2}{\operatorname{argmin}} \int_\Omega \frac{\left(I_1 \circ T_1(y) - I_2 \circ T_2(y) \right)^2}{J_1^{-1}(y) + J_2^{-1}(y)} dy. \quad (4)$$

2.2 Independence from the Mid-Space

Equation (4) is an optimization over both T_1 and T_2, which define the mid-space. Even so, further simplification reveals that the two transformations are redundant. The change of variables $y = T_1^{-1}(x)$, with $dy = dx/J_1 \circ T_1^{-1}(x)$, results in:

$$\hat{T}_1, \hat{T}_2 = \underset{T_1,T_2}{\operatorname{argmin}} \int_\Omega \frac{\left(I_1(x) - I_2 \circ T_2 \circ T_1^{-1}(x) \right)^2}{1 + \dfrac{J_1 \circ T_1^{-1}(x)}{J_2 \circ T_1^{-1}(x)}} dx. \quad (5)$$

---

[1] Regularization terms such as the Tikhonov integrals $\int_\Omega \|\nabla T_1(x) - \mathbb{I}\|_F^2 dx$ and $\int_\Omega \|\nabla T_2(x) - \mathbb{I}\|_F^2 dx$ are also typically included in the cost function to keep the transformations meaningful and penalize excessive distortion. In this section, however, we focus only on the data term. The derivation of Eq. (4) is not impacted by the regularization terms, as they do not depend on A. Please note that anti-drift constraints are needed in addition to the regularization terms.

Recall that the output transformation T is computed as $T(x) = T_2 \circ T_1^{-1}(x)$, the Jacobian determinant of which is $J(x) := \det \partial T(x) = J_2 \circ T_1^{-1}(x)/J_1 \circ T_1^{-1}(x)$. It now becomes clear that the above integral is, remarkably, only a function of T, and that the optimization can be written independently of the individual T_1 and T_2, as:

$$\hat{T} = \underset{T}{\text{argmin}}\, D(I_1, I_2, T),$$

$$D(I_1, I_2, T) := \int_\Omega \left(I_1(x) - I_2 \circ T(x)\right)^2 \frac{J(x)}{1 + J(x)}\, dx. \tag{6}$$

Thus, we can minimize this cost-function data term directly with respect to T, as opposed to the previous methods that optimize their cost functions with respect to both T_1 and T_2, conditioned to constraints that prevent the mid-space drift.

With $D(I_1, I_2, T)$ being independent of T_1 and T_2, the mid-space disappears, eliminating the problem of the mid-space drift as well. We do not need to enforce any anti-drift constraints anymore, hence not biasing the space of possible transformations T by the particular choice of such constraints. This is all while keeping the degrees of freedom of the optimization half of that of the unconstrained problem of solving for both T_1 and T_2. In addition, no transformation needs to be inverted to compute T, as opposed to most existing mid-space approaches that need to invert T_1 to compute $T = T_2 \circ T_1^{-1}$. These advantages are especially valuable for displacement-field parameterized transformations, inverting which is a difficult and inexact task. Lastly, one can verify the expected symmetry of the proposed data term, i.e. $D(I_1, I_2, T) = D(I_2, I_1, T^{-1})$. Note that this symmetry holds only in the continuous domain. In the discrete case, where one image is resampled and the other is not, discretization artifacts produce a bias [19-21].

2.3   Implementation

We implement the proposed registration method via the diffeomorphic demons scheme [22], and minimize $D(I_1, I_2, T)$ of Eq. (6) by gradient descent with line search. Similar to the demons algorithm, T is regularized by Gaussian blurring between each two descent iterations. We use a compositive scheme and update T by composing it with a transformation S, chosen to be the exponential of the update field. At each iteration, we fix T and J, and compute the variation of $D(I_1, I_2, T \circ S)$ with respect to S, with S currently assumed to be the identity transformation. Then, to preserve the diffeomorphism, we initialize $S(x) = x - 2^{-M} \Delta \frac{\delta D}{\delta S}\big|_{S=\mathbb{I}}$ (for a large enough M), with Δ the step size, and compose it with itself ($S \leftarrow S \circ S$) M times, before updating T as $T \leftarrow T \circ S$ [22]. The variation is computed as follows (derivations omitted):

$$\frac{\delta}{\delta S} D(I_1, I_2, T \circ S)\Big|_{S=\mathbb{I}} = -\frac{2(I_1 - I_2 \circ T)J}{(1+J)^2}\left(\nabla I_1 + J\nabla(I_2 \circ T)\right) + \frac{2(I_1 - I_2 \circ T)^2 J}{(1+J)^3} \sum_{k=1}^{d} H^k.\left(C_{k,:}\right)^{\mathrm{T}}, \tag{7}$$

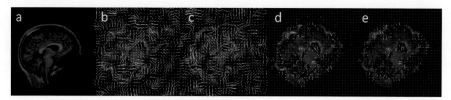

Fig. 1. The original image (a) was deformed by two synthetic random transformations (b,c). The deformed images were then registered with each other, resulting in deformation fields by the proposed (d) and the symmetrization (e) methods.

where C is the cofactor matrix of ∂T with $C_{k,:}$ its kth row, and H^k is the Hessian matrix of the kth element of T. The notation (x) has been dropped for brevity. The last term of Eq. (7) involves the Hessian tensor of the deformation field, which can introduce large discretization error, possibly outweighing the accuracy that this term brings about. In our experiments, ignoring this second-order term improved the optimization of Eq. (6).

3   Experimental Results

We tested the proposed deformable registration method on 2D slices of brain MR images, using our in-house Matlab implementation of the diffeomorphic demons with the compositive scheme [22] (Section 2.3). We compared our symmetric mid-space-independent registration method with the popular symmetrization approach that minimizes the average of the forward and backward cost functions [1-4], simplified in the form of $\int_\Omega \left(I_1(x) - I_2 \circ T(x)\right)^2 \frac{1+J(x)}{2}\,dx$, with $-\left(I_1 - I_2 \circ T\right)\left(J \nabla I_1 + \nabla(I_2 \circ T)\right)$ being its compositive gradient. Each experiment consisted of 2000 gradient descent iterations, and was repeated with the demons regularization parameter taking 22 different values.

3.1   Retrieval of Synthetic Deformations

In the first set of experiments, we compared the two algorithms on the mid-sagittal planes of 20 brain images taken from the publicly available OASIS database [23], which were pre-processed in FreeSurfer [24]. From each intensity-normalized and resampled volume (1-mm³ isotropic voxel), the sagittal slice located four voxels to the right of the mid-sagittal plane was extracted, and resampled to the size 128×128 (Figure 1a). For each subject, two random deformation fields T_1^{synth} and T_2^{synth} were synthesized, spatially low-pass filtered, and applied to the sagittal slice, I, to produce two synthetically deformed images, $I_1 = I \circ T_1^{\text{synth}}$ and $I_2 = I \circ T_2^{\text{synth}}$ (Figure 1b,c), which were then registered with each other using both methods (Figure 1d,e). Ideally, we would expect to retrieve a transformation T satisfying $T_1^{\text{synth}} \approx T_2^{\text{synth}} \circ T$. Accordingly, we computed the error $\int_\Omega \left\| T_1^{\text{synth}}(x) - T_2^{\text{synth}} \circ T(x) \right\|_2^2\,dx$, and for each

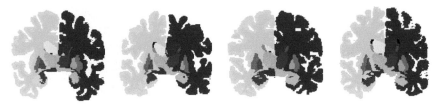

Fig. 2. Examples of the labeled coronal slices used in Section 3.2.

subject and method, chose the best result (with the smallest error) across the experiments with different demons regularization values. Our mid-space-independent registration resulted in lower error than the symmetrization method did in 14 out of the 20 subjects, and the mean error was $0.2\% \pm$ (SE) 0.2% lower for our method. We also ran backward experiments and computed $\int_{\Omega} \|T_{\text{forward}} \circ T_{\text{backward}}(x) - x\|_2^2 dx$ as the inverse-consistency error, which was $4\% \pm 2\%$ lower for our method than for the symmetrization method.

3.2 Cross-Subject Registration of Labeled Images

We performed a second set of experiments on a dataset of brain images with 37 neuroanatomical structures manually labeled [25]. We chose a fixed coronal slice maximizing the number of included distinct labels across the subjects (Figure 2). We randomly selected 40 pairs of subjects, and registered the chosen slices using the two methods. Although cross-sections of labels of 3D structures are not so precise for empirical validation, slice registration, being much faster than volumetric registration, allowed us to run many more experiments with a wide range of regularization.

We first considered 12 key subcortical regions: left/right amygdala, caudate, hippocampus, pallidum, putamen, and thalamus. As a similarity score for comparing the two methods, we computed in the union of these regions the portion of the voxels with matching labels between the two images. For each method and pair of subjects, we chose the maximum score achieved across different values of the demons regularization parameter. When the labels were compared in the native space of I_1, the two methods achieved on average similar scores (difference: $0.0\% \pm 0.2\%$). Alternatively, computing the scores in the native space of I_2 (by nearest-neighbor interpolation), revealed $0.10\% \pm 0.16\%$ higher score for the proposed method than for the symmetrization approach.

In a different comparison, we computed the similarity score for each experiment by averaging the Dice's similarity coefficient across all of the labels. When the label overlaps were computed in the native space of I_1, the symmetrization approach produced a significant $0.7\% \pm 0.2\%$ higher similarity score compared to the proposed method. When the scores were computed in the native space of I_2, however, the two algorithms performed similarly (difference: $0.0\% \pm 0.2\%$).

4   Conclusions

We have demonstrated for the first time that implicit-atlas pairwise registration is inherently independent of the mid-space, which led to deriving a new symmetric data term for deformable image registration. The independence of the cost function from the two image-to-atlas transformations alleviates the need for enforcing anti-drift constraints that can potentially bias the results. Future work includes: comprehensive evaluation of the proposed method on 3D labeled data, extending the proposed framework to group-wise registration, and devising a suitable symmetric regularization scheme.

Acknowledgments: We would like to thank Dr. Ender Konukoglu for his valuable feedback on the evaluation of the method. Support for this research was provided by the National Institutes of Health (U24 RR021382, 8P41 EB015896, R01 EB006758, AG022381, R01 AG008122-22, R01 AG016495-11, RC1 AT005728-01, R01 NS052585-01, 1R21 NS072652-01, 1R01 NS070963, R01 NS083534, 1S10 RR023401, 1S10 RR019307, 1S10 RR023043, 5U01-MH093765, 1K25 EB013649, K25 CA181632). Additional support was provided by the Massachusetts Alzheimer's Disease Research Center (5P50 AG005134), the BrightFocus Foundation (A2012333), the Ellison Medical Foundation (Autism & Dyslexia Project), and the Gipuzkoako Foru Aldundia. BF has a financial interest in CorticoMetrics, a company whose medical pursuits focus on brain imaging and measurement technologies. BF's interests were reviewed and are managed by MGH and Partners HealthCare in accordance with their conflict of interest policies.

References

1. Christensen, G.E., Johnson, H.J.: Consistent image registration. IEEE Transactions on Medical Imaging 20, 568–582 (2001)
2. Cachier, P., Rey, D.: Symmetrization of the non-rigid registration problem using inversion-invariant energies: Application to multiple sclerosis. In: Delp, S.L., DiGoia, A.M., Jaramaz, B. (eds.) MICCAI 2000. LNCS, vol. 1935, pp. 472–481. Springer, Heidelberg (2000)
3. Trouvé, A., Younes, L.: Diffeomorphic matching problems in one dimension: Designing and minimizing matching functionals. In: Vernon, D. (ed.) ECCV 2000. LNCS, vol. 1842, pp. 573–587. Springer, Heidelberg (2000)
4. Tagare, H., Groisser, D., Skrinjar, O.: Symmetric non-rigid registration: A geometric theory and some numerical techniques. J. Mathematical Imaging and Vision 34, 61–88 (2009)
5. Lorenzen, P., Prastawa, M., Davis, B., Gerig, G., Bullitt, E., Joshi, S.: Multi-modal image set registration and atlas formation. Medical Image Analysis 10, 440–451 (2006)
6. Avants, B., Gee, J.C.: Geodesic estimation for large deformation anatomical shape averaging and interpolation. Neuroimage 23(supplement 1), S139–S150 (2004)
7. Yang, D., Li, H., Low, D., Deasy, J., Naqa, I.: A fast inverse consistent deformable image registration method based on symmetric optical flow computation. Phys. Med. Biol. 53 (2008)

8. Noblet, V., Heinrich, C., Heitz, F., Armspach, J.-P.: An efficient incremental strategy for constrained groupwise registration based on symmetric pairwise registration. Pattern Recognition Letters 33, 283–290 (2012)
9. Lorenzi, M., Ayache, N., Frisoni, G.B., Pennec, X.: LCC-Demons: A robust and accurate symmetric diffeomorphic registration algorithm. Neuroimage 81, 470–483 (2013)
10. Ashburner, J., Ridgway, G.R.: Symmetric diffeomorphic modelling of longitudinal structural MRI. Frontiers in Neuroscience 6 (2013)
11. Aganj, I., Reuter, M., Sabuncu, M.R., Fischl, B.: Avoiding symmetry-breaking spatial nonuniformity in deformable image registration via a quasi-volume-preserving constraint. Neuroimage 106, 238–251 (2015)
12. Miller, M., Banerjee, A., Christensen, G., Joshi, S., Khaneja, N., Grenander, U., Matejic, L.: Statistical methods in computational anatomy. Stat. Methods Med. Res. 6, 267–299 (1997)
13. Studholme, C., Cardenas, V.: A template free approach to volumetric spatial normalization of brain anatomy. Pattern Recognition Letters 25, 1191–1202 (2004)
14. Aljabar, P., Bhatia, K.K., Murgasova, M., Hajnal, J.V., et al.: Assessment of brain growth in early childhood using deformation-based morphometry. Neuroimage 39, 348–358 (2008)
15. Grenander, U., Miller, M.I.: Computational anatomy: an emerging discipline. Quarterly of Applied Mathematics LVI, 617-694 (1998)
16. Joshi, S., Davis, B., Jomier, M., Gerig, G.: Unbiased diffeomorphic atlas construction for computational anatomy. Neuroimage 23(supplement 1), S151–S160 (2004)
17. Hart, G.L., Zach, C., Niethammer, M.: An optimal control approach for deformable registration. In: Proc. IEEE CVPR Workshops, pp. 9–16 (2009)
18. Ma, J., Miller, M.I., Trouvé, A., Younes, L.: Bayesian template estimation in computational anatomy. Neuroimage 42, 252–261 (2008)
19. Sabuncu, M.R., Yeo, B.T.T., Van Leemput, K., Vercauteren, T., Golland, P.: Asymmetric image-template registration. In: Yang, G.-Z., Hawkes, D., Rueckert, D., Noble, A., Taylor, C. (eds.) MICCAI 2009, Part I. LNCS, vol. 5761, pp. 565–573. Springer, Heidelberg (2009)
20. Aganj, I., Yeo, B.T.T., Sabuncu, M.R., Fischl, B.: On removing interpolation and resampling artifacts in rigid image registration. IEEE Trans. Image Process. 22, 816–827 (2013)
21. Reuter, M., Rosas, H.D., Fischl, B.: Highly accurate inverse consistent registration: A robust approach. Neuroimage 53, 1181–1196 (2010)
22. Vercauteren, T., Pennec, X., Perchant, A., Ayache, N.: Diffeomorphic demons: Efficient non-parametric image registration. Neuroimage 45, S61–S72 (2009)
23. Marcus, D.S., Wang, T.H., Parker, J., Csernansky, J.G., Morris, J.C., Buckner, R.L.: Open Access Series of Imaging Studies (OASIS): Cross-sectional MRI data in young, middle aged, nondemented, and demented older adults. J. Cognitive Neuroscience 19, 1498–1507 (2007)
24. Fischl, B.: FreeSurfer. Neuroimage 62, 774–781 (2012)
25. Fischl, B., Salat, D.H., Busa, E., Albert, M., Dieterich, M., Haselgrove, C., der van, K.A., Killiany, R., Kennedy, D., Klaveness, S., Montillo, A., Makris, N., Rosen, B., Dale, A.M.: Whole brain segmentation: automated labeling of neuroanatomical structures in the human brain. Neuron 33, 341–355 (2002)

A 2D-3D Registration Framework for Freehand TRUS-Guided Prostate Biopsy

Siavash Khallaghi[1], C. Antonio Sánchez[1], Saman Nouranian[1],
Samira Sojoudi[1], Silvia Chang[2], Hamidreza Abdi[3], Lindsay Machan[2], Alison
Harris[2], Peter Black[3], Martin Gleave[3], Larry Goldenberg[3], and S. Sidney Fels[1],
and Purang Abolmaesumi[1]

Department of Electrical and Computer Engineering, University of British Columbia,
Vancouver, Canada
Vancouver General Hospital, Vancouver, Canada
Department of Urological Sciences, Vancouver, Canada
{siavashk,antonios}@ece.ubc.ca

Abstract. We present a 2D to 3D registration framework that compensates for prostate motion and deformations during freehand prostate biopsies. It has two major components: 1) a trajectory-based rigid registration to account for gross motions of the prostate; and 2) a non-rigid registration constrained by a finite element model (FEM) to adjust for residual motion and deformations. For the rigid alignment, we constrain the ultrasound probe tip in the live 2D imaging plane to the tracked trajectory from the pre-procedure 3D ultrasound volume. This ensures the rectal wall approximately coincides between the images. We then apply a FEM-based technique to deform the volume based on image intensities. We validate the proposed framework on 10 prostate biopsy patients, demonstrating a mean target registration error (TRE) of 4.63 mm and 3.15 mm for rigid and FEM-based components, respectively.

1 Introduction

Prostate biopsy is the gold standard for prostate cancer (PCa) diagnosis. This is typically performed freehand using 2D transrectal ultrasound (TRUS) guidance. Unfortunately, the current systematic biopsy approach is prone to false negatives [9], and patients are frequently asked to repeat the procedure. To improve the cancer yield, 3D biopsy systems have been developed [1,4,12]. In these systems, biopsy locations are planned and recorded with respect to a 3D-TRUS reference volume acquired just prior to the procedure. However, the prostate moves and deforms during the biopsy process, in a way which cannot be compensated for using passive tracking alone [1,4,12]. As a result, slice-to-volume registration is required to maintain alignment of the 2D imaging plane with respect to the pre-procedure 3D-TRUS. The goal of this paper is to provide the registration tools to perform such freehand 3D-guided prostate biopsies.

Robust 2D-3D TRUS registration in a freehand environment is challenging. First, an accurate volume representing the prostate "at rest" must be generated.

© Springer International Publishing Switzerland 2015
N. Navab et al. (Eds.): MICCAI 2015, Part II, LNCS 9350, pp. 272–279, 2015.
DOI: 10.1007/978-3-319-24571-3_33

For freehand biopsies, this volume is typically acquired using a tracked axial sweep from base to apex [7,12]. Unfortunately, due to patient discomfort and inconsistent probe pressure, resulting volumes suffer from deformation artifacts. To reduce these, systems have been developed that use mechanical stabilization [4] or 3D probes [1], ensuring consistent probe pressure. The second challenge relates to the nature of the 2D-3D registration problem. The limited 2D spatial information, low signal-to-noise ratio of TRUS, and varying probe-induced pressures, all make motion and deformation compensation difficult. When the probe is mechanically stabilized, De Silva et al. [4,3] show that rigid 2D-3D registration is sufficient for 3D guidance. They approximate the prostate as rigid, and its motion is learned based on probe positions/orientations [3]. Systems that use 3D probes [1] avoid the 2D-3D registration issue, since the additional out-of-plane information can be used to increase accuracy and robustness [2,7]. However, neither mechanical systems nor 3D probes are widely used in clinics. A solution for freehand 3D-guidance using 2D-TRUS probes, as part of the current standard-of-care, is highly desirable.

In this paper, we provide a solution for freehand TRUS-guided prostate biopsies using a combined rigid and non-rigid 2D-3D registration. The closest works to ours, involving slice-to-volume registration on freehand TRUS data, are by Xu et al. [12] and Khallaghi et al. [7]. The shortcoming in Xu et al. [12] is that their method does not compensate for non-rigid prostate deformations, and target registration error (TRE) is only evaluated on phantom studies. Khallaghi et al. [7] compensate for deformations using a B-spline approach. However, their validation is on axial slices of TRUS images acquired in a similar motion as the pre-procedure sweep, leading to a simpler problem. It has not been applied to TRUS slices obtained from arbitrary orientations.

In the absence of strong prior knowledge of prostate motion, even rigid 2D-3D registration often does not converge. To improve robustness, Baumann et al. [1] constrain the registration using a manually delineated bounding ellipsoid approximating the prostate shape. This provides a boundary condition for rectal probe kinematics. We follow a similar approach. However, in our case the rigid registration is constrained using the trajectory of the tracked probe's tip during the freehand sweep. This ensures that the rectal wall in both the slice and volume are approximately aligned. We then compensate for residual motion and deformation using a non-rigid 2D-3D registration based on a finite element model (FEM). This incorporates physical prior knowledge, since deformations during a prostate biopsy are mostly probe-induced, and therefore biomechanical in nature. FEM-based methods have been previously applied to 3D-3D registration [5,10,11], but these use the FEM as part of a forward transformation model: from source to the target image. When the target is a 2D slice, this requires scattered data interpolation from the warped volume onto the slice plane, which can be computationally expensive. To alleviate this issue, we propose a backward transformation model that maps the regular 2D grid on the slice directly to the 3D volume. To the best of our knowledge, this is the first report of a FEM-based 2D-3D registration for freehand prostate biopsies.

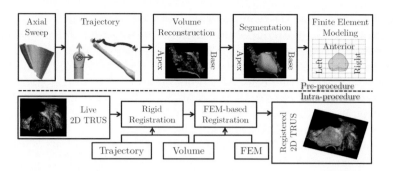

Fig. 1. Clinical workflow. Pre-procedure: The radiologist takes a freehand sweep of the prostate gland from base to apex (frame stack shown in gray). This sweep is used to construct a probe tip trajectory and a 3D volume (sagittal view). This volume is segmented to create a FEM consisting of two regions: the prostate, and the surrounding soft tissue. Intra-procedure: The 2D-TRUS is registered using a rigid transform constrained by the trajectory. Subsequently, a FEM-based non-rigid registration is used to compensate for residual deformations.

2   Methods

2.1   Data Acquisition

The TRUS images in this study were acquired using a magnetically tracked EC9-5/10 probe with a custom data collection software running on a Sonix Touch machine (Ultrasonix Inc., Canada). Prior to the procedure, the probe was calibrated at a depth of 6.0 cm with an N-wire phantom using fCal [8] (calibration accuracy of 0.45 ± 0.2 mm). At the start of the procedure, we asked an interventional radiologist to perform a freehand axial sweep of the prostate gland, from base to apex. We refer to the tracked probe's tip along the sweep as the *trajectory*. This trajectory is shown graphically with red/green/blue axes in Figure 1. Each sweep was obtained at 20 frames/second ($\approx$ 500 frames total), and used to reconstruct a 3D volume of the prostate and surrounding tissue. To account for small fluctuations in probe pressure during the pre-procedure sweep, a moving average with window length of 65 was applied to the transforms. Since the prostate is known to be stiffer than the surrounding tissue [6], we manually segmented the prostate in the 3D-TRUS and created a simplified FEM consisting of two regions: prostate, and the surrounding tissue (see Section 2.2). If desired, segmentation can be automated [13], or skipped and a single homogeneous FEM can be used [10]. Note that commercial 3D-TRUS systems, such as UroNav (Invivo Co., USA) and Artemis (Eigen Inc., USA) already incorporate intra-operative segmentation of the prostate on TRUS images. If elastography becomes part of the prostate biopsy protocol, spatially-varying material properties can also easily be incorporated into the FEM.

Throughout the procedure, tracked TRUS images were obtained continuously at 20 frames/second. At each biopsy location, we asked the radiologist to press a foot-pedal to tag the TRUS image associated with the core. The 2D-TRUS at each biopsy core was used then for off-line validation of our framework. The two major components are the rigid registration, and the FEM-based deformable registration methods, which are discussed in Section 2.2. We refer to the pre-procedure 3D-TRUS and the intra-procedure 2D-TRUS as source and target images, respectively. A full workflow is presented in Figure 1.

2.2   2D-3D Registration

The 2D-3D registration is framed as the minimization of an objective functional between the planar 2D target image, $F(x) : \mathbb{R}^3 \to \mathbb{R}$, and the 3D source, $M(x) : \mathbb{R}^3 \to \mathbb{R}$, where $x \in \Omega$ refers to grid points on the target slice. We denote the number of points in Ω by N and concatenate them into a single $3N \times 1$ vector, $\boldsymbol{x}$. Since the problem is mono-modal, we used the sum-of-squared differences (SSD) for the intensity metric. For rigid registration, the transform is constrained using the probe trajectory. For FEM-based registration, the objective functional is regularized using the total strain energy of the FEM.

Trajectory-Based Rigid Registration: We formulate the rigid registration as the minimization of the objective functional:

$$Q_{\mathrm{r}}(s, \theta_1, \theta_2, \theta_3) = \frac{1}{2N} \left\| F(\boldsymbol{x}) - M(T_{\mathrm{r}}(s, \theta_1, \theta_2, \theta_3, \boldsymbol{x})) \right\|^2, \qquad (1)$$

where $T_{\mathrm{r}}(s, \theta_1, \theta_2, \theta_3, x)$ is a rigid transform. The translation component is restricted to the probe tip trajectory parameterized by $s \in [0, 1]$. This trajectory approximates the rectal wall in the 3D volume, on which the probe tip in the live 2D imaging plane should also fall. Rotation around the probe tip is controlled by the three Euler angles $(\theta_1, \theta_2, \theta_3)$. To initialize the location parameter s, we project the tracked probe tip to the trajectory. The rotation is initialized using the orientation from magnetic tracking. We then used the "pattern search" optimizer in Matlab (MathWorks, USA) to find the optimal rigid parameters $(s, \theta_1, \theta_2, \theta_3)$.

FEM-Based Registration: Central to the deformable registration is a FEM, constructed from the 3D image volume using a $8 \times 8 \times 8$ grid of hexahedral elements. For simplicity, we use a linear material, which depends on a Young's Modulus, E, and Poisson's ratio, ν. Since the prostate more stiff than the surrounding tissue, we increase the Young's Modulus within this region. Similar to [10], we do not assume any boundary conditions; the FEM is freely able to move based on image-driven forces. We systematically compute the stiffness matrix of the FEM, $K_{3J \times 3J}$, where J is the number of FEM nodes in the hexahedral grid. We formulate the objective functional as a regularized SSD metric:

$$Q_{\mathrm{FEM}}(\boldsymbol{u}) = \frac{1}{2N} \left\| F(\boldsymbol{x}) - M(\boldsymbol{x} - \Phi \boldsymbol{u}) \right\|^2 + \frac{\alpha}{2} \left\| \boldsymbol{u} - \boldsymbol{u}^{(p)} \right\|^2 + \frac{\beta}{2} \boldsymbol{u}^{\mathsf{T}} K \boldsymbol{u}, \qquad (2)$$

where $\boldsymbol{u}_{3J \times 1} = (u_{11}, \ldots, u_{13}, \ldots, u_{J3})^{\mathsf{T}}$ is the vector of FEM node displacements. A damping term is added for stability, scaled by a coefficient α, that limits deviation from the previous displacement values, $\boldsymbol{u}^{(p)}$. Deformation is controlled by the strain energy, scaled by regularization weight β. The interpolation matrix, $\Phi_{3N \times 3J}$, is used to represent spatial coordinates $\boldsymbol{x}$ in terms of the FEM node locations. It is constructed by detecting which deformed element contains each point, x, and computing interpolation coefficients based on the element's shape functions (similar to computing barycentric coordinates). Differentiating Equation (2) with respect to the lth coordinate of node k, u_{kl}, yields

$$\frac{\partial Q}{\partial u_{kl}} = \frac{1}{N} \sum_{n=1}^{N} [F_n(\boldsymbol{x}) - M_n(\boldsymbol{y})] \sum_{m=1}^{3} \frac{\partial M_n(\boldsymbol{y})}{\partial y_{nm}} \left(\Phi_{nk} + \sum_{j=1}^{J} \frac{\partial \Phi_{nj}}{\partial u_{kl}} u_{jm} \right)$$

$$+ \alpha \left(u_{kl} - u_{kl}^{(p)} \right) + \beta \sum_{j=1}^{J} \sum_{m=1}^{3} K_{(3k+l)(3j+m)} u_{jm}, \tag{3}$$

where $\boldsymbol{y} = \boldsymbol{x} - \Phi\boldsymbol{u}$ are the mapped coordinates in the moving image volume, n loops over all pixels in the fixed image plane, m loops over the three dimensions, and j loops over all FEM nodes. The derivative of the shape functions with respect to nodal displacements, $\partial\Phi_{nj}/\partial u_{kl}$, can be derived based on the FEM shape functions. By differentiating Equation (2) for all coordinates (k,l) and setting them to zero, we arrive at the sparse linear system:

$$(\Gamma + \alpha I + \beta K)\, \boldsymbol{u} = \Upsilon + \alpha \boldsymbol{u}^{(p)}, \tag{4}$$

where Υ and Γ are defined by collecting the appropriate terms from Equation (3). For the implementation, it is useful to note that if a point $\boldsymbol{x}_n$ falls in an element, then $\Phi_{nk} = \partial\Phi_{nk}/\partial u_{il} = 0$ for all nodes i not belonging to that element. Still, computation of Υ and Γ is the most time-consuming portion of our registration. For each point x, it requires finding the element containing that point, and determining its interpolation functions and their derivatives within the element. We use a bounding volume hierarchy to accelerate the element-detection component. To further improve efficiency, Υ and Γ can be computed in parallel per pixel.

For linear materials, it can be shown that the stiffness matrix scales linearly with the Young's modulus. As a result, the Young's modulus can be factored out and combined with β to create a single free parameter. This means that the proposed registration method has four free parameters: damping coefficient (α), relative soft tissue to prostate elasticity (E_t/E_p), scaled prostate elasticity (βE_p) and Poisson's ratio (ν). Throughout the experiments, we used the following values: $\alpha = 1.0$, $\beta E_p = 0.25 \times 5.0$ kPa [6], $E_t/E_p = 0.2$ [6], $\nu = 0.49$ [10]. The damping parameter, α, prevents large gradients from inducing too strong a force. It should be set large enough to maintain stability, but not too large or it will reduce the convergence rate. The scale parameter, β, controls the relative influence of the image-driven forces and the restoring energy of the FEM. We tuned this parameter to allow realistic deformations. The same parameter values were used for all subjects.

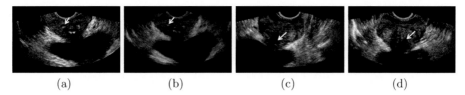

(a)   (b)   (c)   (d)

Fig. 2. Example of a calcification (a) and a cyst (c) on the target slice. The corresponding fiducial on the source volume is shown in (b) and (d), respectively.

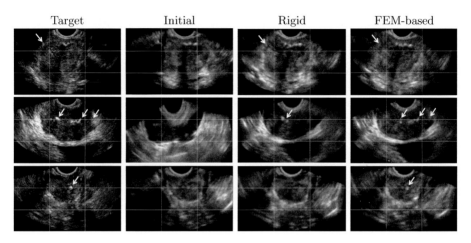

Fig. 3. Typical registration results for three patients (top, middle and bottom rows). The first column denotes the live 2D-TRUS (target) images. The next three columns show the initial alignment using the trajectory, rigid registration, and FEM-based registration results, respectively. White arrows indicate locations where the registration framework shows improvements.

3   Experiments and Results

The proposed 2D-3D registration was evaluated on 10 patients. The systematic sextant biopsy protocol in our hospital requires the acquisition of 8–12 distributed cores, with extra cores in suspicious regions. For the patients in this study, this yielded a total of 10 pre-procedure TRUS volumes and 115 2D TRUS slices at biopsy cores. To quantify registration error, we computed the Euclidean distance between intrinsic fiducials, consisting of micro-calcifications and cysts (Figure 2). A total of 65 fiducials were identified.

Figure 3 shows registration results for three patients. In the top-row, rigid registration performs well, however, there is a slight improvement near the prostate boundary following FEM-based registration. The middle-row shows an example where FEM-based registration corrects for the boundary and brings additional structures into the registration plane. In the bottom-row, FEM-based registration is required to correctly identify the calcification.

Table 1. Registration results and p-value to investigate statistical significance.

TRE, mean $\pm$ s.d. (mm)			$p-$value	
Initial	Rigid	FEM-based	Initial vs. Rigid	Rigid vs. FEM-based
6.31 ± 1.86	4.63 ± 1.05	3.15 ± 0.82	$p < 10^{-4}$	$p < 10^{-5}$

As seen in Table 1, rigid and FEM-based registration reduce the mean TRE from the initial 6.31 mm down to 4.63 mm and 3.15 mm, respectively. This suggests that substantial biomechanical deformations exist and can be compensated for using our FEM-based approach. To investigate the statistical significance of TRE reduction, we first checked if the TREs were normally distributed. Using the one-sample Kolmogorov-Smirnov test, we found that the distribution of the TRE is not normal at the 5% significance level for initial, rigid and FEM-based methods ($p < 10^{-4}$). Therefore, we performed a signed Wilcoxon rank sum test. The $p-$value from this experiment is also shown in Table 1. The test rejected the hypothesis that TREs for initial vs. rigid and rigid vs. FEM-based methods belong to a distribution with equal medians. Therefore, the improvements in mean TRE following rigid and FEM-based registration are statistically significant.

4   Discussion and Conclusions

We presented a novel registration framework for motion and deformation compensation during a freehand TRUS-guided prostate biopsy. The improvement in the TRE using the FEM-based registration should be compared to the acceptable error bounds of a 3D prostate biopsy system. A TRE of 2.5 mm yields a confidence interval in which 95% of registered targets come within the smallest clinically significant tumor [4]. The result of our FEM-based registration (3.15 mm) brings us closer to this acceptable error bound. In our study, no instructions were given to the radiologist to control the probe pressure. If the biopsy protocol is slightly modified to maintain a low probe pressure, it should be possible to decrease the error closer to a clinically acceptable range [4].

Our next steps aim to increase the accuracy of the proposed framework. Since the quality of the pre-procedure volume directly affects registration results [7], we wish to tackle challenges associated with deformation artifacts due to breathing and inconsistent probe pressure, including estimating a "rest shape" of the prostate using shape statistics, and validating the reconstructed volume against magnetic resonance images. Another direction is to perform multi-slice registration, which has been shown to improve the TRE [2,7], and compare our non-rigid registration approach to other methods [7]. The current run-times of the rigid and FEM-based components of our framework are in the order of $\approx$ 30 seconds and $\approx$ 10 minutes, respectively. Decreasing the registration time can be accomplished by calculating the terms in Equation (3) in parallel per pixel on a graphics processing unit, by adopting a multi-resolution approach, and by performing registration continuously during the procedure [4]. This would allow us to integrate the registration framework into the biopsy procedure, so it can be validated on a larger cohort of patients.

Acknowledgments. This work was funded by the Natural Sciences and Engineering Research Council of Canada (NSERC) and the Canadian Institutes of Health Research (CIHR).

References

1. Baumann, M., Mozer, P., Daanen, V., Troccaz, J.: Prostate biopsy tracking with deformation estimation. Medical Image Analysis 16(3), 562–576 (2012)
2. De Silva, T., Cool, D.W., Romagnoli, C., Fenster, A., Ward, A.D.: Evaluating the utility of intraprocedural 3D TRUS image information in guiding registration for displacement compensation during prostate biopsy. Medical Physics 41(8), 082901 (2014)
3. De Silva, T., Cool, D.W., Yuan, J., Romognoli, C., Fenster, A., Ward, A.D.: Improving 2D-3D registration optimization using learned prostate motion data. In: Mori, K., Sakuma, I., Sato, Y., Barillot, C., Navab, N. (eds.) MICCAI 2013, Part II. LNCS, vol. 8150, pp. 124–131. Springer, Heidelberg (2013)
4. De Silva, T., Fenster, A., Cool, D.W., Gardi, L., Romagnoli, C., Samarabandu, J., Ward, A.D.: 2D-3D rigid registration to compensate for prostate motion during 3D TRUS-guided biopsy. Medical Physics 40(2), 022904 (2013)
5. Hu, Y., Ahmed, H.U., Taylor, Z., Allen, C., Emberton, M., Hawkes, D., Barratt, D.: MR to ultrasound registration for image-guided prostate interventions. Medical Image Analysis 16(3), 687–703 (2012)
6. Kemper, J., Sinkus, R., Lorenzen, J., Nolte-Ernsting, C., Stork, A., Adam, G.: MR elastography of the prostate: initial in-vivo application. Fortschr Röntgenstr 176(08), 1094–1099 (2004)
7. Khallaghi, S., Nouranian, S., Sojoudi, S., Ashab, H.A., Machan, L., Chang, S., Black, P., Gleave, M., Goldenberg, L., Abolmaesumi, P.: Motion and deformation compensation for freehand prostate biopsies. In: Proc. SPIE, vol. 9036, pp. 903620–903626 (2014)
8. Lasso, A., Heffter, T., Rankin, A., Pinter, C., Ungi, T., Fichtinger, G.: Plus: Open-source toolkit for ultrasound-guided intervention systems. IEEE Transactions on Biomedical Engineering 61(10), 2527–2537 (2014)
9. Leite, K.R.M., Camara-Lopes, L.H., Dall'Oglio, M.F., Cury, J., Antunes, A.A., Sañudo, A., Srougi, M.: Upgrading the gleason score in extended prostate biopsy: implications for treatment choice. International Journal of Radiation Oncology Biology Physics 73(2), 353–356 (2009)
10. Marami, B., Sirouspour, S., Ghoul, S., Cepek, J., Davidson, S.R., Capson, D.W., Trachtenberg, J., Fenster, A.: Elastic registration of prostate MR images based on estimation of deformation states. Medical Image Analysis 21(1), 87–103 (2015)
11. Wang, Y., Ni, D., Qin, J., Lin, M., Xie, X., Xu, M., Heng, P.A.: Towards personalized biomechanical model and MIND-weighted point matching for robust deformable MR-TRUS registration. In: Luo, X., Reich, T., Mirota, D., Soper, T. (eds.) CARE 2014. LNCS, vol. 8899, pp. 121–130. Springer, Heidelberg (2014)
12. Xu, S., Kruecker, J., Turkbey, B., Glossop, N., Singh, A.K., Choyke, P., Pinto, P., Wood, B.J.: Real-time MRI-TRUS fusion for guidance of targeted prostate biopsies. International Society for Computer Aided Surgery 13(5), 255–264 (2008)
13. Yan, P., Xu, S., Turkbey, B., Kruecker, J.: Adaptively learning local shape statistics for prostate segmentation in ultrasound. IEEE Transactions on Biomedical Engineering 58(3), 633–641 (2011)

Unsupervised Free-View Groupwise Segmentation for M³ Cardiac Images Using Synchronized Spectral Network

Yunliang Cai[1], Ali Islam[3], Mousumi Bhaduri[4], Ian Chan[4], and Shuo Li[2,1]

[1] Department of Medical Biophysics, University of Western Ontario,
London ON, Canada
[2] GE Healthcare, London ON, Canada
[3] St. Joseph's Health Care, London ON, Canada
[4] London Health Sciences Centre, London ON, Canada

Abstract. Image-based diagnosis and population study on cardiac problems require automatic segmentation on increasingly large amount of data from different protocols, different views, and different patients. However, current algorithms are often limited to regulated settings such as fixed view and single image from one specific modality, where the supervised learning methods can be easily employed but with restricted usability. In this paper, we propose the unsupervised free-view groupwise M³ segmentation: a simultaneous segmentation for a group of Multi-modality, Multi-chamber, from Multi-subject images from an arbitrary imaging view. To achieve the segmentation, we particularly develop the Synchronized Spectral Network (SSN) model for the joint decomposing, synchronizing, and clustering the spectral representations of free-view M³ cardiac images. The SSN model generates a set of synchronized superpixels where the corresponding chamber regions share the same superpixel label, which naturally provides simultaneous cardiac segmentation. The segmentation is quantitatively evaluated by more than 10000 images (MR and CT) from 93 subjects and high dice metric ($> 85\%$) is consistently achieved in validation. Our method provides a powerful segmentation tool for cardiac images under non-regulated imaging environment.

1 Introduction

The segmentation of large amount of M³ (Multi-modality, Multi-chamber, Multi-subject) cardiac image data is a clinical routine and notoriously known as tedious and time-consuming. However, most current cardiac segmentations are single modality methods for limited cardiac image views (short-axis/long-axis). These methods require a lot of manual efforts in pre-processing like ROI cropping and view alignments, and need exhaustive conversions in cross-protocol/modality comparison study. A unified segmentation for free-view M³ images is strongly desired in quantitative and population study of cardiac problems which will play an increasingly important role in the practical diagnoses of heart diseases.

The segmentation for M³ images under non-regulated settings, i.e., arbitrary field of views, is a challenging problem. Main difficulties arise from different

© Springer International Publishing Switzerland 2015
N. Navab et al. (Eds.): MICCAI 2015, Part II, LNCS 9350, pp. 280–288, 2015.
DOI: 10.1007/978-3-319-24571-3_34

perspectives: **1)** Image view: cardiac shapes can be completely different in various views, shape-based segmentation could fail easily as unified shape model is difficult to define; **2)** Modality: intensity features in cardiac MR and CT are incompatible, segmentation method in one modality cannot be directly applied to the other; **3)** Joint chamber segmentation: some chamber regions (i.e., RV) are difficult to extract in non-regulated image views due to the edge fuzziness.

The current cardiac segmentation are often performed under regulated settings. As reviewed in [10], most algorithms focused on LV segmentation as RV has more complex motion patterns. Among the LV segmentation, in recent studies, Cousty *et al* [5] used watershed-cut algorithm and incorporated spatio-temporal representation for cardiac segmentation. Pednekar *et al* [9] proposed a intensity-based affinity estimation for LV region and perform segmentation by contour fitting. Deformable models are intensively applied in LV segmentation too. Ben Ayed *et al* [3] followed the level set approach and using overlap LV priors as global constrains to obtain robust segmentation results. In addition, strong shape priors are frequently used in LV-RV segmentation on single MR subject. Zhang et al [11] used a combined active shape and active appearance model (ASM+AAM) for segmentation of 4D MR images. Bai *et al* [1] used multi-atlas approach, applying local classifiers for segmentation LV segmentation. The popular methods in MR segmentation are also frequently used in CT segmentation. Zheng *et al* [12] applied marginal space learning techniques for warping prior control points in CT volumes to perform the model-based segmentation. Isgum *et al* [7] took the multi-atlas approach and perform cardiac and aortic CT segmentation using local label fusion. However, in the above mentioned methods, unregulated M³ segmentation setting (views, modal) were rarely discussed.

To achieve segmentation for M³ images, we propose a free-view groupwise approach which has the following advantages: **1)** Unregulated segmentation setting: our method can be directly applied on standard cardiac views (short-axis, long-axis) and unregulated cardiac views (coronal, axial). There are no shape limits and pre-training steps. **2)** Simultaneous segmentation: our method provides simultaneous segmentation for the set of images from the same arbitrary view. **3)** Multi-modality, Multi-subject, Multi-chamber (M³): our method is independent of image modality, and provides implicit chamber matching between images from the same/different subjects. All chamber regions (i.e., LV/RV, LA+LV/RA+RV) from the input images are jointly extracted. **4)** Automatic ROI localization: our method can be directly apply on raw MR/CT scans without manual ROI cropping. Our method provides a general tool for cardiac segmentation problems.

2   Methodology

2.1   Overview

Our free-view groupwise segmentation is fully unsupervised, whereas the result is only driven by the input images. The segmentation can obtain multi-chamber

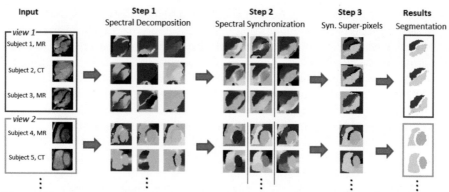

Fig. 1. The overview of our free-view groupwise segmentation. The M^3 images from different views are decomposed and then synchronized using our spectral synchronization network (SSN). The generated synchronized superpixels immediately provide multi-chamber segmentation.

segmentation simultaneously for a group of M^3 images from an unknown view. The overall segmentation process is illustrated in Fig. 1.

1. **Spectral Decomposition.** As Fig. 1 step 1 shows, the input images are decomposed into spectral bases representations. The spectral bases are a set of maps that represent the pairwise pixel similarities in an image, such that smooth regions are enhanced and separated by their in-region similarities. As the similarities only depends on the image itself, spectral bases are modality independent. The spectral bases model [2] is used in our method (see Sec 2.2.1).

2. **Spectral Synchronization.** As illustrated in Fig. 1 step 2, spectral synchronization forces the spectral bases of different images to have similar appearances, so that all spectral representations are jointly matched. *Synchronized Spectral Bases* are obtained by shuffling and recombination of the spectral bases, in which the corresponding regions of different images will have the same positive/negative responses. This provides an implicit registration for the input images without using any explicit alignments (see Sec 2.2.2).

3. **Synchronized Superpixels.** The synchronized spectral bases will serve as image features for clustering the image pixels into superpixels. As shown in Fig. 1 step 3, the synchronized spectral bases expand each pixel to a high-dim feature vector (3d vector in this case). These features are clustered by K-means, sorting all image pixels into a set of synchronized superpixels. These superpixels provide initial over-segmentation for the images, while corresponding image regions are now correlated with same superpixel labels.

4. **Segmentation.** The chamber regions of the input images can be easily identified from the synchronized superpixels of step 3 by their region sizes and the relative positions in images. They are then extracted as the final segmentation.

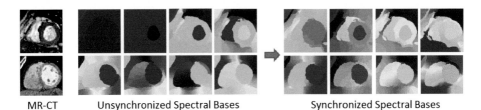

MR-CT   Unsynchronized Spectral Bases   Synchronized Spectral Bases

Fig. 2. The spectral bases versus the proposed synchronized spectral bases. Left to right: The MR-CT images, the unsynchronized spectral bases ([2]), and the synchronized spectral bases (obtained by Eqn (3)).

2.2   Spectral Decomposition and Synchronization Using SSN

The key to provide the spectral synchronization and synchronized superpixels is *Synchronized Spectral Network* (SSN), which is introduced as follows.

1. **Spectral Graph Decomposition.** For an image I, we construct a graph $\mathcal{G} = (V, E)$ such that each edge $e \in E$ that connecting two arbitrary pixels i, j is weighted by $W(i, j)$. The particular weight is determined by the intensities, and the contour interventions (not image gradient) between the two pixels:

$$W(i,j) = \exp\left(-||x_i - x_j||^2/\sigma_x - ||I_i - I_j||^2/\sigma_I - \max_{x \in line(i,j)} ||Edge(x)||^2/\sigma_E\right) \tag{1}$$

where x_i, x_j are the location of the pixels i, j and the I_i, I_j are their intensities respectively. $Edge(x)$ represents an edge detector in location x along line (i, j). $\sigma_x, \sigma_I, \sigma_E$ are constants that will be assigned empirically. In practice, $W(i, j)$ will only be computed in the set of k-nearest neighbors. Suppose image I contains N pixels, then W is a $N \times N$ sparse matrix. Let $\overline{W} = D^{-1/2}WD^{-1/2}$ be the normalized W where D is the diagonal matrix whose elements are the row summations of W. The eigen-decomposition of Laplacian $\mathcal{L} = Id - \overline{W}$ will generate the set of unsynchronized spectral bases $\{\xi_k(\mathcal{G})\}$ (Step 1, Fig. 1).

2. **Synchronization by Joint Diagonalization.** After the spectral decompositions of the original images, spectral synchronization is achieved by applying the joint Laplacian diagonalization [6] [8]. The goal of the joint diagonalization is to obtain a set of qausi-eigenvectors $Y_i = [y_{i,1} \ldots y_{i,K}] \in \mathbb{R}^{N \times K}$ for image I_i:

$$\min_{Y_1,\ldots,Y_M} \sum_{i \in \mathcal{I}} ||Y_i^T \mathcal{L}_i Y_i - \Lambda_i||_F^2 + \mu \sum_{i,j \in \mathcal{I}} ||F(Y_i) - F(Y_j)||^2, \tag{2}$$

where $\mathcal{I}$ is the image set and $\Lambda_i = \text{diag}(\lambda_1, \ldots, \lambda_K)$ is the diagonal matrix for K-largest eigenvalues of $\mathcal{L}_i$. F is an arbitrary feature mapping that maps a spectral map to a fixed dimension feature vector. In other words, Y_i diagonalize the Laplacian $\mathcal{L}_i$ as the ordinary spectral bases do, and its columns are matched implicitly under the feature mapping F. Solving (2) can obtain the demanded synchronized spectral basis (Step 2, Fig. 1).

3. **Fast Computation.** In practice, each $y_{i,k}$ can be approximated by the linear combination of K unsynchronized bases $\{\xi_k(\mathcal{G}_i)\}_{k=1}^K$, which significantly resolves

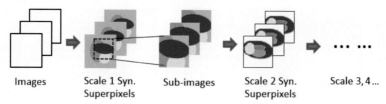

Fig. 3. The hierarchical SSN decomposition. The synchronized superpixels (scale 1) can be sub-decomposed into finer synchronized superpixels (scale 2), and even finer scales (scale 3, 4,...).

the ambiguity of Y_i. We let $Y_i = U_i A_i$ where A_i is a $K \times K'$ matrix variable for $K' \leq K$ and $U_i = [\xi_1(\mathcal{G}_i), \ldots, \xi_K(\mathcal{G}_i)]$, and let F be the matrix of Fourier bases for a Fourier coupling [6]. The optimization (2) is modified as:

$$\min_{A_1,\ldots,A_M} \sum_{i \in \mathcal{I}} ||A_i^T \Lambda_i A_i - \Lambda_i||_F^2 + \mu \sum_{i,j \in \mathcal{I}} ||F U_i A_i - F U_j A_j||^2$$

$$\text{subject to}: A_i^T A_i = Id \quad \text{for all} \quad i \in \mathcal{I} \tag{3}$$

Fig. 2 shows an example of spectral bases for a pair of MR-CT images versus their original spectral basis obtained by using [4].

2.3 Heart Localization Using Hierarchical SSN Decomposition

The SSN decomposition naturally provides the joint extraction of cardiac ROI sub-images from the raw scans (i.e., MR/CT upper body axial scans). This allows us to directly process the raw scans without any manual ROI cropping.

Hierarchical Decomposition. To achieve the ROI extraction, the spectral decomposition and synchronization are applied in multiple scales to perform the hierarchical decomposition as shown in Fig. 3. The subset of particularly identified synchronized superpixels in the Scale 1 decomposition can be extracted for another round of spectral decomposition and synchronization. The results are a new set of finer synchronized superpixels, which provide sub-segmentations of the local image regions and recover more finer details in the images.

Free-View Heart Localization. Fig. 4 shows an representative example of our heart localization. In this example, the two raw images from MR and CT respectively are first taken the SSN decomposition, generating 9 synchronized superpixels. Through the superpixels positions and the imaging protocol, the heart regions are simultaneously identified as the largest superpixels at the centers. The Scale 2 SSN decomposition can then be taken in the heart sub-images, generating a new set of synchronized superpixels for the cardiac segmentation. In practice, the actual number of superpixels of both scales will be determined experimentally. The number will be fixed for the same testing dataset.

3 Experiment

Our segmentation is tested on three M^3 datasets that contain more than 10000 MR+CT images in total from 93 subjects under various views. High dice metric

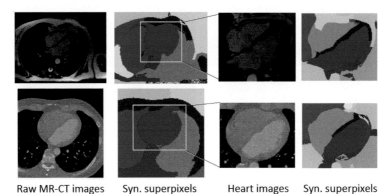

Raw MR-CT images   Syn. superpixels   Heart images   Syn. superpixels

Fig. 4. The simultaneous heart localization in raw axial MR-CT images using hierarchical SSN decomposition. Left to right: the raw axial images; the synchronized superpixels of the raw images; the heart ROI identified from the synchronized superpixels; the scale 2 synchronized superpixels for the heart images.

(DM> 85%) is constantly achieved on both the tests for non-regulated cardiac view images (i.e., 3-chamber coronal view, axial view) and regulated cardiac view images (2/4-chamber view). The tests are arranged in two phases as follows.

Phase 1: Non-Regulated Free-View Evaluation. To evaluate our performance in free-view images, we test our method on a MR+CT dataset which contains 10 MR and 10 CT subjects with non-regulated cardiac views. The representative result of our segmentation on a MR+CT, multi-subject, two-chamber (M³) image set is shown in Fig. 5 and Fig. 6, while the numerical results are summarized in Table 1. During the test, raw images from three views (axial, sagittal, coronal) of each subject are used. Particularly, 3 slices are sampled for each view around the volume center, generating 60 raw images in total for the subject. As the sampled slices are not accurately regulated along the short/long-axis of heart, their views are in fact arbitrary. Images from the same view are then randomly packed up in batches with 4 or 8 images per batch, generating 100 4-image and 100 8-image non-identical batches for testing.

As Fig. 5 shows, our method achieves simultaneous segmentation for the eight MR/CT images (different subjects) in the image batch. LV+LA/RV+RA regions are successfully extracted in the segmentation. Another two successful examples for the segmentation of 4-image batches under non-regulated sagittal and coronal cardiac views are shown in Fig. 6. As the complete evaluation presented in Table 1, the average dice metric on both modalities (MR+CT) for both chambers are 89.2% (4-image batch) and 85.2% (8-image batch) respectively.

Phase 2: Regulated Standard-View Evaluation. To evaluate our robustness performance on larger batches under regulated cardiac image views, we test two MR testsets: the York Cardiac MRI dataset[1] is denoted as testset 1 which contains 33 MR subjects (aligned in two-chamber view); our own collected MR

---

[1] http://www.cse.yorku.ca/mridataset/

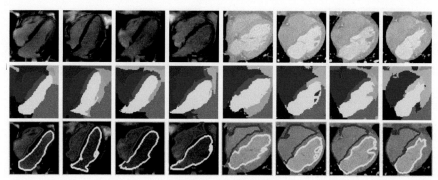

Fig. 5. Example of the unsupervised groupwise segmentation on a 8-image batch (4 MR subjects + 4 CT subjects) under a non-regulated axial view. Row 1: original images; Row 2: synchronized superpixels; Row 3: the LV+LA (**yellow**) and RV+RA (**red**) segmentation.

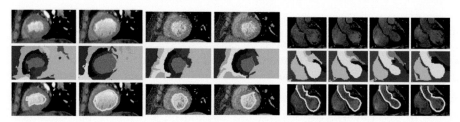

Fig. 6. Examples of the groupwise segmentation on non-regulated image views. Left: CT segmentation for two subjects (2 images/subject) in sagittal view with LV region extracted; Right: MR segmentation for one subject (4 frames) in coronal view with LV/RV (yellow/red, bottom) region extracted.

dataset is denoted as testset 2 which contains 10300 MR images (2740 four-chamber, 7560 two-chamber) from 40 MR subjects. Representative example is shown in Fig. 7 with numerical results are presented in Table 2. Particularly the images are sampled from complete cardiac cycles in order to quantitatively evaluate the robustness of groupwise segmentation. All images from the same cardiac cycles are already well-regulated in short/long-axis views.

As illustrated in Fig. 7, our method has successful simultaneous segmentation on the 20 MR images sampled from a cardiac cycle of one subject. As reported in Table 2, for testset 1, our method achieved average DM 89.1% for the LV segmentation in cardiac cycles under 2-chamber views, and at the same time obtained 85.2% in RV segmentation. For testset2, our segmentation obtain average DM 88.0% (LV) and 84.8% under 2-chamber views, and has 87.6% (LV+LA) and 87.0% (RV+RA) under 4-chamber views. The overall performance in testset 1 and 2 are close and insensitive to view changes.

Table 1. Dice metric (%) and standard derivation on the Free-view M³ data.

	4-image batch			8-image batch		
	LV(+LA)	RV(+RA)	All Chambers	LV(+LA)	RV(+RA)	All Chambers
MR	91.8 ±3.2	90.2 ±3.1	90.4 ±3.3	88.2 ±4.2	87.8 ±4.5	86.8 ±4.2
CT	89.7 ±2.9	88.7 ±3.6	88.6 ±3.5	86.2 ±4.6	84.9 ±4.7	83.8 ±5.1
MR+CT	90.8 ±3.3	89.8 ±3.5	89.2 ±4.1	85.9 ±5.1	84.0 ±5.0	85.2 ±5.2

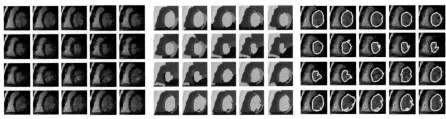

| Images from a cardiac cycle | Synchronized superpixels | LV-RV segmentation |

Fig. 7. Example of the unsupervised groupwise segmentation on 20 images under regulated 2-chamber view. Left to right: MR images from a cardiac cycle; synchronized superpixels; final LV-RV segmentation extracted from superpixels.

Table 2. Dice metric (%) evaluations of the regulated-view testset 1 and 2.

	testset 1			testset 2		
	LV(+LA)	RV(+RA)	All Chambers	LV(+LA)	RV(+RA)	All Chambers
2-Chamb. View	89.1 ±4.1	85.2 ±5.6	87.1 ±5.4	88.0 ±4.0	84.8 ±6.0	86.7 ±5.1
4-Chamb. View	/	/	/	87.6 ±4.6	87.0 ±6.2	87.4 ±3.6

4   Conclusions

In this paper, we proposed an unsupervised segmentation approach for M³ cardiac images (Multi-modality/chamber/subject) under unregulated settings. We developed a synchronized spectral network (SSN) model to conduct hierarchical groupwise segmentation for the input images. The SSN model utilized the robust and modal-independent spectral features to achieve the M³ segmentation. The dice metric of our method constantly larger than 85% in all test datasets.

References

1. Bai, W., Shi, W., Ledig, C., Rueckert, D.: Multi-atlas segmentation with augmented features for cardiac mr images. Medical Image Analysis 19(1), 98–109 (2015)
2. Bart, E., Porteous, I., Perona, P., Welling, M.: Unsupervised learning of visual taxonomies. In: CVPR, pp. 1–8. IEEE (2008)
3. Ayed, I.B., Li, S., Ross, I.: Embedding overlap priors in variational left ventricle tracking. IEEE TMI 28(12), 1902–1913 (2009)
4. Cour, T., Benezit, F., Shi, J.: Spectral segmentation with multiscale graph decomposition. In: CVPR, vol. 2, pp. 1124–1131. IEEE (2005)

5. Cousty, J., Najman, L., Couprie, M., Clément-Guinaudeau, S., Goissen, T., Garot, J.: Segmentation of 4D cardiac mri: Automated method based on spatio-temporal watershed cuts. Image and Vision Computing 28(8), 1229–1243 (2010)
6. Eynard, D., Glashoff, K., Bronstein, M.M., Bronstein, A.M.: Multimodal diffusion geometry by joint diagnoalization of laplacians. arXiv:1209.2295 (2012)
7. Isgum, I., Staring, M., Rutten, A., Prokop, M., Viergever, M.A., van Ginneken, B.: Multi-atlas-based segmentation with local decision fusion–application to cardiac and aortic segmentation in ct scans. IEEE TMI 28(7), 1000–1010 (2009)
8. Kovnatsky, A., Bronstein, M.M., Bronstein, A.M., Glashoff, K., Kimmel, R.: Coupled quasi-harmonic bases. In: EUROGRAPHICS, pp. 439–448. Wiley (2013)
9. Pednekar, A., Kurkure, U., Muthupillai, R., Flamm, S., Kakadiaris, I.A.: Automated left ventricular segmentation in cardiac mri. IEEE Transactions on Biomedical Engineering 53(7), 1425–1428 (2006)
10. Petitjean, C., Dacher, J.N.: A review of segmentation methods in short axis cardiac MR images. Medical Image Analysis 15(2), 169–184 (2011)
11. Zhang, H., Wahle, A., Johnson, R.K., Scholz, T.D., Sonka, M.: 4-D cardiac mr image analysis: left and right ventricular morphology and function. IEEE TMI 29(2), 350–364 (2010)
12. Zheng, Y., Barbu, A., Georgescu, B., Scheuering, M., Comaniciu, D.: Four-chamber heart modeling and automatic segmentation for 3-D cardiac ct volumes using marginal space learning and steerable features. IEEE TMI 27(11), 1668–1681 (2008)

Uncertainty Quantification for LDDMM Using a Low-Rank Hessian Approximation

Xiao Yang[1] and Marc Niethammer[2]

[1] Department of Computer Science,
University of North Carolina at Chapel Hill, USA
[2] Biomedical Research Imaging Center
University of North Carolina at Chapel Hill, USA

Abstract. This paper presents an approach to estimate the uncertainty of registration parameters for the large displacement diffeomorphic metric mapping (LDDMM) registration framework. Assuming a local multivariate Gaussian distribution as an approximation for the registration energy at the optimal registration parameters, we propose a method to approximate the covariance matrix as the inverse of the Hessian of the registration energy to quantify registration uncertainty. In particular, we make use of a low-rank approximation to the Hessian to accurately and efficiently estimate the covariance matrix using few eigenvalues and eigenvectors. We evaluate the uncertainty of the LDDMM registration results for both synthetic and real imaging data.

1 Introduction

Image registration is critical for many medical image analysis systems to provide spatial correspondences. Consequentially, a large number of image registration methods have been developed which are able to produce high-quality spatial alignments of images. However, most image registration approaches do not provide any measures of registration uncertainty and hence do not allow a user to assess if a registration result is locally "trustworthy" or not. This is particularly problematic for highly flexible registration approaches, such as elastic or fluid registration with very large numbers of parameters to model deformations.

Different approaches to address uncertainty quantification in image registration have been proposed. For example, for rigid deformations, physical landmarks have been used to estimate the average registration error for the whole volume. [2]. Non-rigid deformations are challenging as landmarks only capture local aspects of the deformations. Instead, methods have been proposed to assess uncertainty based on probabilistic models of registration and the image itself. For B-spline models, sampling based methods have been proposed for images [5] or the optimal spline parameters [11] to create multiple registrations from which to estimate deformation uncertainty. Simpson [9] uses a variational Bayesian approach to infer the posterior distribution of B-spline parameters. Monte-Carlo sampling methods have also been explored in the context of elastic registration [8] and for LDDMM [12].

Existing methods mainly focus on parametric non-rigid registration methods such as the B-spline model or require large computational effort to sample over

© Springer International Publishing Switzerland 2015
N. Navab et al. (Eds.): MICCAI 2015, Part II, LNCS 9350, pp. 289–296, 2015.
DOI: 10.1007/978-3-319-24571-3_35

high-dimensional parameter spaces [8,12] as for LDDMM [1]. Here, we develop a method to estimate uncertainty in the deformation parameters of the shooting formulation [10] of LDDMM.

We assume a local multivariate Gaussian distribution at the optimal solution, and approximate the covariance matrix through the inverse of the approximated energy Hessian to quantify uncertainty of the registration parameters. Using the Hessian of the energy to estimate the covariance matrix of parameters has been discussed for large-scale inverse problems in other application domains [3,4]. For high dimensional parameter spaces, computing the full Hessian is prohibitive due to large memory requirements. Therefore, we develop a method to compute Hessian vector products for the LDDMM energy. This allows us to efficiently compute and store an approximation of the Hessian. In particular, we directly approximate the covariance matrix by exploiting the low-rank structure of the image mismatch Hessian. Our framework therefore allows uncertainty analysis for LDDMM at a manageable computational cost.

Sec. 2 discusses the relationship of the covariance matrix of the parameter distribution and the Hessian of the energy function. Sec. 3 introduces our framework to compute the Hessian and to estimate the covariance matrix. Sec. 4 shows experimental results for both synthetic and real data, and discusses how our method extends to other registration models and its potential applications.

2   Covariance Matrix and Hessian of the Energy

Consider a Gaussian random vector θ of dimension N_θ with mean value θ^* and covariance matrix Σ_θ. Its joint probability density function can be written as

$$P(\theta) = (2\pi)^{-\frac{N_\theta}{2}} |\Sigma_\theta|^{-\frac{1}{2}} \exp\left[-\frac{1}{2}(\theta - \theta^*)^T \Sigma_\theta^{-1} (\theta - \theta^*)\right]. \tag{1}$$

In image registration one typically minimizes the energy given by the negative log-likelihood of the posterior distribution. As the negative log-likelihood of the multivariate Gaussian is given by

$$E(\theta) = -\ln(P(\theta)) = \frac{N_\theta}{2}\ln 2\pi + \frac{1}{2}\ln|\Sigma_\theta| + \frac{1}{2}(\theta - \theta^*)^T \Sigma_\theta^{-1}(\theta - \theta^*), \tag{2}$$

computing the Hessian of $E(\theta)$ with respect to θ results in $H_{E(\theta)} = \Sigma_\theta^{-1}$ and directly relates the covariance matrix of the multivariate Gaussian model to the Hessian of the energy through its inverse.

In our method, we assume that at optimality the LDDMM energy can be locally approximated by a second order function and hence by a multivariate Gaussian distribution. In particular, we make use of the shooting based formulation of LDDMM [10] which parameterizes the spatial deformation by an initial momentum (or equivalently by an initial velocity field) and associated evolution equations describing the space deformation over time. Specifically, the registration parameter in shooting based LDDMM is the initial momentum m, which is the dual of the initial velocity v, an element in a reproducing kernel Hilbert space V. The initial momentum belongs to V's dual space V^*, and it is connected with v via a positive-definite, self-adjoint differential operator $L : V \to V^*$ such that $m = Lv$ and $v = Km$. Here the operator K denotes the inverse of L. The energy of LDDMM with the dynamic constraints [10] can then be written as

$$E(m_0) = \langle m_0, Km_0 \rangle + \frac{1}{\sigma^2}||I(1) - I_1||^2, \tag{3}$$

$$m_t + \text{ad}_v^* m = 0, \ m(0) = m_0, \qquad I_t + \nabla I^T v = 0, \ I(0) = I_0 \qquad m - Lv = 0, \tag{4}$$

where the operator ad^* is the dual of the negative Jacobi-Lie bracket of vector fields: $\text{ad}_v w = -[v, w] = Dvw - Dwv$, $\sigma > 0$, and I_0 and I_1 are the source and the target images for registration respectively. The Hessian of this energy is

$$H_{m_0} = 2K + \frac{\partial^2 \frac{1}{\sigma^2}||I(1) - I_1||^2}{\partial m_0^2}. \tag{5}$$

Computing this Hessian is not straightforward, because $I(1)$ only indirectly depends on m_0 through the dynamic constraints and m_0 can become very high-dimensional, making computation and storage challenging. Sec. 3 therefore discusses how to compute the Hessian and its inverse in practice.

3   Hessian Calculation and Covariance Estimation

3.1   Calculating Hessian-Vector Products Using the Adjoint Method

To avoid computation of the full Hessian we instead compute Hessian-vector products. This enables us to make use of efficient iterative methods (such as the Lanczos method) to perform eigen-decomposition of the Hessian, which we exploit to compute an approximation of the Hessian and the covariance matrix.

The equivalent of Hessian-vector products for LDDMM can be computed using the second variation of the LDDMM energy. Specifically, the second variation in the direction δm_0 can be written as

$$\delta^2 E(m_0; \delta m_0) := \frac{\partial^2}{\partial \epsilon^2} E(m_0 + \epsilon \delta m_0)|_{\epsilon=0} = \langle \delta m_0, \nabla^2 E \delta m_0 \rangle. \tag{6}$$

Here $\nabla^2 E$ denotes the Hessian of $E(m_0)$. Using this formulation, we can read off the Hessian-vector product $\nabla^2 E \delta m_0$ from the second variation. Computing this second variation of the LDDMM shooting energy can be accomplished by linearizing both the forward equations for shooting as well as the associated adjoint equations around the optimal solution (the solution of the registration problem). Solving these equations for a given initial condition δm_0 then allows the computation of the Hessian vector product (in a functional sense) as

$$\nabla^2 E \delta m_0 = 2K \delta m_0 - \delta \hat{m}(0). \tag{7}$$

Here, $2K \delta m_0$ can be computed directly and $\delta \hat{m}(0)$ is the perturbation of the adjoint of the momentum propagation constraint at $t = 0$, which is obtained efficiently through a forward-backward sweep through the linearized forward and adjoint equations. Please refer to the supplementary material for details.

3.2   Covariance Estimation Using Low-Rank Hessian

To estimate the covariance, a straightforward way is inverting the Hessian of the full energy. This is not feasible for standard LDDMM because the number of parameters is so large that saving or computing the inverse of the full Hessian is prohibitive[1]. Another possibility is to approximate the full energy Hessian. Note that the Hessian of the LDDMM energy can be separated into the Hessian of the regularization energy and the Hessian of the image mismatch energy. Thus we can separately calculate Hessian vector products for these two parts based on Eq. 7 as:

$$H_m^{\text{regularization}} \delta m_0 = 2K\delta m_0, \quad H_m^{\text{mismatch}} \delta m_0 = -\delta \hat{m}(0).$$

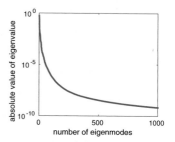

A simple low-rank pseudoinverse as an approximation of the Hessian would result in approximation errors for both $H_m^{\text{regularization}}$ *and* H_m^{mismatch}. This can be partially avoided by using the *exact* inverse of the Hessian of the regularization combined with an *approximation* for the image mismatch Hessian. To compute the covariance matrix, we realize that for many ill-posed inverse problems, the spectrum of the absolute values of the eigenvalues of the image mismatch Hessian decays rapidly to zero. Fig. 1 shows an example of the largest 1000 absolute values of the eigenvalues for a 2D 100×140 pixels heart registration case for initial momentum LDDMM. By computing only a few dominant eigenmodes (using an iterative eigensolver such as the Lanczos method) of the image mismatch Hessian with respect to initial momentum, we can ac-

Fig. 1. First 1000 largest absolute eigenvalues of image mismatch Hessian for a 100×140 pixels heart registration case using initial momentum LDDMM.

curately approximate the Hessian with much less memory and computational effort. Suppose we approximate the image mismatch Hessian with k dominating eigenmodes as

$$H_{m(k)}^{\text{mismatch}} \approx V_{m(k)}^T D_{m(k)} V_{m(k)}.$$

Here $D_{m(k)}$ is a $k \times k$ diagonal matrix, where the diagonal elements are the eigenvalues; $V_{m(k)}$ is a $k \times n$ matrix, where n is the number of all parameters, and each row of V_k is an eigenvector. For simplicity we write $H_m^{\text{regularization}}$ as H_m^{reg}. We can then approximate the covariance matrix Σ_m as

$$\Sigma_m = (H_m^{\text{reg}} + H_m^{\text{mismatch}})^{-1} \approx (H_m^{\text{reg}} + V_{m(k)}^T D_{m(k)} V_{m(k)})^{-1}. \qquad (8)$$

Since we have a closed-form solution for the inverse of H_m^{reg}, we can directly apply the Woodbury identity to the right hand side of equation 8 and obtain

$$\Sigma_m \approx (H_m^{\text{reg}})^{-1} - (H_m^{\text{reg}})^{-1} V_{m(k)}^T (D_{m(k)}^{-1} + V_{m(k)}(H_m^{\text{reg}})^{-1} V_{m(k)}^T)^{-1} V_{m(k)} (H_m^{\text{reg}})^{-1}. \qquad (9)$$

---

[1] Note that this would be possible when using a landmark-based LDDMM variant where the parameterization of the deformation becomes finite-dimensional.

The advantage of this formulation is that $D_{m(k)}^{-1} + V_{m(k)}(H_m^{\text{reg}})^{-1}V_{m(k)}^T$ is a small $k \times k$ matrix, and its inverse can be computed easily using dense algebra.

In LDDMM we could quantify the uncertainty through the covariance with respect to either the initial momentum or its corresponding initial velocity. If we use the initial momentum, the approximation of $(D_{m(k)}^{-1}+V_{m(k)}(H_m^{\text{reg}})^{-1}V_{m(k)}^T)^{-1}$ will be accurate for small k, because the image mismatch Hessian for the initial momentum has a rapidly decreasing eigen-spectrum. However, the inverse of the regularization kernel would be $(H_m^{\text{reg}})^{-1} = (2K)^{-1} = \frac{1}{2}L$, which is a rough kernel. In experiments, using the rough kernel significantly increases the difference between approximations for different k's. On the other hand, in the initial velocity formulation, $(H_m^{\text{reg}})^{-1}$ is a smoothing kernel, and it further decreases the approximation difference for different k's. Unfortunately, the image mismatch Hessian with respect to the initial velocity does not have a fast-decreasing spectrum due to the implicit smoothness of the initial velocity.

We want to use the rapidly decreasing eigen-spectrum of the momentum-based formulation, but at the same time we want to avoid its rough kernel when calculating the covariance matrix. Our solution is to use the low-rank approximation of the initial *momentum* image mismatch Hessian to approximate the covariance with respect to the initial *velocity*. Recall the relation between momentum and velocity: $v = Km$. This means the Jacobian of v with respect to m is $J_{\frac{v}{m}} = K$. Thus by change of variables, we can obtain our final approximation of the covariance with respect to the initial velocity as

$$\Sigma_v = J_{\frac{v}{m}} \Sigma_m J_{\frac{v}{m}}^T \approx \frac{K}{2} - \frac{1}{4}V_{m(k)}^T (D_{m(k)}^{-1} + V_{m(k)}\frac{L}{2}V_{m(k)}^T)^{-1}V_{m(k)}. \tag{10}$$

4   Experiments and Discussions

We evaluate our proposed model using synthetic and real data. In the following experiments, L corresponds to the invertible and self-adjoint Sobolev operator, $L = a\Delta^2 + b\Delta + c$, with $a = 9 \times 10^{-4}$, $b = -6 \times 10^{-2}$, and $c = 1$; $\sigma = 0.1$. For the eigen-decomposition we use PROPACK [6], which uses a Lanczos bidiagonalization method. Computing 200 dominant eigenvectors for the 2D synthetic example, which gives a very accurate Hessian estimation, requires less than 3 min in Matlab; however computing the full Hessian requires more than 30 min. Hence, our method is an order of magnitude faster. All images below are rescaled to a $[0, 1]$ space range.

Synthetic Data. The synthetic example is a simple registration of an expanding square. Figure 3 shows the source image, the target image, and the final registration result. The size of the image is 51×51 pixels, thus the size of the Hessian is 5202×5202. Since this Hessian is small, we compute the full covariance matrix using finite differences as the ground truth for our covariance estimation. We compare our method with the low rank pseudoinverse using both the initial momentum Hessian and the initial velocity Hessian.

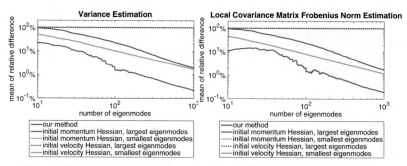

Fig. 2. Relative low-rank approximation differences for synthetic data.

We approximate two uncertainty measures: the variance of each parameter, and the spatially localized covariance matrix for each image pixel[2]. Fig. 2 shows the mean of relative differences with respect to the ground truth for different methods. Our method outperforms the other methods even with very few eigenmodes selected. In some test cases (see supplementary material) when only a few eigenmodes are selected (e.g., 10), the pseudoinverse of the Hessian achieves relatively better accuracy than our method, but in those cases, the relative difference can be up to

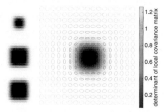

Fig. 3. Square registration case. Left: top to bottom: source image, target image, warped result. Right: Uncertainty visualization by ellipses, mapped on source image.

100%, making the approximation unusable. For reasonable numbers of eigenmodes (e.g., larger than 100), our method is always better. E.g., in Fig 2, while 100 eigenmodes result in a relative error of around 1% for our method, around 1000 are required for the other approaches for similar accuracy.

To visualize the uncertainty information, we extract the local covariance matrices from the approximated covariance matrix and visualize these matrices as ellipses on the source image. Fig. 3 shows the uncertainty visualization for the synthetic data. The ellipses are estimated using 200 dominant eigenmodes from the image mismatch Hessian. The color indicates the determinant of local covariance matrices. The closer to the center of the square, the smaller the determinant is, meaning a more confident registration result closer to the center. Furthermore, the uncertainty along the edge is larger than the uncertainty perpendicular to the edge, indicating the aperture problem of image registration.

2D Heart Image. We use cardiac data from the Sunnybrook cardiac MR database [7]. The image corresponds to a beating heart of a 63 years normal individual at two different time points.

---

[2] In 2D this amounts to computing $\begin{pmatrix} \sigma_{xx}^2(i,j) & \sigma_{xy}^2(i,j) \\ \sigma_{xy}^2(i,j) & \sigma_{yy}^2(i,j) \end{pmatrix}$ for each pixel location (i,j), i.e., not considering non-local cross-variances.

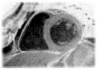
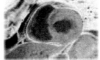
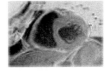

(a) Source image   (b) Target image   (c) Warped result

Fig. 4. Heart registration test case.

We cropped the axial images to a common 2D rectangular region around the heart. Fig. 4 shows the heart image and registration result. The size of the heart image is 100×140 pixels, resulting in a 28000×28000 Hessian. We select the top 500 eigenmodes for approximation and achieve a mean relative difference for variance of 1.13%, and for the Frobenius norm of the local covariance matrix of 0.94%. Using the pseudoinverse of the full Hessian gives a mean relative difference of 6.81% and 6.27% for the initial velocity Hessian, and 31.17% and 30.04% for the initial momentum Hessian.

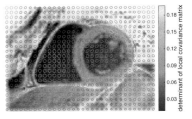

Fig. 5. Uncertainty visualization of heart test case mapped on source image.

Fig. 5 shows the uncertainty visualization for the initial velocity on the source image. From the image we see that the area inside the ventricle has high uncertainty, indicating low deformation confidence in the isotropic area. Also, there exists high uncertainty at the upper right edge of the atrium. This indicates high uncertainty for shifting along the edge.

3D Brain Image. Here our data is two MR images ($75 \times 90 \times 60$ voxels) of a macaque monkey at 6 months and 12 months of age. The size of this Hessian is $1,215,000 \times 1,215,000$. We calculate the largest 1000 eigenmodes for covariance approximation. For visualization of uncertainty, we use the trace of the local covariance matrix. Fig. 6 shows the 3D test case as well as the uncertainty visualization. We can see that although the deformation is very small despite of

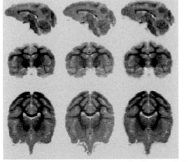
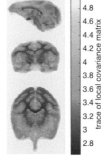

Fig. 6. 3D monkey brain test case. Left to right: source image, target image, warped result, visualization of trace of local covariance matrix on the source image.

overall intensity change, our method can still capture isotropic areas that have very small changes. These areas have a higher uncertainty compared to others.

Discussions. Although we focus on LDDMM, our method has much wider applicability. Using the Hessian-vector product for efficient low-rank Hessian optimization is relevant for many other non-parametric registration approaches formulated with similar regularization and image similarity measures, such as optic flow and registration by stationary velocity fields, since they are usually over-parameterized. Even for low-dimensional parameterization methods such as landmark LDDMM, our method could be used to compute the full Hessian. Our method could also be used as in [9] for uncertainty-based smoothing, and for surgical- or radiation-treatment planning to inform margins. Finally, comparing our method with sampling-based methods for LDDMM [12] will be useful.

Support. This research is supported by NSF EECS-1148870 and EECS-0925875.

References

1. Beg, M., Miller, M., Trouvé, A., Younes, L.: Computing large deformation metric mappings via geodesic flows of diffeomorphisms. IJCV 61(2), 139–157 (2005)
2. Fitzpatrick, J., West, J.: The distribution of target registration error in rigid-body point-based registration. IEEE Trans. Med. Imaging 20(9), 917–927 (2001)
3. Flath, H.P., Wilcox, L.C., Akçelik, V., Hill, J., van Bloemen Waanders, B., Ghattas, O.: Fast algorithms for Bayesian uncertainty quantification in large-scale linear inverse problems based on low rank partial Hessian approximations. SISC 33(1), 407–432 (2011)
4. Kalmikov, A.G., Heimbach, P.: A hessian-based method for uncertainty quantification in global ocean state estimation. SISC 36(5), S267–S295 (2014)
5. Kybic, J.: Bootstrap resampling for image registration uncertainty estimation without ground truth. IEEE Trans. Med. Imaging 19(1), 64–73 (2010)
6. Larsen, R.: Lanczos bidiagonalization with partial reorthogonalization. DAIMI Report Series 27(537) (1998)
7. Radau, P., Lu, Y., Connelly, K., Paul, G., Dick, A., Wright, G.: Evaluation framework for algorithms segmenting short axis cardiac MRI. The MIDAS Journal 49 (2009)
8. Risholm, P., Janoos, F., Norton, I., Golby, A.J., Wells, W.M.: Bayesian characterization of uncertainty in intra-subject non-rigid registration. Medical Image Analysis 17(5), 538–555 (2013)
9. Simpson, I.J.A., Woolrich, M.W., Groves, A.R., Schnabel, J.A.: Longitudinal brain MRI analysis with uncertain registration. In: Fichtinger, G., Martel, A., Peters, T. (eds.) MICCAI 2011, Part II. LNCS, vol. 6892, pp. 647–654. Springer, Heidelberg (2011)
10. Vialard, F.X., Risser, L., Rueckert, D., Cotter, C.J.: Diffeomorphic 3D image registration via geodesic shooting using an efficient adjoint calculation. IJCV 97(2), 229–241 (2012)
11. Watanabe, T., Scott, C.: Spatial confidence regions for quantifying and visualizing registration uncertainty. In: Dawant, B.M., Christensen, G.E., Fitzpatrick, J.M., Rueckert, D. (eds.) WBIR 2012. LNCS, vol. 7359, pp. 120–130. Springer, Heidelberg (2012)
12. Zhang, M., Singh, N., Fletcher, P.T.: Bayesian estimation of regularization and atlas building in diffeomorphic image registration. In: Gee, J.C., Joshi, S., Pohl, K.M., Wells, W.M., Zöllei, L. (eds.) IPMI 2013. LNCS, vol. 7917, pp. 37–48. Springer, Heidelberg (2013)

A Stochastic Quasi-Newton Method for Non-Rigid Image Registration

Yuchuan Qiao[1], Zhuo Sun[1], Boudewijn P.F. Lelieveldt[1,2], and Marius Staring[1]

[1] Division of Image Processing (LKEB) Department of Radiology,
Leiden University Medical Center, Leiden, The Netherlands
{Y.Qiao,Z.Sun,B.P.F.Lelieveldt,M.Staring}@lumc.nl
[2] Department of Intelligent Systems,
Delft University of Technology, Delft, The Netherlands

Abstract. Image registration is often very slow because of the high dimensionality of the images and complexity of the algorithms. Adaptive stochastic gradient descent (ASGD) outperforms deterministic gradient descent and even quasi-Newton in terms of speed. This method, however, only exploits first-order information of the cost function. In this paper, we explore a stochastic quasi-Newton method (s-LBFGS) for non-rigid image registration. It uses the classical limited memory BFGS method in combination with noisy estimates of the gradient. Curvature information of the cost function is estimated once every L iterations and then used for the next L iterations in combination with a stochastic gradient. The method is validated on follow-up data of 3D chest CT scans (19 patients), using a B-spline transformation model and a mutual information metric. The experiments show that the proposed method is robust, efficient and fast. s-LBFGS obtains a similar accuracy as ASGD and deterministic LBFGS. Compared to ASGD the proposed method uses about 5 times fewer iterations to reach the same metric value, resulting in an overall reduction in run time of a factor of two. Compared to deterministic LBFGS, s-LBFGS is almost 500 times faster.

1 Introduction

Image registration is important in the field of medical image analysis. However, this process is often very slow because of the large number of voxels in the images and the complexity of the registration algorithms [1,2]. A powerful optimization method is needed to shorten the time consumption during the registration process, which would benefit time-critical intra-operative procedures relying on image guidance.

The stochastic gradient descent method is often used to iteratively find the optimum [3]. This method is easy to implement and fast because at each iteration only a subset of voxels from the fixed image is evaluated to obtain gradients. Although it obtains a good accuracy, its convergence rate is poor since only first order derivatives are used. A preconditioning matrix can be used to improve the convergence rate of (stochastic) gradient descent, but this was only proposed in

© Springer International Publishing Switzerland 2015
N. Navab et al. (Eds.): MICCAI 2015, Part II, LNCS 9350, pp. 297–304, 2015.
DOI: 10.1007/978-3-319-24571-3_36

a mono-modal setting [4]. The quasi-Newton method also has a better convergence rate than deterministic gradient descent, but comes at a higher cost in computation time and large memory consumption. Limited memory Broyden-Fletcher-Goldfarb-Shanno (LBFGS) takes an advantage in the storage of only a few previous Hessian approximations, however, the computation time is still very long as all voxels are needed for new Hessian approximations [2].

Some approaches to create a stochastic version of the quasi-Newton method are proposed in a mathematical setting, such as online LBFGS [5], careful quasi-Newton stochastic gradient descent [6], regularized stochastic BFGS [7] and stochastic LBFGS [8]. However, there is no application in the image registration field, and applying the stochastic quasi-Newton method to non-rigid image registration is still a challenge. All of the previous methods either used a manually selected constant step size or a fixed decaying step size, which are not flexible when switching problem settings or applications. Moreover, the uncertainty of gradient estimation introduced by the stochastic gradient for Hessian approximation is still a problem. Although Byrd [8] used the exact Hessian to compute curvature updates, which is still difficult to calculate for high dimensional problems. For careful QN-SGD [6], the average scheme may be useless in case of an extremely large or small scaling value for H_0. Mokhtari [7] used a regularized term like Schraudolph [5] did to compensate the gradient difference y from the parameter difference s and introduced a new variable δ, which is not only complex, but also needs to store all previous curvature pairs.

In this paper, we propose a stochastic quasi-Newton method specifically for non-rigid image registration inspired by Byrd et al. [8]. Different from Byrd's method, the proposed method employs only gradients and avoids computing second order derivatives of the cost function to capture the curvature. Secondly, we employ an automatic and adaptive scheme for optimization step size estimation instead of a fixed manual scheme. Finally, we propose a restarting mechanism where the optimal step size is recomputed when a new Hessian approximation becomes available, i.e. every L iterations. The proposed method and some variations are validated using 3D lung CT follow-up data using manually annotated corresponding points for evaluation.

2 Methods

Non-rigid image registration aims to align images following a continuous deformation strategy. The optimal transformation parameters are the solution that minimizes the dissimilarity between fixed I_F and moving image I_M:

$$\widehat{\boldsymbol{\mu}} = \arg\min_{\boldsymbol{\mu}} \mathcal{C}(I_F, I_M \circ \boldsymbol{T_\mu}), \tag{1}$$

in which $\boldsymbol{T_\mu}(\boldsymbol{x})$ is a coordinate transformation parameterized by $\boldsymbol{\mu}$.

2.1   Deterministic Quasi-Newton

The deterministic quasi-Newton method employs the following iterative form:

$$\boldsymbol{\mu}_{k+1} = \boldsymbol{\mu}_k - \gamma_k \boldsymbol{B}_k^{-1} \boldsymbol{g}_k, \tag{2}$$

where $\boldsymbol{B}_k$ is a symmetric positive definite approximation of the Hessian matrix $\nabla^2 \mathcal{C}(\boldsymbol{\mu}_k)$. Quasi-Newton methods update the inverse matrix $\boldsymbol{H}_k = \boldsymbol{B}_k^{-1}$ directly using only first order derivatives, and have a super-linear rate of convergence. Among many methods to construct the series $\{\boldsymbol{H}_k\}$, Broyden-Fletcher-Goldfarb-Shanno (BFGS) tends to be efficient and robust in many applications. It uses the following update rule for $\boldsymbol{H}_k$:

$$\boldsymbol{H}_{k+1} = \boldsymbol{V}_k^T \boldsymbol{H}_k \boldsymbol{V}_k + \rho_k \boldsymbol{s}_k \boldsymbol{s}_k^T, \tag{3}$$

in which

$$\rho_k = \frac{1}{\boldsymbol{y}_k^T \boldsymbol{s}_k}, \quad \boldsymbol{V}_k = \boldsymbol{I} - \rho_k \boldsymbol{y}_k \boldsymbol{s}_k^T, \quad \boldsymbol{s}_k = \boldsymbol{\mu}_{k+1} - \boldsymbol{\mu}_k, \quad \boldsymbol{y}_k = \boldsymbol{g}_{k+1} - \boldsymbol{g}_k. \tag{4}$$

Since the cost of storing and manipulating the inverse Hessian approximation $\boldsymbol{H}_k$ is prohibitive when the number of the parameters is large, a frequently used alternative is to only store the latest M curvature pairs $\{\boldsymbol{s}_k, \boldsymbol{y}_k\}$ in memory: limited memory BFGS (LBFGS). The matrix $\boldsymbol{H}_k$ is not calculated explicitly, and the product $\boldsymbol{H}_k \boldsymbol{g}_k$ is obtained based on a 2-rank BFGS update, which uses a two loop recursion [8]. The initial inverse Hessian approximation usually takes the following form, which we also use in this paper:

$$\boldsymbol{H}_k^0 = \theta_k \boldsymbol{I}, \quad \theta_k = \frac{\boldsymbol{s}_{k-1}^T \boldsymbol{y}_{k-1}}{\boldsymbol{y}_{k-1}^T \boldsymbol{y}_{k-1}}. \tag{5}$$

2.2   Stochastic Quasi-Newton

A large part of the computation time of quasi-Newton methods is in the computation of the curvature pairs $\{\boldsymbol{s}_k, \boldsymbol{y}_k\}$. The pairs are computed deterministically using all samples from the fixed image. A straightforward way to obtain a stochastic version of the quasi-Newton method is to construct the curvature pairs using stochastic gradients, using only a small number of samples at each iteration. This however introduces too much noise in the curvature estimation, caused by the fact that stochastic gradients are inherently noisy and for each iteration are also evaluated on different subsets of image voxels, both of which may yield a poor Hessian approximation. This leads to instability in the optimization.

To cope with this problem, Byrd *et al.* [8] proposed a scheme to eliminate the noise by averaging the optimization parameters for a regular interval of L iterations and obtain the curvature through a direct Hessian calculation on a random subset $\mathcal{S}_2$. This is combined with a series of L iterations performing LBFGS using the thus obtained inverse Hessian estimate together with *stochastic* gradients (using a small random subset $\mathcal{S}_1$). Inspired by this scheme, we propose a method suitable for medical image registration and avoiding manual tuning the step size. First, more samples are used for the curvature pair update than for the stochastic gradient evaluation. Second, the curvature information is obtained using a gradient difference instead of second order derivatives evaluated at an identical subset of samples, i.e. $\boldsymbol{y}_t = \boldsymbol{g}(\bar{\boldsymbol{\mu}}_I; \mathcal{S}_2) - \boldsymbol{g}(\bar{\boldsymbol{\mu}}_J; \mathcal{S}_2)$ and the curvature condition $\boldsymbol{y}^T \boldsymbol{s} > 0$ is checked to ensure positive definiteness of the LBFGS update [8]. Finally, the initial step size at the beginning of each L iterations is automatically determined, with or without restarting. Restarting is a recent development [9] showing improved rate of convergence, which in this paper we apply to the step size selection.

Instead of manual constant step size selection as in [8], we employ an automatic method. A commonly used function for the step size which fulfils the convergence conditions [10] is $\gamma_k = \eta a/(t_k + A)^\alpha$, with $A \geq 1$, $a > 0$, $0 \leq \eta \leq 1$ and $0 \leq \alpha \leq 1$. The step size factor a and the noise compensation factor η are automatically determined through the statistical distribution of voxel displacements [11], while $A = 20$ according to [3] and $\alpha = 1$ is theoretically optimal [3]. Different strategies for the artificial time parameter t_k are tested: a constant step size $t_k = 0$, a regularly decaying step size $t_k = k$, and an adaptive step size $t_k = f(\cdot)$. Here, f is a sigmoid function with argument of the inner product of the gradients $\tilde{\boldsymbol{g}}_k^T \cdot \tilde{\boldsymbol{g}}_{k-1}$ for gradient descent. For s-LBFGS, it can be derived that the search direction is needed as argument, i.e. $\boldsymbol{d}_k^T \cdot \boldsymbol{d}_{k-1}$ with $\boldsymbol{d}_k = \boldsymbol{B}_k^{-1} \boldsymbol{g}_k$.

An overview of the proposed s-LBFGS method is given in Algorithm 1.

3   Experiment

The proposed method was integrated in the open source software package elastix [12]. The experiments were performed on a workstation with 8 cores running at 2.4 GHz and 24 GB memory, with an Ubuntu Linux OS.

3D lung CT scans of 19 patients acquired during the SPREAD study [13] were used to test the performance. Each patient had a baseline and a follow-up scan with an image size around $450 \times 300 \times 150$ and the voxel size around $0.7 \times 0.7 \times 2.5$ mm. For each image, one hunred anatomical corresponding points were chosen semi-automatically using Murphy's method in consensus by two experts, to obtain a ground truth.

To evaluate the method, each follow-up image was registered to the baseline image using mutual information and a B-spline transformation model. The maximum number of iterations for each resolution was 500. A three-level multi-resolution framework was employed using a Gaussian smoothing filter with standard deviations of 2, 1 and 0.5 mm for each resolution. The grid spacing of the B-spline control points was halved between each resolution resulting in a final grid spacing of 10 mm in each direction. After initial testing, we chose the update frequency $L = 10, 20, 40$ for each resolution, respectively, the memory $M = 5$ from [2,8], the number of samples for stochastic gradient computation $|S_1| = 5000$, and the number of samples for the curvature pair update $|S_2| = 50000$.

To measure the registration accuracy, the anatomical points from each baseline image were transformed using the obtained transformation parameters and

---

Algorithm 1. Stochastic LBFGS (s-LBFGS) with and without restarting

---

Require: initial parameters $\boldsymbol{\mu}_0$, memory size M, update frequency L, iteration number K

1: Set $t = 0$, $\bar{\boldsymbol{\mu}}_J = \boldsymbol{\mu}_0$, $\bar{\boldsymbol{\mu}}_I = \mathbf{0}$
2: Automatically estimate the initial step size λ_0 ▷ According to [11]
3: **for** $k = 1, 2, 3, \ldots, K$ **do**
4:     Compute $\tilde{\boldsymbol{g}}_k(\boldsymbol{\mu}_k; \mathcal{S}_1)$ ▷ stochastic gradient
5:     $\bar{\boldsymbol{\mu}}_I = \bar{\boldsymbol{\mu}}_I + \boldsymbol{\mu}_k$ ▷ Update the mean parameters
6:     **if** $k <= 2L$ **then**   ▷ ASGD update
7:        Update the step size λ_k ▷ According to [11]
8:        $\boldsymbol{\mu}_{k+1} = \boldsymbol{\mu}_k - \lambda_k \tilde{\boldsymbol{g}}_k$
9:     **else**   ▷ s-LBFGS update
10:        Compute $\boldsymbol{d}_k = \boldsymbol{H}_t \tilde{\boldsymbol{g}}_k$ ▷ s-LBFGS search direction, see [8] and (2)
11:        **if** $\mod (k, L) = 0$ and restarting **then**
12:           Automatically estimate the initial step size λ'_0
13:           Reset $\lambda_k = \lambda'_0$
14:        Update the step size λ_k ▷ According to [11] but using $\boldsymbol{d}_k^T \cdot \boldsymbol{d}_{k-1}$
15:        $\boldsymbol{\mu}_{k+1} = \boldsymbol{\mu}_k - \lambda_k \boldsymbol{d}_k$
16:     **if** $\mod (k, L) = 0$ **then**   ▷ Curvature pairs update
17:        $\bar{\boldsymbol{\mu}}_I = \bar{\boldsymbol{\mu}}_I / L$ ▷ Update the mean parameters
18:        $\boldsymbol{s}_t = \bar{\boldsymbol{\mu}}_I - \bar{\boldsymbol{\mu}}_J$, $\boldsymbol{y}_t = \boldsymbol{g}(\bar{\boldsymbol{\mu}}_I; \mathcal{S}_2) - \boldsymbol{g}(\bar{\boldsymbol{\mu}}_J; \mathcal{S}_2)$ ▷ New curvature pair
19:        $\bar{\boldsymbol{\mu}}_J = \bar{\boldsymbol{\mu}}_I$, $\bar{\boldsymbol{\mu}}_I = \mathbf{0}, t = t + 1$
20: **return** $\boldsymbol{\mu}_K$

---

then compared to the corresponding points of the follow-up image. We used the Euclidean distance between the corresponding points $\boldsymbol{p}_F \in \Omega_F$ and $\boldsymbol{p}_M \in \Omega_M$ to measure the accuracy using the following equation: $ED = \frac{1}{n} \sum_{i=1}^{n} \|\boldsymbol{T}(\boldsymbol{p}_F^i) - \boldsymbol{p}_M^i\|$. For 19 patients, we first obtained the mean distance error of 100 points for each patient then performed Wilcoxon signed rank test to these mean errors. For convergence testing we computed the cost function value after each iteration deterministically, i.e. based on full sampling. The registration time in the first resolution is presented to compare the algorithm speeds.

4 Results

To gain insight in the proposed method, we investigated some aspects that influence registration performance. The restarting scheme (Restart) was compared with a scheme without restarting. We evaluated different step size selection strategies all based on automatic initial step size selection [11]: a constant scheme (Constant, $t_k = 0$), a regularly decaying scheme (Decaying, $t_k = k$), and the proposed adaptive scheme (Adaptive, $t_k = f(\cdot)$). The proposed method is further compared with the ASGD method [3] and with deterministic LBFGS [2].

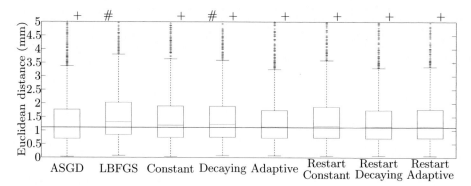

Fig. 1. Euclidean distance error in mm. The symbols # and + indicate a statistically significant difference with ASGD and LBFGS, respectively.

Table 1. Run time in the first resolution. I indicates how many iterations are needed to reach the same metric value as ASGD after 500 iterations. s-LBFGS and s-LBFGS-NR are with and without restarting, both using adaptive step sizes. The speed-up is relative to ASGD.

	Time at $k = 500$	I	Time (s) at $k = I$	Speed-up
ASGD	27.2 ± 0.7	500	-	-
LBFGS	26838 ± 9965	21 ± 1	8081 ± 1580	0.004 ± 0.0005
s-LBFGS-NR	74.3 ± 4.8	190 ± 93	30.6 ± 13.9	1.0 ± 0.4
s-LBFGS	75.8 ± 1.0	107 ± 17	18.1 ± 2.6	1.5 ± 0.2

From Fig. 1 we can see that all methods have very similar final registration error, for LBFGS regularization may improve the results [14]. Fig. 2 shows the convergence plots of the methods for several patients. Comparing the three step size strategies in Fig. 2a and 2b, the regularly decaying method has suboptimal convergence, while the constant and the adaptive scheme behave similarly. The restarting scheme shows a substantial improvement in convergence rate, therefore in Fig. 2c~2f we only show the result of restarting scheme with adaptive step size (s-LBFGS). Some small spikes are visible in Fig. 2b and Fig. 2f, which we attribute to noise in the curvature pair estimation: an experiment using 1.5 million samples for the curvature estimation yielded smooth results (not shown). In terms of iterations, s-LBFGS always obtains faster convergence than ASGD, but slower than LBFGS. The registration time of ASGD, LBFGS and s-LBFGS is shown in Table 1. The LBFGS method is very costly, as expected. To obtain the same metric value as ASGD at iteration 500, the proposed method always takes fewer iterations resulting in an average speedup of two, while the proposed method without restarting requires more iterations and therefore more time.

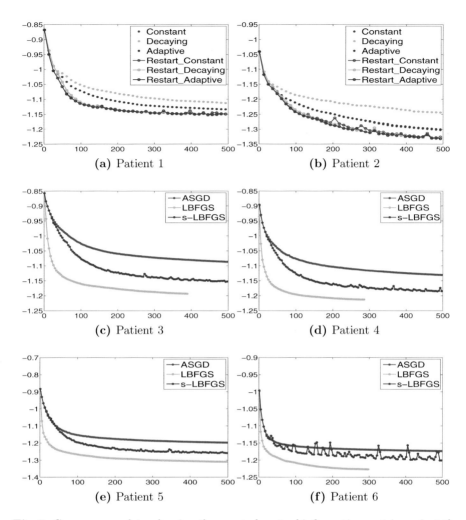

Fig. 2. Convergence plots, showing the negated mutual information metric against the iteration number.

5   Conclusion

In this paper, we present for the first time a stochastic quasi-Newton optimization method (s-LBFGS) for non-rigid image registration. It uses the classical limited memory BFGS method in combination with noisy estimates of the gradient. Curvature information of the cost function is estimated robustly once every L iterations and then used for the next L iterations in combination with stochastic gradients. A novel restarting procedure, automatically selecting the optimization step size, is shown to be beneficial for accelerated convergence. The new optimization routine is validated on follow-up data of 3D chest CT scans (19 patients).

Compared to ASGD the proposed method uses about 5 times fewer iterations to reach the same metric value, resulting in an overall reduction in run time of a factor of two. Compared to deterministic LBFGS, s-LBFGS is almost 500 times faster. Future work will focus on developing a stopping condition for stochastic second order procedures, on a more robust estimation of the initial approximation of H_0 more resilient against noise, on alterative quasi-Newton schemes such as the symmetric rank-one update [15], and more extensive validation.

References

1. Sotiras, A., Davatzikos, C., Paragios, N.: Deformable medical image registration: A survey. IEEE Transactions on Medical Imaging 32(7), 1153–1190 (2013)
2. Klein, S., Staring, M., Pluim, J.P.: Evaluation of optimization methods for nonrigid medical image registration using mutual information and B-splines. IEEE Transactions on Image Processing 16(12), 2879–2890 (2007)
3. Klein, S., Pluim, J., Staring, M., Viergever, M.: Adaptive stochastic gradient descent optimisation for image registration. International Journal of Computer Vision 81(3), 227–239 (2009)
4. Klein, S., Staring, M., Andersson, P., Pluim, J.P.W.: Preconditioned stochastic gradient descent optimisation for monomodal image registration. In: Fichtinger, G., Martel, A., Peters, T. (eds.) MICCAI 2011, Part II. LNCS, vol. 6892, pp. 549–556. Springer, Heidelberg (2011)
5. Schraudolph, N., Yu, J., Günter, S.: A stochastic quasi-Newton method for online convex optimization (2007)
6. Bordes, A., Bottou, L., Gallinari, P.: SGD-QN: Careful quasi-Newton stochastic gradient descent. The Journal of Machine Learning Research 10, 1737–1754 (2009)
7. Mokhtari, A., Ribeiro, A.: RES: Regularized stochastic BFGS algorithm. IEEE Transactions on Signal Processing 62(23), 6089–6104 (2014)
8. Byrd, R.H., Hansen, S., Nocedal, J., Singer, Y.: A stochastic quasi-Newton method for large-scale optimization. arXiv preprint arXiv:1401.7020 (2014)
9. O'Donoghue, B., Candés, E.: Adaptive restart for accelerated gradient schemes. Foundations of Computational Mathematics, 1–18 (2013)
10. Kiefer, J., Wolfowitz, J.: Stochastic estimation of the maximum of a regression function. The Annals of Mathematical Statistics 23(3), 462–466 (1952)
11. Qiao, Y., Lelieveldt, B., Staring, M.: Fast automatic estimation of the optimization step size for nonrigid image registration. In: SPIE Medical Imaging, International Society for Optics and Photonics, pp. 90341A–90341A (2014)
12. Klein, S., Staring, M., et al.: Elastix: a toolbox for intensity-based medical image registration. IEEE Transactions on Medical Imaging 29(1), 196–205 (2010)
13. Stolk, J., Putter, H., Bakker, E.M., et al.: Progression parameters for emphysema: a clinical investigation. Respiratory Medicine 101(9), 1924–1930 (2007)
14. Sun, W., Niessen, W., van Stralen, M., Klein, S.: Simultaneous multiresolution strategies for nonrigid image registration. IEEE Transactions on Image Processing 22(12), 4905–4917 (2013)
15. Modarres Khiyabani, F., Leong, W.: Limited memory methods with improved symmetric rank-one updates and its applications on nonlinear image restoration. Arabian Journal for Science and Engineering 39(11), 7823–7838 (2014)

Locally Orderless Registration for Diffusion Weighted Images

Henrik G. Jensen, Francois Lauze, Mads Nielsen, and Sune Darkner

Department of Computer Science, University of Copenhagen
Universitetsparken 1, DK-2100 Copenhagen, Denmark
{henne,madsn,francois,darkner}@di.ku.dk

Abstract. Registration of Diffusion Weighted Images (DWI) is challenging as the data, in contrast to scalar-valued images, is a composition of both directional and intensity information. The DWI signal is known to be influenced by noise and a wide range of artifacts. Therefore, it is attractive to use similarity measures with invariance properties, such as Mutual Information. However, density estimation from DWI is complicated by directional information. We address this problem by extending Locally Orderless Registration (LOR), a density estimation framework for image similarity, to include directional information. We construct a spatio-directional scale-space formulation of marginal and joint density distributions between two DWI, that takes the projective nature of the directional information into account. This accounts for orientation and magnitude and enables us to use a wide range of similarity measures from the LOR framework. Using Mutual Information, we examine the properties of the scale-space induced by the choice of kernels and illustrate the approach by affine registration.

1 Introduction

The registration of Diffusion Weighted Images (DWI) is interesting as it contains information about the fibrous micro-architecture otherwise invisible to structural MRI. Registration of these structures enables us to compare connectivity within and across subjects. However, registration is challenging due to the inherent geometry of DWI; notably high-angular resolution diffusion imaging (HARDI) which models more complex displacement profiles. We extend the Locally Orderless Registration (LOR) [2] density estimation framework for image similarity from scalar-valued images to DWI. The LOR is a scale-space framework for image density estimation that allows us to employ a wide range of similarity measures for registration, including MI. By introducing a spatio-directional kernel, thus including the space of gradient directions, we model the relationship between direction and measurements as histograms. The histograms are mapped to probability density estimates by normalization and marginalization over the deformed space.

Our contribution is a full LOR scale-space formulation for DWI, offering explicitly control of orientation, image, intensity and integration scale. We examine

© Springer International Publishing Switzerland 2015
N. Navab et al. (Eds.): MICCAI 2015, Part II, LNCS 9350, pp. 305–312, 2015.
DOI: 10.1007/978-3-319-24571-3_37

306 H.G. Jensen et al.

the effects of the scale-space and illustrate the application of the density estimate by affine image registration of DWI data using Mutual Information.

2 Previous Work and Background

Locally Orderless Images (LOI) [6] is a scale-space representation of intensity distributions in images modeling three inherent scales: the image scale (i.e. image smoothing), the integration scale (local histogram), and the intensity scale (soft bin width). The first mention of LOI in the context of image registration was in by Hermosillo et al. [4] where a variational approach to image registration was presented. The LOR framework [2], an extension of [1], generalized a range of similarity measures as linear and non-linear functions of density estimates for scalar-valued images. One such non-linear similarity measure is Mutual Information (MI) [13]. MI is one of the most frequently used similarity measures in image registration and was introduced as a multi-modal similarity measure. MI is frequently used in MRI due to its invariance properties with respect to intensity values and is associated with scalar-valued images. It is used in the context of DWI for distortion-correction [9] on e.g. b_0 or individual DWI directions. Van Hecke et al. [12] used MI for non-rigid registration of DWI. Under an assumption of alignment, each gradient direction was evaluated separately as well as in a pooled fashion to form a joint density distribution. Interpolation of directional information in DWI was introduced by Tao and Miller [10] for affine registration using SSD and extended by Duarte-Carvajalino et al. [3] to non-rigid B-spline registration. The angular interpolation was extended with a Watson distribution by Rathi et al. [8]. Raffelt et al. [7] used SSD after spherical deconvolution for fiber modeling (FODs), while others, like Yap et al. [14], compared the coefficients of the spherical harmonics.

Image registration is the process of spatially aligning (two) images (I and J) under some transformation Φ given some regularity condition $\mathcal{S}(\Phi)$ and similarity $\mathcal{F}(I \circ \Phi, J)$ such that $\mathcal{M}(I, J, \Phi)$ is minimized

$$\mathcal{M}(I, J, \Phi) = \mathcal{F}(I \circ \Phi, J) + \mathcal{S}(\Phi) \tag{1}$$

In this paper we address the estimation of $\mathcal{F}$ of single shell DWI as an extension of LOR with application to MI. DWI MR attenuation signals at location $\boldsymbol{x}$, for a gradient direction $\boldsymbol{v}$, are modeled by $S(\boldsymbol{x}, \boldsymbol{v}) = S_0(\boldsymbol{x})e^{-bI(\boldsymbol{x},\boldsymbol{v})}$ [10] and apparent diffusion coefficients volumes are given by $I(\boldsymbol{x}, \boldsymbol{v}) = -\frac{1}{b}\log\frac{S(\boldsymbol{x},\boldsymbol{v})}{S_0(\boldsymbol{x})}$. Gradient directions $\boldsymbol{v}$ are taken on the unit sphere $\mathbb{S}^2$ although diffusion are orientation-free and have $I(\boldsymbol{x}, \boldsymbol{v}) \approx I(\boldsymbol{x}, -\boldsymbol{v})$, i.e., with antipodal symmetry. Such a symmetric function $I(\boldsymbol{x}, -)$ on the sphere can be represented by a function on the projective space $\mathbb{P}^2$ of directions of $\mathbb{R}^3$, $\mathbb{P}^2 \simeq \mathbb{S}^2/\{\pm 1\}$.

We start by defining the type of transformation considered for the LOR density estimates for single shell DWI presented in this paper. For any transformation ϕ of a point $\boldsymbol{x}$, we consider only diffeomorphic mappings $\phi(\boldsymbol{x})\colon \mathbb{R}^3 \to \mathbb{R}^3$. Under this assumption, ϕ is invertible and its differential, or Jacobian $d_{\boldsymbol{x}}\phi$ at

$\boldsymbol{x}$, gives naturally rise to a projective transformation on $\mathbb{P}^2$: $t\boldsymbol{v} \mapsto t d_{\boldsymbol{x}}\phi(\boldsymbol{v}), t \in \mathbb{R}\backslash\{0\}$. We drop $\boldsymbol{x}$ and simply write $d\phi$. Its representation over $\mathbb{S}^2$ is $\boldsymbol{v} \in \mathbb{S}^2 \mapsto \pm\frac{d\phi(\boldsymbol{v})}{|d\phi(\boldsymbol{v})|}$. This term appears within a spherical kernel Γ_κ with antipodal symmetry, making the sign irrelevant. Setting $\psi(\boldsymbol{v}) = \frac{d\phi(\boldsymbol{v})}{|d\phi(\boldsymbol{v})|}$, it corresponds to the transformation proposed by [10]. We therefore extend our transformation to $\tilde{\Phi} : (\boldsymbol{x}, \boldsymbol{v}) \mapsto (\phi(\boldsymbol{x}), \psi(\boldsymbol{v}))$. This type of transformation is also argued in [7], although neither [10] nor [7] did consider its projective nature. We proceed to describe the LOR.

The LOR framework defines the similarity over three scales: The image scale σ, the intensity scale β, and the integration scale α. In registration, for a transformation ϕ, we get

$$h_{\beta\alpha\sigma}(i,j|\phi,\boldsymbol{x}) = \int_\Omega P_\beta(I_\sigma(\phi(\boldsymbol{x})) - i)P_\beta(J_\sigma(\boldsymbol{x}) - j)W_\alpha(\boldsymbol{\tau} - \boldsymbol{x})d\boldsymbol{\tau} \qquad (2)$$

$$p_{\beta\alpha\sigma}(i,j|\phi,\boldsymbol{x}) \simeq \frac{h_{\beta\alpha\sigma}(i,j|\phi,\boldsymbol{x})}{\int_{\Lambda^2} h_{\beta\alpha\sigma}(k,l|\phi,\boldsymbol{x})dk\,dl} \qquad (3)$$

where $i,j \in [a_1, a_2]$ are values in the image intensity range, $I_\sigma(\phi(\boldsymbol{x})) = (I * K_\sigma)(\phi(\boldsymbol{x}))$ and $J_\sigma(\boldsymbol{x}) = (J * K_\sigma)(\boldsymbol{x})$ are images convolved with the kernel K_σ with standard deviation σ, P_β is a Parzen-window of scale β, and W_α is a Gaussian integration window of scale α. The marginals are trivial and obtained by integration over the appropriate variable. The LOR-approach to similarity lets us use a set of generalized similarity measures, the linear and non-linear

$$\mathcal{F}_{lin} = \int_{\Lambda^2} f(i,j)p(i,j)di\,dj \qquad \mathcal{F}_{non-lin} = \int_{\Lambda^2} f(p(i,j))di\,dj \qquad (4)$$

where the linear measure $f(i,j)$ includes e.g. sum of squared differences and Huber, and the non-linear $f(p(i,j))$ includes e.g. MI, NMI, see [2] for details.

3   Locally Orderless DWI

To extend the density estimates of LOR to include directional information, we introducing a kernel on the sphere to account for directional smoothing. With that in mind, we extend spatial smoothing to be spatio-directional, where the directional smoothing preserves this symmetry, and thus the projective structure, via a symmetric kernel $\Gamma_\kappa(\boldsymbol{\nu}, \boldsymbol{v})$ on $\mathbb{S}^2$. We define the smoothed signal $I_{\sigma,\kappa}$ at scales (σ, κ) by

$$I_{\sigma\kappa}(\boldsymbol{x}, \boldsymbol{v}) = \int_{S^2} \left(\int_\Omega I(\boldsymbol{\tau}, \boldsymbol{\nu})K_\sigma(\boldsymbol{\tau} - \boldsymbol{x})d\boldsymbol{\tau} \right) \Gamma_\kappa(\boldsymbol{\nu}, \boldsymbol{v})d\boldsymbol{\nu} = (I * (K_\sigma \otimes \Gamma_\kappa))(\boldsymbol{x}, \boldsymbol{v}) \qquad (5)$$

where $K_\sigma(\boldsymbol{x})$ is a Gaussian kernel with σ standard deviation. We use a symmetric Watson distribution [5] as $\Gamma_\kappa(\boldsymbol{\nu}, \boldsymbol{v})$ for directional smoothing on $\mathbb{S}^2$, given by

$$\Gamma_\kappa(\boldsymbol{\nu}, \boldsymbol{v}) = Ce^{\kappa(\langle\boldsymbol{\nu},\boldsymbol{v}\rangle)^2}, \qquad C = M(\frac{1}{2}, \frac{1}{d}, \kappa) = \sum_{i=0...\infty} \frac{\kappa^n}{(\frac{3}{2})^n n!} \qquad (6)$$

where M is the Kummer function for a d-dimensional unit vector $\boldsymbol{\nu}$, (in this case $d = 3$), $\pm\boldsymbol{v}$ the center of the distribution, and κ the concentration parameter, which is roughly inverse proportional to the variance on the sphere. As one alternative, a symmetrized von Mises-Fisher [5] distribution could be considered.

In order to use the similarity measures provided by the LOR framework, we extend the LOR formulation from scalar-valued images to DWI. The joint histogram, that is, the contribution to $h(i,j)\colon \Lambda^2 \to \mathbb{R}_+$ of the joint histogram and normalization can be written as

$$h_{\beta\alpha\sigma\kappa}(i,j|\boldsymbol{x}) = \int_{\Omega \times S^2} P_\beta(I_{\sigma\kappa}(\boldsymbol{x},\boldsymbol{v}) - i)P_\beta(J_{\sigma\kappa}(\boldsymbol{x},\boldsymbol{v}) - j)W_\alpha(\boldsymbol{\tau} - \boldsymbol{x})d\boldsymbol{x} \times d\boldsymbol{v}$$

(7)

$$p_{\beta\alpha\sigma\kappa}(i,j|\boldsymbol{x}) = \frac{h_{\beta\alpha\sigma\kappa}(i,j|\boldsymbol{x})}{\int_{\Lambda^2} h_{\beta\alpha\sigma\kappa}(k,l|\boldsymbol{x})dk\ dl}$$

(8)

where $I_{\sigma\kappa}(\boldsymbol{x},\boldsymbol{v})$ and $J_{\sigma\kappa}(\boldsymbol{x},\boldsymbol{v})$ are defined as in Equation (5), P is a Gaussian Parzen-window with standard deviation β, and W a Gaussian window of integration around $\boldsymbol{x}$ with standard deviation α. The marginals are trivial and obtained by integration over the appropriate variable. The joint and marginal probability densities allow us to apply the generalized similarity measures in Equation (4). In this paper, we use the non-linear MI.

4 Image Registration

We write the joint histogram and density for similarity in image registration as

$$h_{\beta\alpha\sigma\kappa}(i,j|\tilde{\Phi},\boldsymbol{x}) =$$

(9)

$$\int_{\Omega \times S^2} P_\beta(I_{\sigma\kappa}(\phi(\boldsymbol{x}),\psi(\boldsymbol{v})) - i)P_\beta(J_{\sigma\kappa}(\boldsymbol{x},\boldsymbol{v}) - j)W_\alpha(\boldsymbol{\tau} - \boldsymbol{x})d\boldsymbol{\tau} \times d\boldsymbol{v}$$

$$p_{\beta\alpha\sigma\kappa}(i,j|\tilde{\Phi},\boldsymbol{x}) = \frac{h_{\beta\alpha\sigma\kappa}(i,j|\tilde{\Phi},\boldsymbol{x})}{\int_{\Lambda^2} h_{\beta\alpha\sigma\kappa}(i,j|\tilde{\Phi},\boldsymbol{x})dl\ dk}$$

(10)

Most similarity measures are global measures, including MI. To make the density estimate global, we let $\alpha \to \infty$ such that W becomes constant. The first-order structure of the similarity (1) is derived following the approach of [2], denoting differentials as $dg = Dg(\boldsymbol{x})d\boldsymbol{x}$, where D is the partial derivative operator and $d\boldsymbol{x}$ a vector of differentials. We seek $d\mathcal{M}$, the derivative of (1), ignoring the regularization term and omitting irrelevant parameters in the notation. The derivative of MI with respect to $h(i,j)$ is found in [2]. Thus, we seek $dh(i,j)$

$$dh(i,j) = \int_{\Omega \times S^2} dP_\beta(I_{\sigma\kappa}(\phi(\boldsymbol{x}),\psi(\boldsymbol{v})) - i)P_\beta(J_{\sigma\kappa}(\boldsymbol{x},\boldsymbol{v}) - j)W_\alpha(\boldsymbol{\tau} - \boldsymbol{x})d\boldsymbol{\tau} \times d\boldsymbol{v}$$ (11)

with $\quad dP_\beta(I_{\sigma\kappa}(\phi(\boldsymbol{x}),\psi(\boldsymbol{v})) - i) = DP_\beta(I_{\sigma\kappa}(\phi(\boldsymbol{x}),\psi(\boldsymbol{v})) - i)dI_{\sigma\kappa}(\phi(\boldsymbol{x}),\psi(\boldsymbol{v}))$

$DP_\beta(I_{\sigma\kappa}(\phi(\boldsymbol{x}), \psi(\boldsymbol{v})) - i)$ can be found in [1,2]. Inserting (5), we get

$$dI_{\sigma\kappa}(\phi(\boldsymbol{x}), \psi(\boldsymbol{v})) = d\int_{S^2}\left(\int_\Omega I(\boldsymbol{\tau}, \boldsymbol{\nu})K_\sigma(\boldsymbol{\tau} - \phi(\boldsymbol{x}))d\boldsymbol{\tau}\right)\Gamma_\kappa(\boldsymbol{\nu}, \psi(\boldsymbol{v}))d\boldsymbol{\nu}. \quad (12)$$

and using the Leibniz integration rule and the product rule, we get

$$dI_{\sigma\kappa}(\phi(\boldsymbol{x}), \psi(\boldsymbol{v})) = \int_{S^2}\left(d\int_\Omega I(\boldsymbol{\tau}, \boldsymbol{\nu})K_\sigma(\boldsymbol{\tau} - \phi(\boldsymbol{x}))d\boldsymbol{\tau}\right)\Gamma_\kappa(\boldsymbol{\nu}, \psi(\boldsymbol{v}))d\boldsymbol{\nu}+$$
$$\int_{S^2}\left(\int_\Omega I(\boldsymbol{\tau}, \boldsymbol{\nu})K_\sigma(\boldsymbol{\tau} - \phi(\boldsymbol{x}))\boldsymbol{\tau}\right)d\Gamma_\kappa(\boldsymbol{\nu}, \psi(\boldsymbol{v}))d\boldsymbol{\nu} \quad (13)$$

We consider each of the terms on the sum separately. Using Leibniz integration rule on the first term of the sum, we get

$$\int_{S^2}\left(\int_\Omega I(\boldsymbol{\tau}, \boldsymbol{\nu})dK_\sigma(\boldsymbol{\tau} - \phi(\boldsymbol{x}))\boldsymbol{\tau}\right)\Gamma_\kappa(\boldsymbol{\nu}, \psi(\boldsymbol{v}))d\boldsymbol{\nu} \quad (14)$$

where $dK_\sigma(\boldsymbol{\tau} - \phi(\boldsymbol{x})) = DK_\sigma(\boldsymbol{\tau} - \phi(\boldsymbol{x}))d\phi(\boldsymbol{x})$ which is trivial in the context of registration. From the second term we get $d\Gamma_\kappa(\boldsymbol{\nu}, \psi(\boldsymbol{v})) = D\Gamma_\kappa(\boldsymbol{\nu}, \psi(\boldsymbol{v}))d\psi(\boldsymbol{v})$ and specifying $\Gamma_\kappa(\boldsymbol{\nu}, \psi(\boldsymbol{v}))$ as a Watson distribution gives

$$D\Gamma_\kappa(\boldsymbol{\nu}, \psi(\boldsymbol{v})) = Ce^{\kappa(\langle\boldsymbol{\nu}, \psi(\boldsymbol{v})\rangle)^2}2\kappa\langle\boldsymbol{\nu}, \psi(\boldsymbol{v})\rangle d\psi(\boldsymbol{v}) \quad (15)$$

which leaves $d\phi(\boldsymbol{x})$ and $d\psi(\boldsymbol{v})$. The first term $d\phi$ is the Jacobian of ϕ and classical in registration literature. The first-order information on spherical reorientation $d\psi(\boldsymbol{v})$ is more complicated, as with our definition of $\psi(\boldsymbol{v})$ as $\frac{d\phi(\boldsymbol{v}}{|d\phi(\boldsymbol{v})|}$, this leads to second-order information of ϕ, which is complex but trivial.

5   Experiments and Results

A series of experiments was conducted to illustrate the scales introduced (spatial, intensity, and directional) with respect to MI. We computed the MI between two subjects and plotted the MI as a function of global rotation and translation (Figure 1) as well as local rotation of three random patches of $10 \times 10 \times 10$ voxels (Figure 2). In addition, we performed a few affine registrations of DWI data using the proposed extension of LOR to DWI and MI. We used data from the Human Connectome Project (HCP) database, release Q3, structurally aligned to the MNI-152 template [11], with 90 gradient directions and a b-value of 3000.

The locally orderless structure introduces four explicit scales on DWI: Image K_σ, intensity P_β, and integration W_α, as well as the extension to orientation Γ_κ. To examine the effect of the scales (ignoring integration scale W_α, i.e. $\alpha \to \infty$), we use Mutual Information, which in itself is a complicated measure. Mutual Information of two observations A, B can be interpreted as the capability of A to encode B. We use this notion of MI to examine the properties of the proposed extension of density estimation to DWI. As a first observation from Figure 1

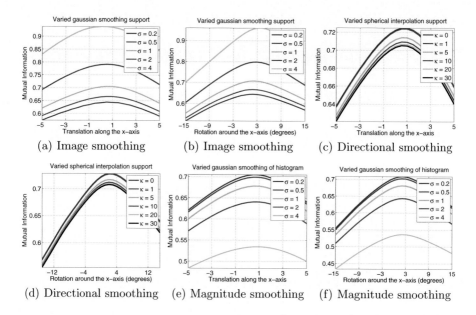

Fig. 1. MI as a function of translation and rotation at different scales. As shown, smoothing in $\mathbb{R}^3$ (a & b) moves the optima, while the change in the angular or diffusion scale (c & d) preserves the MI, despite increased the angular information. This is a good indication of a substantial information in the directions. Smoothing of diffusion magnitudes (e & f) has a similar effect to that observed for scalar-valued images.

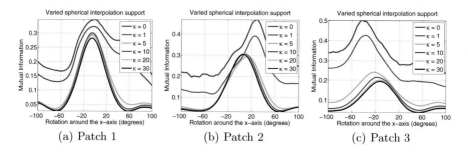

Fig. 2. We computed the MI between to DWI volumes within three random patches of $10 \times 10 \times 10$ voxels as a function of rotation and directional smoothing. This clearly illustrates the change in optima as a function of the directional scale. As the images are reasonably well-aligned, this is a strong indication that directional information is required for proper local alignment

it is clear that the DWI optima does not correspond to the structural optima of the registration (to MNI) provided by the HCP. This is illustrated by the fact that the maxima of Figure 1 are not at 0.

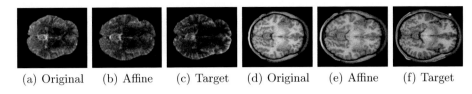

(a) Original   (b) Affine   (c) Target   (d) Original   (e) Affine   (f) Target

Fig. 3. Two DWI images registered using affine transformation and MI for DWI. (left) b=0 gradient images. (Right) T1-weighted images.

The Image Scale influences the MI significantly. Smoothing in the individual directions increases the MI (Figures 1(a) and 1(b)). This increase is not surprising as this smoothing of the intensities will transform the distribution of observed intensities towards the mean of the image. **The Intensity Scale** (i.e. Parzen-window) behaves as reported in [2] where the optima displaces with increased kernel size (Figures 1(e) and 1(f)). Increasing the size of the Parzen-window corresponds to reducing the number of bins. **The Orientation Scale** has an effect similar to image smoothing (Figures 1(c) and 1(d)). We observe that smoothing results in increased Mutual Information as the diffusion measurements of all 90 directions converge towards the rotation-invariant *mean diffusivity* for $\kappa \to 0$. Note that the corresponding curves of MI using small kernels, i.e. higher angular resolution, only results in a small decrease in the MI. Figures 1(c) and 1(d) shows preservation of the slope of MI towards the optima is observed, revealing a well-defined optima. Locally, Figure 2, we observe a dramatic shift in optima from mean diffusivity $\kappa = 0$ to high directional resolution $\kappa = 30$. As illustrated, the local optima shifts 30-40 degrees as a function of scale, which justify the need for our proper scale-space formulation for similarity of DWI. **To Illustrate** the LOR for DWI with MI, we performed a few affine registrations using MI, $\kappa = 30$, a cubic B-spline Parzen-window with 200 bins, and B-Spline image interpolation. A registration can be seen in Figure 3.

6   Discussion and Conclusion

The LOR for DWI includes directional information and so first-order information of the deformation is required. We therefore restrict the deformation model to diffeomorphisms to ensure well-defined derivatives. For gradient-based optimization, this implies that the second-order information of the deformation is required, which severely complicates any implementation. We have chosen the Watson distribution for its simplicity compared to e.g. a symmetrized von Mises-Fisher kernel or symmetrized geodesic distances.

We have presented an extension of the Locally Orderless Registration for DWI by introducing a scale-space which accounts for the projective nature of DWI in a theoretically sound manner. Our experiments show that directional resolution is important in order to obtain proper local alignment in registration. Our formulation allows us to directly control the scales of the information from which we estimate the similarity. By extending the LOR framework, we can easily apply a wide range of similarity measures. We provided the first-order information of the densities, briefly reviewed the effects of the scales, and illustrated the approach by affine registration of DWI using Mutual Information.

References

1. Darkner, S., Sporring, J.: Generalized partial volume: An inferior density estimator to parzen windows for normalized mutual information. In: Székely, G., Hahn, H.K. (eds.) IPMI 2011. LNCS, vol. 6801, pp. 436–447. Springer, Heidelberg (2011)
2. Darkner, S., Sporring, J.: Locally Orderless Registration. IEEE Transactions on Pattern Analysis and Machine Intelligence 35(6), 1437–1450 (2013)
3. Duarte-Carvajalino, J.M., Sapiro, G., Harel, N., Lenglet, C.: A framework for linear and non-linear registration of diffusion-weighted mris using angular interpolation. Frontiers in Neuroscience 7 (2013)
4. Hermosillo, G., Chefd'Hotel, C., Faugeras, O.: Variational methods for multimodal image matching. International Journal of Computer Vision 50(3), 329–343 (2002)
5. Jupp, P.E., Mardia, K.: A unified view of the theory of directional statistics, 1975-1988. International Statistical Review, 261–294 (1989)
6. Koenderink, J., Van Doorn, A.: The structure of locally orderless images. International Journal of Computer Vision 31(2), 159–168 (1999)
7. Raffelt, D., Tournier, J., Fripp, J., Crozier, S., Connelly, A., Salvado, O., et al.: Symmetric diffeomorphic registration of fibre orientation distributions. NeuroImage 56(3), 1171–1180 (2011)
8. Rathi, Y., Michailovich, O., Shenton, M.E., Bouix, S.: Directional functions for orientation distribution estimation. Medical Image Analysis 13(3), 432–444 (2009)
9. Rohde, G., Barnett, A., Basser, P., Marenco, S., Pierpaoli, C.: Comprehensive approach for correction of motion and distortion in diffusion-weighted mri. Magnetic Resonance in Medicine 51(1), 103–114 (2004)
10. Tao, X., Miller, J.V.: A method for registering diffusion weighted magnetic resonance images. In: Larsen, R., Nielsen, M., Sporring, J. (eds.) MICCAI 2006. LNCS, vol. 4191, pp. 594–602. Springer, Heidelberg (2006)
11. Van Essen, D.C., Smith, S.M., Barch, D.M., Behrens, T.E., Yacoub, E., Ugurbil, K.: The wu-minn human connectome project: an overview. Neuroimage 80, 62–79 (2013)
12. Van Hecke, W., Leemans, A., D'Agostino, E., De Backer, S., Vandervliet, E., Parizel, P.M., Sijbers, J.: Nonrigid coregistration of diffusion tensor images using a viscous fluid model and mutual information. IEEE Transactions on Medical Imaging 26(11), 1598–1612 (2007)
13. Wells, W.M., Viola, P., Atsumi, H., Nakajima, S., Kikinis, R.: Multi-modal volume registration by maximization of mutual information. Medical Image Analysis 1(1), 35–51 (1996)
14. Yap, P.T., Chen, Y., An, H., Yang, Y., Gilmore, J.H., Lin, W., Shen, D.: Sphere: Spherical harmonic elastic registration of hardi data. NeuroImage 55(2), 545–556 (2011)

Predicting Activation Across Individuals with Resting-State Functional Connectivity Based Multi-Atlas Label Fusion

Georg Langs[1,2], Polina Golland[2], and Satrajit S. Ghosh[3,4]

[1] Department of Biomedical Imaging and Image-guided Therapy,
CIR Lab, Medical University of Vienna, Vienna, Austria
[2] CSAIL, MIT
[3] McGovern Institute for Brain Research, MIT, Cambridge, MA, USA
[4] Department of Otology and Laryngology, Harvard Medical School,
Boston, MA, USA

Abstract. The alignment of brain imaging data for functional neuroimaging studies is challenging due to the discrepancy between correspondence of morphology, and equivalence of functional role. In this paper we map functional activation areas across individuals by a multi-atlas label fusion algorithm in a functional space. We learn the manifold of resting-state fMRI signals in each individual, and perform manifold alignment in an embedding space. We then transfer activation predictions from a source population to a target subject via multi-atlas label fusion. The cost function is derived from the aligned manifolds, so that the resulting correspondences are derived based on the similarity of intrinsic connectivity architecture. Experiments show that the resulting label fusion predicts activation evoked by various experiment conditions with higher accuracy than relying on morphological alignment. Interestingly, the distribution of this gain is distributed heterogeneously across the cortex, and across tasks. This offers insights into the relationship between intrinsic connectivity, morphology and task activation. Practically, the mechanism can serve as prior, and provides an avenue to infer task-related activation in individuals for whom only resting data is available.

1   Introduction

Establishing functional correspondence across the brains of individuals is a central prerequisite for neuroimaging group studies. Standard approaches rely on brain morphology to perform group-wise registration, and their improvement has brought a substantial boost to the specificity of neuroimaging results and their interpretation in light of neuroscientific questions. Recent results indicate that the variability of the functional architecture across individuals makes the concept of correspondence more challenging to grasp. Specifically, the link between anatomical location and functional role can be weak. This results in the decrease of specificity in group studies, and potential bias. In this paper we propose multi-atlas label fusion based on functional alignment. The method establishes correspondence of cortical positions based on resting-state functional magnetic resonance imaging (rs-fMRI) signals. Using this functional alignment with label-fusion of activations

© Springer International Publishing Switzerland 2015
N. Navab et al. (Eds.): MICCAI 2015, Part II, LNCS 9350, pp. 313–320, 2015.
DOI: 10.1007/978-3-319-24571-3_38

observed during task fMRI (t-fMRI) in a population of source subjects, we predict task activations in a target, aligned subject. Transferring information using functional connectivity alignment results in higher accuracy of transferring task activation compared to morphological alignment. This method extends functional region based analyses [2] to functional networks.

Alignment of function across individuals. Neuroimaging group-studies typically rely on registering structural imaging data of all subjects to a common template using software such as FreeSurfer [5], FSL [8], or SPM [1]. This establishes spatial correspondence across the population, and allows for local comparison of activation, or connectivity. However, function exhibits a high degree of variability [12] and is not necessarily tightly linked to anatomy [2]. Approaches to match function across individuals beyond relying on anatomy have been proposed before. In [14] the cortical surfaces were aligned by maximizing the correlation among fMRI signals recorded in different subjects during watching synchronized movies. A common space representing visual stimulus responses was used to establish correspondence across individuals in [7]. In [10] a joint manifold representing the functional connectivity patterns recorded during language experiments in multiple individuals was used to align function across subjects independent of the anatomical anchors of functional units. Instead of using across-subject correlation, it relies on the within-subject correlation patterns to match shared network architecture across the population.

Contribution. In this paper we extend the functional connectivity alignment proposed in [10] to "resting state" data and multi-atlas label fusion. First, we establish correspondence between cortical surface points across individuals by functional connectivity alignment. Then, we predict task activations in a target subject, by evaluating the similarity of the matched embedding maps of all source subjects, and the target. Finally, we transfer predictions by selecting the most similar subject on a voxel-by-voxel basis. In the absence of any ground truth on functional connectivity, evaluating task-based correspondence by measuring the Dice coefficient between predicted and actual task-based activation provides an objective way to evaluate the alignment. The proposed approach can cope with variability, since it selects the most similar individual in the source population, based on functional connectivity, for activation label prediction. Furthermore, we can use it to study and compare the discrepancy between functional transfer of activation areas, and morphological transfer across the cortex. Finally, we gain insights into the relationship between the embedding structure, and the correspondence across the cortex.

Related work. The work is closely linked to surface matching algorithms based on curvature [11]. However, instead of relying on morphological features, we inject functional information to map similarity across the cortex. Multi-atlas label fusion transfers information such as labels from a set of atlases to target data. Instead of building a single model from the atlas population, it first fits all atlas templates to the target data. Then it transfers labels from atlases, or groups of atlases to the target based on a similarity function that reflects the suitability of an atlas for predicting the labeling of the target [15,9,18]. Reducing the dimensionality of data can capture underlying structure that is not apparant in its native space. It can be achieved through linear models (e.g., PCA [13], ICA [3]) or using non-linear embedding approaches. The latter assume that the data of interest *lives* on a low dimensional nonlinear manifold and estimate its intrinsic coordinate structure by *embedding* the data.

2   Method

The proposed method first performs embedding of individual resting state functional connectivity graphs. The embedding maps are aligned and labels are transferred from a source population to a target individual based on their fit in the embedding space after alignment in a multi-atlas label fusion approach.

Embedding the Intrinsic Connectivity Structure of rs-fMRI Data. We view an fMRI sequence $\mathbf{I} \in \mathbb{R}^{T \times N}$ as a graph of N voxels (or cortical surface vertices). Each voxel (vertex) $\mathbf{v}_i$ carries an fMRI signal over T time points. We calculate a pairwise similarity matrix $\mathbf{W} \in \mathbb{R}^{+N \times N}$ that assigns the correlation $\mathbf{W}(i,j)$ of the time-courses to each pair of voxels (i,j) (edge) [4]. Following [4] this graph defines a Markov chain with transition matrix $\mathbf{P} = \mathbf{D}^{-\frac{1}{2}} \mathbf{W} \mathbf{D}^{-\frac{1}{2}}$, where $\mathbf{D}$ is a diagonal normalization matrix such that $d_i = \mathbf{D}(i,i) = \sum_j w(i,j)$ is the strength of node i. The eigenvectors of the transition matrix scaled by their eigenvalues (λ^t) define an embedding that results in a representation of each voxel as a point in the embedding space: $i \mapsto \Phi_i$ [10] (where t is the diffusion time parameter). To capture positive and negative correlations and to create an affinity matrix, the correlation matrix was scaled between 0 and 1 and then converted to a sparse graph representation (A) using a nearest neighbor approach. The 100 closest neighbors of each vertex were retained. The graph was checked to ensure that it was a connected graph. The diffusion map embedding was then computed on the normalized Laplacian of this graph. The eigenvalues λ are divided by $1 - \lambda$. The division of the λ parameter provides noise robustness and allows variation from the standard form potentially eliminating the use of the diffusion time (t) parameter. In many empirically tested cases, where the embedding is known, setting $t = 0$ returns a result that is close to using the optimal diffusion time parameter. Given that the optimal solution is generally unknown, setting ($t = 0$) is often a practical choice. The resulting embedding is a lower dimensional representation of the intrinsic functional connectivity of the brain.

Aligning Embeddings. For a target $\mathbf{I}^T$ and each source $\mathbf{I}_s^S$, we find a orthonormal alignment via Procrustes analysis [16]: $\mathbf{Q}_{S,T}$. Given target- $\Phi^T = [\phi_1^T, \ldots, \phi_N^T]^\top$ and source embedding coordinates $\Phi^S = [\phi_1^S, \ldots, \phi_1^S]^\top$, $\mathbf{Q}_{S,T} = \mathbf{V}\mathbf{U}^\top$, where $\mathbf{U}$ and $\mathbf{V}$ are constructed via the singular value decomposition $\mathbf{U}\Sigma\mathbf{V}^\top = \Phi^{T^\top} \mathrm{diag}(\mathbf{w}_m)\Phi_{r_m}^S$. See [10] for detailed description of the approach. Figure 1 shows each of the first 5 individual components of the average embedding from 40 participants and the same components from 3 individual participants (we enlarge one for better visibility in the bottom row). We hypothesise

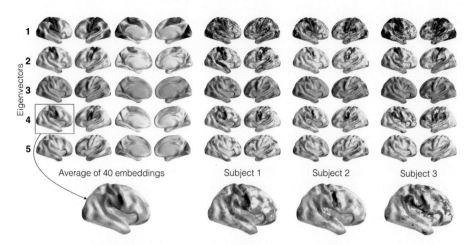

Fig. 1. The first 5 components of an average embedding computed from the 40 participants and three individual embeddings. The differences across individuals reflect different spatial distributions of resting state functional networks. We use the similarity of these surface markers to (locally) select the best source subjects during prediction by label fusion.

that these components form an intrinsic functional basis of brain activity and show aligned embedding coordinates on the cortical surface. The coefficients of the first 5 eigenvectors projected to the surface after functional alignment in the embedding space mark comparable systems on the cortex. Their fine-grained cortical distribution varies across individuals. The proposed label transfer is based on the assumption that activation can be transferred among individuals with similar cortical functional eigenvector profiles.

Predicting Activation. The proposed multi-atlas label fusion method chooses source subjects for the prediction of activation on each cortical vertex based on how similar those eigenvector coefficients (Figure 1) are at the vertex location. That is, we select source subjects based on how similar their resting-state connectivity aligns with the target subject connectivity. The alignment in the embedding space enables a straight-forward calculation of this similarity. Specifically, we predict activation maps in a target subject based on the known activation in a set of source subjects. We know the activation $f(\mathbf{v}_{i,s}^S)$ of each voxel $\mathbf{v}_{i,s}^S$ in each source volume s. Given the target embedding $\mathbf{\Phi}^T$ and all aligned source embeddings $\mathbf{\Phi}_s^{AS}$ for each voxel (or surface vertex) we calculate a score by the Euclidean distance between the target point ϕ_i^T and the anatomically corresponding source point $\phi_{i,s}^{AS}$ in the embedding space: $k_{i,s} = \|\phi_i^T - \phi_{i,s}^{AS}\|$. Then the predictor for the activation $f(\mathbf{v}_i^T)$ at voxel $\mathbf{v}_i^T$ is

$$\forall i : f(\mathbf{v}_i^T) = f(\mathbf{v}_{i,s^*}^S), \text{ where } \quad s^* = \operatorname*{argmin}_{s=1,\ldots,S} k_{i,s}. \tag{1}$$

We compare this prediction guided by the functional alignment to two alternatives that are based solely on the anatomical position. As a first comparison, we predict $f(\mathbf{v}_i^T) = \text{mean}_{s=1,\dots,S}\, f(\mathbf{v}_{i,s}^S)$, i.e., the average activation f at the anatomically corresponding positions in the source subjects. Secondly, we predict $f(\mathbf{v}_i^T) = f(\mathbf{v}_{i,s}^S)$, where s is chosen randomly. For the evaluation, we average this prediction-accuracy over all individuals.

3   Experiments

Data We used data from 40 randomly selected participants from the Human Connectome Project (HCP; [17]) 500-Subject data release. For each participant, we used the data from one of the preprocessed functional runs [6] together with FIX cleanup. For each rs-fMRI run, data projected onto the average cortical surface (59412 vertices × 1200 timepoints) were used to construct a correlation matrix (59412 × 59412). This matrix is the basis for the embedding and functional alignment. We used task fMRI data of 7 paradigms from the same participants (motor, language, working memory, social, gambling relational, emotion). For each paradigm we used z-score maps calculated for each contrast within each paradigm. We evaluated the accuracy of the activation prediction by leave-one-out cross validation across 40 subjects. During each prediction by label fusion, we chose one contrast, and predicted the Z-score on a hold-out target subject. The prediction was performed by label-fusion from the Z-scores of the remaining source subjects. We calculated the Dice coefficient between predicted-, and actual activation region in the target subject using a Z-score cutoff of $Z > 3.09$, corresponding to $p < 0.001$ as a marker for *activation region*.

Impact of Embedding Parameters. To evaluate the effect of embedding parameters of the diffusion map embedding, on the prediction accuracy, two of the embedding parameters were varied: diffusion time was set to 0 and 5, while the number of nearest neighbors was varied across 50, 100, and 500. In our experiments, these parameters had a minimal effect on the Dice coefficients, with variations ($\sigma > 0.01$) being observed only at values of $Z > 5$ for the emotion and gambling tasks.

Comparison of Prediction Accuracy. We compare the proposed label-fusion with functional alignment based prediction with an approach that does not take the functional rs-fMRI information into account. Figure 2 provides an overview of prediction accuracy with functional alignment label-fusion versus the average accuracy when predicting the activation based on the anatomical position. Each row corresponds to one of 7 paradigms, and each column to one of the contrasts in these paradigms. We only show the first 6 contrasts for each paradigm. Label-fusion that takes the distance in the functional embedding map into account when choosing a source subject for each vertex, consistently yields higher accuracy than uninformed transfer. We observe similar differences when comparing the label-fusion with prediction based on the average Z-score in the population. Note that the proposed approach primarily improves accuracy, if the anatomical mapping accuracy is poor. Figure 3 provides a detailed comparison for 4 illustrative paradigms, and a range of Z-score cut-off values. The plots show the

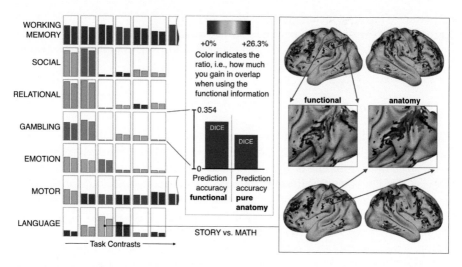

Fig. 2. Improvement of accuracy by functional alignment label-fusion over anatomical alignment varies across different experiment conditions. For 7 tasks, we show the prediction accuracy for the first 6 contrasts. On the right the actual individual activation and predictions based on functional multi-atlas fusion (green) is shown in comparison to prediction based on the average activation in the source subjects (blue).

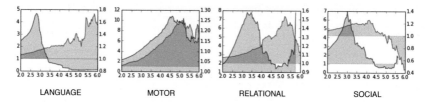

Fig. 3. Ratio between functional alignment label-fusion and predictions based on anatomy for example contrasts for 4 tasks: (1) averaged accuracy when transferring from random individuals (red, right scale), (2) transferring the average Z-score of the source population (blue, left scale).

ratio between the proposed alignment accuracy and the two morphology based comparison methods. Values higher than 1 mean that label-fusion accuracy is higher. Results show that the improvement varies across paradigms and Z-score cut-offs, but that the majority of contrasts exhibit improvement for the proposed label-fusion.

The Heterogeneous Distribution of the Impact across the Cortex. Is the advantage of the functional alignment label-fusion clustered in certain areas? Figure 4 shows the average ratio between prediction accuracy (Dice of $p < 0.001$ areas) of the proposed approach and anatomical alignment mapped to the cortical surface. We only provide values in those areas where the 7 available paradigms exhibit any activation (we chose a more liberal $p < 0.01$ to allow for estimates of this ratio in larger areas). The ratio is different across the cortex, and exhibits strong

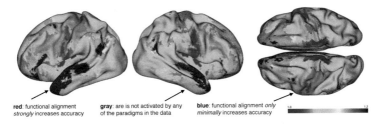

red: functional alignment *strongly* increases accuracy   **gray**: are is not activated by any of the paradigms in the data   **blue**: functional alignment *only minimally* increases accuracy

Fig. 4. Improvement by functional alignment label-fusion varies across the cortex. Only areas that are covered by at least one of the 7 paradigms with $p < 0.01$ are plotted.

symmetry across the two hemispheres. Areas such as motor cortex, and visual cortex show little improvement by functional alignment, indicating that the location of function varies little across the population. In contrast specifically those areas close to language network, and temporal regions exhibit the most gain.

4   Conclusion

In this paper we propose the prediction of the areas active during a task response in a target subject by multi-atlas label fusion from a source population based on functional alignment. The label-fusion algorithm selects predictors for the Z-score in a target subject among the Z-score at the corresponding position in a population of source subjects. The selection is based on the fit between the aligned target and the source in the embedding space, and extends the rationale behind alignment across individuals using functional regions to functional networks. The embedding represents the functional connectivity observed during rs-fMRI. Results suggest that the resting-state functional connectivity structure is a reliable basis to guide the mapping of task response activations across individuals. It highlights the strong link between the functional connectivity architecture of the brain, and the location of specific functional units that serve individual tasks. The distribution of this gain across the cortex enables insights into the locally varying link between morphology and function.

Acknowledgments. Data provided by the Human Connectome Project, WU-Minn Consortium (1U54MH091657) funded by NIH Blueprint for Neuroscience Research, and McDonnell Center for Systems Neuroscience at WU. Work was partly supported by CDMRP grant PT100120 (SG), by NIH NICHD R01HD067312 and NIH NIBIB NAC P41EB015902, OeNB 14812 and 15929, and EU FP7 2012-PIEF-GA-33003.

References

1. Ashburner, J.: Computational anatomy with the spm software. Magnetic Resonance Imaging 27(8), 1163–1174 (2009)
2. Brett, M., Johnsrude, I.S., Owen, A.M.: The problem of functional localization in the human brain. Nat. Rev. Neurosci. 3(3), 243–249 (2002)

3. Cardoso, J.F.: Source separation using higher order moments. In: 1989 International Conference on Acoustics, Speech, and Signal Processing, ICASSP 1989, pp. 2109–2112. IEEE (1989)
4. Coifman, R.R., Lafon, S.: Diffusion maps. App. Comp. Harm. An. 21, 5–30 (2006)
5. Fischl, B., Salat, D., Busa, E., Albert, M., Dieterich, M., Haselgrove, C., van der Kouwe, A., Killiany, R., Kennedy, D., Klaveness, S., et al.: Whole Brain Segmentation: Automated Labeling of Neuroanatomical Structures in the Human Brain. Neuron 33(3), 341–355 (2002)
6. Glasser, M.F., Sotiropoulos, S.N., Wilson, J.A., Coalson, T.S., Fischl, B., Andersson, J.L., Xu, J., Jbabdi, S., Webster, M., Polimeni, J.R., Van Essen, D.C., Jenkinson, M.: WU-Minn HCP Consortium: The minimal preprocessing pipelines for the human connectome project. NeuroImage 80, 105–124 (2013). http://europepmc.org/articles/PMC3720813
7. Haxby, J.V., Guntupalli, J.S., Connolly, A.C., Halchenko, Y.O., Conroy, B.R., Gobbini, M.I., Hanke, M., Ramadge, P.J.: A common, high-dimensional model of the representational space in human ventral temporal cortex. Neuron 72(2), 404–416 (2011)
8. Jenkinson, M., Beckmann, C.F., Behrens, T.E., Woolrich, M.W., Smith, S.M.: FSL. NeuroImage 62(2), 782–790 (2012)
9. Langerak, T.R., van der Heide, U.A., Kotte, A.N., Viergever, M.A., van Vulpen, M., Pluim, J.P.: Label fusion in atlas-based segmentation using a selective and iterative method for performance level estimation (simple). IEEE Transactions on Medical Imaging 29(12), 2000–2008 (2010)
10. Langs, G., Sweet, A., Lashkari, D., Tie, Y., Rigolo, L., Golby, A.J., Golland, P.: Decoupling function and anatomy in atlases of functional connectivity patterns: Language mapping in tumor patients. NeuroImage 103, 462–475 (2014)
11. Lombaert, H., Sporring, J., Siddiqi, K.: Diffeomorphic spectral matching of cortical surfaces. In: Gee, J.C., Joshi, S., Pohl, K.M., Wells, W.M., Zöllei, L. (eds.) IPMI 2013. LNCS, vol. 7917, pp. 376–389. Springer, Heidelberg (2013)
12. Mueller, S., Wang, D., Fox, M.D., Yeo, B.T.T., Sepulcre, J., Sabuncu, M.R., Shafee, R., Lu, J., Liu, H.: Individual variability in functional connectivity architecture of the human brain. Neuron 77(3), 586–595 (2013)
13. Pearson, K.: Principal components analysis. The London, Edinburgh, and Dublin Philosophical Magazine and Journal of Science 6(2), 559 (1901)
14. Sabuncu, M., Singer, B., Conroy, B., Bryan, R., Ramadge, P., Haxby, J.: Function-based intersubject alignment of human cortical anatomy. Cerebral Cortex 20(1), 130–140 (2010)
15. Sabuncu, M., Yeo, B., Van Leemput, K., Fischl, B., Golland, P.: A generative model for image segmentation based on label fusion. IEEE Transactions on Medical Imaging 29(10), 1714–1729 (2010)
16. Scott, G., Longuet-Higgins, H.: An algorithm for associating the features of two images. Proceedings: Biological Sciences 244(1309), 21–26 (1991)
17. Van Essen, D.C., Smith, S.M., Barch, D.M., Behrens, T.E., Yacoub, E., Ugurbil, K.: The wu-minn human connectome project: an overview. Neuroimage 80, 62–79 (2013)
18. Wachinger, C., Golland, P.: Spectral label fusion. In: Ayache, N., Delingette, H., Golland, P., Mori, K. (eds.) MICCAI 2012, Part III. LNCS, vol. 7512, pp. 410–417. Springer, Heidelberg (2012)

Crossing-Lines Registration for Direct Electromagnetic Navigation

Brian J. Rasquinha, Andrew W.L. Dickinson, Gabriel Venne,
David R. Pichora, and Randy E. Ellis

Queen's University, Kingston, Canada

Abstract. Direct surgical navigation requires registration of an intraoperative imaging modality to a tracking technology, from which a patient image registration can be found. Although electromagnetic tracking is ergonomically attractive, it is used less often than optical tracking because its lower position accuracy offsets its higher orientation accuracy.

We propose a crossing-lines registration method for intraoperative electromagnetic tracking that uses a small disposable device temporarily attached to the patient. The method exploits the orientation accuracy of electromagnetic tracking by calculating directly on probed lines, avoiding the problem of acquiring accurately known probed points for registration. The calibration data can be acquired and computed in less than a minute (50 s $\pm$ 12 s). Laboratory tests demonstrated fiducial localization error with sub-degree and sub-millimeter means for 5 observers. A pre-clinical trial, on 10 shoulder models, achieved target registration error of 1.9 degree $\pm$ 1.8 degree for line directions and 0.8 mm $\pm$ 0.6 mm for inter-line distance. A Board-certified orthopedic surgeon verified that this accuracy easily exceeded the technical needs in shoulder replacement surgery.

This preclinical study demonstrated high application accuracy. The fast registration process and effective intraoperative method is promising for clinical orthopedic interventions where the target anatomy is small bone or has poor surgical exposure, as an adjunct to intraoperative imaging.

1 Introduction

Direct surgical navigation is a subset of image-guided surgery where the guidance image is acquired intraoperatively, using modalities such as MRI, 3D fluoroscopy or ultrasound [9,12,4]. A limiting constraint on direct navigation is the registration of the image to the 3D tracking system, for which simultaneous tracking of the imaging device and the patient has proven so cumbersome as to prevent widespread adoption. Although preoperative calibration is an effective option for floor-mounted imaging [11], mobile-imaging devices remain a challenge.

The most used tracking technology for direct navigation is optical localization. Major drawbacks are maintaining a line of sight – the principal reason that direct navigation is not more prevalent – and, for small or deep anatomy such as the bones of the shoulder, the optical devices are too large to be rigidly affixed to thin fragile bone. Another prevalent tracking technology uses electromagnetic

© Springer International Publishing Switzerland 2015
N. Navab et al. (Eds.): MICCAI 2015, Part II, LNCS 9350, pp. 321–328, 2015.
DOI: 10.1007/978-3-319-24571-3_39

(EM) physics. EM is superior to optical technology by being very lightweight –
a sensor is an antenna with electrical leads, often sub-millimeter in diameter –
and avoiding line-of-sight problems. The major drawback is that, even when used
far from conductive materials, EM has less positional accuracy than optical
tracking [6,8], in some cases with errors increasing by an order of magnitude
between laboratory and clinical settings [7]. Intriguingly, EM appears to have
high inherent orientation accuracy for common two-coil 6DOF trackers [10] that
might be useful for a novel kind of image-tracking registration.

The method is a fast, accurate intraoperative registration method for EM-
tracking that needs no preoperative calibration or anatomical probing. The
mathematics are an adaptation of X-ray source localization by computation of
lines that cross in space. The concept is to affix a small, lightweight plastic device to the target anatomy, then probe linear paths to achieve a registration. An
example application is reverse shoulder replacement surgery, where the tip of a
drill is visible to the surgeon and the drill orientation is critically important but
difficult to achieve without image-based navigation. The technique was tested
on 10 models of cadaveric shoulders and produced sub-millimeter accuracy.

2   Materials and Methods

Two kinds of methods were used: computational and empirical. Materials were
manufactured by the authors; some were derived from CT scans of cadaveric
donations, the latter approved by the relevant Institutional Review Board.

The fundamental datum was a line, which was a point $\vec{p}$ and a signed direction vector $\vec{d}$ (i.e., a spatial point on the unit sphere). A previous registration
method [5] uses line data to establish correspondences, but not as registration
features. The fundamental sources were EM tracking of a pointed cylindrical
surgical probe and the planned directions of linear holes in a calibration device.

2.1   Computational Methods

Our registration problem was estimation of a rigid transformation from the electromagnetic coordinate frame $\boldsymbol{E}$ to the calibrator coordinate frame $\boldsymbol{C}$. As is
usual, we separated this into orientation estimation and translation estimation.
Each estimate was found using a somewhat novel variant of previous methods.

For orientation, we paired a tracked probe direction $^{E}\vec{d}$ with a planned calibrator hole direction $^{C}\vec{d}$. Rather than thinking of these as direction vectors,
we interpreted them as points on the unit sphere; n of these spherical points
could be registered using Arun's method [3]. A least-squares registration trans-
formation $^{C}_{E}R$ from frame $\boldsymbol{E}$ to frame $\boldsymbol{C}$, which minimizes the residual distances
between the sets of points, can be computed from Sibson's 3×3 data matrix
H [13] using the singular-value decomposition (SVD) as

$$H = \sum_{i=1}^{n} \left(^{C}\vec{d_i}\,^{E}\vec{d_i}^{\,T} \right) = U\Sigma V^T$$

$$\Rightarrow \quad ^{C}_{E}R = VU^T \tag{1}$$

Cases with $\det(VU^T) \neq 1$ were rejected as geometric singularities [3]. This solved the orientation problem without using points, needing only directions $\vec{d}_i$.

To estimate the translation component, a variant of "crossing-lines" was used. Crossing-lines has been used extensively in 2D virtual fluoroscopy to determine the X-ray source location from an image that contains tiny fiducial markers; this is illustrated in Figure 1(a) and a corresponding calibration device, with holes that guide 7 lines, is shown in Figure 1(b). The mathematics are straightforward: let $\vec{c}$ be the nominal crossing point of n lines in space. Minimization of the distance between $\vec{c}$ and the ith line $\vec{l}(\lambda) = \vec{p}_i + \lambda \vec{d}_i$, over all n lines, can be found in the least-squares sense by solving the overdetermined linear equation

$$\left(\sum_{i=1}^{n}\left(I - \vec{d}_i\vec{d}_i^T\right)\right)\vec{c} = \sum_{i=1}^{n}\left(\left(I - \vec{d}_i\vec{d}_i^T\right)\vec{p}_i\right) \qquad (2)$$

The value $\vec{c}$ in Equation 2 was computed from the QR decomposition. Together, $_E^C R$ and $\vec{c}$ constituted a least-squares registration solution that depended primarily on the direction vectors $\vec{d}_i$ and to a lesser degree on the point positions $\vec{p}_i$; this took great advantage of the orientation accuracy of EM sensing.

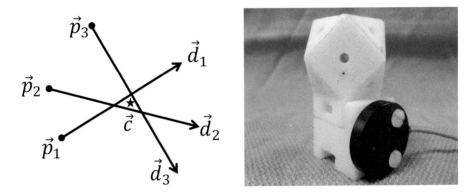

Fig. 1. Crossing-lines for registration. (left) From lines that contain points $\vec{p}_i$ and have corresponding directions $\vec{d}_i$, the center of crossing $\vec{c}$ can be estimated in a least-squares sense. (right) A device was additively manufactured to constrain 7 such lines.

2.2   Calibration Device

A cuboctahedral calibration device was additively manufactured in ABS plastic, shown in Figure 1(b). Seven tantalum beads, for CT verification in subsequent work, were fixed in dimples in the device faces: three in the top face and one in each vertical face. The device included 7 through holes that physically provided 7 crossing lines. The design files were used to establish the calibrator coordinate frame C, with each hole axis giving a direction vector $^C\vec{d}_i$.

An Aurora 6-DOF disc EM sensor (NDI, Waterloo, CA) was fixed to the device using two nylon 4-40 machine screws. The disc was used to establish the EM coordinate frame $\boldsymbol{E}$, in which pointer directions $^{E}\vec{d_i}$ were measured.

2.3   Tracking Hardware and Software

During EM tracking, a manufacturer's standard surgical probe was used to gather position data from its tip and direction data from its axis. Custom C++ software gathered data at $\approx$ 45 Hz, averaging 45 consecutive readings as unsigned axial means [1]. Translations were averaged linearly. All tests representing intra-operative activities (Sections 2.5 and 2.6) were conducted in a surgical operating room, thus reproducing representative sources of EM interference. Cone beam computed tomography (CBCT) scans in these sections were performed using an Innova 4100 (General Electric, Waukesha, US) at a 0.46 mm voxel size.

2.4   Fiducial Localization Error (FLE)

Because registration was computed from paired lines, the Fiducial Localization Error (FLE) was also calculated from the lines. The paired lines were, respectively, sensed by the EM tracker and derived from the calibrator design file. Each angular FLE was the angular difference between each matched pair of skew lines. The distance FLE was the minimal normal distance between the infinitely long skew lines, which was the formulation used in the registration algorithm.

Using a consistent experimental setup in a laboratory environment, five subjects (the co-authors) collected data for FLE assessment. For one trial, each subject probed each hole of the calibrator for approximately 1 s; this produced 7 lines per subject. Each subject performed 5 trials, totalling 35 lines per subject.

The line FLEs of each subject were pooled to find mean and standard deviations. Subject performance was assessed by comparing the pooled line FLEs to the best accuracies found in the literature, which were $1°$ in direction and 0.5 mm in translation. The line FLEs of all subjects were further pooled.

Based on the line FLE findings, we conducted a detailed accuracy assessment using data collected by one investigator (DRP, an orthopedic surgeon).

2.5   Point Target Registration Error (Point TRE)

Point-to-point positioning was assessed using a custom accuracy apparatus, which was an additively manufactured ABS plate that incorporated a dovetail for mounting the calibrator. Fourteen 0.8 mm tantalum beads were fixed in a planar spiral, at $60°$ with 5 mm spacing; the apparatus is pictured in Figure 2.

Point target registration error (point-TRE) was assessed in an operating room with the calibrator fixed to the apparatus. Each bead was probed for $\approx$ 1 s with the 6DOF probe by one subject (author DRP). The position and direction of the probe were recorded relative to the calibrator-fixed EM sensor. After EM collection, CBCT images of the point-TRE apparatus were acquired and the beads were manually segmented.

EM measurements were transformed to the CBCT frame using the calibrator transform and the residuals between paired features were used as the point-TRE measurement. This represented an end-to-end system accuracy, incorporating the errors in segmentation, calibration, and tracking of a surgical work-flow.

2.6   Line Target Registration Error (Line-TRE)

Line target registration error (line-TRE) was assessed using preparations from shoulder arthroplasty. Ten cadaveric shoulders, with no specimen having a history of surgical intervention, were scanned using axial CT at 0.49 mm resolution and 0.63 mm slice spacing. Each scapula scan was manually segmented and a Board-certified surgeon planned paths for a reverse shoulder arthroplasty baseplate peg and four implanting screws; this produced five target lines in each cadaver image volume. Each line was modeled as a 3 mm diameter cylinder that was subtracted from the segmented scapula. Previous studies using this workflow and equipment replicated bony geometry to submillimeter accuracy as compared to laser scans of dry bones [2].

A male dovetail was added to the coracoid process of each scapula for calibrator fixation. Each modified scapula was additively manufactured in ABS plastic. An example line-TRE scapula is pictured in Figure 2.

For each scapula, two titanium screws were placed in the dovetail to allow for EM tracking alterations that might occur during clinical fixation. The calibrator was affixed and each drill path was probed by the planning surgeon using the 6DOF EM probe. As in Section 2.5, ≈ 1 s of relative pose measurements were collected in an operating room and the probe position and direction relative to the calibrator were averaged. The scapula and affixed calibrator were then scanned with CBCT and manually segmented. Each original 3D design file was registered to the segmented CBCT models using an ICP algorithm. This registration transformed the planned screw and base-plate peg lines to the CBCT coordinate frame. The transformed planned lines were compared to the EM probed lines.

The line-TRE was assessed using the line-FLE methods, which were the angles between paired direction vectors and the minimum paired line-line distance. These measurements represented an end-to-end error assessment that closely simulated the error expected in surgical navigation.

3   Results

Paired line calibrations were performed with an average time of 50 s ± 12 s, including data collection and calculating the calibrator transform; each of 5 observers acquired 7 consecutive lines, 5 times each. Fiducial localization errors (FLEs) from these calibrations are presented in Table 1. The FLEs were consistently below manufacturer reported errors, which were $1°$ in orientation accuracy and 0.5 mm in position accuracy. Based on these excellent results, a single observer was chosen for the TRE experiments.

A single observer, highly experienced in data acquisition and use of computer-assisted surgery, touched each of the 14 beads in the point-TRE apparatus with

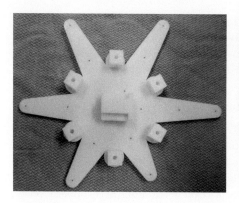 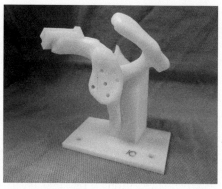

Fig. 2. Point TRE device (left) and Line TRE device (right); no calibrator present.

Table 1. Summary of Fiducial Localization Error (FLE) for each investigator and with all investigators pooled. None of these error groups were found to be statistically significantly higher than $1°$ or 0.5 mm using a one-sided, one sample t-test ($\alpha = 0.95$).

Observers, by alphabetic code; 35 lines per observer

	A	B	C	D	E	Pooled
Angular FLE (°)	0.7 ± 0.3	0.8 ± 0.3	0.4 ± 0.2	0.8 ± 0.4	0.8 ± 0.4	0.7 ± 0.4
Distance FLE (mm)	0.3 ± 0.2	0.3 ± 0.3	0.3 ± 0.2	0.3 ± 0.2	0.4 ± 0.3	0.3 ± 0.2

the pointed EM-tracked probe. After transforming the EM readings into a CT-derived coordinate frame, the residual point-TRE experiment had an accuracy of 2.3 mm $\pm$ 0.8 mm.

The same single observer later acquired 5 lines for each line-TRE scapula, the lines being preoperatively planned drill holes that were manufactured into each scapula. Detailed line-TRE results are presented in Table 2. In summary, the line-TRE, pooling all 5 lines of 10 scapular models, had an overall angular error

Table 2. Summary of Line Target Registration Errors (Line-TRE). For each line-TRE scapula, line-line angles were assessed using the skew angle between the lines; means (μ) and standard deviations (σ) are reported for the 5 lines used for each scapula. Likewise, line-line distances were assessed using the minimum normal distance between the 5 lines for each scapula. Pooled results are for all 50 lines.

Line-TRE scapula, by code; 5 lines per scapula

	S01	S02	S03	S04	S05	S06	S07	S08	S09	S10	Pooled
Angular TRE μ (°)	2.4	1.1	1.6	0.8	2.8	3.3	2.4	2.0	0.9	1.3	1.9
Angular TRE σ (°)	1.6	1.3	0.6	0.8	4.0	2.7	1.4	0.3	1.3	0.3	1.8
Distance TRE μ (mm)	1.2	1.5	0.4	0.8	0.5	1.2	1.1	1.2	1.3	1.4	1.1
Distance TRE σ (mm)	0.7	0.4	0.3	0.5	0.3	1.0	0.5	0.9	1.0	0.9	0.7

of $1.9°\pm 1.8°$ of skew angle between the actual EM probe line and the physical hole in CT-derived coordinates. The line-line distance was 1.1 mm $\pm$ 0.7 mm, assessed as being the minimum normal distance between the two lines.

4   Discussion

Electromagnetic tracking for surgical navigation is ergonomically preferred over optical tracking in procedures where sensor size and line-of-sight are major concerns. One impediment of EM has been its relatively poor point-localization accuracy, which precludes the use of surface-based registration algorithms on small anatomical targets. Poor localization leads to poor registration, which may have limited the adoption of EM technology in high-accuracy surgical applications.

This work largely avoids the potentially poor point localization of EM by instead relying on its superior orientation accuracy. Decoupling a rigid registration into an orientation problem and a translation problem, the orientation problem was solved by interpreting directions as points on a sphere and adapting previous point-based methods to estimate a least-squares orientation. The translation problem was solved by modifying a method from X-ray calibration to register multiple lines that cross in space, combining direction and position measurements so that positions were relied on as little as possible.

The point-based FLE was consistently below 0.5 mm and 1°, which suggests an excellent match between the sensed axis of a tracked EM probe and its CT-based location. Conventional measurement of TRE was 2.3 mm $\pm$ 0.8 mm, which is consistent with the literature [6,10].

The line-TRE, pooling 50 acquisitions by a single observer, was $1.9° \pm 1.8°$ in angle and 1.1 mm $\pm$ 0.7 mm in distance. The angular accuracy is close to what is found in surgical navigation based on optical tracking, where orientation must be inferred from a rigid array of markers. The distance accuracy is also close to optical tracking, with the caution that this measures line-line distances whereas most navigation work reports point-point distances.

This work suggests that EM tracking can provide excellent accuracy from intraoperative data collection and calibration that requires less than a minute to perform. Future developments of this system towards clinical practice include automating the current manual segmentation step of the workflow and verifying the results on these phantoms with drilling tasks on cadaveric specimens.

Although EM navigation has fundamental physics limitations, such as field alteration by external objects, this work is an example of how relatively low positioning accuracy can be overcome by using the relatively high orientation accuracy of EM tracking in a disciplined registration framework. A crossing-lines registration apparatus can be temporarily added to an electromagnetic surgical tracking device that is already affixed to a patient, solving an existing problem in direct surgical navigation with a simple combination of hardware and software. Further, this registration technique can be applied to any tracking modality with a calibrated probe, including optical tracking.

The prominent surgical opportunity is for direct navigation of small orthopedic targets, for which optical devices are too large or heavy to be practical.

An example is the shoulder glenoid, where perforation of the thin scapula when drilling presents considerable risk of post-surgical complications. Such an application exploits the main accuracy of EM – direction determination – and supplements a surgeon's conventional positioning accuracy within a clear surgical exposure. Future work may include clinical trials of the device, particularly in the shoulder and wrist, for treatment of early-onset arthritis or to repair poorly healed fractures in or around a joint.

References

1. Amaral, G.J.A., Dryden, I.L., Wood, A.T.A.: Pivotal bootstrap methods for k-sample problems in directional statistics and shape analysis. J. Am. Stat. Assoc. 102(478), 695–707 (2007)
2. Anstey, J.B., Smith, E.J., Rasquinha, B., Rudan, J.F., Ellis, R.E.: On the use of laser scans to validate reverse engineering of bony anatomy. Stud. Health Technol. Inform., 18–24 (2011)
3. Arun, K.S., Huang, T.S., Blostein, S.D.: Least-squares fitting of two 3-D point sets. IEEE Trans. Pattern Anal. Mach. Intell. 9(5), 698–700 (1987)
4. Chopra, S.S., Hünerbein, M., Eulenstein, S., Lange, T., Schlag, P.M., Beller, S.: Development and validation of a three dimensional ultrasound based navigation system for tumor resection. Eur. J. Surg. Oncol. 34(4), 456–461 (2008)
5. Deguchi, D., Feuerstein, M., Kitasaka, T., Suenaga, Y., Ide, I., Murase, H., Imaizumi, K., Hasegawa, Y., Mori, K.: Real-time marker-free patient registration for electromagnetic navigated bronchoscopy: a phantom study. Int. J. Comput. Assist. Radiol. Surg. 7(3), 359–369 (2012)
6. Frantz, D.D., Wiles, A.D., Leis, S.E., Kirsch, S.R.: Accuracy assessment protocols for electromagnetic tracking systems. J. Phys. Med. Biol. 48(14), 2241–2251 (2003)
7. Franz, A.M., Haidegger, T., Birkfellner, W., Cleary, K., Peters, T.M., Maier-Hein, L.: Electromagnetic tracking in medicine-a review of technology, validation and applications. IEEE. Trans. Med. Imag. 33(8), 1702–1725 (2014)
8. Hummel, J.B., Bax, M.R., Figl, M.L., Kang, Y., Maurer Jr., C., Birkfellner, W., Bergmann, H., Shahidi, R.: Design and application of an assessment protocol for electromagnetic tracking systems. J. Med. Phys. 32(7), 2371–2379 (2005)
9. Jolesz, F.A., Navabi, A., Kikinis, R.: Integration of interventional MRI with computer- assisted surgery. J. Magn. Reson. Imaging 13(1), 69–77 (2001)
10. Lugez, E., Sadjadi, H., Pichora, D.R., Ellis, R.E., Akl, S.G., Fichtinger, G.: Electromagnetic tracking in surgical andinterventional environments: usability study. Int. J. Comput. Assist. Radiol. Surg. 10(3), 253–262 (2014)
11. Oentoro, A., Ellis, R.E.: High-accuracy registration of intraoperative CT imaging. In: SPIE Med. Imaging, pp. 762505–762505 (2010)
12. Smith, E.J., Al-Sanawi, H., Gammon, B., Ellis, R.E., Pichora, D.R.: Volume rendering of 3D fluoroscopic images forpercutaneous scaphoid fixation: An in vitro study. Proc. Inst. Mech. Eng. H 227(4), 384–392 (2013)
13. Sibson, R.: Studies in the robustness of multidimensional scaling: Procrustes statistics. J. Royal. Stat. Soc. B 40(2), 234–238 (1978)

A Robust Outlier Elimination Approach for Multimodal Retina Image Registration

Ee Ping Ong[1], Jimmy Addison Lee[1], Jun Cheng[1], Guozhen Xu[1],
Beng Hai Lee[1], Augustinus Laude[2], Stephen Teoh[2], Tock Han Lim[2],
Damon W.K. Wong[1], and Jiang Liu[1]

[1]Institute for Infocomm Research, Agency for Science, Technology and Research, Singapore
{epong,jalee,jcheng,benghai,xug,wkwong,jliu}@i2r.a-star.edu.sg
[2]National Healthcare Group (NHG), Eye Institute, Tan Tock Seng Hospital, Singapore
{laude_augustinus,stephen_teoh,tock_han_lim}@ttsh.com.sg

Abstract. This paper presents a robust outlier elimination approach for multimodal retina image registration application. Our proposed scheme is based on the Scale-Invariant Feature Transform (SIFT) feature extraction and Partial Intensity Invariant Feature Descriptors (PIIFD), and we combined with a novel outlier elimination approach to robustly eliminate incorrect putative matches to achieve better registration results. Our proposed approach, which we will henceforth refer to as the residual-scaled-weighted Least Trimmed Squares (RSW-LTS) method, has been designed to enforce an affine transformation geometric constraint to solve the problem of image registration when there is very high percentage of incorrect matches in putatively matched feature points. Our experiments on registration of fundus-fluorescein angiographic image pairs show that our proposed scheme significantly outperforms the Harris-PIIFD scheme. We also show that our proposed RSW-LTS approach outperforms other outlier elimination approaches such as RANSAC (RANdom SAmple Consensus) and MSAC (M-estimator SAmple and Consensus).

1 Introduction

Image registration is the process of aligning an image to another image taken from the same scene/object but in different situations [7, 10, 15]. Image registration is an important prior processing step before other processes such as image mosaicking [2], image fusion [7], and retina verification etc. can be carried out. Image registration approaches can be classified into two different types: unimodal and multimodal [7, 15]. Multimodal image registration approaches are designed for registering pairs of images from different imaging modalities, such as attempting to register a retina color fundus image with a retina fluorescein angiographic (FA) image. The purpose of such multimodal retina image registration is to assist eye doctors to automatically register fundus and FA images captured from the retina of the same person to enable the doctor to more easily diagnose eye problems and diseases. The registered fundus-FA image pair and their fusion can aid the doctor in planning treatment and surgery for their patients.

© Springer International Publishing Switzerland 2015
N. Navab et al. (Eds.): MICCAI 2015, Part II, LNCS 9350, pp. 329–337, 2015.
DOI: 10.1007/978-3-319-24571-3_40

On the other hand, unimodal image registration approaches are designed for registering pairs of images from the same imaging modality. Generally, unimodal image registration approaches do not work on multimodal image registration.

One of the better known multimodal image registration approach in recent year is the Harris-partial intensity invariant feature descriptor (Harris-PIIFD) approach proposed by Chen et al. [3]. In [3], they proposed a scheme to register multimodal images by extracting corner points using the Harris-Stephen corner detector, estimate the main orientation of each corner point, followed by computing a partial intensity invariant feature descriptor (PIIFD) for each point. Then, they match the PIIFDs using a nearest-neighbor criterion with a pre-determined threshold to obtain the putative matches. Thereafter, they attempt to remove any incorrect matches (i.e. outliers) by applying 2 different pre-determined thresholds to the 2 criteria: the difference in main orientations and the ratio of geometric distances between corner points. Then, they try to refine the locations of the matches. Thereafter, they apply a particular transformation mode to register the pair of multimodal images to be registered. Chen et al. [3] showed that their proposed Harris-PIIFD approach performs better than SIFT [8] and GDB-ICP [12, 13] algorithms for registering multimodal image pairs.

In [6], the authors proposed the use of uniform robust scale invariant feature transform (UR-SIFT) features (instead of Harris corner feature points as used by [3]) together with PIIFD for improved multimodal image registration. Incorrect matches (i.e. outliers) are eliminated by checking each matched pair against the global transformation and those which have highest geometric errors are removed one by one until achieving a root mean square error less than a certain threshold.

In both approaches proposed in [3] and [6], the outliers elimination step appears weak and are not robust enough when there are very high percentage of incorrect matches present in the putatively matched feature points. An alternative robust outlier elimination approach that is widely used in the computer vision community is the RANdom SAmple Consensus (RANSAC) algorithm [5]. The goal of RANSAC is to find a model that maximizes the number of data points with error smaller than a user defined threshold t. One of the problems with the RANSAC approach is that in many real-life problems, it might not be possible to know the error bound t for inlier data beforehand. As pointed out in [14], the choice of the threshold is a sensitive parameter and can affect the performance dramatically. In [4], the authors conducted a performance evaluation of the various robust outlier elimination methods in the RANSAC family (such as RANSAC, MSAC, MLESAC, LO-RANSAC, R-RANSAC, MAPSAC, AMLESAC, GASAC, u-MLESAC, and pbM-estimator) for a range of outlier ratiso from 10% to 70%. They found that many methods do not perform well when the outlier ratio was increased to 70% despite the fact that various thresholds associated with the respective methods were tuned and the authors only report the best results obtained. The authors [4] showed that at outlier ratio of 70%, MSAC (M-estimator SAmple and Consensus) [14] and pbM-estimator give the best results.

Our contributions are as follow: We propose a robust outlier elimination approach, which hereby we will refer to as the residual-scaled-weighted Least Trimmed Squares (RSW-LTS). We will show how we can adapt the Least Trimmed Squares estimator (using our proposed formulation of weights estimate and iteratively re-weighted least squares procedure) to apply an affine transformation geometric constraint for robust pruning of putatively matched feature points (to remove the wrong matches or outliers) and to estimate the affine transformation model's parameters. We show that we are able to achieve the goal of obtaining improved performance over the original Harris-PIIFD multimodal scheme in [3], as well as improved performance over other outlier elimination approaches such as RANSAC [5] and MSAC [4, 14].

2   Proposed Method

Our proposed scheme operates as follow:

1. Extract salient feature points using the scale-invariant feature transform (SIFT) algorithm [8].
2. Compute the partial intensity invariant feature descriptor (PIIFD) [3] for each salient feature point (using the method in [3]).
3. Putative matching of the PIIFDs using a nearest-neighbor criterion (following the method described in [3]).
4. Outlier elimination and affine transformation parameter estimation using our proposed approach.
5. Perform image registration using the estimated transformation parameters.

The details of our proposed outlier elimination approach are as described below.

2.1   Outlier Elimination and Transformation Parameter Estimation

The putative matches obtained in earlier stage may have many wrong matches (or outliers), depending on the complexity and difficulty of the matching due to the underlying differences between the pair of images to be registered. As such, a robust outlier elimination step is required. Here, we proposed the residual-scaled-weighted Least Trimmed Squares (RSW-LTS) estimator with affine transformation to perform outlier elimination. In essence, we are trying to apply an affine transformation geometric constraint on the putative matches and remove those matched points that do not satisfy the same geometric constraint. The robust estimator we proposed here is basically a Least Trimmed Squares (LTS) estimator with residual-scaled-weights and followed by an iteratively re-weighted Least Squares estimation process.

The original Least Trimmed Squares (LTS) estimate [11] is given by:

$$\hat{\Theta} = \arg\min_{\Theta} \sum_{i=1}^{h} \hat{r}_i(\mathbf{x}, \Theta)^2 \tag{1}$$

where Θ is the set of model parameters, $\mathbf{x} \in R$, R being the neighborhood used for the transformation computation, $\hat{r}_1 <= \ldots <= \hat{r}_n$ are the ordered squared residuals, n is the total number of data in the dataset, and h denotes the hth ranked residual above which the rest of the residuals representing $(n-h)$ will be trimmed (i.e. removed from consideration in the estimation of the model parameters). Rousseeuw and Leroy [11] states that h should be more than $[n/2]+1$, giving the LTS estimator a maximum outlier breakdown point of 50%.

The residual-scaled-weighted Least Trimmed Squares affine transformation estimation method that we proposed here has the advantage that it does not need a predefined threshold t for inliers (in contrast to the RANSAC method). Without the need
for a pre-defined t, the proposed method is very flexible and is able to handle different
data, and hence has clear advantage over the standard RANSAC method. In addition,
contrary to the value of h advocated in [11], we found that we are able to obtain good
results with our proposed scale estimate, residual-scaled weights, and iteratively re-
weighted least-squares procedure for our adapted LTS method even when we have
chosen a value of h less than $[n/2]+1$. This means that our proposed RSW-LTS with
the associated scale estimate and weights computation coupled with the iteratively re-
weighted least squares computation can give an outlier rejection ratio of more than
50%. By using a value of h equals to $n/10$, our experiments show that we are able to
achieve up to about 90% of outlier rejection. The details of the residual-scaled-
weighted Least Trimmed Squares affine transformation estimator are as follow.

An affine transformation model that describes the affine transformation of a point
$\mathbf{x}=(x,y)^T$ to $\mathbf{u}=(u,v)^T$, in the x and y directions, can be defined as:

$$\mathbf{u}(\mathbf{x},\boldsymbol{\Theta}) = \mathbf{A}\mathbf{x}+\mathbf{b} \tag{2}$$

where $A=\begin{pmatrix} a_0 & a_1 \\ a_2 & a_3 \end{pmatrix}$ and $\mathbf{b}=(b_0,b_1)^T$, and we can denote the transformation parameters

as: $\boldsymbol{\Theta}=(b_o,a_1,a_1,b_1,a_2,a_3)^T$. Let the residual in modelling the transformation (with

transformation parameters $\boldsymbol{\Theta}$) at a point $\mathbf{x}$ be $r(\mathbf{x},\boldsymbol{\Theta})$, where:

$$r(\mathbf{x},\boldsymbol{\Theta}) = \|\mathbf{u}(\mathbf{x},\boldsymbol{\Theta})-\mathbf{u}\| \tag{3}$$

Given a data set of n observations, the algorithm repeatedly draws m sub-samples
each of p different observations from the data set using a Monte-Carlo type technique,
where p is the number of parameters in the model ($p = 3$ for the affine transformation
model). For each sub-sample, indexed by J, $1 \leq J \leq m$, the corresponding parameters
(denoted by $\hat{\boldsymbol{\Theta}}_J$) are estimated from the p observations. In addition, the sum of the
least trimmed squared residuals, denoted by M_J, is also determined, where:

$$M_J = \sum_{i=1}^{h} \bar{r}_i(\mathbf{x},\hat{\boldsymbol{\Theta}}_J)^2 \tag{4}$$

The LTS solution is the $\hat{\boldsymbol{\Theta}}$ for which the corresponding M_J is the minimum among
all the m different M_Js, i.e.:

$$\hat{\boldsymbol{\Theta}} = \arg\min_{\boldsymbol{\Theta}_J} \sum_{i=1}^{h} \bar{r}_i(\mathbf{x},\boldsymbol{\Theta}_J)^2 \tag{5}$$

The minimum number of sub-samples, m, required is given by:

$$m = \frac{\log(1-P)}{\log[1-(1-\varepsilon)^p]} \tag{6}$$

where P is the probability that at least one of the m sub-samples consists of p good
observations, and ε is the fraction of outliers that may be present in the data.

We proposed the following to estimate the initial scale estimate of RSW-LTS:

$$\sigma^0 = c.\frac{1}{h}\sum_{i=1}^{h}\bar{r}_i(\mathbf{x},\hat{\Theta}) \tag{7}$$

where $h = n/10$ (so as to be able to handle up to 90% of outliers), and c is a constant and is merely a correction factor used to achieve consistency at Gaussian error distributions. The initial scale estimate is used to determine an initial weight $w(\mathbf{x})$ for each observation using the following formulation:

$$w(\mathbf{x}) = \begin{cases} \left(e^{-(r(\mathbf{x},\hat{\Theta})/\sigma^0)^2/2}\right)\Big/\sqrt{2\pi}\sigma^0 & \text{if } \left|r(\mathbf{x},\hat{\Theta})/\sigma^0\right| \le d \\ 0 & \text{otherwise} \end{cases} \tag{8}$$

where d is a constant and determines the percentage of Gaussian inliers that may be incorrectly rejected. We have used a value of 1.96 for d so that Gaussian inliers are only incorrectly rejected 5% of the time. Note that in our case, the weights used are scaled using the scale estimate with respect to the residual values. The reason we used residual-scaled weights is because doing so will remove the data dependency and enable the method to handle different data (in contrast to, for example, RANSAC which uses a fixed pre-defined threshold to filter the residuals, and resulted in needing to use different threshold for different data in order to get optimal results).

Thereafter, we proposed an iterative re-weighted least squares procedure to iteratively estimate the transformation parameters $\hat{\Theta}^j$ by solving:

$$\hat{\Theta}^j = \underset{\Theta}{\operatorname{argmin}}\sum_{\mathbf{x}} w^j(\mathbf{x})r^j(\mathbf{x},\Theta^{j-1})^2 \tag{9}$$

We performed the iterative re-weighted least squares computation (according to equation (9)) for 10 iterations (for $j = 1, ..., 10$) using updated σ^j (according to equation (7) by replacing σ^0 by σ^j) and updated $w^j(\mathbf{x})$ (according to equation (8) and with σ^0 replaced by σ^j) for each of the jth iteration. In our experiments, we found that σ^j will usually converge after 4-6 iterations.

3   Results

Our proposed method has been evaluated on a dataset collected by clinicians from a Hospital. It contains a total of 200 retina images (100 pairs of corresponding color fundus and fluorescein angiographic (FA) images). These are real-life fundus-FA image pairs of patients showing symptoms of severe macula edema and staphyloma that necessitate retinal photocoagulation or photodynamic therapy. These fundus-FA image pairs are referred to by doctors in the pre-treatment stage to guide them in their planning of treatments for their patients. This dataset is very challenging because they are retina images of real-life diseased eyes and is a particular dataset considered by the doctors as most challenging ones compared to other retinal abnormalities.

To illustrate the operations of our proposed retina image registration scheme, we show the original color fundus and FA images in Figure 1, while Figure 2 shows the feature points extracted from both the fundus and FA images using the Scale-Invariant

Feature Transform (SIFT) algorithm. Figure 3 shows the results of the putative feature point matching step using the Partial Intensity Invariant Feature Descriptors (PIIFD), while Figure 4 shows the results of pruned matched feature points after outlier elimination using our proposed RSW-LTS approach. From this example, you can see that there are a total of 143 putatively matched feature points (see Figure 3). However, a very large percentage of these putative matches are incorrect. After applying our proposed RSW-LTS outlier elimination approach, we obtained only 10 matched feature points which are all correctly matched (see Figure 4). In this example, the outlier rejection ratio is about 93%. Theoretically, our RSW-LTS approach has been designed to handle up to 90% of outliers. However, in practice, our proposed approach has been shown to work for slightly more than 90% of outliers, as in this example (due to the combinations of scale estimate, residual-scaled weights and the iteratively re-weighted least squares procedure). (Note that this example shows the image pair that the Harris-PIIFD scheme [3] is unable to register successfully, and both the RANSAC [5] and MSAC [14] methods also failed.)

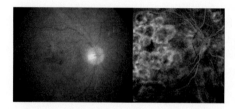
Fig. 1. riginal fundus-FA image pair.

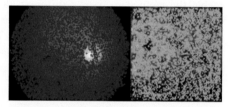
Fig. 2. Extracted SIFT feature points.

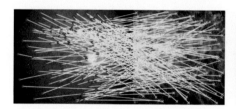
Fig. 3. Results of PIIFD putative matching.

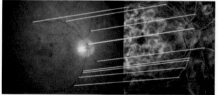
Fig. 4. Pruned matches using RSW-LTS.

In order to objectively evaluate the fundus-FA image registration results, we have adopted the root-mean-squared error (RMSE) [6, 9], the median error (MEE) [3, 6], and the maximal error (MAE) [3, 6] as the objective error measurements. These objective error measures are computed from the ground truth data generated for all the fundus-FA image pairs. We obtained the ground truth data by manually selecting 10 corresponding points that are distributed uniformly in each of the corresponding fundus and FA image pair. The ground truth and their localization are then double-checked by another group of team members to verify the correctness of the manually marked corresponding points. The process to generate the ground truth data is tedious and time consuming but necessary so that we are able to compute the objective error measures for different image registration techniques. Following [6], we consider an image pair to have been successfully registered when its RMSE is below 5 pixels, since RMSE less than 5 pixels have been found to be acceptable for clinical purposes [9]. We adopted the definition of the "success rate" to be the ratio of the number of successfully registered image pairs to the total number of image pairs being registered [6, 12]. The average objective error measures are then computed only for those image pairs with successful registration.

Table 1 shows the results of Harris-PIIFD scheme [3] and our proposed scheme for successful fundus-FA image registration. It can be seen that our proposed scheme with 83% successful registration rate significantly outperforms the original Harris-PIIFD scheme [3] (which only has a 22% successful registration rate). Also, our proposed scheme gives lower objective measurement errors (in terms of average RMSE, MAE, and MEE) compared to the Harris-PIIFD scheme. We found that we are unable to obtain 100% successful registration rate because some of these images are of very poor visual quality and/or correspondence for the purpose of image registration.

In order to verify that our RSW-LTS approach contributes to the significant improvements in successful registration rate and lower objective measurement errors (and not because of the SIFT+PIIFD combination), we had conducted several other experiments where we replaced our RSW-LTS algorithm with the well-known robust estimator, RANSAC [5], while keeping all other processes the same as in our proposed scheme with RSW-LTS. (We used publicly available RANSAC implementation to generate our results here). The number of random sub-samples used for RANSAC has been set to very large in all RANSAC experiments in order to reduce the effect of error due to sampling (We used a value of 9000 in all our experiments, thus the confidence of finding a good sub-sample and parameter estimate here is about 99.9%). Note that the main parameters that control the performance of the RANSAC method are the number of random sub-samples used and the threshold applied (which determines the error tolerance allowed in considering whether a matched point is an inlier). We experimented with numerous well-spaced threshold values for RANSAC and we only present the best RANSAC result (obtained with a specific threshold value) in Table 1. From Table 1, it can be seen that the RANSAC approach only has a successful registration rate of 32%. We analyzed the results and found that in many cases, the percentage of the putative feature point matches that is wrong is quite large, and there are significant number of cases where the outlier ratio range from 70% to more than 90%. This could be the reason why RANSAC did not perform well in our case here, despite the tuning of the parameters.

Table 1. Comparison of results.

Method	Success rate (%)	Average RMSE	Average MAE	Average MEE
Harris-PIIFD scheme [3]	22%	3.40	8.22	3.93
Our proposed scheme (with RSW-LTS)	83%	3.08	7.80	3.50
Our scheme but with LTS replaced by RANSAC	32%	3.23	8.12	3.64
Our scheme but with LTS replaced by MSAC	34%	3.16	7.81	3.71

Since MSAC [14] has been reported in [4] to be one of the two best methods at outlier ratio of 70%, we also presented the image registration results obtained by replacing the RSW-LTS with MSAC. (We used publicly available MSAC implementation to generate the results here). The results of the approach with the RSW-LTS replaced with MSAC (and with a threshold that gives the best results) are shown in Table 1, where it only gives a successful registration rate of 34%. From the above, we found that our proposed RSW-LTS approach when applied for fundus-FA image registration gives the best results (in terms of significantly higher successful registration rate and lower objective measurement errors) when compared to using RANSAC [5], MSAC [14], and the Harris-PIIFD scheme [3]. The computational time for Harris-PIIFD [3] is about 3.9s, our proposed scheme is 34.0s, using RANSAC is 36.1s, and using MSAC is 52.2s (when running all methods on the same Intel i7-4470 3.40GHz PC with 8GB RAM in Matlab). However, as our proposed approach is for the purpose of multimodal retina image registration application that doctors may use during pre-planning stage for planning of treatment and surgery for their patients, real-time computation is not necessary. Hence, our study here is primarily focused on the robustness and increasing the accuracy and successful registration rate of the multimodal image registration application.

4   Conclusions

In this paper, we present a robust outlier elimination approach for multimodal retina fundus-fluorescein angiographic image registration. Our main contribution here is a novel outlier elimination method, the residual-scaled-weighted Least Trimmed Squares (RSW-LTS), to robustly eliminate incorrectly matched putative feature point matches. We showed that our proposed scheme provides significant improvement over the original Harris-PIIFD scheme [3]. The improvement in performance is mainly due to our outlier elimination method. We also showed that our proposed RSW-LTS approach outperforms other outlier elimination approaches such as RANSAC (RANdom SAmple Consensus) and MSAC (M-estimator SAmple and Consensus).

Acknowledgement. The authors are grateful to Jian Chen for providing his codes that implement [3].

References

1. Brown, M., Lowe, D.G.: Recognising panoramas. In: Int. Conf. Comp. Vis, pp. 1218–1225 (2003)
2. Cattin, P.C., Bay, H., Van Gool, L., Székely, G.: Retina mosaicing using local features. In: Larsen, R., Nielsen, M., Sporring, J. (eds.) MICCAI 2006. LNCS, vol. 4191, pp. 185–192. Springer, Heidelberg (2006)
3. Chen, J., Tian, J., Lee, N., Zheng, J., Smith, R.T., Laine, A.F.: A Partial Intensity Invariant Feature Descriptor for Multimodal Retinal Image Registration. IEEE T. on Biomedical Engineering 57, 1707–1718 (2010)

4. Choi, S., Kim, T., Yu, W.: Performance evaluation of RANSAC family. In: Proc. British Machine Conference, pp. 81.1–81.12 (2009)
5. Fischler, M.A., Bolles, R.C.: Random Sample Consensus: A Paradigm for Model Fitting with Applications to Image Analysis and Automated Cartography. Comm. of the ACM 24(6), 381–395 (1981)
6. Ghassabi, Z., Shanbehzadeh, J., Sedaghat, A., Fatemizadeh, E.: An efficient approach for robust multimodal retinal image registration based on UR-SIFT features and PIIFD descriptors. EURASIP J. on Image and Video Processing, 25 (2013)
7. Laliberte, F., Gagnon, L., Sheng, Y.: Registration and Fusion of Retina Images – An Evaluation Study. IEEE T. Medical Imaging 22(5), 661–673 (2003)
8. Lowe, D.: Distinctive Image Features from Scale-Invariant Keypoints. Int. J. of Computer Vision 60(2), 91–110 (2004)
9. Matsopoulos, G.K., Asvestas, P.A., Mouravliansky, N.A., Delibasis, K.K.: Multimodal registration of retinal images using self organizing maps. IEEE T. on Med. Imaging 23(12), 1557–1563 (2004)
10. Ritter, N., Owens, R., Cooper, J., Eikelboom, R., van Saarloos, P.P.: Registration of stereo and temporal images of the retina. IEEE T. Medical Imaging 18, 404–418 (1999)
11. Rousseeuw, P.J., Leroy, A.M.: Robust regression and outlier detection. John Wiley & Sons, New York (1987)
12. Stewart, C.V., Tsai, C.L., Roysam, B.: The dual-bootstrap iterative closest point algorithm with application to retinal image registration. IEEE T. Med. Imaging 22(11), 1379–1394 (2003)
13. Stewart, C.V., Yang, G.: The generalized dual bootstrap-ICP executable (2008). http://www.vision.cs.rpi.edu/download.html
14. Torr, P.H.S., Zisserman, A.: MLESAC: A new robust estimator with application to estimating image geometry. J. Computer Vis. & Image Understanding 78(1), 138–156 (2000)
15. Zitova, B., Flusser, J.: Image registration methods - A survey. IVC 21, 977–1000 (2003)

Estimating Large Lung Motion in COPD Patients by Symmetric Regularised Correspondence Fields

Mattias P. Heinrich[1], Heinz Handels[1], and Ivor J.A. Simpson[2]

[1] Institute of Medical Informatics, University of Lübeck, Germany
[2] Centre for Medical Image Computing, University College London, UK
heinrich@imi.uni-luebeck.de
www.mpheinrich.de

Abstract. This paper presents a new and highly efficient approach for finding correspondences across volumes with large motion. Most existing registration approaches are set in the continuous optimisation domain, which has severe limitations for estimating larger deformations. Feature-based approaches that rely on finding corresponding keypoints have been proposed, but they are prone to erroneous matching due to repetitive features and low contrast areas. This can be overcome by using a discrete optimisation approach. However, finding a constrained search space and regularisation strategy is still an open problem. Our method calculates a dissimilarity distribution over a densely sampled space of displacements for a small number of distinctive keypoints (found in only one volume). A parts-based model is used to infer smooth motion of connected keypoints and regularise the correspondence field. This effective and highly accurate approach is further improved by enforcing the symmetry of uncertainty estimates of displacements. Our method ranks first on one of the most challenging medical registration benchmarks for breath-hold CT scan-pairs of COPD patients, where accurate motion estimation is important for diagnosis.

Keywords: Deformable registration, Parts-based model, Discrete optimisation.

1 Introduction

Finding correspondences between scans is a fundamental process in medical image analysis. In particular, in the diagnosis of COPD (Chronic Obstructive Pulmonary Disease), the detection of air trapped in localised malfunctioning regions of the lung can be assisted by registering an inhale and exhale CT scan pair. Motion of small amplitude can be robustly estimated with widely studied intensity-based continuous optimisation approaches, which often use coarse-to-fine schemes. However, such approaches are severely limited when the expected motion vectors are of larger scale than the image features (>40 mm for respiration). The difficulty of registering inhale and exhale images is highlighted in a comparison of many state-of-the-art methods for deformable registration of

N. Navab et al. (Eds.): MICCAI 2015, Part II, LNCS 9350, pp. 338–345, 2015.
DOI: 10.1007/978-3-319-24571-3_41

lung motion [19]. Discrete optimisation registration strategies have been demonstrated to be helpful in the estimation of larger scale deformation in computer vision [16] and recently also for medical image registration [15,11,13]. However, choosing an appropriate search space of deformations and regularisation strategy are still open problems for efficient, accurate and plausible registration.

In feature-based matching, the search space is restricted and correspondences across images are only seeked for sparse keypoints. These discrete matches can act as constraints in a continuous motion estimation [3]. However, it may be difficult in many applications to find enough corresponding features that can be reliably detected directly in both images. Feature matching has also been used in [20], where additionally the mutual saliency of interest points was optimised. In [14], 3D volumes were represented by supervoxels and used together with a graphical model to match corresponding feature regions across images. Block-matching is an alternative solution to find correspondence fields for medical scans [4,8]. It has, however, two main disadvantages. First, no spatial regularity between matches of neighbouring patches is enforced, so unrealistic deformations from these point matches have to be compensated for. Second, usually only the best match is retained (with the exception of e.g. [23] who use a small set of possible correspondences), and a following smoothing step of the motion field usually ignores any probabilistic information from the initial discrete search.

In this work, we present a novel framework that addresses these limitations using the following three steps. First, we extract features from one image using a keypoint operator. Second, a similarity measure is calculated over a densely quantised space of displacements, which translate to potentially corresponding locations in the other image (in contrast to previous work using only sparse samples [3,14,23]). Third, we exploit contextual information by using a parts-based model in order to regularise the differences of neighbouring displacements vectors using a Markov Random Field (MRF). Inference of regularisation for general MRFs is NP-hard, however, tree approximations have been shown to produce accurate and fast solutions [24]. Parts-based models [10], which employ interactions between different parts of an object to stabilise their localisation, have so far only been employed for landmark localisation in medical images [22]. We evaluate our method in Sec. 3 on the challenging COPD dataset.

2   Method

We aim to find a dense correspondence field between a fixed volume F and a moving volume M. Our method consists of three main steps, which are detailed below. First, a set of distinctive keypoints $\mathbf{k}_F \in K$ with spatial coordinates (k_x, k_y, k_z) are extracted from F, the inhale scan (total lung capacity) and a graph is built that uses edges $e_{ij} \in \mathcal{E}$ to connect nodes i and j with similar coordinates and intensities. Second, a similarity metric is calculated for voxels within a small patch around the keypoint $\mathbf{k}_F$ in the fixed volume and a corresponding patch displaced by a 3D motion vector $\mathbf{d} = (d_x, d_y, d_z)$. This is repeated for every displacement in the set $\mathcal{L}$ yielding a 3D distribution of similarity energies. Third, spatial regularity is inferred over the full displacement distributions of all keypoints together using belief propagation with a squared penalty for deviations of displacements, which yields an exact solution in linear time (c.f.[10]).

Keypoint Detection: Following previous work in lung registration [21], we employ the Foerstner operator to find keypoints in the 3D intensity volumes. After smoothing the volume with a Gaussian kernel G_σ the spatial gradients ∇F are calculated. A distinctiveness $D(\mathbf{x}) = 1/\operatorname{trace}\left((G_\sigma * (\nabla F \nabla F^T))^{-1}\right)$ can then be determined for each voxel $\mathbf{x}$, where a high response indicates good candidates (see Fig. 1). In order to obtain a good dispersion of points over the whole volume of interest, we apply a grey-value dilation over a 3D cubic region G_M with side-length c_D to the Foerstner response and obtain $D^* = \max_{\mathbf{y} \in G_M} D(\mathbf{y})$. Only points with equal response in D and D^* are added to K.

Similarity Evaluation over Search Space: The aim of image registration is to find a correspondence (or displacement) field, which assigns a motion vector to every control point: $\mathbf{u}(\mathbf{k}_F) \leftarrow \mathbf{d}$. The new location $\mathbf{l} = (l_x, l_y, l_z) = (k_x + d_x, k_y + d_y, k_z + d_z)$ is chosen to maximise the similarity between images. We define the space of potential displacements for every keypoint $\mathbf{k}_F$ to be the densely sampled 3D set $\mathbf{d} \in \mathcal{L} = \{0, \pm q, \pm 2q, \ldots, \pm l_{\max} q\}^3$, where q is a very small quantisation step and $l_{\max} q$ large enough to cover all potential motion between both images. Note, that in contrast to previous work on medical image registration [11] the motion is not decoupled into 1D displacements, as this may lead to inferior matching. Since, medical volumes with large motion are often also degraded by local intensity variations and influenced by strong noise, we use the self-similarity descriptors (SSC) proposed in [12] for matching. The dissimilarity metric $\mathcal{D}$, the L_1 norm between 64 bit binary descriptor representations SSC_F and SSC_M at locations $\mathbf{k}$ and $\mathbf{l}$, can be efficiently calculated in the Hamming space: $\mathcal{D}(\mathbf{k}, \mathbf{l}) = 1/|\mathcal{P}| \sum_{p \in \mathcal{P}} \Xi\{SSC_F(\mathbf{k} + p) \oplus SSC_M(\mathbf{l} + p)\}$, where $\oplus$ defines an exclusive OR, Ξ a bit-count, and $\mathcal{P}$ a local patch.

Parts-Based Model for Inference of Regularisation: In traditional block-matching approaches [4,8] or hybrid approaches [3], the motion vector corresponding to the minimum dissimilarity is selected and a heuristic or variational regularisation is then applied to the correspondence field. It is, however, beneficial

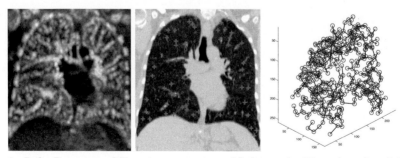

Fig. 1. Left: Response of Foerstner operator with log scale. Keypoints found in the respective coronal plane of the CT volume (and 3 neighbouring slices each) are marked with red crosses. Right: Minimum-spanning-tree, which connects keypoints.

to evaluate the spatial regularity of the correspondence field over the whole space
of displacements as done in MRF-based medical image registration [11,13]. While
the previous approaches use a regular grid of equally spaced control points, we
employ only a very sparse set of keypoints. Building a graph on this irregular set
of points is not straightforward. While a general k-nearest neighbour graph would
be possible, it is not necessarily spanning. Following parts-based models [10], we
opt to use a minimum-spanning-tree (MST) to define the set of edges $\mathcal{E}$ in our
model. MSTs have been used for inference in many applications including stereo
estimation [24] and 3D registration [13] on regular grids. The regularisation cost
assigns a penalty $\mathcal{R}$ for every pair of keypoints, which is connected in the graph
by an edge e_{ij} and has unequal displacements:

$$\mathcal{R}(\mathbf{d}_i, \mathbf{d}_j) = \frac{||\mathbf{d}_i - \mathbf{d}_j||^2}{\sqrt{||\mathbf{x}_i - \mathbf{x}_j||^2 + |I(\mathbf{x}_i) - I(\mathbf{x}_j)|/\sigma_I}} \qquad (1)$$

This term encourages smoothly varying displacements in the estimated correspondence field and makes our method robust against missing correspondences
or image artefacts. The denominator accounts for different lengths of edges,
which includes both their spatial Euclidean distance and the absolute difference
of their local intensity means. Combining the regularisation penalty with the
self-similarity based dissimilarity (weighted by α) yields the total energy of a
certain correspondence field $\mathbf{u}$: $E(\mathbf{u}) = \alpha \sum_{\mathbf{k} \in K} \mathcal{D}(\mathbf{k}, \mathbf{d}_\mathbf{k}) + \sum_{e_{ij} \in \mathcal{E}} \mathcal{R}(\mathbf{d}_i, \mathbf{d}_j)$.

Belief propagation can be used to obtain exact marginal distributions after
two passes of messages. Starting from the leaf nodes, messages $\mathbf{m}$ are passed
along the edges e_{ij} of the tree and updated with the following computation for
a node i and its parent j [10]:

$$\mathbf{m}_i(\mathbf{d}_j) = \min_{\mathbf{d}_i} \left(\alpha \mathcal{D}(\mathbf{d}_i) + \mathcal{R}(\mathbf{d}_i, \mathbf{d}_j) + \sum_c \mathbf{m}_c(\mathbf{d}_i) \right), \qquad (2)$$

where c are the children of i. The evaluation of Eq. 2 is particularly efficient
(linear in $|\mathcal{L}|$), when using distance transforms.

Symmetry of Marginal Distribution: After globally optimising the regu-
larised cost function, there may still be spurious errors. To reduce their influence we make use of the estimated marginal energies. An additional estimation
of the marginal distribution is performed in opposite direction (from moving to
fixed volume) using the translated keypoints of the first optimisation as control
points. Ideally, the forward estimate was correct and so the energies of the back-
wards displacement space are symmetrical to the forward ones and averaging
re-enforces them. If the correspondence from fixed to moving image pointed to
a close neighbour of the correct displacement and the motion in a small neighbourhood is smooth the backward search can improve the match. Forward and
backward marginal energies are averaged as follows. Let $M_{\mathbf{k}_F}^f$ by a vector of
marginal energies of length $|\mathcal{L}|$ using the forward search for a certain point $\mathbf{k}_F$
and $M_{\mathbf{k}_M}^b$ the marginals from the backward search of the translated control point

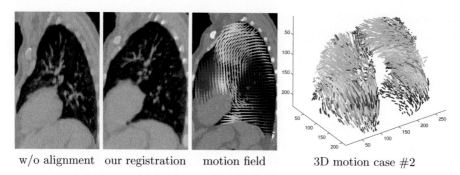

w/o alignment   our registration   motion field   3D motion case #2

Fig. 2. Visual results of dense correspondence fields using our proposed method for case #4. Colour overlay of inhale (green) and exhale (magenta) sagittal slices. 3D motion vectors (magnitude from blue to red) are shown for the most challenging case #2.

in the moving volume $\mathbf{k}_M$. The symmetric marginal energies $M_{\mathbf{k}}^s$ are then defined as $M_{\mathbf{k}}^s(i) = \frac{1}{2}(M_{\mathbf{k}_F}^f(i) + M_{\mathbf{k}_M}^b(|\mathcal{L}| - i))$.

Dense Field from Sparse Matches: In the previous steps, we have described how an accurate, sparse correspondence field can be established by minimising the registration cost function. We estimate the marginal distributions for every displacements and node, so a first refinement of the integer motion vectors to sub-voxel precision can be obtained by a parabolic fit around the minimum. We employ thin-plate splines (TPS) [2] to interpolate motion vectors between known keypoints. This approach yields a smooth dense displacement field.

Refinement of Correspondences: A further improvement in accuracy can be obtained by refinement of the correspondence field. Using the dense displacement field, the moving volume is warped towards the fixed volume. A new displacement space $\mathcal{L}_{\text{refine}}$ with a smaller search range and quantisation q is then defined. We increase the number of keypoints, since this second optimisation will be of much lower complexity due to the reduced label space. In order to correctly regularise the combined motion, the concept of offsets in the message computation [13] is employed. As before, first forward and then backward correspondence fields are estimated for improved accuracy and robustness.

3   Experiments and Results

To evaluate our method for very large 3D motion, we use the recently published dataset of [6]. It consists of ten inhale and exhale scan pairs of patients from the COPDgene study, with severe breathing disorders. One difficulty is the poor SNR of the exhale scan due to an ultra-low dose CT protocol. The lung volume change between full exhalation and inhalation can be more than 100 % and the motion magnitude of individual features within the lungs is much larger than in other medical image registration benchmarks (4DCT motion [5] or inter-subject brain mapping), where the performance of new algorithms has nearly converged. The challenges of the COPD dataset have been highlighted by a comparison of three of the most widely used medical registration tools in [18]. The quantitative

Table 1. Results for 3D registration of 10 inhale and exhale CT scan pairs of COPD data set. The average TRE in mm is evaluated for 300 expert selected landmark pairs per case as defined by [6]. The p-values show the statistical significance of the difference in landmark error from the proposed method (calculated with Wilcoxon rank-sum test).

case #	initial	gsyn [1]	LMP [21]	MILO [6]	SGM [15]	without inference	Laplacian [7]	uniform points	asym-metric	proposed
1	26.3	1.21	1.26	**0.93**	1.22	5.86	2.90	1.13	1.10	**1.00±0.93**
2	21.8	3.01	2.02	1.77	2.48	8.39	6.70	2.27	2.10	**1.62±1.78**
3	12.6	1.24	1.14	**0.99**	1.01	4.18	1.41	1.22	1.08	**1.00±1.06**
4	29.6	1.38	1.62	1.14	2.42	7.85	2.24	1.39	1.20	**1.08±1.05**
5	30.1	1.31	1.47	1.02	1.93	6.36	2.61	1.21	1.15	**0.96±1.13**
6	28.5	1.49	1.39	**0.99**	1.45	4.49	2.30	1.03	1.20	**1.01±1.25**
7	21.6	1.24	1.22	**1.03**	1.05	5.13	2.11	1.09	1.07	**1.05±1.07**
8	26.5	2.09	1.63	1.31	1.16	5.29	1.74	1.35	1.15	**1.08±1.24**
9	14.9	1.18	1.12	0.86	0.81	5.29	1.37	1.16	0.84	**0.79±0.80**
10	21.8	1.63	1.45	1.23	1.28	7.98	4.40	1.47	1.47	**1.18±1.31**
avg	23.4	1.58	1.43	1.13	1.48	6.08	2.78	1.33	1.24	**1.08**
std	10.1	1.93	1.45	1.29	2.19	7.00	4.57	1.67	1.60	**1.21**
time		>30 m	-	>10 m	1.5 m	1.5 m	3.5 m	3 m	1.8 m	3 m
p-val		$6 \cdot 10^{-4}$	$1 \cdot 10^{-3}$	0.45	0.03	$9 \cdot 10^{-5}$	$2 \cdot 10^{-4}$	$6 \cdot 10^{-3}$	0.03	-

evaluation revealed errors of 1.79±2.1 mm, 2.19±2.0 mm and 4.68±4.1 mm for the ANTS gsyn [1], NiftyReg [17] and DROP [11] methods, respectively (results are after applying the boosting method of [18]).

Implementation Details: The original size of a voxel is between 0.586 and 0.742 mm in-plane and 2.5 mm in z-direction. The fixed volume was manually cropped to include the full lung and resampled to an isotropic voxel-size of 1 mm. The moving volume is also cropped and then resampled to match the dimensions of the fixed volume. A lung segmentation of the fixed volume is automatically obtained using thresholding and morphological filters. This mask is only used to restrict keypoint detection to the inner lung volume. The following parameters were used for the initial correspondence search: $G_\sigma = 1.4$, $c_D = 6$, $\sigma_I = 150$, $l_{max}q=32$, $q = 2$, which yielded $\approx$3000 keypoints and $|\mathcal{L}| = 35'937$ displacement labels. The regularisation weight was manually tuned for one case (#4) to $\alpha = 1$ and left unaltered for all other cases. For the refinement stage we reduce $c_D = 3$, $l_{max}=8$, $q = 1$. Computation times for the dissimilarity calculation are 60 sec. and 32 sec. for inference (per direction using one CPU core). Our source code is made publicly available at http://mpheinrich.de/software.html.

Discussion of Results: Table 1 (right) lists the obtained target registration error (TRE) of 1.08 mm for our proposed method over 300 manual selected landmark pairs per case [6]. Visualisations of the outcome for two cases are shown in Fig. 2. The obtained deformations have a small amount, 0.14% on average, of voxels with negative Jacobians, and the average deformation Jacobian std. dev. is 0.26. We also evaluated the TRE for the following four variants of our algorithm to show the usefulness of our algorithmic choices. No inference or regularisation (classical block-matching) leads to 6.08 mm; random-walk regularisation with the graph Laplacian as used in [7] to 2.78 mm; belief propagation without symmetric constraint to 1.24 mm; and uniform keypoint sampling without Foerstner operator to a TRE of 1.33 mm.

The task of aligning COPD breath-hold scans has been addressed by the following methods. In [21] a block-matching approach is used for keypoints, but without MRF regularisation, and a TPS transform to initialise a variational optimisation method (LMP). The TPS has an accuracy of 3.20 mm, the refinement reduces this to 1.43 mm. Hermann [15] used a discrete optimisation (semi-global matching, SGM), with a coarse-to-fine multi resolution scheme, and Census cost function and reached a TRE of 1.48 mm. Finally, Castillo et al. [4] used a very large number of control points (every 2nd voxel in each dimension) for block-matching followed by an optimisation based filtering of outliers (MILO). They obtained a TRE of 1.13 mm, which is slightly inferior to our results of 1.08 mm, and they report relatively high computation times of 10 to 20 minutes per case. For the more commonly used 4DCT data of [5], we achieve an average TRE of 0.97 mm, which compares well with [15]: 0.95mm, [13]: 1.43mm and [21]: 1.10mm.

4   Conclusion

We have presented a new MRF-based approach to estimate accurate correspondence fields for images with large motion. Our main contribution is a sparse, but informative, sampling of keypoints locations for which motion vectors are determined from a large set of displacements. The regularity of the displacements is enforced by inference over all pair-wise combinations of close locations using a parts-based model. Devoting much effort only to interesting positions in the image, yields both accurate and fast results. Our method currently achieves the lowest registration error of 1.08 mm on the public COPD dataset of [6]. Future work, will include the application to whole-body registration using organ-surface keypoints and comparisons to graph matching [9].

References

1. Avants, B., Epstein, C., Grossman, M., Gee, J.: Symmetric diffeomorphic image registration with cross-correlation: Evaluating automated labeling of elderly and neurodegenerative brain. Med. Imag. Anal. 12(1), 26–41 (2008)
2. Bookstein, F.L.: Principal warps: Thin-plate splines and the decomposition of deformations. IEEE Trans. Pat. Anal. Mach. Intel. 11(6), 567–585 (1989)
3. Brox, T., Malik, J.: Large displacement optical flow: descriptor matching in variational motion estimation. IEEE Pattern Anal. Mach. Intell. 33(3), 500–513 (2011)
4. Castillo, E., Castillo, R., Fuentes, D., Guerrero, T.: Computing global minimizers to a constrained B-spline image registration problem from optimal L1 perturbations to block match data. Med. Phys. 41(4), 041904 (2014)
5. Castillo, R., Castillo, E., Guerra, R., Johnson, V., McPhail, T., Garg, A., Guerrero, T.: A framework for evaluation of deformable image registration spatial accuracy using large landmark point sets. Phys. Med. Biol. 54(7), 1849 (2009)
6. Castillo, R., Castillo, E., Fuentes, D., Ahmad, M., Wood, A.M., Ludwig, M.S., Guerrero, T.: A reference dataset for deformable image registration spatial accuracy evaluation using the COPDgene study archive. Phys. Med. Biol. 58(9) (2013)

7. Cobzas, D., Sen, A.: Random walks for deformable image registration. In: Fichtinger, G., Martel, A., Peters, T. (eds.) MICCAI 2011, Part II. LNCS, vol. 6892, pp. 557–565. Springer, Heidelberg (2011)
8. Commowick, O., Arsigny, V., Isambert, A., Costa, J., Dhermain, F., Bidault, F., Bondiau, P.Y., Ayache, N., Malandain, G.: An efficient locally affine framework for the smooth registration of anatomical structures. Med. Imag. Anal. 12(4) (2008)
9. Duchenne, O., Bach, F., Kweon, I.S., Ponce, J.: A tensor-based algorithm for high-order graph matching. IEEE Pattern Anal. Mach. Intell. 33(12), 2383–2395 (2011)
10. Felzenszwalb, P.F., Huttenlocher, D.P.: Pictorial structures for object recognition. Int. J. Comp. Vis. 61(1), 55–79 (2005)
11. Glocker, B., Komodakis, N., Tziritas, G., Navab, N., Paragios, N.: Dense image registration through MRFs and efficient linear programming. Med. Imag. Anal. 12(6), 731–741 (2008)
12. Heinrich, M.P., Jenkinson, M., Papież, B.W., Brady, S.M., Schnabel, J.A.: Towards realtime multimodal fusion for image-guided interventions using self-similarities. In: Mori, K., Sakuma, I., Sato, Y., Barillot, C., Navab, N. (eds.) MICCAI 2013, Part I. LNCS, vol. 8149, pp. 187–194. Springer, Heidelberg (2013)
13. Heinrich, M., Jenkinson, M., Brady, M., Schnabel, J.: MRF-based deformable registration and ventilation estimation of lung CT. IEEE Trans. Med. Imag. 32(7), 1239–1248 (2013)
14. Heinrich, M.P., Jenkinson, M., Papież, B.W., Glesson, F.V., Brady, S.M., Schnabel, J.A.: Edge- and detail-preserving sparse image representations for deformable registration of chest MRI and CT volumes. In: Gee, J.C., Joshi, S., Pohl, K.M., Wells, W.M., Zöllei, L. (eds.) IPMI 2013. LNCS, vol. 7917, pp. 463–474. Springer, Heidelberg (2013)
15. Hermann, S.: Evaluation of scan-line optimization for 3D medical image registration. In: CVPR 2014, pp. 1–8 (2014)
16. Liu, C., Yuen, J., Torralba, A.: SIFT flow: Dense correspondence across scenes and its applications. IEEE Pattern Anal. Mach. Intell. 33(5), 978–994 (2011)
17. Modat, M., Ridgway, G.R., Taylor, Z.A., Lehmann, M., Barnes, J., Hawkes, D.J., Fox, N.C., Ourselin, S.: Fast free-form deformation using graphics processing units. Comp. Meth. Prog. Bio. 98(3), 278–284 (2010)
18. Muenzing, S.E., van Ginneken, B., Viergever, M.A., Pluim, J.P.: DIRBoost–an algorithm for boosting deformable image registration: Application to lung CT intrasubject registration. Med. Imag. Anal. 18(3), 449–459 (2014)
19. Murphy, K., et al.: Evaluation of registration methods on thoracic CT: The EMPIRE10 challenge. IEEE Trans. Med. Imag. 30(11), 1901–1920 (2011)
20. Ou, Y., Sotiras, A., Paragios, N., Davatzikos, C.: DRAMMS: deformable registration via attribute matching and mutual-saliency weighting. Med. Imag. Anal. 15(4), 622–639 (2011)
21. Polzin, T., Rühaak, J., Werner, R., Strehlow, J., Heldmann, S., Handels, H., Modersitzki, J.: Combining automatic landmark detection and variational methods for lung CT registration. In: MICCAI Workshop: Pulmonary Image Analysis (2013)
22. Potesil, V., Kadir, T., Platsch, G., Brady, M.: Personalization of pictorial structures for anatomical landmark localization. In: Székely, G., Hahn, H.K. (eds.) IPMI 2011. LNCS, vol. 6801, pp. 333–345. Springer, Heidelberg (2011)
23. Taquet, M., Macq, B., Warfield, S.K.: Spatially adaptive log-euclidean polyaffine registration based on sparse matches. In: Fichtinger, G., Martel, A., Peters, T. (eds.) MICCAI 2011, Part II. LNCS, vol. 6892, pp. 590–597. Springer, Heidelberg (2011)
24. Veksler, O.: Stereo correspondence by dynamic programming on a tree. In: CVPR 2005, vol. 2, pp. 384–390 (2005)

Combining Transversal and Longitudinal Registration in IVUS Studies

G.D. Maso Talou[1,2], P.J. Blanco[1,2], I. Larrabide[3], C. Guedes Bezerra[4,5],
P.A. Lemos[4,5], and R.A. Feijóo[1,2]

[1] Laboratório Nacional de Computação Científica, LNCC-MCTI, Av. Getúlio Vargas
333, 25651-075 Petrópolis, Brazil
[2] Instituto Nacional de Ciência e Tecnologia em Medicina Assistida por Computação
Científica, INCT-MACC, Petrópolis, Brazil
[3] Comisión Nacional de Investigaciones Científicas y Técnicas, Pladema - CONICET,
UNICEN, Tandil, Argentina
[4] Instituto do Coração (InCor), São Paulo, SP, 05403-904, Brazil
[5] Universidad de São Paulo, Faculdade de Medicina, São Paulo, SP, 05403-904, Brazil

Abstract. Intravascular ultrasound (IVUS) is a widely used imaging
technique for atherosclerotic plaque assessment, interventionist guidance,
stent deploy visualization and, lately, as tissue characterization tool.
Some IVUS applications solve the problem of transducer motion by gating a particular phase of the study while others, such as elastography or
spatio-temporal vessel reconstruction, combine image data from different cardiac phases, for which the gating solution is not enough. In the
latter, it is mandatory for the structures in different cardiac phases to be
aligned (cross-sectional registration) and in the correct position along the
vessel axis (longitudinal registration). In this paper, a novel method for
transversal and longitudinal registration is presented, which minimizes
the correlation of the structures between images in a local set of frames.
To assess the performance of this method, frames immediately after carina bifurcation were marked at different cardiac phases and the error
between registrations was measured. The results shown a longitudinal
registration error of 0.3827 ± 0.8250 frames.

Keywords: IVUS, transversal registration, longitudinal registration, cardiac phases.

1 Introduction

Intravascular ultrasound (IVUS) is an imaging technique widely used for atherosclerotic plaque assessment. During its acquisition, the heart contraction imprints
a motion pattern on the transducer and the vessel (referred to as cardiac dynamic component), misleading the identification of frame spatial location at
non-diastolic phases. The transducer motion can be decomposed in two spatial
components, the transversal motion and the longitudinal motion. The former
produces a translation and rotation of the structures from one image to the

© Springer International Publishing Switzerland 2015
N. Navab et al. (Eds.): MICCAI 2015, Part II, LNCS 9350, pp. 346–353, 2015.
DOI: 10.1007/978-3-319-24571-3_42

next, while the latter produces a proximal/distal displacement additional to the pullback [3,4].

The transversal motion component has been widely treated by rigid [13,8,14,9,6,16,15,5] and non-rigid [2,7] registration approaches. In contrast, the longitudinal motion component is usually neglected even though [3] reported an average axial displacement of 1.5 ± 0.8 mm in 0.016 mm interframe acquisitions. Due to the catheter migration, the transversal region observed in systolic phases is much more proximal than expected (mean offset of 93.75 frames). As a consequence the wall strain estimation from the IVUS images along the cardiac phases is not necessarily valid. In [12] a method for rigid longitudinal motion is proposed which aligns each cardiac phase against the diastolic phase of the study. A more complete scheme is proposed in [10] performing longitudinal prior transversal registration of two cardiac phases of the study.

In our work, we present a method to treat both motion components involved in the transducer displacement after the gating process. The goal here is to improve the registration accuracy by identifying both motion components in a fully coupled manner. To measure the accuracy of the methods, bifurcations carina locations are identified manually across different cardiac phases of in-vivo studies. After the registration process, it is expected that bifurcations are registered at the same longitudinal position. Then, the difference in the spatial position is computed as the longitudinal registration error.

2   Methodology

2.1   IVUS Pre-processing

A region of interest (ROI) for the k-th frame $J_k(x, y)$ of the original IVUS sequence, is defined as the non-zero values of the binary mask $M_k(x, y)$ with the same size of the IVUS frame. Similarly, we define $M_{\mathrm{DR}}(x, y)$ and $M_{\mathrm{GW}}^k(x, y)$ as the binary masks associated to the down-ring and the guidewire artifacts regions. Then, the image mask in the k-th frame is defined as $M_k = \neg(M_{\mathrm{DR}} \vee M_{\mathrm{GW}}^k)$ where $\neg$ and $\vee$ stand for NOT and OR boolean operators, respectively. The ROI described by M_k is artifact free and will be used to assess similarity between vessel structures of two different IVUS frames. $M_{\mathrm{DR}}(x, y)$ and $M_{\mathrm{GW}}^k(x, y)$ can be obtained semi-automatically as described in [11].

2.2   Cross-Sectional Registration

Let us define a similarity function, c, that measures alignment of structures between two frames. For the given IVUS frames J_n and J_m and the corresponding ROIs M_n and M_m, we define a common ROI as $M_{n,m} = M_n \wedge M_m$ where $\wedge$ is the AND boolean operator. Pixel set $\mathscr{R}^{n,m} = \{(x, y), M_{n,m}(x, y) = 1\}$ is used to construct a normalized cross-correlation function that compares pixels in $\mathscr{R}^{n,m}$ as follows

$$c(J_n, J_m)|_{\mathscr{R}} = \frac{\displaystyle\sum_{(x,y)\in\mathscr{R}^{n,m}} (J_n(x, y) - \mu_n)(J_m(x, y) - \mu_m)}{\sigma_n \, \sigma_m} \tag{1}$$

where μ_n and σ_n are the mean and standard deviation of the $\mathscr{R}^{n,m}$ values of frame J_n. Cross-correlation provides a fair comparison of the vessel structures due to the correlation between noise pattern and tissue micro-structure [1].

Thus, we search for the rigid motion that maximizes the similarity function c between the two frames. The rigid motion, called Ξ, is described by the horizontal and vertical displacements, τ_x and τ_y, and a rotation around the center of the frame θ. Then, Ξ that maps J_m onto J_n, is defined as

$$\Xi_m^n = \arg\max_{\Xi^* \in \mathscr{U}} \mathscr{F}(J_n, J_m, \Xi^*) = \arg\max_{\Xi^* \in \mathscr{U}} c(J_n, J_m(x(\Xi^*), y(\Xi^*)))|_{\mathscr{R}} \quad (2)$$

where $\mathscr{U}$ is the space of admissible rigid motions of the transducer and $J_m(x(\Xi^*), y(\Xi^*))$ is the frame J_m after applying the rigid motion Ξ^* through which the coordinate (x, y) is displaced. Because of the acquisition sampling, the space $\mathscr{U}$ is discrete and translations and rotations only make sense for multiples of one pixel and $\frac{2\pi}{256}$ radians, respectively. Also, the transducer is confined to the lumen restricting horizontal and vertical displacements. Thus, we characterize $\mathscr{U} = \{\Xi = (\tau_x, \tau_y, \theta)\}$, where $\theta = i\frac{\pi}{128}, i = 0, \ldots, 255$, $\tau_x \in [\tau_x^m, \tau_x^M] \subset \mathbb{Z}$ and $\tau_y \in [\tau_y^m, \tau_y^M] \subset \mathbb{Z}$ being $\tau_{(\cdot)}^M$ and $\tau_{(\cdot)}^m$ the maximum and minimum admissible displacement in $(\cdot)$ direction.

Equation 2 involves the maximization of a not necessarily convex functional. Then, we propose a novel heuristic approach called multi-seed gradient ascend (MSGA) method to account for the non-convexity of the problem. Here, multiple initializations are used to ascend and the instance that reaches maximum functional cost value is considered to be the solution. A suitable trade-off between accuracy and performance is found for an initialization with 5 equidistant seeds.

2.3   Longitudinal Registration

Longitudinal registration is performed between volumes of different cardiac phases. For this, IVUS studies are recorded synchronously with the patient ECG. Then, a specialist indicates in the ECG the R-wave peak moment identifying the first cardiac phase volume. Other P cardiac phase volumes are extracted by picking the $1, \ldots, P$ next frames of the original IVUS volume. Although the images within each set are ordered longitudinally, displacements between frames may not necessarily be homogeneous because of the large variability in the transducer motion throughout the cardiac cycle. Particularly, a diastolic phase before cardiac contraction, referred to as *steady phase*, is assumed to feature homogeneous displacement field as a result of the reduced cardiac motion. Then, from the $\mathscr{I}_i$, $i = 1, \ldots, P$ cardiac phases, we define the steady phase $\mathscr{I}_{st}$ as

$$\mathscr{I}_{st} = \arg\min_{i=1,\ldots,P} \mathscr{P}_{motion}(\mathscr{I}_i) = \arg\min_{i=1,\ldots,P} \left\{ -\frac{1}{N_i} \sum_{j=1}^{N_i} \sum_{y=1}^{H} \sum_{x=1}^{W} |\nabla I_j^i(x, y)| \right\} \quad (3)$$

where I_j^i denotes the j-th study frame in the i-th phase, N_i is the number of frames for that i-th cardiac phase, and H and W are the study frame dimensions and ∇ is the gradient operator. Steady phase frames will be denoted as I_j^{st}.

With motionless assumption at the steady phase, the longitudinal location of its frames along the catheter is characterized as $r(I_j^{\text{st}}) = r_0 + \frac{j\,v_p}{f_s}$ where I_j^{st} is the j-th study frame in the phase $\mathscr{I}_{\text{st}}$, r_0 is the transducer initial position over the longitudinal axis, v_p is the pullback velocity in $mm \cdot s^{-1}$ and f_s is the acquisition framerate in $frame \cdot s^{-1}$.

The steady phase $\mathscr{I}_{\text{st}}$, and the known spatial location of the corresponding frames I_j^{st}, $j = 1, \ldots, N_{\text{st}}$, is used to perform a non-linear longitudinal registration of the remaining phases, hereafter referred to as *non-steady phases*. The registration process consists in assessing the similarity of each non-steady phase frame against the steady phase frames. The most similar steady phase is used to place the non-steady one. For the i-th cardiac phase, the degree of similarity between j-th frame I_j^i and I_k^{st}, $k = 1, \ldots, N_{\text{st}}$, is measured through a neighborhood correlation defined as follows

$$c_w(I_j^i, I_k^{\text{st}}) = \frac{\sum\limits_{d=-w}^{w} \phi(d, \sigma_G)\, c(I_{j+d}^i, I_{k+d}^{\text{st}})|_{\mathscr{R}}}{\sum\limits_{d=-w}^{w} \phi(d, \sigma_G)}, \qquad (4)$$

where w is the frame neighborhood width and ϕ is a Gaussian weight function with σ_G standard deviation. The parameter w is defined as $w(\sigma, T) = \left\lfloor \sigma(-2\ln(T))^{\frac{1}{2}} \right\rfloor$ to neglect the contributions from frames with weights that are smaller than $T\ \phi(0, \sigma_G)$ (with $T = 10^{-1}$). The parameter σ_G should be small enough to be representative of the local structures and large enough to incorporate information about the longitudinal structure to achieve robustness (Section 3.2). Finally, the position in space of the frame I_j^i, which belongs to a *non-steady phase*, i.e. $i \neq \text{st}$, is defined as $r(I_j^i) = r(I_m^{\text{st}})$ where $m = \underset{k=1,\ldots,N_{\text{st}}}{\arg\max}\, c_w(I_j^i, I_k^{\text{st}})$. A formal definition for the set of frames located at the n-th frame position of the steady phase, is given by $\mathscr{X}_n = \{I_j^i;\ r(I_j^i) = r(I_n^{\text{st}}), j = 1, \ldots, N_i, i = 1, \ldots, P\}$.

The estimated transducer motion (Figure 1) resembles the motion pattern experimentally observed in medical practice. Specifically, the pseudo-periodic proximal-distal oscillations and their amplitudes obtained here, are within the ranges reported experimentally in [3].

2.4   Coupling Transversal and Longitudinal Registration

Cross-sectional registration is performed prior the comparison presented in (4). In that manner, the position in space of the frame I_j^i, which belongs to a *non-steady phase* and the applied transversal rigid motion Ξ_j^i to that frame are defined as $r(I_j^i(x(\Xi_j^i), y(\Xi_j^i))) = r(I_m^{\text{st}})$, where

$$m = \underset{k=1,\ldots,N_{\text{st}}}{\arg\max}\, c_w(I_j^i(x(\Xi_j^i), y(\Xi_j^i)), I_k^{\text{st}}) \qquad (5)$$

and

$$\Xi_j^i = \underset{\Xi^* \in \mathscr{U}}{\arg\max}\, \sum_{d=-w}^{w} \mathscr{F}(I_{k+d}^{\text{st}}, I_{j+d}^i, \Xi^*). \qquad (6)$$

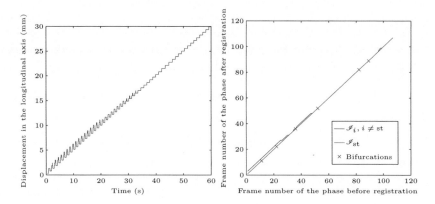

Fig. 1. Longitudinal registration process in-vivo using $\sigma_G = 0.4$: (Left) Transducer longitudinal displacement; (Right) Registration of a non-steady cardiac phase against $\mathscr{I}_{st}$.

Note that the transversal registration performed in (6) is now coupled with the longitudinal registration due to (5). Although, this implementation models a more suitable scheme for the longitudinal comparison due to the alignment of the structures, it also increases the computational cost. Finally, the aligned set of frames located at the n-th frame position of the steady phase, is given by $\mathscr{X}_n^C = \{I_j^i(x(\Xi_j^i), y(\Xi_j^i)); \ r(I_j^i(x(\Xi_j^i), y(\Xi_j^i))) = r(I_n^{st}), \ j = 1, \ldots, N_i, i = 1, \ldots, P\}$.

3 Results and Discussion

3.1 IVUS Data

The IVUS studies were acquired with the Atlantis™SR Pro Imaging Catheter at 40 MHz synchronized with an ECG signal and connected to an iLab™ Ultrasound Imaging System (both by Boston Scientific Corporation, Natick, MA, USA), at the Heart Institute (InCor), University of São Paulo Medical School and Sírio-Libanês Hospital, São Paulo, Brazil. The procedure was performed during a diagnostic or therapeutic percutaneous coronary procedure. Vessels were imaged using automated pullback at 0.5 mm/s. Overall, 30 IVUS studies with synchronized ECG signal were performed on different patients.

3.2 Validation Using Bifurcation Sites

Bifurcation sites, more precisely the first frame of anastomosis, were used as landmark points to assess the longitudinal misalignment between two phase image volumes. Then, we define longitudinal registration error as $\varepsilon^k = \frac{1}{NB} \sum_{j=1}^{NB} |B^{st}(j) - B^k(j)|$ where NB is the number of bifurcations in the study, $B^k(j)$ is the frame at the j-th bifurcation in the k-th cardiac phase.

Table 1 presents ε^k for different values of σ_G which determines the frames neighborhood (w). Values for σ_G where chosen such as w differs by 1 between

Table 1. Mean ($E(\varepsilon^k)$) and standard deviation ($s(\varepsilon^k)$) of the longitudinal registration error in frames for different values of σ_G for 30 IVUS studies.

w	0	1	2	3	4
σ_G	0.4	0.8	1.2	1.6	2.0
$E(\varepsilon^k)) \pm s(\varepsilon^k)$	0.383 ± 0.825	0.506 ± 1.48	0.630 ± 2.009	0.605 ± 1.991	0.470 ± 1.532

1

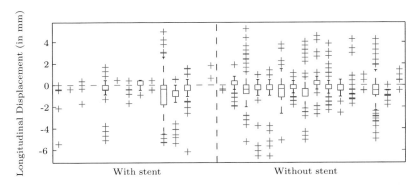

Fig. 2. Box plot presenting the transducer longitudinal displacements at each heartbeat for all the studies, dividing them as patients with or without stent deployment.

comparisons, evidencing the neighbor contribution. The registration process rendered the lowest discrepancy against the specialist identification for $\sigma_G = 0.4$ (error of 0.3827 ± 0.8250 frames). This means that the usage of adjacent frames data does not improve the registration and this is because of two factors: i) the presence of adventitia and luminal areas with decorrelated noise within the ROI; ii) the variation of the motion pattern in successive heartbeats. In the following sections σ_G is fixed to 0.4.

3.3 Correlation between Longitudinal Motion and Stent Deployment

IVUS studies were divided in 2 groups of cases: studies with stent (N=14) and without stent (N=16). Using the longitudinal displacement applied for longitudinal registration of the systolic and diastolic phase (phases with highest and lowest values of $\mathscr{P}_{\text{motion}}$) of each study, we measure the amplitude of the transducer migration during the cardiac cycle. In Figure 2 a reduction of the longitudinal displacements amplitude can be noticed for cases with stent deployment. A longitudinal displacement of 0.283 ± 0.739 mm and 0.519 ± 0.785 (absolute value of displacements) for cases with and without stent deployment is observed, respectively. These results confirm the previous findings reported in [3].

For further analysis, the longitudinal displacement was calculated in an artery before and after stent deployment (Figure 3). As result, the method shows reproducibility, i.e., it delivers a close displacement pattern at the stent distal

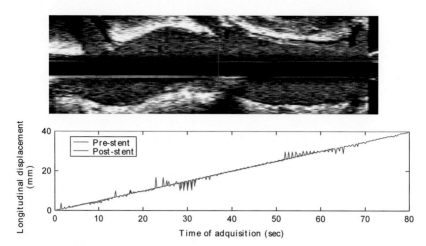

Fig. 3. Estimation of the transducer longitudinal displacement before and after stent deployment: (top) longitudinal view at $\mathscr{I}_{st}$ phase (left is the distal position); (bottom) Transducer longitudinal displacement. The red line marks the distal point of the stent.

positions in both cases (before and after stenting). Also, a complete attenuation of the longitudinal displacement upstream the stent area is observed. Hence, downstream displacements are slightly larger after the stenting procedure.

4   Conclusions

A novel method for longitudinal and transversal registration of IVUS studies was presented. It is concluded that the optimal longitudinal registration is performed when only local cross sectional data are used. Comparisons against a specialist shows an error of 0.3827 ± 0.8250 frames at the bifurcation sites. The inclusion of neighbor frames at the registration deteriorates the block matching with a ROI of the full image (excluding image artifacts). Further works, may include the use of different ROIs excluding the adventitia and lumen areas where the data is not reliable for matching the vessel wall structures. Performance issues must be further explored, although the present strategy allows a parallelization at frame comparison level that is well suited for GP-GPU implementations.

The motion estimated by the longitudinal registration has also been used to study the association of the transducer longitudinal displacement and stenting. Remarkably, the proposed method estimates larger motion in non-stented vessels, while smaller displacements are observed in stented vessels confirming previous findings. Future work will include larger patient populations.

Acknowledgements. This research was partially supported by the Brazilian agencies CNPq, FAPERJ and CAPES. The support of these agencies is gratefully acknowledged. Also, the authors would like to thank the anonymous reviewers for their valuable comments and suggestions to improve the quality of the paper.

References

1. Abbott, J.G., Thurstone, F.L.: Acoustic speckle: Theory and experimental analysis. Ultrason. Imag. 324(4), 303–324 (1979)
2. Amores, J., Radeva, P.: Retrieval of IVUS images using contextual information and elastic matching. Int. J. Intell. Syst. 20(5), 541–559 (2005)
3. Arbab-Zadeh, A., DeMaria, A.N., Penny, W.F., Russo, R.J., Kimura, B.J., Bhargava, V.: Axial movement of the intravascular ultrasound probe during the cardiac cycle: implications for three-dimensional reconstruction and measurements of coronary dimensions. Am. Heart J. 138(5 Pt 1), 865–872 (1999)
4. Bruining, N., von Birgelen, C., de Feyter, P.J., Ligthart, J., Li, W., Serruys, P.W., Roelandt, J.R.: Ecg-gated versus nongated three-dimensional intracoronary ultrasound analysis: implications for volumetric measurements. Cathet. Cardiovasc. Diagn. 43(3), 254–260 (1998)
5. Danilouchkine, M.G., Mastik, F., van der Steen, A.F.: Improving IVUS palpography by incorporation of motion compensation based on block matching and optical flow. IEEE Trans. Ultrason. Ferroelectrics Freq. Contr. 55(11), 2392–2404 (2008)
6. Hernandez-Sabate, A., Gil, D., Fernandez-Nofrerias, E., Radeva, P., Marti, E.: Approaching artery rigid dynamics in IVUS. IEEE Trans. Med. Imag. 28(11), 1670–1680 (2009)
7. Katouzian, A., Karamalis, A., Lisauskas, J., Eslami, A., Navab, N.: IVUS-histology image registration. In: Dawant, B.M., Christensen, G.E., Fitzpatrick, J.M., Rueckert, D. (eds.) WBIR 2012. LNCS, vol. 7359, pp. 141–149. Springer, Heidelberg (2012)
8. Leung, K.Y.E., Baldewsing, R., Mastik, F., Schaar, J.A., Gisolf, A., van der Steen, A.F.W.: Motion compensation for intravascular ultrasound palpography. IEEE Trans. Ultrason. Ferroelectrics Freq. Contr. 53(7), 1269–1280 (2006)
9. Liang, Y., Zhu, H., Friedman, M.H.: Estimation of the transverse strain tensor in the arterial wall using IVUS image registration. Ultrasound Med. Biol. 34(11), 1832–1845 (2008)
10. Liang, Y., Zhu, H., Gehrig, T., Friedman, M.H.: Measurement of the transverse strain tensor in the coronary arterial wall from clinical intravascular ultrasound images. J. Biomech. 41(14), 2906–2911 (2008)
11. Maso Talou, G.D.: IVUS images segmentation driven by active contours and spaciotemporal reconstruction of the coronary vessels aided by angiographies. Master's thesis, National Laboratory for Scientific Computing, Petrópolis, Brazil (2013)
12. Matsumoto, M.M.S., Lemos, P.A., Furuie, S.S.: Ivus coronary volume alignment for distinct phases. In: SPIE Medical Imaging, p. 72650X. International Society for Optics and Photonics (2009)
13. Mita, H., Kanai, H., Koiwa, Y.: Cross-sectional elastic imaging of arterial wall using intravascular ultrasonography. Jpn. J. Appl. Phys. 40(7), 4753–4762 (2001)
14. Oakeson, K.D., Zhu, H., Friedman, M.H.: Quantification of cross-sectional artery wall motion with ivus image registration. In: Medical Imaging 2004, pp. 119–130. International Society for Optics and Photonics (2004)
15. Rosales, M., Radeva, P., Rodriguez-Leor, O., Gil, D.: Modelling of image-catheter motion for 3-D IVUS. Medical Image Analysis 13(1), 91–104 (2009)
16. Zheng, S., Jianjian, W.: Compensation of in-plane rigid motion for in vivo intracoronary ultrasound image sequence. Comput. Biol. Med. 43(9), 1077–1085 (2013)

Interpolation and Averaging
of Multi-Compartment Model Images

Renaud Hédouin[1], Olivier Commowick[1], Aymeric Stamm[2],
and Christian Barillot[1]

[1] VISAGES: INSERM U746, CNRS UMR6074, INRIA, Univ. of Rennes I, France
[2] CRL, Children's Hospital Boston, Harvard Medical School, Boston, USA

Abstract. Multi-compartment diffusion models (MCM) are increasingly
used to characterize the brain white matter microstructure from diffusion
MRI. We address the problem of interpolation and averaging of MCM
images as a simplification problem based on spectral clustering. As a
core part of the framework, we propose novel solutions for the averaging
of MCM compartments. Evaluation is performed both on synthetic and
clinical data, demonstrating better performance for the "covariance analytic" averaging method. We then present an MCM template of normal
controls constructed using the proposed interpolation.

1 Introduction

Diffusion Weighted Imaging (DWI) is a unique MRI acquisition strategy, which
can provide invaluable insights into the white matter architecture in-vivo and
non-invasively. A number of diffusion models have been devised, with the aim to
characterize the underlying tissue microstructure. The most widespread model
is known as Diffusion Tensor Imaging (DTI) [3] which, under the assumption
of homogeneous diffusion in each voxel, describes the random motion of water
as a single Gaussian process with a diffusion tensor. However, many regions
of crossing fibers exist in low-resolution clinical DWI and the DTI model fails
at correctly representing them. Multi-compartment models (MCM) have been
extensively proposed and studied as alternative diffusion models to cope with
the intrinsic voxelwise diffusion heterogeneity [4]. The key principle of MCM
is to explicitly model the diffusion in a number of pre-specified compartments
akin to groups of cells inducing similar diffusion properties. MCMs may have
a great impact on patient care, as they allow for a better characterization of
brain tissue microstructure, which enables the identification of more specific
biomarkers such as proportion of free water (edema), proportion of water in
axons (partial disruption or complete loss of axons, axonal injury), etc.

A critical step to identify relevant biomarkers on a large database is the creation of an atlas from individual estimated MCM images. This is achieved using registration and interpolation of MCMs. To date, only few approaches have
addressed this issue. Among them, Barmpoutis et al. [2] or Geng et al. [5] introduced registration methods specifically tuned for Orientation Distribution Functions (ODF) on the sphere. Goh et al. [6] introduced an interpolation method

© Springer International Publishing Switzerland 2015
N. Navab et al. (Eds.): MICCAI 2015, Part II, LNCS 9350, pp. 354–362, 2015.
DOI: 10.1007/978-3-319-24571-3_43

for ODFs in a spherical harmonics basis as a Riemannian average. However, this approach does not apply to MCMs as they are not expressed in the same basis. Taquet et al. [13] proposed an interpolation approach seen as a simplification problem of all weighted compartments from a set of voxels into a smaller set of compartments. However, they assume that a single compartment belongs to the exponential family which is not the case for all MCMs.

We introduce a new interpolation method for MCM images also as a simplification problem. It relies on the fuzzy spectral clustering [9] of input compartments, from MCMs provided e.g. from trilinear interpolation, into a predefined number of output compartments. Then, each cluster is used to compute an interpolated compartment, providing an output MCM. This method is very generic as it relies only on the definition of a similarity measure between compartments and of a weighted averaging scheme for compartments. It can therefore be applied to any MCM as long as those two components may be defined.

In the following, we present MCM interpolation / averaging as a simplification problem based on spectral clustering (Section 2.1). Then, we define 4 possible compartment averaging methods for the Diffusion Directions Imaging (DDI) model [11] in Section 3 and similarity measures related to each of those averaging schemes. We demonstrate qualitatively and quantitatively the interest of both the averaging schemes and interpolation framework on simulated and in vivo data. We finally apply this framework to compute an atlas of DDI (Section 3) which clearly highlights average crossing fiber regions.

2 Theory

2.1 Model Interpolation as a Simplification Problem

We consider m MCM $M^i (i = 1, ..., m)$ each containing $c(i)$ compartments of constrained water diffusion and a free water compartment describing isotropic unconstrained water diffusion. We note F_j^i the j-th compartment of M^i and F_{free}^i its free water compartment, their respective weights being w_j^i and w_{free}^i and sum to 1. Each of these M^i has an associated weight α^i. For example, in the case of a trilinear interpolation, we have 8 MCM with spatial weights α^i. We formulate the interpolation problem as merging the M^i into one MCM with a predetermined number of compartments q and one free water compartment. There are therefore two different averaging parts: compartments and free water compartment.

The averaging of all compartments coming from M^i into q compartments is performed using spectral clustering [9]. Having defined a similarity matrix S between compartments, spectral vectors are extracted from S. These spectral vectors are then clustered using fuzzy C-Means. Hence, we obtain q sets of n weights (n being the total number of compartments) $\beta_{j,k}^i$ that are probabilities for the j-th compartment of M^i to belong to the k-th cluster. We define $\theta_{j,k}^i$ the weight of the j-th compartment of M^i in the k-th cluster and θ_i the weight of the free water compartment of M^i:

$$\theta^i_{j,k} = \alpha^i w^i_j \beta^i_{j,k}, \qquad \theta_i = \alpha^i w^i_{\text{free}} \tag{1}$$

From $\theta^i_{j,k}$ and θ_i, we compute weights ϕ_k and ϕ_{free} of the output compartments.

$$\forall k = 1, ..., q \quad \phi_k = \sum_{i=1}^{m} \sum_{j=1}^{c(i)} \theta^i_{j,k}, \qquad \phi_{\text{free}} = \sum_{i=1}^{m} \theta_i \tag{2}$$

We also define $\hat{\theta}^i_{j,k}$ and $\hat{\theta}_i$ two different sets of normalized weights from $\theta^i_{j,k}$ and θ_i. This framework is very generic and can be applied to any MCM as long as we provide a way to compute a similarity matrix between compartments. Free water averaging is common to any MCM and is described in Section 2.2. We derive MCM compartments averaging for DDI in Section 2.3 and similarity matrix computation in Section 2.4.

2.2   Free Water Compartments Averaging

We estimate from the isotropic diffusivities d^i_{free} of M^i the diffusivity d_{free} of the average model associated to weight ϕ_{free}. Free diffusion follows an isotropic Gaussian distribution with covariance matrix $D^i_{\text{free}} - d^i_{\text{free}} I_3$ (where I_3 is the identity matrix). The averaging is performed using the log-Euclidean framework [1]:

$$D_{\text{free}} = \exp(\sum_{i=1}^{m} \hat{\theta}_i \log(D^i_{\text{free}})) \quad \Rightarrow \quad d_{\text{free}} = \exp(\sum_{i=1}^{m} \hat{\theta}_i \log(d^i_{\text{free}})) \tag{3}$$

2.3   MCM Compartments Averaging

We propose four different methods to average DDI compartments into a single one: classic, tensor, log VMF, and covariance analytic. For each cluster k, we wish to average the set of F^i_j with weights $\hat{\theta}^i_{j,k}$ into a compartment C_k with weight ϕ_k. To simplify notations, we now just consider n compartments $F_i(i = 1, ..., n)$ with their corresponding weights w_i.

2.3.1   Specification of the DDI Model
Each MCM has specific parameters and models for compartments. The compartment averaging part therefore cannot be exactly similar for any MCM. We choose to detail several compartments averaging methods for one particular MCM: the DDI model.

In addition to the free water compartment, a number of axonal compartments can be added to DDI to model how water molecules diffuse in axonal bundles with various orientations. Diffusing water molecules in a particular axonal compartment are assumed to undergo a random displacement that is the independent sum of a von Mises & Fisher (VMF) vector on S^2 of radius r and a

Gaussian vector on $\mathbb{R}^3$. Hence, the resulting diffusion probability density function describing this random displacement is given by the 3D convolution of the VMF distribution with the Gaussian distribution:

$$p_{\mu,\kappa,d,\nu} = \text{Convolution}(\text{VMF}(\mu,\kappa,r), \text{Gaussian}(0, \frac{(1-\nu)d}{\kappa+1}[I_3 + \kappa\mu\mu^T]) \quad (4)$$

where $\mu \in S^2$ is the principal axis of diffusion, κ an index of the concentration of diffusion around μ, d the diffusivity along μ, ν the proportion of extra-axonal space in the compartment, r the radius of the VMF sphere given by $r = \sqrt{\nu d}$. Σ is the covariance matrix of the Gaussian part. Let $\mu_i, \kappa_i, \nu_i, d_i$ be the parameters of F_i and μ, κ, ν, d be the parameters of the average compartment F.

2.3.2 Common Part of Compartment Averaging

We choose to average the sphere of radius r as the one whose surface is the average of the input sphere surfaces. This corresponds to a Euclidean average of the individual r_i^2: $r^2 = \sum_{i=1}^{n} w_i r_i^2$. This also gives us a direct relation between ν and d leading to only 3 parameters to estimate (μ, κ and ν), d being computed as $d = r^2/\nu$.

2.3.3 Simple Averaging

The simplest approach performs a weighted Euclidean averaging on each parameter except μ. Each μ_i is a direction in S^2. However, for the DDI model, they do not represent a direction but an orientation. The simplest way to solve this problem (as two opposite directions) is to put all μ_i in the top hemisphere and average them on the sphere to obtain μ.

2.3.4 Tensor Averaging

The simple averaging is however only a partial solution, especially for directions close to the sphere equator. We now consider μ_i as orientations instead of directions. μ_i is represented as a cigar-shaped tensor $T_i \in \mathcal{S}_3^+(\mathbb{R})$ defined as:

$$T_i = \mu_i \mu_i^T + \varepsilon I_3 \quad (5)$$

With ε small to have non degenerated tensors. Then, we can average T_i using the log-Euclidean framework similarly to Eq. (3). We define the average μ as the principal direction of T (eigenvector with the largest eigenvalue). The other parameters are obtained as for simple averaging.

2.3.5 Covariance Analytic

Another approach uses information from covariance matrices Σ_i of DDI compartments. These Σ_i matrices belong to $S_3^+(\mathbb{R})$ and can be averaged into Σ similarly to Eq. (3). We wish to extract all parameters from the average Σ. We start by approximating Σ by a cigar-shaped tensor to match the DDI compartment model. To do that, we need to enforce two equal secondary eigenvalues $\lambda_\perp$. In the log-Euclidean framework, this amounts to compute $\lambda_\perp$ as $\lambda_\perp = \sqrt{\lambda_2\lambda_3}$ where λ_2, λ_3 are the two lowest eigenvalues of Σ. We now have $\hat{\Sigma}$ the cigar-shaped tensor of F:

$$\hat{\Sigma} = \frac{(1-\nu)d}{\kappa+1}[I_3 + \kappa\mu\mu^T] \quad (6)$$

Proceeding by identification and given that $r^2 = \nu d$, we obtain that μ is the principal eigenvector of $\hat{\Sigma}$. ν and κ are given by:

$$\nu = \frac{r^2}{\lambda + r^2}, \quad \kappa = 2\frac{\lambda - \lambda_\perp}{\lambda_\perp} \tag{7}$$

2.3.6   Log VMF

We now explore the option to use the VMF to compute μ and κ and recover only ν from $\hat{\Sigma}$. We consider a VMF distribution as a point in a Riemannian manifold, similarly to the approach presented by McGraw et al. [8]. To interpolate several points, a geodesic on these manifolds is defined (refer to [8] for details). Orientation averaging is similar to tensor averaging as in Section 2.3.4. The interpolation of κ is done recursively by projection as in McGraw et al. Letting $\kappa = \kappa_1$, repeat until convergence (i.e until $l_\kappa < \varepsilon$):

$$l_\kappa = \sum_{i=1}^{n} w_i \log(\frac{\kappa_i}{\kappa}) \tag{8}$$

$$\kappa = \kappa \exp(l_\kappa) \tag{9}$$

Knowing all parameters except ν, we obtain it from $\hat{\Sigma}$ as:

$$\nu = \frac{r^2[2r^2 + \lambda + \lambda_\perp(1 + \kappa)]}{2(r^2 + \lambda)[r^2 + \lambda_\perp(1 + \kappa)]} \tag{10}$$

2.4   Similarity Measure between Compartments

To perform spectral clustering, we need a similarity measure between compartments. To stay coherent with the compartment averaging part, they are defined following metrics associated with each method. In each case except covariance analytic, we compute separately the distance between μ, κ, r and add them with normalization terms α, β to give each parameters the same influence. For two compartments F_1 and F_2, the similarity measures are defined as follows:

$$\begin{cases} d_{\text{simple}}(F_1, F_2) = <\mu_1, \mu_2>^2 + \alpha|\kappa_1 - \kappa_2| + \beta|r_1 - r_2| \\ d_{\text{tensor}}(F_1, F_2) = ||\log(T_1) - \log(T_2)|| + \alpha|\kappa_1 - \kappa_2| + \beta|r_1 - r_2| \\ d_{\text{logVMF}}(F_1, F_2) = ||\log(T_1) - \log(T_2)|| + \alpha|\log(\kappa_1) - \log(\kappa_2)| + \beta|r_1 - r_2| \\ d_{\text{covariance analytic}}(F_1, F_2) = ||\log(\Sigma_1) - \log(\Sigma_2)|| \end{cases} \tag{11}$$

3   Experiments and Results

3.1   Compartment Averaging Evaluation on Simulated Data

We first evaluate compartment averaging into a single one. To do so, we simulate random DDI compartments by drawing parameter values from uniform distribution between different bounds depending on the parameter: 0 and 20 for κ,

$5.10^{-4}m.s^{-2}$ and $5.10^{-3}m.s^{-2}$ for d, 0 and 1 for ν, and random orientation on S^2 for μ. Four random DDI compartments are computed, they correspond to the four corners of a grid of size 11×11 that we want to extrapolate. To perform a robust experiment, we created a database of 500 sets of 4 corners. The reference is a grid containing 4 compartments per pixel with a weight proportional to the position of the voxel with respect to each corner (see Fig. 1.e). For each method, we average each pixel of the reference image into only one DDI compartment. To quantitatively evaluate DDI averaging, we simulate, for each method and the reference, a DWI signal from DDI models following Eq. (6) in [11] on 60 directions for each of 3 different b-values. A Euclidean distance between simulated DWIs of the 4 methods and the reference provides quantitative results.

The Euclidean distances on the 500 random images are normalized so that the simple error mean is 100. The result for the different methods are: simple: 100, tensor: 31.6, log VMF: 28.0, covariance analytic: 11.1. We present in Fig. 1 representative images from averaged DDI models superimposed on the corresponding error maps. The simple method has a large error explained by direction averaging. The tensor method is better: thanks to the orientation averaging part. However, there are still large errors which can be explained by large κ values in regions averaging orthogonal directions, which is not realistic. log VMF suffers from the same problem as tensor. Covariance analytic performs much better than all other methods. This is mainly due to smaller errors in crossing fibers. This is logical as when two orthogonal compartments are averaged, the best single compartment representing them is almost spherical, meaning a low κ value. The Euclidean distance map in the DWI signal confirms this idea.

3.2   MCM Extrapolation on Real Data

The second experiment was to test the entire MCM interpolation pipeline including spectral clustering and free water compartment averaging. We tested methods on a set of 20 real DDI images estimated from DWI with $128 \times 128 \times 55$ voxels with a $2 \times 2 \times 2mm^3$ resolution, 30 gradient directions with one b-value $= 1000$ s.mm^{-2}. In order to assess the quality of interpolation, we extrapolate voxels from their neighborhood. To do so, one in every two voxels are removed and extrapolated from the known remaining values. Input DDI models have three compartments, and so will the extrapolated DDI. Again we compute the Euclidean distance between extrapolated DDI and the original one on the DWI corresponding images. Means are respectively simple: 100, tensor: 84.6, log VMF: 107.0, covariance analytic: 66.2. These results show that covariance analytic performs significantly better than all other methods (paired t-test, $p < 1.0 \times 10^{-5}$) also when used in the complete MCM interpolation framework on real data.

3.3   DDI Atlas Construction

The ultimate step of registration of MCM images is the production of an average atlas of the white matter microstructure. We computed an atlas from the 20 DDI images following Guimond et al. atlas construction method [7]. This atlas

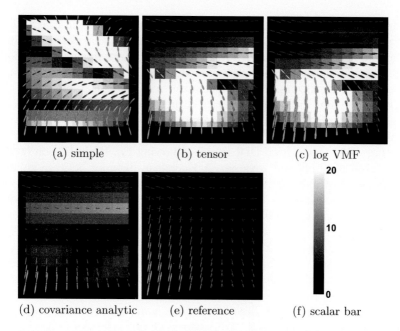

(a) simple   (b) tensor   (c) log VMF

(d) covariance analytic   (e) reference   (f) scalar bar

Fig. 1. First four images (a-d) illustrate DDI averaging using the four methods superimposed on their local error maps. Image (d) is the reference.

construction was performed using non linear DTI registration as proposed by Suarez et al. [12]. Then, the obtained transformations were applied to the DDI models. We interpolated the DDI models using our clustering approach with the covariance analytic averaging. In addition, when applying a transformation to oriented models, it is necessary to apply the local linear part of the transformation to the interpolated models. We used a technique similar to finite-strain reorientation for tensors [10] by applying the local rotation to the μ_i directions of each compartment of the interpolated DDI. We present the visual result of the atlas and a zoomed area in Fig. 2. This atlas provides a clear distinction of crossing fibers and will be of great interest in future studies for example of white matter microstructure destruction in diseases.

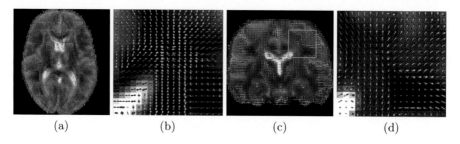

(a)   (b)   (c)   (d)

Fig. 2. Example of a DDI atlas superimposed on the average B0 image.

4   Conclusion

We have addressed the problem of interpolation and averaging of MCM images. As MCMs become increasingly popular and used, the issue of interpolation (e.g. for a registration purpose) or averaging (e.g. for atlas creation) becomes acute in the absence of relevant dedicated solutions yet. We have proposed to perform interpolation as a MCM simplification problem, relying on spectral clustering and compartment averaging methods handling both free water and compartment parameters. For this latter part, we have proposed and compared four different alternatives, these methods being evaluated with synthetic and real data. According to these different experimental conditions, the covariance analytic solution exhibits significantly better performance than the others. This can be explained by its capability to better handle the diffusion dispersion parameter (κ) around each compartment principal orientation. Although this study has been validated on one MCM model (DDI), the method proposed is generic and may be extended to all currently available MCMs.

References

1. Arsigny, V., Fillard, P., Pennec, X., Ayache, N.: Log-Euclidean metrics for fast and simple calculus on diffusion tensors. MRM 56(2), 411–421 (2006)
2. Barmpoutis, A., Vemuri, B.C., Forder, J.R.: Registration of high angular resolution diffusion MRI images using 4th order tensors. In: Ayache, N., Ourselin, S., Maeder, A. (eds.) MICCAI 2007, Part I. LNCS, vol. 4791, pp. 908–915. Springer, Heidelberg (2007)
3. Basser, P.J., Pierpaoli, C.: Microstructural and physiological features of tissues elucidated by quantitative diffusion-tensor MRI. Journal of Magnetic Resonance, Series B 111(3), 209–219 (1996)
4. Ferizi, U., Schneider, T., et al.: A ranking of diffusion MRI compartment models with in vivo human brain data. MRM 72(6), 1785–1792 (2014)
5. Geng, X., et al.: Diffusion MRI registration using orientation distribution functions. In: Prince, J.L., Pham, D.L., Myers, K.J. (eds.) IPMI 2009. LNCS, vol. 5636, pp. 626–637. Springer, Heidelberg (2009)
6. Goh, A., Lenglet, C., Thompson, P.M., Vidal, R.: A nonparametric Riemannian framework for processing high angular resolution diffusion images and its applications to ODF-based morphometry. Neuroimage 56, 1181–1201 (2011)
7. Guimond, A., Meunier, J., Thirion, J.P.: Average brain models: A convergence study. Computer Vision and Image Understanding 77(2), 192–210 (2000)
8. McGraw, T., Vemuri, B.: Von mises-fisher mixture model of the diffusion ODF. In: IEEE ISBI, pp. 65–68 (2006)
9. Ng, A.Y., Jordan, M.I., Weiss, Y., et al.: On spectral clustering: Analysis and an algorithm. Advances in Neural Information Processing Systems 2, 849–856 (2002)
10. Ruiz-Alzola, J., Westin, C.F., et al.: Nonrigid registration of 3D tensor medical data. Medical Image Analysis 6(2), 143–161 (2002)
11. Stamm, A., Pérez, P., Barillot, C.: A new multi-fiber model for low angular resolution diffusion mri. In: ISBI, pp. 936–939. IEEE (2012)

12. Suarez, R.O., Commowick, O., et al.: Automated delineation of white matter fiber tracts with a multiple region-of-interest approach. Neuroimage 59(4), 3690–3700 (2012)

13. Taquet, M., Scherrer, B., Commowick, O., Peters, J., Sahin, M., Macq, B., Warfield, S.K.: Registration and analysis of white matter group differences with a multi-fiber model. In: Ayache, N., Delingette, H., Golland, P., Mori, K. (eds.) MICCAI 2012, Part III. LNCS, vol. 7512, pp. 313–320. Springer, Heidelberg (2012)

Structured Decision Forests for Multi-modal Ultrasound Image Registration

Ozan Oktay[1], Andreas Schuh[1], Martin Rajchl[1], Kevin Keraudren[1],
Alberto Gomez[3], Mattias P. Heinrich[2], Graeme Penney[3], and Daniel Rueckert[1]

[1] Biomedical Image Analysis Group, Imperial College London, UK
o.oktay13@imperial.ac.uk
[2] Institute of Medical Informatics, University of Lübeck, Germany
[3] Imaging Sciences and Biomedical Engineering Division, King's College London, UK

Abstract. Interventional procedures in cardiovascular diseases often require ultrasound (US) image guidance. These US images must be combined with pre-operatively acquired tomographic images to provide a roadmap for the intervention. Spatial alignment of pre-operative images with intra-operative US images can provide valuable clinical information. Existing multi-modal US registration techniques often do not achieve reliable registration due to low US image quality. To address this problem, a novel medical image representation based on a trained decision forest named probabilistic edge map (PEM) is proposed in this paper. PEMs are generic and modality-independent. They generate similar anatomical representations from different imaging modalities and can thus guide a multi-modal image registration algorithm more robustly and accurately. The presented image registration framework is evaluated on a clinical dataset consisting of 10 pairs of 3D US-CT and 7 pairs of 3D US-MR cardiac images. The experiments show that a registration based on PEMs is able to estimate more reliable and accurate inter-modality correspondences compared to other state-of-the-art US registration methods.

1   Introduction

In cardiovascular minimally invasive procedures such as mitral valve repair and aortic valve implantation [12], pre-operative surgical plans and roadmaps may be complemented by intra-operative image guidance provided by ultrasound (US) and fluoroscopy. Computed tomography (CT) and magnetic resonance imaging (MRI) are widely used for planning of cardiovascular interventions since they can provide detailed images of the anatomy which are not usually visible in intra-operative cardiac US images. As the shape and pose of the heart changes over time during the intervention (e.g. due to respiration and patient motion), registration and fusion of pre- and intra-operative images can be a useful technology to improve the quality of image guidance during the intervention and subsequent clinical outcome. However, the difference in appearance of the heart in the different image modalities makes multimodal US image registration a challenging problem. In particular, the choice of an appropriate multimodal image similarity metric can be considered as the main challenge.

© Springer International Publishing Switzerland 2015
N. Navab et al. (Eds.): MICCAI 2015, Part II, LNCS 9350, pp. 363–371, 2015.
DOI: 10.1007/978-3-319-24571-3_44

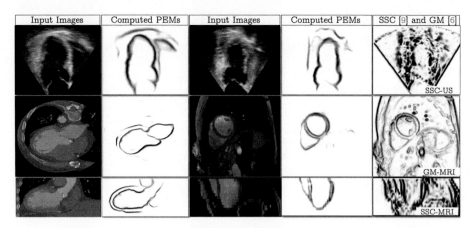

| Input Images | Computed PEMs | Input Images | Computed PEMs | SSC [9] and GM [6] |

Fig. 1. Example of PEMs, obtained from cardiac images of different modalities, are compared to gradient magnitude (GM) and self-similarity descriptors (SSC). Since SSC is a vectorial descriptor, only a single component of SSC is visualized.

Related Work: Current approaches for multi-modal US registration can be classified into two categories: (i) those using global and local information theoretic measures, and (ii) those reducing the multi-modal problem to a mono-modal problem. Early approaches in the first category suggested the use of normalized mutual information (NMI) [16] as a multimodal similarity metric. Recently, local similarity measures were proposed as an alternative to the global similarity measures. This reflects the fact that the US image characteristics show local variations due to wave reflections at tissue boundaries. Measures such as local NMI (LNMI) [10] and local correlation coefficient (LCC) [6] are designed to deal with this non-stationary behaviour. The second category of approaches converts the images from different modalities into a common feature space so that a mono-modal registration can be performed. In [11], fetal US and MR brain images are registered by generating pseudo-US images from MRI tissue segmentations. Other approaches, such as local phase [17], gradient orientations [4], and self-similarity descriptors (SSC) [9], generate similar structural representations from images to find correspondences between different imaging modalities.

Contributions: This paper proposes the use of probabilistic edge map (PEM) image representation for multi-modal US image registration. In contrast to local phase, SSC and gradient magnitude [6] (GM) representations, PEMs highlight only the image structures that are relevant for the image registration. This is because some of the anatomical structures visible in US images may not be visible in CT/MR images and vice versa, e.g. endocardial trabeculae, clutter, and shadowing artefacts. Therefore, extracting and registering only the left ventricle (LV) and atrial boundaries is a more robust approach than registering every voxel in the images. Moreover, PEMs generate a clear and accurate tissue boundary delineations, Fig. 1, in comparison to other image representations. This improvement produces better spatial alignment and increases the

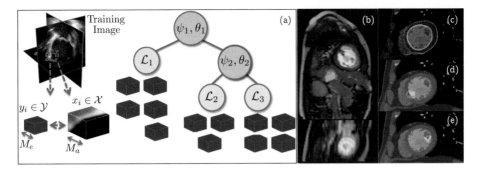

Fig. 2. Structured decision tree training procedure, label patches are clustered at each node split (a). Mid-ventricle (b), mid-septal (d) and mid-lateral (e) wall landmark localization by using PEMs (in green)(c) and regression nodes.

robustness to noise which is important in US image registration. Additionally, PEMs are invariant under rigid transformations, unlike SSC descriptors. Thus they can cope with large rotational differences between images. Lastly, the proposed approach does not require tissue segmentations and can be generalized to other organs and modalities differing from the simulation based registration methods.

The proposed generic and modality independent representation is generated by a structured decision forest [5]. PEMs from different modalities are aligned with a block matching algorithm based on robust statistics followed by a deformable registration. The proposed registration framework is evaluated on US/CT and US/MR image pairs acquired from different pathological groups. The results show that PEM achieves lower registration errors compared to other image similarity metrics. This observation shows that PEM is a well-suited image representation for multimodal US image registration.

2   Methods

Probabilistic Edge Map (PEM) Representation: Cardiac US images mainly show the anatomy of the cardiac chambers and less detail of soft tissues. Therefore, further processing of these images, e.g. registration, requires a structural representation of the cardiac chamber boundaries such as the left ventricle (LV). In this work, a structural representation, PEM, is generated from a structured decision forest (SDF). Learning the image representation from training data increases the robustness in US images and allows the registration to focus on the organs of interest. As can be seen in Fig. 1, the PEMs outline only the LV and atrium while ignoring irrelevant anatomical boundaries. In addition the generated boundaries are cleaner and smoother.

PEMs are modality independent; as such the same representation can be generated from different modalities. More importantly, a single training configuration can be applied to train SDFs for all modalities, including the same image feature types and patch sizes. While SDFs are very similar to decision forests, they possess several unique properties. In particular, in SDFs the output space $\mathcal{Y}$ is defined by structured segmentation labels $\boldsymbol{y}_i \in \mathcal{Y}$ rather than a single label $y_i \in \{0,1\}$. SDF decision trees can be trained as long as the high-dimensional structural labels can be clustered into two or more subgroups at each tree node split ψ_j as illustrated in Fig. 2. This is achieved by mapping each patch label to an intermediate space $(\Theta : \mathcal{Y} \rightarrow \mathcal{Z})$ where label clusters can be generated based on their pairwise Euclidean distances in $\mathcal{Z}$ (cf. [5]). Once the training is completed, each leaf node $\mathcal{L}_j$ stores a segmentation patch label $\boldsymbol{y}_i \in \mathbb{Z}^{(M_e)^3}$ of size $(M_e)^3$. Additionally, the corresponding edge map $\boldsymbol{y}_i' \in \{0,1\}^{(M_e)^3}$ is stored as well. This allows predictions to be combined simply by averaging during inference.

Similar to decision forests, the input space $\mathcal{X}$ for the SDFs is characterized by the high dimensional appearance features $(\boldsymbol{x}_i \in \mathcal{X})$ extracted from image patches of fixed size $(M_a)^3$. These features are computed in a multi-scale fashion and correspond to intensity values, gradient magnitudes, six HoG-like channels, and local phase features. The weak learner parameters $(\boldsymbol{\theta}_j)$, e.g. stump threshold value and selected feature channel id, are optimized to maximize Shannon entropy $\mathcal{H}_1$ based information gain $\mathcal{I}(S_j) = \mathcal{H}_1(S_j) - \sum_{k \in \{L,R\}} \frac{|S_j^k|}{|S_j|} \mathcal{H}_1(S_j^k)$ at each node split. Here $S_j = \{\mathcal{T}_i = (\boldsymbol{x}_i, \boldsymbol{y}_i)\}$ is a set of patch labels and features reaching node j. During the PEM generation (testing time), each input voxel accumulates $N_t \times (M_e)^3$ overlapping binary edge votes $\boldsymbol{y}_i'$ from N_t number of trained decision trees. These predictions are later averaged to yield a probabilistic edge response. Spatial aggregation of a large number of edge votes results in a smoother and accurate delineation of the structures of interest.

Structured Regression Forest Based Initialization: The presented SDF can be modified to allow additionally for simultaneous voting for predefined landmark locations such as the apex, mid-lateral and mid-septal walls, as shown in Fig. 2. Each landmark point is detected independently in both target and source images. This can be used to obtain an initial rigid alignment as a starting point for the registration. Similar to Hough forests [7], classification nodes ψ_j are combined with regression nodes Λ_j in the tree structure. In this way, in addition to the patch labels $\boldsymbol{y}_i$, each leaf node contains an average location offset $\boldsymbol{d}_i^n$ and confidence weight σ_i^n for each landmark $n \in \{1, \ldots, N\}$ (cf. [3]). Inclusion of these nodes does not introduce any significant computational cost at testing time but adds additional information about the location of the landmarks.

The set of offsets $\mathcal{D}_i = (\boldsymbol{d}_i^1, \ldots, \boldsymbol{d}_i^N)$ in the training samples $\mathcal{T}_i = (\boldsymbol{x}_i, \boldsymbol{y}_i, \mathcal{D}_i)$, is defined only for the voxels close to the boundaries of the ventricle. At each regression node Λ_j, the offset distributions are modelled with a multivariate Gaussian. The differential entropy of these distributions [3] is used as the uncertainty measure $\mathcal{H}_2$ in the training of Λ_j. In training, classification and regression nodes are selected randomly [7]. During testing, landmark location votes are weighted by the confidence weights and edge probabilities of the voxels.

Global Alignment of PEMs: Similar to [11], a block matching approach is used to establish spatial correspondences between the PEMs (Fig. 3), where

Input cardiac images CT and 3D-US	Generated PEMs	Initial spatial overlay of intensity images and PEMs	Spatial overlay after PEM – Linear block matching	Final overlay after PEM – LCC Non-rigid registration

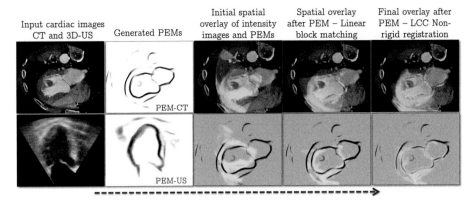

Fig. 3. A block diagram of the proposed multi-modal image registration method.

the normalized cross correlation (NCC) is used as a measure of similarity. As suggested in [13], the set of displacement vectors computed between the corresponding PEM blocks are regularized with least-trimmed squared regression before estimating the global rigid transformation R. In this way, the influence of image blocks with no correspondences is removed, reducing the potential registration error introduced by shadowing or limited field-of-view in US images.

Non-rigid Alignment of PEMs: To correct for the residual misalignment, due to cardiac and respiratory motion, between target (P^T) and source (P^S) PEMs, B-spline FFD [14] based non-rigid alignment follows the global rigid registration. The total energy function, minimized with conjugate-gradient descent optimization, is defined as: $E(T) = -LCC(P^T, P^S \circ T \circ R) + \lambda BE(T)$, where λ is the trade-off between the local correlation coefficient [2] (LCC) similarity metric and bending energy regularization (BE). As the SDF classifier makes use of intensity values, local intensity variations in US images influence the edge probabilities in PEMs. For this reason, a local similarity measure is more suitable for PEMs than a global measure such as sum of squared differences. For similar reasons, LCC was used in [6] to align US-MR gradient magnitude images.

3   Experiments and Results

The proposed PEM registration framework is evaluated on 3D US-CT (10 pairs) and 3D US-MR (7 pairs) cardiac images. The CT images were acquired pre-operatively from adults after a contrast injection. The corresponding trans-esophageal US images were acquired during the cardiac procedure. In the second dataset, lower quality trans-thoracic US acquisitions are registered with multi-slice, cine-MR images (slice thickness 8 mm). Five of these pairs were acquired from children diagnosed with hypoplastic left heart syndrome and the rest from healthy adults. As a preprocessing step, all the images are denoised using non-local means [1] and resampled to isotropic voxel size of 0.80 mm per dimension.

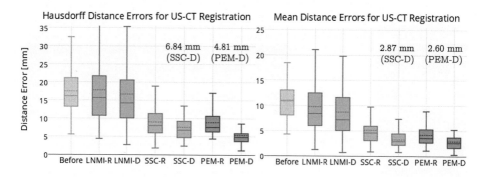

Fig. 4. US/CT registration errors after rigid (R) and deformable (D) alignment. The mean and median values are shown in dashed and solid lines respectively.

In both experiments, PEM-LCC registration performance is compared with LNMI [10] and SSC [9] similarity based registration methods. Implementations of these methods were obtained from their corresponding authors. Particularly, in the SSC method, linear registration of the descriptors is performed by using least-trimmed squares of point-to-point correspondences for improved robustness. In the local alignment of SSC, a discrete optimization scheme (deeds [8]) is used to optimize SSC energy function. In LNMI, histograms with 64 bins are built locally and the registration is optimized using stochastic gradient descent. The number of bins is optimized for best performance.

In all three modalities, PEMs are generated and evaluated with the same training, testing and registration parameters. A PEM-SDF classifier was trained for each modality with set of cardiac images (50-80 images/modality) that is disjoint from the test set (17 pairs). It is important to highlight that the images from different modalities are not required to be spatially registered or come from the same subjects because the classifiers are trained separately for each modality. This significantly increases the availability of training data. The training data contains labels for myocardium, LV endocardium and atrium. The registration results are evaluated based on mean and Hausdorff distances of seven landmark points in the US images to closest points on the manually annotated LV endo-cardial surface in CT and MR images. The landmark points correspond to: apex, apical (2), basal (2), and mid-ventricle (2). For each method, the distances are computed after rigid and deformable alignment, and they are reported together with their values before the registration. For each image pair, 10 different registrations were performed with random global transformations for initialization.

US/CT Evaluation Results: The registration errors, provided in Fig. 4, show that local intensity statistics based similarity measures do not perform consistently and in some cases the registration fails to converge to the correct solution. This suggests that structural representation methods, such as PEMs and SSC,

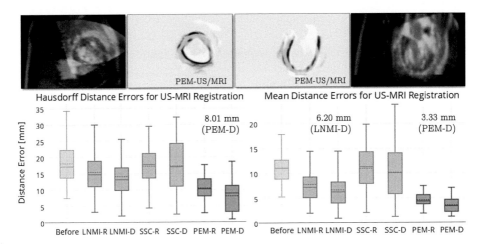

Fig. 5. Global alignment of US/MR images (top). The boxplot shows the US/MR landmark distance errors after rigid (*R*) and deformable (*D*) alignment.

are more reliable measures in US/CT image registration. On the other hand, after local alignment, PEMs achieve lower registration errors compared to SSC, which can be linked to the accurate and smooth boundary representation provided by PEMs. As shown in Fig. 1, PEMs are less sensitive to noise and follow the anatomical boundaries more accurately.

US/MRI Evaluation Results: It is observed that the SSC descriptors do not provide enough guidance in alignment of MR images acquired from children. As shown in Fig. 5, the images contain more texture due to smaller size of the heart and trabeculae in transthoracic acquisitions. In contrast to this, PEM relies on annotations of the boundaries used in the training. It is able to generate a more accurate structural representation that is better matching with the myocardial boundary in MR images. The performance difference, shown in Fig. 5, is explained with this observation.

Experimental Details: All experiments were carried out on a 3.00 GHz quad-core CPU. The average computation time per registration was 73s for non-rigid registration, 21s for rigid alignment and 20s to compute each PEM. The training of the SDFs (70 min/tree) was performed offline prior to the registrations.

Discussion: In the experiments, after spatially aligning US/CT and US/MR images, we observed that the endocardial annotations in US images underestimate the LV volume compared to the annotated CT and MR images. In a clinical study [15], US volume measurement errors and underestimation were linked to the visible endocardial trabeculae. Therefore, to obtain matching PEM correspondences between the modalities, the US annotations are morphologically dilated before the training of the SDF. In contrast, the other structural representation techniques are expected to fail to achieve optimal local alignment accuracy as these tissues are not visible in CT and MR images (Fig. 5).

4   Conclusion

In this paper, a novel PEM image representation technique and its application on US multi-modality image registration has been presented. The experimental results show that PEM provides a more accurate and consistent registration performance between different modalities compared to the state-of-the-art methods. Therefore, we can conclude that PEM is more suitable for image-guided cardiac interventions where alignment of pre-operative images to inter-operative images is required. Moreover, PEM is a generic and modular image representation method; it can be applied to any other US, CT and MR image analysis problem.

References

1. Buades, A., Coll, B., Morel, J.M.: A non-local algorithm for image denoising. In: IEEE Conference on Computer Vision and Pattern Recognition, pp. 60–65 (2005)
2. Cachier, P., Pennec, X.: 3D non-rigid registration by gradient descent on a Gaussian windowed similarity measure using convolutions. In: IEEE Workshop on Mathematical Methods in Biomedical Image Analysis, pp. 182–189 (2000)
3. Criminisi, A., Shotton, J., Robertson, D., Konukoglu, E.: Regression forests for efficient anatomy detection and localization in CT studies. In: Menze, B., Langs, G., Tu, Z., Criminisi, A. (eds.) MICCAI 2010 Workshop MCV. LNCS, vol. 6533, pp. 106–117. Springer, Heidelberg (2011)
4. De Nigris, D., Collins, D.L., Arbel, T.: Multi-modal image registration based on gradient orientations of minimal uncertainty. IEEE TMI 31(12), 2343–2354 (2012)
5. Dollár, P., Zitnick, C.L.: Structured forests for fast edge detection. In: IEEE International Conference on Computer Vision, pp. 1841–48 (2013)
6. Fuerst, B., Wein, W., Müller, M., Navab, N.: Automatic ultrasound - MRI registration for neurosurgery using the 2D and 3D LC^2 metric. MedIA (2014)
7. Gall, J., Lempitsky, V.: Class-specific hough forests for object detection. In: IEEE Conference on Computer Vision and Pattern Recognition (2009)
8. Heinrich, H., Jenkinson, M., Brady, M., Schnabel, J.A.: MRF-based deformable registration and ventilation estimation of lung CT. IEEE TMI, 1239–48 (2013)
9. Heinrich, M.P., Jenkinson, M., Papież, B.W., Brady, S.M., Schnabel, J.A.: Towards realtime multimodal fusion for image-guided interventions using self-similarities. In: Mori, K., Sakuma, I., Sato, Y., Barillot, C., Navab, N. (eds.) MICCAI 2013, Part I. LNCS, vol. 8149, pp. 187–194. Springer, Heidelberg (2013)
10. Klein, S., van der Heide, U.A., Lips, I.M., van Vulpen, M., Staring, M., Pluim, J.P.: Automatic segmentation of the prostate in 3D MR images by atlas matching using localized mutual information. Medical Physics 35(4), 1407–1417 (2008)
11. Kuklisova-Murgasova, M., Cifor, A., Napolitano, R., Papageorghiou, A., Quaghebeur, G., Rutherford, M.A., Hajnal, J.V., Noble, J.A., Schnabel, J.A.: Registration of 3D fetal neurosonography and MRI. MedIA 17(8), 1137–1150 (2013)
12. Nguyen, C.T., Lee, E., Luo, H., Siegel, R.J.: Echocardiographic guidance for diagnostic and therapeutic percutaneous procedures. Cardiovasc. Diagn. Ther. (2011)
13. Ourselin, S., Roche, A., Pennec, X., Ayache, N.: Reconstructing a 3D structure from serial histological sections. Image and Vision Computing 19(1), 25–31 (2001)
14. Rueckert, D., Sonoda, L., Hayes, C., Hill, D.L., Leach, M., Hawkes, D.J.: Nonrigid registration using free-form deformations: Application to breast MR images. IEEE T. Med. Imaging 18(8), 712–721 (1999)

15. Shernand, S.: Evaluation of the left ventricular size and function. In: Comprehensive Atlas of 3D Echocardiography. Lippincott Williams and Wilkins (2012)
16. Studholme, C., Hill, D.L., Hawkes, D.J.: An overlap invariant entropy measure of 3D medical image alignment. Pattern Recognition 32(1), 71–86 (1999)
17. Zhang, W., Noble, J.A., Brady, J.M.: Spatio-temporal registration of real time 3D ultrasound to cardiovascular MR sequences. In: Ayache, N., Ourselin, S., Maeder, A. (eds.) MICCAI 2007, Part I. LNCS, vol. 4791, pp. 343–350. Springer, Heidelberg (2007)

A Hierarchical Bayesian Model for Multi-Site Diffeomorphic Image Atlases

Michelle Hromatka[1], Miaomiao Zhang[1], Greg M. Fleishman[2,3],
Boris Gutman[2], Neda Jahanshad[2], Paul Thompson[2], and P. Thomas Fletcher[1]

[1] School of Computing, University of Utah, Salt Lake City, UT, USA
[2] Imaging Genetics Center, University of Southern California,
Marina del Rey, CA, USA
[3] Dept. of Bioengineering, University of California, Los Angeles, CA, USA

Abstract. Image templates, or atlases, play a critical role in imaging studies by providing a common anatomical coordinate system for analysis of shape and function. It is now common to estimate an atlas as a deformable average of the very images being studied, in order to provide a representative example of the particular population, imaging hardware, protocol, etc. However, when imaging data is aggregated across multiple sites, estimating an atlas from the pooled data fails to account for the variability of these factors across sites. In this paper, we present a hierarchical Bayesian model for diffeomorphic atlas construction of multi-site imaging data that explicitly accounts for the inter-site variability, while providing a global atlas as a common coordinate system for images across all sites. Our probabilistic model has two layers: the first consists of the average diffeomorphic transformations from the global atlas to each site, and the second consists of the diffeomorphic transformations from the site level to the individual input images. Our results on multi-site datasets, both synthetic and real brain MRI, demonstrate the capability of our model to capture inter-site geometric variability and give more reliable alignment of images across sites.

1 Introduction

Recent years have seen a movement towards combining neuroimaging data collected across multiple sites. Such multi-site data has the potential to accelerate scientific discovery by providing increased sample sizes, broader ranges of participant demographics, and publicly available data. Different approaches include large, coordinated multi-site neuroimaging studies, such as the Alzheimer's Disease Neuroimaging Initiative (ADNI) [7], as well as data sharing initiatives that combine multiple independent single-site studies, such as the Autism Brain Imaging Data Exchange (ABIDE) [3]. Larger sample sizes are especially critical in genome-wide association studies (GWAS), in order to provide sufficient statistical power to test millions of genetic variants. This requires aggregation across a broad range of neuroimaging studies, such as those involved in the Enhancing NeuroImaging Genetics through Meta-Analysis (ENIGMA) consortium [10]. Analysis using these multi-site data sets, however, is not straightforward. Styner

© Springer International Publishing Switzerland 2015
N. Navab et al. (Eds.): MICCAI 2015, Part II, LNCS 9350, pp. 372–379, 2015.
DOI: 10.1007/978-3-319-24571-3_45

et al. [9] compared intra- and inter-site variability by analyzing variability of tissue and structural volumes of the same subject imaged twice at each of five sites. This analysis showed that, regardless of segmentation approach, there was always higher inter-site variability, most notably when those sites used different brands of MRI scanner. In large multi-site studies, there are possibly multiple confounding factors across sites, including different MRI scanners, protocols, populations, and diagnosis techniques.

A common first step in neuroimage analysis is to register all images to a common coordinate system, or atlas, often generated as an unbiased deformable average of the input images themselves. When dealing with multi-site image data, one possibility is to pool the images from all of the sites and estimate an atlas. However, treating multi-site data as a single, homogeneous dataset fails to account for the variability across sites, which can be detrimental to the statistical power and counteract the gains made by increasing the sample size. Another option is to carry out individual image processing and statistical analyses at each site, and combine the statistical results in a post hoc meta-analysis. While this can be an effective way to combine statistical tests of low-dimensional summary measures, it is not applicable to problems on high-dimensional data, such as images, without first learning and establishing a common coordinate frame between the pooled datasets.

We present a hierarchical Bayesian model to estimate atlases on multi-site imaging data, which controls for the inter-site variability, while providing a common coordinate system for analysis. This builds on methods presented in [12], where the large deformation diffeomorphic metric mapping (LDDMM) problem is formulated as a probabilistic model, and the transformations between the atlas and individual images are considered random variables. To build an atlas from multi-site image data, we propose to add an additional layer in this probabilistic model to account for systematic geometric differences between imaging sites, resulting in concatenated transformations, one site-specific, one subject-specific, which describe the deformation of a subject's image to the estimated atlas. Bayesian inference is performed through an iterative, *maximum a posteriori* (MAP) estimate of the random variables until convergence conditions are met. We demonstrate that the resulting model reduces the confounding inter-site variability, and results in improved statistical power in a statistical analysis of brain shape.

2   Background

Single Site Bayesian Atlas Building. We will work within the framework of large deformation diffeomorphic metric mapping (LDDMM) [1], as it provides a rigorous setting for defining a distance metric on deformations between images. The atlas building problem in LDDMM can be phrased as a minimization of the sum-of-squared distances function from the atlas to the input images. Images are treated as L^2 functions on a compact image domain Ω. The diffeomorphism registering the atlas image $A \in L^2(\Omega, \mathbb{R})$ to the input image $I_k \in L^2(\Omega, \mathbb{R})$

will be denoted $\phi_k \in \mathrm{Diff}(\Omega)$. It is given by the flow of a time-varying velocity field, $v_k(t) \in C^\infty(T\Omega)$. In the geodesic shooting framework, this velocity field is governed by the geodesic shooting equation on $\mathrm{Diff}(\Omega)$. As such, it is sufficient to represent a geodesic by its velocity at $t = 0$. Thus, we will simplify notation by excluding the time variable, and write $v_k = v_k(0)$. Given this setup, the atlas building problem seeks to minimize the energy

$$E(v_k, A) = \sum_{k=1}^{N}(Lv_k, v_k) - \frac{1}{\sigma^2}\sum_{k=1}^{N}\|A \circ \phi_k^{-1} - I_k\|_{L^2}^2, \tag{1}$$

where L is a Riemannian metric on velocities, given by a self-adjoint differential operator that controls the regularity of the transformations, and σ^2 is the image noise variance.

Zhang et al. [12] describe a Bayesian interpretation of this diffeomorphic atlas building problem, where the initial velocities, v_k, become latent random variables. In the Bayesian setting, the regularization term on v_k is the log-prior and the image match term is the log-likelihood. We will adopt this probabilistic interpretation, as it allows us to define a hierarchical Bayesian model for multi-site atlas building.

Geodesic Shooting of Diffeomorphisms. In the interest of space, we will give a very brief description of geodesic shooting in the space of diffeomorphisms. Given an initial velocity $v \in C^\infty(T\Omega)$, the evolution of the velocity along a geodesic path is given by the Euler-Poincaré equations (EPDiff) [6],

$$\frac{\partial v}{\partial t} = -K\,\mathrm{ad}_v^*\,m = -K\left[(Dv)^T m + Dm\,v + m\,\mathrm{div}\,v\right], \tag{2}$$

where D denotes the Jacobian matrix, and $K = L^{-1}$. The operator ad^* is the dual of the negative Lie bracket of vector fields,

$$\mathrm{ad}_v\,w = -[v, w] = Dvw - Dwv.$$

The EPDiff equation (2) results in a time-varying velocity $v_t : [0, 1] \to V$, which is integrated in time by the rule $(d\phi_t/dt) = v_t \circ \phi_t$ to arrive at the geodesic path, $\phi_t \in \mathrm{Diff}^s(\Omega)$.

3   Hierarchical Bayesian Model

We now present our hierarchical Bayesian model for multi-site atlas estimation. The input are images I_{ik}, where $i = 1, \ldots, S$ represents the site index and $k \in 1, \ldots, N_i$ represents the subject index at site i. The goal is to estimate a common atlas image for all sites, $A \in L^2(\Omega, \mathbb{R})$, and simultaneously capture the geometric differences between sites. We represent the inter-site variability as a set of site-specific deformations, ϕ_i, which, when composed with A, describe site-specific atlases, $A \circ \phi_i^{-1}$. The site-specific atlas is then deformed by the

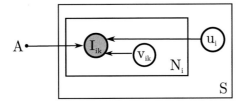

Fig. 1. The hierarchical Bayesian model for multi-site atlas estimation.

individual-level diffeomorphism, ψ_{ik}, to arrive at the final registration of the atlas, $A \circ \phi_i^{-1} \circ \psi_{ik}^{-1}$, to the input image I_{ik}. As above, we will use the initial geodesic velocity to capture a diffeomorphism: denote u_i for the intial velocity of ϕ_i and v_{ik} for that of ψ_{ik}. This approach gives rise to a hierarchical Bayesian model, shown in Figure 1, which decomposes the diffeomorphic transformation from the atlas A to the individual image I_{ik} into the site-specific initial velocity, u_i, and the subject-specific initial velocity, v_{ik}.

In order to estimate the u_i, v_{ik} in the Bayesian setting, we need to define priors on our random variables:

$$u_i \sim N(0, L^{-1})$$
$$v_{ik} \sim N(0, L^{-1}),$$

where $L = (-\alpha \Delta + I)^c$, the same value discussed in Section 2.

Our model assumes i.i.d. Gaussian image noise, yielding the likelihood:

$$p(I_{ik}|v_{ik}, u_i, A) \sim \prod_{k \in N_i} N(A \circ \phi_i^{-1} \circ \psi_{ik}^{-1}, \sigma^2). \tag{3}$$

While it is not readily apparent that v_{ik}, u_i are related in the priors, these two variables are conditionally dependent, as seen in the head-to-head nature of the sub-model involving v_{ik}, I_{ik}, u_i. When I_{ik} are also random variables, v_{ik} and u_i are independent; when I_{ik} is observed, this introduces a link between v_{ik}, u_i and they are now dependent in their respective posterior distributions:

$$\ln \; p(v_{ik}|I_{ik}, A, u_i; \sigma) \propto -(Lv_{ik}, v_{ik}) - \frac{1}{2\sigma^2}\|A \circ \phi_i^{-1} \circ \psi_{ik}^{-1} - I_{ik}\|^2, \tag{4}$$

$$\ln \; p(u_i|I_{ik}, A, v_{ik}; \sigma) \propto -(Lu_i, u_i) - \frac{1}{2\sigma^2}\sum_{k=1}^{N_i}\|A \circ \phi_i^{-1} - I_{ik} \circ \psi_{ik}\|^2|D\psi_{ik}|. \tag{5}$$

Performing Bayesian inference on the system described above could be done in several ways. We have chosen a *maximum a posteriori* (MAP) optimization that alternates between maximizing the posterior equations given in (4) and (5) over v_{ik}, u_i, and the closed-form maximization for A given in (6). Alternatively, we could sample the v_{ik}, u_i using Gibbs sampling on the posteriors in a Monte Carlo expectation maximation (MCEM) procedure. However, the MAP estimate is a mode approximation to the full EM algorithm and sufficient to show the utility of our hierarchical Bayesian model for estimating multi-site image atlases.

We compute the MAP estimates through a gradient ascent procedure in which we alternate between updating the v_{ik} and the u_i, then updating the atlas, A, using an adaptation of the closed form MAP update derived in [12]:

$$A = \frac{\sum_{i \in S} \sum_{k \in N_i} (I_{ik} \circ \psi_{ik} \circ \phi_i) |D(\psi_{ik} \circ \phi_i)|}{\sum_{i \in S} \sum_{k \in N_i} |D(\psi_{ik} \circ \phi_i)|}. \tag{6}$$

This is done iteratively until the energy, $E(v_{ik}, u_i, A)$ converges within reasonable tolerance. In our model, we fix the parameters $\sigma = 0.05$, $\alpha = 3$ and $c = 3$. To compute the gradient w.r.t. the initial velocity v_{ik}, we follow the geodesic shooting algorithm and reduced adjoint Jacobi fields from Bullo [2]. We first forward integrate the geodesic evolution equation (2) along time points $t \in [0, 1]$, and generate the diffeomorphic deformations by $(d/dt)\phi(t, x) = v(t, \phi(t, x))$. The gradient at $t = 1$ is computed as

$$\nabla_{v_{ik}} \ln p(v_{ik} | I_{ik}, A, u_i; \sigma) = -K \left[\frac{1}{\sigma^2} (A \circ \phi_i^{-1} \circ \psi_{ik}^{-1} - I_{ik}) \cdot \nabla (A \circ \phi_i^{-1} \circ \psi_{ik}^{-1}) \right].$$

We then integrate the gradient above backward to time point $t = 0$ by reduced adjoint Jacobi fields to update the gradient w.r.t. the initial velocity v_{ik}. Similarly for u_i, we compute the gradient at $t = 1$ by

$$\nabla_{u_i} \ln p(u_i | I_{ik}, A, v_{ik}; \sigma) = -K \left[\frac{1}{\sigma^2} (A \circ \phi_i^{-1} - I_{ik} \circ \psi_{ik}) \cdot |D\psi_{ik}| \cdot \nabla (A \circ \phi_i^{-1}) \right].$$

4   Results

We present results from a multi-site neuroimaging dataset as a demonstration of the hierarchical model's ability to capture inter-site variability. Furthermore, we show that controlling for this inter-site variability results in improved statistical characterization of the underlying shape variability due to factors of interest, such as age and diagnosis.

Data. The Autism Brain Imaging Data Exchange (ABIDE) database is an online consortium of MRI and resting-state fMRI data from 17 international sites, resulting in brain imaging data for 539 individuals with an autism spectrum disorder (ASD) and 573 typically developing (TD) controls [3]. These sites vary in scanner type and imaging protocol, among many other variables. From three sites with different scanner brands, we selected 45 age and group matched subjects (15 from each site), including 27 TD and 18 ASD subjects. The MRIs for these subjects were then skull stripped, motion corrected, bias field corrected, rigidly registered, and intensity normalized prior to analysis.

Statistical Comparison. We compared our hierarchical multi-site atlas to a single atlas computed from the pooled data. The results are shown in Figure 2. Notice that the top-level atlas A estimated in the multi-site model is similar to

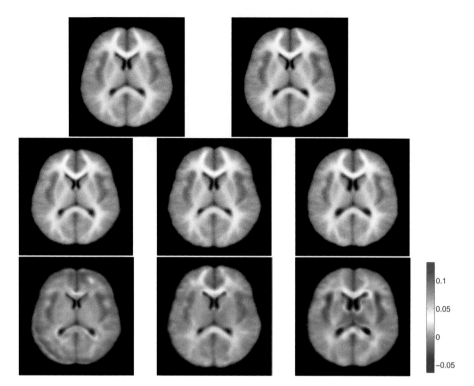

Fig. 2. Axial slices of the estimated atlases: pooled (top left), multi-site (top right), site-specific (middle) and the site-specific atlases overlaid with the log-determinant Jacobian of the site-specific deformations (bottom). A negative value (blue) denotes shrinkage and positive value (red) denotes expansion from the site level to the estimated atlas.

the single atlas from the pooled data. However, our model captures differences between the site-specific atlases, as can be seen in the log-determinant Jacobian maps of the site-specific diffeomorphisms. Similar analysis was performed on the pooled results, using the estimated initial velocities within each site for the estimated pooled atlas to generate the site deformations. This analysis showed that just pooling the data and estimating site-specific deformations yields smaller differences across sites in terms of magnitude and average deformation.

In order to focus on biological shape variability, we can control for the confounding inter-site variability by "removing" the estimated site-specific transformations from our multi-site approach. We do this by adjoint transport of the initial velocity fields, v_{ik}, from the site atlas back to the top-level atlas coordinates, giving transported velocities, $\tilde{v}_{ik} = \mathrm{Ad}_{\phi_i^{-1}} v_{ik}$.

To test if our multi-site atlas is better able to capture age-related and diagnosis-related shape variability, we use partial least squares (PLS) regression on the diagnosis (ASD or TD) and age versus the initial velocity fields $\tilde{v}_{ik}$. PLS seeks to predict a set of dependent variables from a set of independent variables,

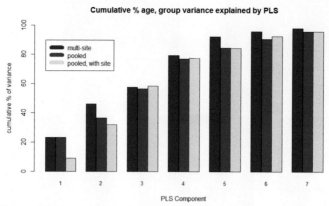

Fig. 3. The cumulative age and group variance (blue, red) or age, group and site (gold) accounted for by each PLS component of the velocity fields.

yielding, among other analyses, what percentage of the variance with respect to the independent variables is accounted for by the dependent variables [11]. In our case, the dependent variables for analyzing the multi-site method are age and diagnosis, and for the pooled method are age, diagnosis and site versus the initial velocity fields. Figure 3 shows that variance in the multi-site velocity field data is able to explain age and diagnosis in fewer PLS components than in the velocities estimated by pooling the data, even when site is included as a dependent variable. Of course with enough dimensions, both methods are able to fully explain the responses, but our hierarchical model explains the variance more efficiently. Additionally, the total variance of the system described by PLS on the multi-site data was nearly 14% lower than the total variance on pooled data, for totals of 1129056 and 1305985 respectively. This shows that our proposed hierarchical model is able to more efficiently capture biological variability in shape of the multi-site ABIDE dataset by reducing the overall inter-site variance.

5   Conclusion

We have presented a novel approach to the problem of multi-site atlas estimation and shown its utility in reducing the variability of high-dimensional, multi-site imaging data. Our hierarchical Bayesian model captures inter-site variability in site-specific diffeomorphisms which, when composed with diffeomorphisms at the individual level, achieve the final diffeomorphic transformations between the atlas and input images. Our multi-site model was able to reduce overall variability and capture the relevant variability of the data, i.e., that due to age or diagnosis, in fewer PLS components than its pooled atlas counterpart.

We chose to compare our approach to a single atlas on the pooled data due to the prevalence of this approach in the literature, e.g., [4], [8]. An alternative comparison would be to use a multi-atlas [5] on the pooled data to determine if our decrease in variance is due solely to the fact that we are estimating multiple atlases. The difference is that our multi-site atlas directly models and controls for the inter-site variance. We leave comparison to a multi-atlas as future work.

Acknowledgements. This work was supported by NIH Grant R01 MH084795, NSF Grant 1251049, and NSF CAREER Grant 1054057.

References

1. Beg, M.F., Miller, M.I., Trouvé, A., Younes, L.: Computing large deformation metric mappings via geodesic flows of diffeomorphisms. International Journal of Computer Vision 61(2), 139–157 (2005)
2. Bullo, F.: Invariant affine connections and controllability on lie groups. Tech. rep., Geometric Mechanics, California Institute of Technology (1995)
3. Di Martino, A., Yan, C.G., Li, Q., Denio, E., Castellanos, F.X., Alaerts, K., Anderson, J.S., Assaf, M., Bookheimer, S.Y., Dapretto, M., et al.: The autism brain imaging data exchange: towards a large-scale evaluation of the intrinsic brain architecture in autism. Molecular Psychiatry (2013)
4. Jahanshad, N., Kochunov, P.V., Sprooten, E., Mandl, R.C., Nichols, T.E., et al.: Multi-site genetic analysis of diffusion images and voxelwise heritability analysis: a pilot project of the enigma–dti working group. Neuroimage 81, 455–469 (2013)
5. Leporé, N., Brun, C., Chou, Y.Y., Lee, A., Barysheva, M., De Zubicaray, G.I., et al.: Multi-atlas tensor-based morphometry and its application to a genetic study of 92 twins. In: 2nd MICCAI Workshop on Mathematical Foundations of Computational Anatomy, pp. 48–55 (2008)
6. Miller, M.I., Trouvé, A., Younes, L.: Geodesic shooting for computational anatomy. Journal of Mathematical Imaging and Vision 24(2), 209–228 (2006)
7. Mueller, S.G., Weiner, M.W., Thal, L.J., Petersen, R.C., Jack, C.R., Jagust, W., Trojanowski, J.Q., Toga, A.W., Beckett, L.: Ways toward an early diagnosis in Alzheimer's disease: The Alzheimer's Disease Neuroimaging Initiative (ADNI). Alzheimer's & Dementia 1(1), 55–66 (2005)
8. Qiu, A., Miller, M.I.: Multi-structure network shape analysis via normal surface momentum maps. NeuroImage 42(4), 1430–1438 (2008)
9. Styner, M.A., Charles, H.C., Park, J., Gerig, G.: Multisite validation of image analysis methods: assessing intra-and intersite variability. In: Medical Imaging 2002, pp. 278–286. International Society for Optics and Photonics (2002)
10. Thompson, P.M., Stein, J.L., Medland, S.E., Hibar, D.P., Vasquez, A.A., Renteria, M.E., Toro, R., Jahanshad, N., Schumann, G., Franke, B., et al.: The ENIGMA Consortium: large-scale collaborative analyses of neuroimaging and genetic data. Brain Imaging and Behavior 8(2), 153–182 (2014)
11. Wold, H.: Partial least squares. Encyclopedia of Statistical Sciences (1985)
12. Zhang, M., Singh, N., Fletcher, P.T.: Bayesian estimation of regularization and atlas building in diffeomorphic image registration. In: Gee, J.C., Joshi, S., Pohl, K.M., Wells, W.M., Zöllei, L. (eds.) IPMI 2013. LNCS, vol. 7917, pp. 37–48. Springer, Heidelberg (2013)

Distance Networks for Morphological Profiling and Characterization of DICCCOL Landmarks

Yue Yuan[1,*], Hanbo Chen[2,*], Jianfeng Lu[1], Tuo Zhang[2,3], and Tianming Liu[2]

[1] School of Computer Science, Nanjing University of Science and Technology, China
[2] Cortical Architecture Imaging and Discovery, Department of Computer Science and Bioimaging Research Center, The University of Georgia, Athens, GA, USA
[3] School of Automation, Northwestern Polytechnical University, Xi'an, China

Abstract. In recent works, 358 cortical landmarks named Dense Individualized Common Connectivity based Cortical Landmarks (DICCCOLs) were identified. Instead of whole-brain parcellation into sub-units, it identified the common brain regions that preserve consistent structural connectivity profile based diffusion tensor imaging (DTI). However, since the DICCCOL system was developed based on connectivity patterns only, morphological and geometric features were not used. Thus, in this paper, we constructed distance networks based on both geodesic distance and Euclidean distance to morphologically profile and characterize DICCCOL landmarks. Based on the distance network derived from 10 templates subjects with DICCCOL, we evaluated the anatomic consistency of each DICCCOL, identified reliable/unreliable DICCCOLs, and modeled the distance network of DICCCOLs. Our results suggested that the most relative consistent connections are long distance connections. Also, both of the distance measurements gave consistent observations and worked well in identifying anatomical consistent and inconsistent DICCCOLs. In the future, distance networks can be potentially applied as a complementary metric to improve the prediction accuracy of DICCCOLs or other ROIs defined on cortical surface.

Keywords: cortical landmark, DICCCOL, geodesic distance, Euclidean distance, ROIs

1 Introduction

In a previous work, Zhu *et al.* identified 358 brain landmarks that are consistently preserved across individuals named Dense Individualized Common Connectivity based Cortical Landmarks (DICCCOLs) [1]. Instead of whole-brain parcellation into sub-units, these DICCCOLs landmarks aim to identify the common brain regions that preserve consistent structural connectivity profile based diffusion tensor imaging (DTI) (section 2.2). It has been shown that these landmarks can be applied as network nodes that possess correspondence across individuals to investigate brain functional/structural networks [2]. However, despite that it is an important contribution to

---

[*] Co-first authors.

© Springer International Publishing Switzerland 2015
N. Navab et al. (Eds.): MICCAI 2015, Part II, LNCS 9350, pp. 380–387, 2015.
Doi: 10.1007/978-3-319-24571-3_46

human brain mapping field, several limitations of current DICCCOL framework had also been identified [3]. Firstly, different brain anatomic regions may also generate similar DTI derived axonal fiber connection profiles and the proposed tracemap descriptor [1] might not be able to differentiate these brain regions in such cases. Secondly, since DICCCOL is obtained by data driven approaches and the training process only searches the neighbor regions for the optimal locations of DICCCOLs (section 2.2), some DICCCOLs may converge to the local minimum during the search process. Due to these limitations, the same DICCCOL may converge to different anatomical locations during training and prediction process. Though three experts visually inspect the results to eliminate those connectionally or anatomically inconsistent landmarks before generating the finalized DICCCOLs, due to the unavoidable subjective judgments and the experts' possible mistakes, there still might be unreliable ROIs embedded in the template of the current DICCCOL system.

In the literature, distance measurement has been shown to be promising in characterizing brain anatomies. In [4], the geodesic distances (GDs) between landmarks were applied to characterize and extract structures on the cortex. In [5], the authors extracted sulci fundi on cerebral cortex based on the geodesic characteristics. In [6] and [7], the Euclidean distance (ED) was applied to investigate and characterize the spatial relationships between the brain's functional regions. GD is powerful in describing anatomical correlations between cortical landmarks since the neocortex of human brain is highly convoluted and the brain anatomy also correlates with cortical folding patterns in a certain degree (**Fig. 1**(a)). Meanwhile, ED is simple to compute and does not rely on surface reconstruction quality (**Fig. 1**(a)). Since the DICCCOL system was developed mainly based on the connectivity patterns, morphological and geometric features were not used. Therefore, GDs and EDs between DICCCOLs can be possibly applied to construct distance networks as a complementary metric to improve DICCCOL.

By constructing distance networks of DICCCOLs in the 10 templates subjects and comparing the variability and regularity of these 10 networks, we evaluate the anatomical consistency of each DICCCOL, identify reliable/unreliable DICCCOLs, and model the distance network of DICCCOLs. Intriguingly, our result showed that the most consistent distance edges are the long global distance connections while the most inconsistent edges are local connections. Also, the distance networks based ED and GD gave quite similar observations and performed accurately in identifying anatomical consistent or inconsistent DICCCOLs. By adding this distance network as a new constraint of DICCCOL, the reliability of DICCCOL system could be increased in the future in both modeling common cortical landmarks and predicting these landmarks in new subject's brain.

2   Method

2.1   Experimental Data

The DTI data downloaded from DICCCOL website (http://dicccol.cs.uga.edu/) which was applied in the development and the definition of DICCCOLs was applied in this study. As described in Zhu *et al.*'s paper [1], the scans were performed on a GE 3T Sigma MRI system using an 8-channel head coil. The acquisition parameters are: matrix size = 128×128, 60 slices, image resolution = 2×2×2mm isotropic, TR=15s, ASSET=2, 3 B0 images, 30 optimized gradient directions, b-value=0/1000. Acquired data were preprocessed via the preprocessing pipeline of DICCCOL as described in [1] which includes eddy current correction, skull removal, computing FA image [8], GM/WM segmentation [9], WM surface reconstruction [10], and streamline fiber tracking [11].

2.2   DICCCOL

DICCCOLs were originally developed by data-driven approaches [1]. In brief, training subjects were aligned to the same space by linear image registration. 2056 vertices on the reconstructed cortical surfaces were randomly selected as initial ROIs and the correspondence was assigned to the vertices from different subjects that are spatially close to each other. Then each initial ROI was moved around to maximize the similarity of its DTI connection profile to the profile of corresponding ROIs. By doing so iteratively, all those ROIs finally converged to a location that the similarity was maximized. Such process was performed in two groups of subjects independently. Then by comparing the converged ROIs in these two groups based on the quantitative measurement and the advice from three experts, the ones with similarity in both spatial location and connection profile were picked as DICCCOLs. Finally, 358 DICCCOLs were picked and the 10 subjects used for training were taken as the template [1].

To predict DICCCOLs on new individuals, the brain of the individual were rigidly aligned to the templates' space. The location of each DICCCOL in the template brains were taken as the initial location. Then a search was run in its neighborhood [1] on the cortical surface and the location of DICCCOL on the new subject was determined as the region that most resemble the connection profile of the template.

2.3   Geodesic Distance

We applied the method based on fast matching proposed in [5, 12] to find the shortest path between DICCCOLs on the reconstructed cortical surface and estimate geodesic distance between them. Generally, by assigning speed $F(x)$ to each vertex x on surface, a closed curve evolves and expands on the surface starting from a source vertex in a manner of 'wave'. During this procedure, we record the arrival time $T(x)$ of a vertex x that the 'wave' takes to travel from the source vertex. This problem is solved by equation in [2]:

$$|\nabla T(x)|F(x) = 1, x \in S \tag{1}$$

where S represents the surface. In this paper, we set $F(x)$ to be '1' for all vertices, so that arrival time $T(x)$ is equivalent to the geodesic distance between the two vertices.

2.4   Distance Network Variability

For each pair of DICCCOLs, the GD and ED between them were computed. By taking DICCCOLs as network nodes and GD/ED as the edges between nodes, a distance network can be constructed for DICCCOLs in each individual's brain. By examining the consistency of this network between templates, we could evaluate the anatomical consistency of each DICCCOL, identify reliable/unreliable DICCCOLs, and model the distance network of DICCCOLs. The evaluation was performed based on GD network and ED network separately and by comparing the outcome of each network, the performance of ED/GD as distance constrain for cortical landmarks will be discussed. Specifically, the mean value of each edge among 10 template subjects and the corresponding standard deviations were obtained. Intuitively, since GD is larger than ED, the standard deviation of GD is also larger than ED on average which makes it difficult to compare these two measurements. Thus in this paper, we applied relative standard deviation as a measurement of the variability of edges:

$$Var(E) = E_{std}/\overline{E} \qquad (2)$$

where E is the edge to measure, Estd and $\overline{E}$ are the standard deviation and mean of its length.

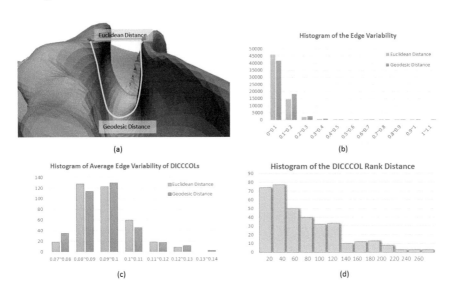

(a)

(b)

(c)

(d)

Fig. 1. (a) Illustration of geodesic distance (GD) and Euclidean distance (ED) between two ROIs. (b) Histogram of the variability of the edges in 10 templates' brains. (c) Histogram of the average edge variability of the DICCCOLs among templates. (d) Histogram of the distance between DICCCOL consistency ranks.

3   Results

Firstly, we compute the DICCCOLs' distance network in the brains of templates. The distributions of the variability of GD and ED are quite similar (Fig. 1(b)). Intriguingly, the most consistent edges are long distance connections while (Fig. 2(a)-(b)) the most inconsistent edges are local connections (Fig. 2(c)-(d)). This is partially due to the relative deviation we applied for analysis. Moreover, the spatial distributions of consistent/inconsistent GD/ED edges are quite similar (Fig. 2, Table 1, Table 2). The edges within occipital lobes are the most inconsistent while the edges between occipital lobes and frontal lobes are the most consistent.

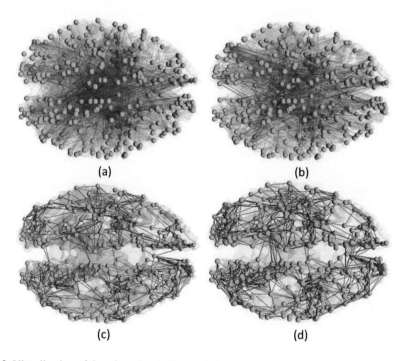

Fig. 2. Visualization of the edges that (a) have relatively small ED variability (<0.04); (b) have relatively small GD variability (<0.04); (c) have relatively large ED variability (>0.3); (d) have relatively large GD variability (>0.3).

Then for each DICCCOL, the average variability of the edges ($\overline{E_{var}}$) connected to it were calculated (Fig. 3). By assuming that the DICCCOLs with consistent anatomy should stay at the same location across brains and thus the edges connected to it should be similar across individuals, those DICCCOLs with smaller $\overline{E_{var}}$ could be more reliable than those with larger $\overline{E_{var}}$. We ranked the DICCCOLs in ascending order based on $\overline{E_{var}}$ of GD and Ed separately. The ranking results are quite similar between two different measurements as revealed by the histogram in Fig. 1(d). To examine and compare the performance of GD and ED in identifying the anatomy consistent and the reliable DICCCOLs, we visualized certain DICCCOLs that are agreed or disagreed by GD/ED on 10 templates' cortical surfaces in **Fig. 4**. DICCCOL #245 is agreed by both measurements to be one of the most consistent landmarks while #290 is agreed to be one of the most inconsistent one. By visual check, #290's location truly varies across templates as highlighted by arrows with different colors, while #245 is relatively consistent across templates. #312/#4 was indicated to be inconsistent by ED/GD only. However, as highlighted by the arrows with different colors, these DICCCOLs are also relatively anatomically inconsistent across templates. These observations suggested that both GD and ED can be applied as distance constraints for brain landmarks and they are complementary to each other.

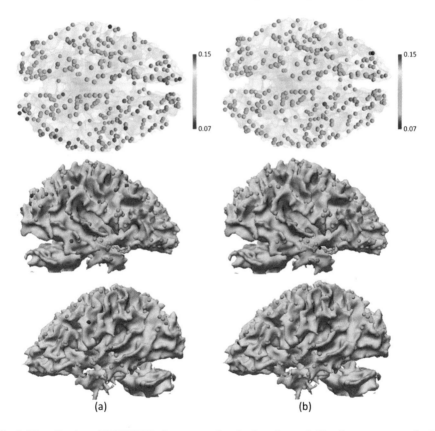

(a)   (b)

Fig. 3. Visualization of DICCCOLs in one template brain color-coded by the average standard deviations of (a) ED or (b) GD from each DICCCOL to the rest DICCCOLs in 10 template subjects.

386   Y. Yuan et al.

Table 1. Average standard deviations of the ED between DICCCOLs within or between lobes.

	Frontal	Parietal	Temporal	Limbic	Occipital
Frontal	0.1130	0.0820	0.0798	0.0952	0.0659
Parietal	0.0820	0.1245	0.0972	0.0839	0.1090
Temporal	0.0798	0.0972	0.1184	0.0960	0.0891
Limbic	0.0952	0.0839	0.0960	0.1497	0.0846
Occipital	0.0659	0.1090	0.0891	0.0846	0.1683

Table 2. Average standard deviations of the GD between DICCCOLs within or between lobes.

	Frontal	Parietal	Temporal	Limbic	Occipital
Frontal	0.1240	0.0898	0.0860	0.0966	0.0720
Parietal	0.0898	0.1412	0.1081	0.0949	0.1314
Temporal	0.0860	0.1081	0.1282	0.1011	0.1020
Limbic	0.0966	0.0949	0.1011	0.1482	0.0993
Occipital	0.0720	0.1314	0.1020	0.0993	0.2029

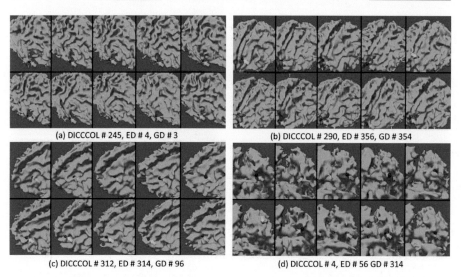

(a) DICCCOL # 245, ED # 4, GD # 3   (b) DICCCOL # 290, ED # 356, GD # 354

(c) DICCCOL # 312, ED # 314, GD # 96   (d) DICCCOL # 4, ED # 56 GD # 314

Fig. 4. Visualization of four DICCCOLs (bubble) on the cortical surfaces of 10 templates. The DICCCOL ID and its consistency rank by different distance measurement are listed below each sub-figure.

4   Conclusion

In this paper, we analyzed the morphological profile and character of DICCCOL landmarks based on distance networks. The distance network based on different distance measurements gave similar observations in our experiments. Intriguingly, the long distance connections are more reliable than local connections. By comparing the consistency of distance networks, the errors and anatomical inconsistent DICCCOLs in the templates were also identified. Since DICCCOL system was developed based on the structural connectivity network, our results showed that distance network could be a useful, complementary metric of the DICCCOL system. In the future, we will improve the reliability of DICCCOL models and the accuracy of DICCCOL prediction by integrating distance network into the DICCCOL framework. And the improved framework will be applied to analyze brain diseases.

Acknowledgements. This research was supported in part by Jiangsu Natural Science Foundation (Project No. BK20131351), by the 111 Project (No.B13022), by National Institutes of Health (R01DA033393, R01AG042599), by the National Science Foundation Graduate Research Fellowship (NSF CAREER Award IIS-1149260, CBET-1302089, BCS-1439051).

References

1. Zhu, D., Li, K., Guo, L., Jiang, X., Zhang, T., Zhang, D., Chen, H., Deng, F., Faraco, C., Jin, C., Wee, C.-Y., Yuan, Y., Lv, P., Yin, Y., Hu, X., Duan, L., Hu, X., Han, J., Wang, L., Shen, D., Miller, L.S., Li, L., Liu, T.: DICCCOL: Dense Individualized and Common Connectivity-Based Cortical Landmarks. Cereb. Cortex (2012)
2. Chen, H., Li, K., Zhu, D., Jiang, X., Yuan, Y., Lv, P., Zhang, T., Guo, L., Shen, D., Liu, T.: Inferring group-wise consistent multimodal brain networks via multi-view spectral clustering. IEEE Trans. Med. Imaging 32, 1576–1586 (2013)
3. Chen, H., Li, K., Zhu, D., Guo, L., Jiang, X., Liu, T.: Group-wise optimization and individualized prediction of structural connectomes. In: ISBI, pp. 742–745. IEEE (2014)
4. Datar, M., Lyu, I., Kim, S., Cates, J., Styner, M.A., Whitaker, R.: Geodesic distances to landmarks for dense correspondence on ensembles of complex shapes. In: Mori, K., Sakuma, I., Sato, Y., Barillot, C., Navab, N. (eds.) MICCAI 2013, Part II. LNCS, vol. 8150, pp. 19–26. Springer, Heidelberg (2013)
5. Li, G., Guo, L., Nie, J., Liu, T.: An automated pipeline for cortical sulcal fundi extraction. Med. Image Anal. 14, 343–359 (2010)
6. Vértes, P.E., Alexander-Bloch, A.F., Gogtay, N., Giedd, J.N., Rapoport, J.L., Bullmore, E.T.: Simple models of human brain functional networks. Proc. Natl. Acad. Sci. U. S. A. 109, 5868–5873 (2012)
7. Alexander-Bloch, A.F., Vértes, P.E., Stidd, R., Lalonde, F., Clasen, L., Rapoport, J., Giedd, J., Bullmore, E.T., Gogtay, N.: The anatomical distance of functional connections predicts brain network topology in health and schizophrenia. Cereb. Cortex 23, 127–138 (2013)
8. Jenkinson, M., Beckmann, C.F., Behrens, T.E., Woolrich, M.W., Smith, S.M.: FSL. Neuroimage 62, 782–790 (2012)
9. Liu, T., Li, H., Wong, K., Tarokh, A., Guo, L., Wong, S.T.C.: Brain tissue segmentation based on DTI data. Neuroimage 38, 114–123 (2007)
10. Liu, T., Nie, J., Tarokh, A., Guo, L., Wong, S.T.C.: Reconstruction of central cortical surface from brain MRI images: method and application. Neuroimage 40, 991–1002 (2008)
11. Toussaint, N., Souplet, J., Fillard, P.: MedINRIA: Medical image navigation and research tool by INRIA. In: MICCAI, pp. 1–8 (2007)
12. Kimmel, R., Sethian, J.A.: Computing geodesic paths on manifolds. Proc. Natl. Acad. Sci. 95, 8431–8435 (1998)

Which Metrics Should Be Used in Non-linear Registration Evaluation?

Andre Santos Ribeiro[1], David J. Nutt[1], and John McGonigle[1]

Centre for Neuropsychopharmacology, Division of Brain Sciences,
Department of Medicine, Imperial College London, UK
j.mcgonigle@imperial.ac.uk

Abstract. Non-linear registration is an essential step in neuroimaging, influencing both structural and functional analyses. Although important, how different registration methods influence the results of these analyses is poorly known, with the metrics used to compare methods weakly justified. In this work we propose a framework to simulate true deformation fields derived from manually segmented volumes of interest. We test both state-of-the-art binary and non-binary, volumetric and surface -based metrics against these true deformation fields. Our results show that surface-based metrics are twice as sensitive as volume-based metrics, but are typically less used in non-linear registration evaluations. All analysed metrics poorly explained the true deformation field, with none explaining more than half the variance.

1 Introduction

Analysis of medical data often requires a precise alignment of subjects' scans with a common space or atlas. This alignment allows the comparison of data across time, subject, image type, and condition, while also allowing its segmentation into different anatomical regions, or find meaningful patterns between different groups [7]. Due to high inter-subject variability, a non-linear deformation of a subject's scan is typically applied to best conform this image to a reference standard. This type of deformation allows for complex modulation, such as elastic or fluid deformations.

The quantification of the accuracy of a non-linear registration is intrinsically complex. The main reason being the lack of a ground truth for the validation of different methods [8]. While in a rigid registration only three non-colinear landmarks are required, in non-linear registration a dense mesh of landmarks is needed [12]. To provide ground truth data the EMPIRE 10 challenge [9] provided correspondences of 100 annotated landmark pairs to distinguish between registration algorithms. However, the precision of the evaluation is still limited by the number of correspondence points. Furthermore, this study focused on intra-subject thoracic CT which may not fully apply across inter-subject studies or other modalities and structures.

Two other main approaches exist to evaluate non-linear registration methods: one based on the simulation of deformation fields; and the other in the evaluation of manually segmented regions in different subjects.

© Springer International Publishing Switzerland 2015
N. Navab et al. (Eds.): MICCAI 2015, Part II, LNCS 9350, pp. 388–395, 2015.
DOI: 10.1007/978-3-319-24571-3_47

In the former, several types of deformation field simulations are suggested, based in the deformation of control points, biomechanical models [2],[3],[13] or Jacobian maps [6],[11]. These techniques can struggle in that they are not capable of simulating the totality of inter-subject variation, nor the artefacts present in medical images.

In the latter, a database of different subjects with both an anatomical image and manually segmented volumes of interest (VOI) is typically used, in which each subject is registered to a randomly chosen subject, or average image, and the calculated deformation applied to the VOI map [4],[15]. In this way, the registered VOI map of the source subject can be compared with the VOIs of the target subject. Typically, to evaluate the different methods a labelling metric is used: Dice coefficients [7]; volume overlap [7],[14]; Jaccard index [10],[12]. This analysis assumes that the metrics evolve in the same way as the unknown deformation field. To our knowledge no study has been performed that effectively compare such metrics with a ground truth such as the true deformation field.

In this study we simulate pairs of deformation fields target images, and evaluate the relation between the different similarity metrics and the true deformation field. We explore what proportion of the variance of the ground truth can be explained by each metric, and which is more suitable when ground truth is not available (such as in inter-subject registration).

2   Methods

2.1   Data Acquisition

20 individual healthy T1 weighted brain images along with cortical and sub-cortical manual segmentations were obtained from the Open Access Series of Imaging Studies (OASIS) project[1]. The manually edited cortical labels follow sulcus landmarks according to the Desikan-Killiany-Tourville (DKT) protocol, with the sub-cortical labels segmented using the NVM software[2]. The resulting maps provide a maximum of 105 regions for each individual.

2.2   True Deformation Field Simulation

The first step of the framework is the simulation of the true deformation field. This field should attempt to maintain the characteristics of the native image such as the overall shape of the head, and absent of foldings. The former is required to remove the effect of global transformations such as affine or purely rigid transformations, while the latter is important as current methods limit the Jacobian determinants (here on referred to as Jacobian) to be positive to provide reasonable fields.

To generate the ground truth deformation fields used in this work the manually segmented images were used to provide an anatomically driven deformation.

---

[1] http://mindboggle.info/data.html
[2] http://neuromorphometrics.org:8080/nvm/

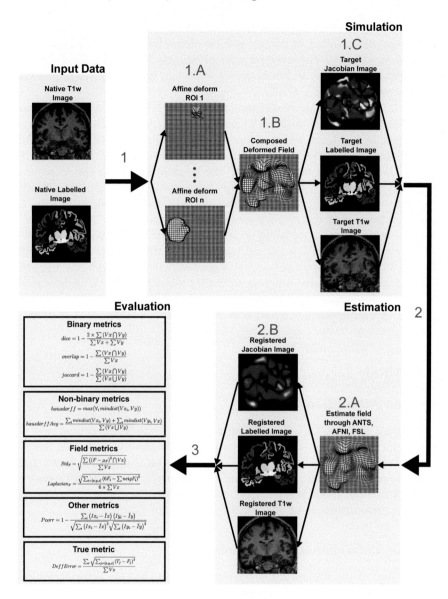

Fig. 1. Scheme of the proposed evaluation framework. 1 - The manually labelled images are input to the simulation block to derive the ground truth deformation fields (1.B), target T1 images and target labelled images (1.C). To generate this field the labels are affine transformed (1.A), combined and regularized (1.B). 2 - The T1 native and target images are passed to the estimation block to estimate the deformation field (2.A), and registered T1 and labelled images (2.B). 3 - The registered and target images are finally given to the evaluation block to evaluate the different metrics against the true deformation field error metric - DeffError. $mindist(x_i, y)$ - minimum Euclidean distance between point x_i and set y. Note that the deformations shown were greatly enhanced for visualization purposes only.

As such, for each segmented image, each of the VOIs was allowed to randomly deform in an affine manner with 12 degrees of freedom. The affine transform of each VOI was normally distributed and centred at the identity transform. The variance for the translation, rotation, scale, and shear parameters were respectively, 1, 1, 0.1, and 0.1. Due to the free deformation of each VOI, the resulting field was regularized by locally smoothing the image such that every voxel presented a Jacobian within a range between 0.125 and 8, with a maximum deformation gradient of 0.5 in every direction. The deformation fields were further limited to retain skull invariance.

For each subject, 20 different ground truth deformation fields were produced, for a total of 400 simulations. For each deformation field a target T1 weighted image was created by deforming the original acquired image with the simulated field.

2.3   Estimation of the Deformation Field

To generate expected deformation fields through non-linear registration algorithms, ANTS-SyN, FSL-FNIRT, and AFNI-3dQwarp were used to register the original T1 to the simulated T1 image.

It should be noted that these methods are being used solely in the evaluation of the different metrics and no comparison between them is made in this work.

For each simulation, a registration was performed by each method and the resulting deformed T1 image and respective segmentation obtained, for a total of 1200 simulations. The Jacobian for each obtained deformation field was also calculated.

2.4   Evaluation of Registration Metrics

For each VOI of the simulations, each metric is calculated to investigate the similarity between the estimated and simulated fields.

Due to their popularity in the evaluation of registration the following metrics were analysed[3]: Dice coefficients (Figure 1 - Dice); Jaccard index (Figure 1 - Jaccard); target overlap (Figure 1 - overlap); Hausdorff distance (Figure 1 - Hausdorff); and Pearson correlation (Figure 1 - Pcorr). Due to the sensitivity of the Hausdorff distance [5], a modified average Hausdorff distance, also called Mean Absolute Distance - MAD [1], is further analysed (Figure 1 - Hausdorff average). This metric uses the average of all the closest distances from the registered to the target VOI, and the target to the registered VOI, instead of relying on a single point to derive the distance metric.

Although not generally used to compare different methods, field smoothness metrics are used to assess whether a particular method provides reasonable deformation fields. The standard deviation, and the Laplacian of both the deformation field, and the derived Jacobian (Figure 1 - std and laplacian) were further calculated. Landmark-based metrics were not included due to the lack of annotations (one-to-one correspondences) in the analysed dataset.

---

[3] All metrics were transformed such as the best value is 0.

Due to the highly folded nature of cortical gray matter, a good surface overlap is usually required. Volume-based metrics may not be suitable for this particular problem. Therefore, all the previously described metrics, with the exception of the Pearson correlation, were further applied to the surfaces of each VOI (i.e. the boundary voxels of the VOI).

For each metric (M) the resultant similarity values were randomly divided into 50 sub-groups (G) of $X = 2000$ VOIs, and linearly and non-linearly correlated with the true deformation field metric (T) (Figure 1 - DeffError) as described below:

1. Select a random subset of X VOIs from the total pool of VOIs;
2. Extract the analysed metrics (M), and the true metric (T), for each X;
3. Apply Pearson's linear correlation (r), and Spearman's rank correlation (ρ) between each M and T;
4. Square both r and ρ to obtain the proportion of shared variance in a linear fit and between the two ranked variables, respectively.
5. Repeat 1 to 4 for each of G sub-groups.
6. Compare the distribution of r^2 and ρ^2 for each M.

In this work the total number of VOIs was (number of subjects × number of simulations per subject × number of regions per subject × number of registration methods) $\approx$ 126,000.

Pearson's r was calculated as it provides a view of the linear relation between the metrics and the true field, while Spearman's ρ only assumes monotonicity and therefore extends the analysis to non-linear correlations.

A full schematic of the proposed framework is presented in Figure 1.

3   Results

In Figure 2 the explained variance (r^2 and ρ^2) of the ground truth deformation field for each of the analysed metrics is shown. All the metrics explain only a fraction (all below 50% for both r^2 and ρ^2) of the total variance present in the true deformation field. Specifically, the surface-based metrics were around twice as sensitive as their volume-based equivalents.

From the binary metrics the Jaccard index showed the highest r^2 (volume: $r^2 = 0.17 \pm 0.02$, surface: $r^2 = 0.32 \pm 0.02$), while in the non-binary metrics the Hausdorff average showed the highest r^2 (volume: $r^2 = 0.29 \pm 0.03$, surface: $r^2 = 0.40 \pm 0.04$). The original Hausdorff distance showed much lower results for both volume and surface metrics (volume: $r^2 = 0.11 \pm 0.02$, surface: $r^2 = 0.11 \pm 0.02$).

For the field metrics, all poorly explained the variance, with the best metric being the standard deviation of the deformation field ($r^2 = 0.08 \pm 0.01$). ρ^2 presented a similar trend to r^2, except between volume and surface versions of the Dice and Jaccard indexes. For these metrics the same ρ^2 was observed (volume: $\rho^2 = 0.22$, surface: $\rho^2 = 0.43$).

Paired t-tests, corrected for multiple comparisons (Bonferroni), were further performed between all metrics. This test was performed as the samples are not independent (i.e. the methods were applied over the same regions), making the distribution seen on Figure 2 only an indication of the difference between methods. The results were in agreement with the previous figure, suggesting that the Hausdorff average is more sensitive overall to changes in the deformation field. The only tests that did not presented significant differences were between the surface Jaccard and Pearson corr, and between the surface Dice and volume Hausdorff average.

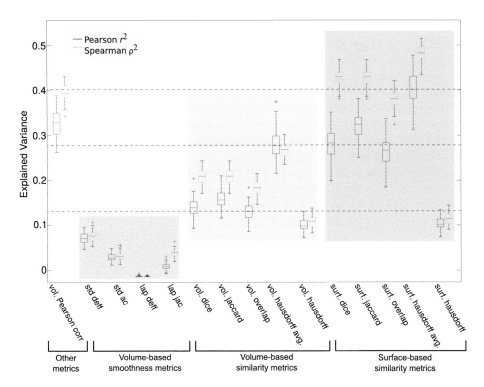

Fig. 2. Boxplot of the explained variance (derived through r^2 and ρ^2) of the true deformation field for each of the analysed metrics. Dark blue boxes - Pearson r^2; Light bashed blue boxes - Spearman ρ^2. Dashed lines serve as reference for the r^2 of the volume overlap metric presented in [7], the best volume-based metric, and the best surface-based metric.

4   Discussion

These results suggest that surface-based metrics are more sensitive to the true deformations than volume-based metrics, both for binary and non-binary metrics. One explanation for such behaviour is that the volume enclosed by a surface does not provide sufficient additional information regarding whether the region is overlapping or not, yet decreases the sensitivity of the metric.

Binary surface metrics are more prone to erroneous evaluations, as a simple shift of the two surfaces (still maintaining a high volume overlap) will lead to an almost null surface overlap.

Non-binary/distance metrics attempt to solve this problem by calculating the distance between the two sets, with the small shift identified either by the distance of each voxel in one set to the closest voxel in the other set, or simply by the center of mass of both sets. This leads to typically more robust metrics than binary ones, as is seen by the Hausdorff average distance. The original Hausdorff distance, however, showed low results for both volume and surface metrics, yet this was expected due to its sensitivity to outliers [5].

Although the Dice and Jaccard indexes differ in the r^2 they showed the same results for the ρ^2. This was also expected as they have the same monotonicity, yet differ in how they are normalized. As a linear trend is usually desirable, the Jaccard index should be used instead of the Dice coefficients.

Interestingly, in these results the Pearson correlation (applied only to the volume-based metrics) showed a much higher sensitivity compared to the volume-based metrics, and was similar to surface-based metrics. Yet this metric may be influenced by noise in the T1 images, and may not be suitable in registering images of different contrasts, such as in inter-modality analysis.

In general these results show that none of the metrics examined here explain more than 50% of the variance of the deformation field. Further, the best metric observed was the Hausdorff average distance (a modified version of the original Hausdorff distance). This poses the question of whether current assumptions based on these metrics hold true with regard to the evaluation of non-linear registration methods.

5   Conclusion

In this work we presented a framework to evaluate currently accepted metrics for comparison of non-linear registration algorithms, and showed that they perform poorly at estimating the true deformation field variance. These results suggest that current assumptions regarding "good" and "bad" methods may not be applicable. Furthermore, although surface-based metrics seem to perform better than volume-based metrics, they are typically less used in non-linear registration comparisons.

References

1. Babalola, K., Patenaude, B., Aljabar, P., Schnabel, J., Kennedy, D., Crum, W., Smith, S., Cootes, T., Jenkinson, M., Rueckert, D.: An evaluation of four automatic methods of segmenting the subcortical structures in the brain. NeuroImage 47, 1435–1447 (2009)
2. Camara, O., Scahill, R., Schnabel, J., Crum, W., Ridgway, G., Hill, D., Fox, N.: Accuracy assessment of global and local atrophy measurement techniques with realistic simulated longitudinal data. Med. Image Comput. Comput. Assist. Interv. 10(2), 785–792 (2007)

3. Camara, O., Schweiger, M., Scahill, R., Crum, W., Sneller, B., Schnabel, J., Ridgway, G., Cash, D., Hill, D., Fox, N.: Phenomenological model of diffuse global and regional atrophy using finite-element methods. IEEE Trans. Med. Imag. 25(11), 1417–1430 (2006)

4. Hellier, P., Barillot, C., Corouge, I., Gibaud, B., Le Goualher, G., Collins, D., Evans, A., Malandain, G., Ayache, N., [...], Johnson, H.: Retrospective evaluation of intersubject brain registration. IEEE Trans. Med. Imag. 22, 1120–1130 (2003)

5. Hyder, A.K., Shahbazian, E., Waltz, E. (eds.): Multisensor Fusion. Springer Science & Business Media (2002)

6. Karaali, B., Davatzikos, C.: Simulation of tissue atrophy using a topology preserving transformation model. IEEE Trans. Med. Imag. 25(5), 649–652 (2006)

7. Klein, A., Andersson, J., Ardekani, B., Ashburner, J., Avants, B., Chiang, M., Christensen, G., Louis Collinsi, D., Geef, J., [...], Parsey, R.: Evaluation of 14 nonlinear deformation algorithms applied to human brain MRI registration. NeuroImage 46, 786–802 (2009)

8. Murphy, K., van Ginneken, B., Klein, S., Staring, M., de Hoop, B.J., Viergever, M.A., Pluim, J.P.W.: Semi-automatic construction of reference standards for evaluation of image registration. Medical Image Analysis 15(1), 71–84 (2011)

9. Murphy, K., Ginneken, B., Reinhardt, J., Kabus, S., Ding, K., Deng, X., Cao, K., Du, K., Christensen, G., [...], Pluim, J.: Evaluation of Registration Methods on Thoracic CT: The EMPIRE10 Challenge. IEEE Trans. Med. Imag. 30(11), 1901–1920 (2011)

10. Ou, Y., Akbari, H., Bilello, M., Da, X., Davatzikos, C.: Comparative evaluation of registration algorithms in different brain databases with varying difficulty: results and insights. IEEE Trans. Med. Imag. 33(10), 2039–2065 (2014)

11. Pieperhoff, P., Sdmeyer, M., Hmke, L., Zilles, K., Schnitzler, A., Amunts, K.: Detection of structural changes of the human brain in longitudinally acquired MR images by deformation field morphometry: methodological analysis, validation and application. NeuroImage 43(2), 269–287 (2008)

12. Rohlfing, T.: Image similarity and tissue overlaps as surrogates for image registration accuracy: widely used but unreliable. IEEE Trans. Med. Imag. 31(2), 153–163 (2012)

13. Schnabel, J., Tanner, C., Castellano-Smith, A., Degenhard, A., Leach, M., Hose, D., Hill, D., Hawkes, D.: Validation of nonrigid image registration using finite-element methods: application to breast MR images. IEEE Trans. Med. Imag. 22(2), 238–247 (2003)

14. Wu, G., Kim, M., Wang, Q., Shen, D.: S-HAMMER: hierarchical attribute-guided, symmetric diffeomorphic registration for MR brain images. Hum. Brain Mapp. 35(3), 1044–1060 (2014)

15. Yassa, M.A., Stark, C.E.L.: A quantitative evaluation of cross-participant registration techniques for MRI studies of the medial temporal lobe. NeuroImage 44, 319–327 (2009)

Modelling and Simulation for Diagnosis and Interventional Planning

Illustrative Visualization of Vascular Models for Static 2D Representations

Kai Lawonn[1,2], Maria Luz[3], Bernhard Preim[1], and Christian Hansen[1]

[1] Otto-von-Guericke University, Germany
[2] TU Delft, Netherlands
[3] TU Berlin, Germany
{lawonn,preim,hansen}@isg.cs.uni-magdeburg.de,
mluz@zmms.tu-berlin.de

Abstract. Depth assessment of 3D vascular models visualized on 2D displays is often difficult, especially in complex workspace conditions such as in the operating room. To address these limitations, we propose a new visualization technique for 3D vascular models. Our technique is tailored to static monoscopic 2D representations, as they are often used during surgery. To improve depth assessment, we propose a combination of supporting lines, view-aligned quads, and illustrative shadows. In addition, a hatching scheme that uses different line styles depending on a distance measure is applied to encode vascular shape as well as the distance to tumors. The resulting visualization can be displayed on monoscopic 2D monitors and on 2D printouts without the requirement to use color or intensity gradients. A qualitative study with 15 participants and a quantitative study with 50 participants confirm that the proposed visualization technique significantly improves depth assessment of complex 3D vascular models.

Keywords: Line and Curve Generation, Visualization, Evaluation, Planning and Image Guidance of Interventions.

1 Introduction

During surgery it is often important to understand the morphology of vascular structures and its spatial relation to surrounding risk structures such as tumors. Therefore, high-quality vascular 3D models, reconstructed from CT, are applied using direct or indirect volume rendering techniques. The vascular models often portray complex geometries and therefore demand cognitive effort and user interaction. Physicians request a visualization technique that can encode essential information such as the location, spatialness, and distances to important anatomical structures. The ideal solution might be to provide one or more static images that encode all relevant information at a glance. These static images might be printed out or displayed on a monitor in order to provide decision support during surgery.

The work of Ritter et al. [7] is closest to our work and is guided by a similar set of requirements and application scenarios. They evaluated non-photorealistic rendering techniques for vascular structures and showed that these techniques facilitate shape and depth assessment. Wang et al. [10] presented a method for depth perception on interventional X-ray images. They improved the rendering scheme and used depth cues that

© Springer International Publishing Switzerland 2015
N. Navab et al. (Eds.): MICCAI 2015, Part II, LNCS 9350, pp. 399–406, 2015.
DOI: 10.1007/978-3-319-24571-3_48

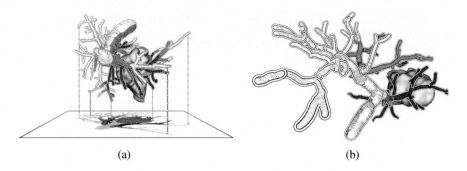

Fig. 1. Our visualization technique applied to hepatic vasculature with a tumor obtained by using [3]. In (a), we use illustrative shadows, supporting lines, and contours as depth cues. In (b), different hatching styles and a decent gray tone emphasize vessels at risk around the tumor.

preserve the original X-ray intensities. Furthermore, methods for depth-based color-coding were proposed, e.g., pseudo-chromadepth by Ropinski et al. [9]. Kersten-Oertel et al. [4] investigated the effect of different perceptual cues for vascular volume visualization and showed that pseudo-chromadepth cues were stronger cues than stereopsis. Because color-coding of depth is not always applicable (e.g. printouts or AR projections on the organ surface) a color-sparse representation of spatial information would be beneficial. We propose a visualization technique that uses as few colors as possible, see Fig. 1. To assess the benefit of our visualization technique, we performed a qualitative study. In addition, a subsequent quantitative study compared our approach with Phong shading [6] and pseudo-chromadepth rendering [9], as it was rated best of different depth cues in previous studies, c.f. [4, 9].

2   Method

To improve depth assessment of 3D vascular models, we present a combination of illustrative shadows, supporting lines and view-aligned quads. A hatching scheme that uses different stroke styles depending on a distance measure is described.

• *Illustrative shadows:* Inspired by Ritter et al. [8], we employed illustrative shadows. For this, we placed a plane under the vascular model. The position of the plane is determined by the center point of the vascular model and it is shifted along the up-vector of the camera such that it does not intersect the model. The up-vector of the camera serves also as the normal of the plane. Afterwards, we place a camera on the opposite direction of the plane to create shadows by an orthographic projection. Frame buffer objects were used to save the scene of the camera and to texture the underlying plane. For the vessel shadows, we use the same grey values as for distance encoding between vessel and tumor in the 3D model in order to illustrate the spatial relations on the plane. We apply hatched strokes to emphasize the projected tumor.

• *Supporting Lines:* As an additional depth cue and reference for the shadows, we introduce supporting lines. Here, we used the idea by Glueck et al. [2] to generate lines from the objects of interest to the plane. The medical expert can select a point on the

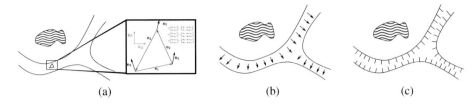

(a)   (b)   (c)

Fig. 2. Overview of the *ConFIS* method. In the first step, the curvature tensor per triangle is determined, see (a). This is used to calculate the principle curvature directions per vertex, see (b). Afterwards, the streamlines are determined, see (c).

surface by picking, and a supporting line is generated that connects the point and the corresponding intersection point of the plane. Along the line, a view-aligned quad is provided. On this quad, we generate texture coordinates to draw a ruler-like illustration. Finally, we generate (x,y) coordinates, where x represents the width of the quad and y lies in the range $[0, L_{line}]$ with L_{line} representing the length of the quad and starting from the plane with $y = 0$. The ruler-like illustration may serve as an indicator for the distance to the plane. Here, we draw a white line with a black contour such that it can be perceived independent of the background color. Therefore, if x lies in a margin around zero, the fragments are drawn white, and for a larger margin, the black color is used. Conceptually, we generated the coordinate system (x, y) by:

$$x' = \text{fract}(d \cdot x) - 0.5, \quad y' = d \cdot y, \tag{1}$$

where fract computes the fractional part of the argument and d is a value that specifies how many glyphs are drawn in the interval $[0, 1]$. Then, the coordinate system can be used to draw white squares with a black contour around it. The ruler-like supporting lines can also be used for precise depth comparisons. The more squares are under the back line of the plane, the closer is the corresponding point.

• *Depth-Dependent Contour:* To further support depth assessment, we utilized a depth-dependent halo contour inspired by Bruckner and Gröller [1]. First, we determine the shading by multiplying the normals of the vascular with the view vector. We use these values as a scalar field: $\varphi = \langle \mathbf{n}, \mathbf{v} \rangle$, where $\mathbf{n}$ is the normal and $\mathbf{v}$ is the normalized view vector. Afterwards, we determine the position of the zero-crossing of φ on the edges per triangle, which are denoted by $\mathbf{p}_i$ and $\mathbf{p}_{i+1}$. Finally, we use these positions to generate a view-aligned quad with their endpoints $\mathbf{p}_{out1/2/3/4}$ in the *Geometry Shader*. For this, we use the *width* as well as the normal vector at the zero-crossing:

$$\mathbf{p}_{out1/2} = \mathbf{p}_i \pm width \cdot \mathbf{n}_i, \quad \mathbf{p}_{out3/4} = \mathbf{p}_{i+1} \pm width \cdot \mathbf{n}_{i+1}. \tag{2}$$

Note that $\mathbf{n}_i$ is the interpolated and normalized normal vector of the triangle at the zero-crossing at position $\mathbf{p}_i$. As vascular models are usually based on world space coordinates, the perceived thickness of the contour is a measure for the distance between vessel and camera position. For this purpose, we linearized the *depth* ranging from 0 to 1 in the near and far plane. Afterwards, the *width* is computed by: $width = 2 \cdot (1 - depth^2)$. This allows a better assessment of the depth by using quadratic function.

• *Shape Cues and Distance Encoding:* To provide recognizable shape cues, we employed the *ConFIS* method by Lawonn et al. [5], see Fig. 2 for an overview of this method. The distance of the vascular structure to the tumor determines the strokes of the streamlines. Therefore, we need to determine the distances of the vascular structures to the tumor. As the tumor is given as a triangulated surface mesh, the triangles of the tumor are used to generate an infinite prism along the normal. Then, we iterate over the generated prisms of the tumor and test if the vertices of the vascular structure lie inside the prism. If this is the case, we determine the distance of the triangle with the vertex. Furthermore, we calculate the distance between the vessel vertices and the tumor vertices. Finally, we compare all distances and associate the shortest distance to the vertex of the vessel. This yields tessellation-independent distances of the vascular structure with the tumor.

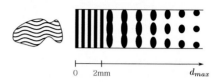

Fig. 3. For the risk zones, streamlines are used for illustration. The more distant from the tumor the more the α increases.

To enhance vessel parts at risk zones, we alter the *ConFIS* visualization at potentially affected vessels. Instead of generating streamlines, we generated quads as described in Eq. 2 with a corresponding coordinate system (recall Eq. 1). Then, we use implicit ellipses which are drawn on the quad: $\alpha \cdot x'^2 + y'^2 \leq r^2$. Whenever this inequality is fulfilled, the fragments are drawn, where r specifies the radius and α is a distance-dependent value that describes the width of the ellipse. The values of α are set as:

$$\alpha(dist) = \begin{cases} 0 & \text{if } dist \leq 2mm \\ \frac{dist}{dist_{max}} & \text{otherwise,} \end{cases} \tag{3}$$

where *dist* describes the distance from the tumor and $dist_{max}$ is the maximum distance. We used 2mm as a threshold as this describes the risk zone and set α such that the streamlines are fully drawn at the risk zone. In addition, the glyphs continuously change from ellipses to circles depending on the distance to the tumor, see Fig. 3.

• *Evaluation:* To assess our visualization concept, we started with a *qualitative study*. The study was performed with 10 researchers who are familiar with medical visualization and 5 physicians with a focus on surgery. First, we showed the subjects our visualization technique with different vascular models. Then, they could explore the model, until they were ready for the next task. Second, we explained them our new visualization technique and showed them how to place the supporting lines. Finally, we presented 12 printed scenes with 3D vascular models rendered using our approach. The models were generated out of 6 liver CT datasets including 12 vascular trees – portal vein and hepatic vein for each dataset. In addition, red points were placed on different branches of each tree. We presented the scenes to the subjects and asked them to order the labeled branches according to the distance from the viewing plane, and asked them how they assessed the distances.

Based on the results of the qualitative evaluation, we conducted a *quantitative study* using a web-based questionnaire. Because in [4], pseudo-chromadepth rendering was

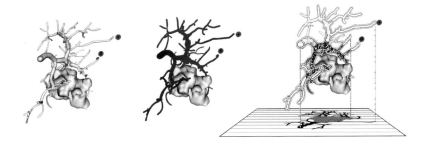

Fig. 4. A scene with a tumor and liver vessel is illustrated using different renderings styles. From left to right: Phong shading, pseudo-chromadepth, and our technique.

rated as the best depth cue for vascular visualization, we compared our illustrative visualization technique with pseudo-chromadepth rendering [9], and Phong shading [6] (no explicit depth cue). Our subject pool consists of 50 subjects (19 female, 31 male, age M=30.9y, range 17-48y). 24 subjects are computer scientists, others are physicians (8), engineers (6), natural scientists (5), and others (7). Most of them (31) have no experience with vascular visualizations.

To probe the subjects assessment of relative depth distances, we designed 24 tasks that require a precise judgment of depth. For each task, subjects had to sort the correct depth order of two labeled branches, see Fig. 4. The models were presented to the subjects in pseudo-randomized order to minimize learning effects. Because we wanted to assess the effect of our illustration technique, 8 visualizations of vascular models using the new techniques had to be compared with 8 pseudo-chromadepth renderings and 8 Phong renderings of the same model identical in every major aspect, except for the display algorithm. We defined four conditions: FF, FN, NF, and NN to specify the positions of the labels, where F means *far* and N means *near*. The first capital describes the pixels' distance of the labeled branches in the image space. We consider the maximum distance D connecting branches that are furthest away from each other. If the distance d of the labeled branches fulfills $d < \frac{D}{2}$ then it is defined as N, otherwise as F. For the second capital we use the z distance of the near and far plane. If the z distance of the labeled branches is greater than half of the distance of the far and near plane it is denoted as F, otherwise as N.

The quantitative investigation included a training phase, in which all 3 modalities were explained and subjects were asked to perform two test tasks (not included in the evaluation) for each modality. They were also informed that time is measured after the training phase. After completing a task, subjects were asked to rate their confidence on a 5-point Likert confidence scale where 5 means very confident and 1 very unconfident, and to press a button to start the next task.

3   Results

In the *qualitative study*, subjects stated that a mix of illustrative shadows and supporting lines was the most useful combination. Contours were rarely used, as the differences in width were hard to perceive. Three subjects stated that the contour supports a spatial impression and supports the depth assessment, but it depends on the distance of labeled branches. If the points were placed on supporting lines the subjects could order the depth correctly. Four subjects asked for a grid on the floor to easily see the intersection point of the supporting line with the plane. They stated that this would enhance and fasten the sorting process of the supporting lines. We added this feature for the quantitative study. If no supporting lines were placed, the result strongly depends on the complexity of the vascular tree. Therefore, the more complex the vascular structure the more supporting lines are needed to assess the correct depth.

For the *quantitative study*, the data was analyzed by a 3 (visualization techniques: illustrative, pseudo-chromadepth, and Phong) $\times$ 2 (*xy* distance: F far, N near) $\times$ 2 (*z* distance: F far, N near) ANOVA for repeated measurements (see Table 1 for the statistical results).

Table 1. ANOVA results of different effects.

*p <0.05 and **p <0.01			Assessment		Confidence		Time	
Effect	df1	df2	F	η^2	F	η^2	F	η^2
Visualization techniques	2	98	93.25**	.66	118.61**	.71	16.71**	.25
xy distances	1	49	22.86**	.32	.77	.02	2.62	.05
z distances	1	49	27.31**	.36	110.43**	.69	1.90	.04
Visualization techniques * *xy*	2	98	4.42*	.08	7.05**	.13	.37	.01
Visualization techniques * *z*	2	98	20.16**	.29	85.94**	.64	2.00	.04
xy * *z*	1	49	.03	.00	12.92**	.21	4.12*	.08
Visualization techniques * *xy* * *z*	2	98	2.12	.04	16.38**	.25	28.38**	.37

• *Distance Assessment:* Subjects were able to assess the relative distances more precisely with the illustrative visualization, followed by pseudo-chromadepth (Fig. 5). The given answers for Phong seem to be randomly; only $\approx$48% of the distance estimation tasks were performed correctly. With Phong, subjects achieved better results when the distance in the *xy* plane was small. For the illustrative visualization, the same but weaker effect could be assumed, while for pseudo-chromadepth rendering the *xy* distance seems to have no effect. The opposite effect was observed for *z* distance: while subjects could perform the pseudo-chromadepth tasks significantly better in case the *z* distance was large, this effect was not observed for Phong and the illustrative visualization.

• *Confidence:* Subjects were most confident with the illustrative visualization, followed by pseudo-chromadepth, and most unconfident with Phong (Fig. 6). They were more confident with conditions FF and NF. The significant triple interaction shows, that subjects are most confident with condition FF using illustrative visualization or pseudo-chromadepth, and condition NN using illustrative visualization. Subjects were most unconfident with condition NN using pseudo-chromadepth, and with Phong in general.

• *Time:* As shown in Fig. 7, subjects decided significantly faster using pseudo-chromadepth (M = 10.95 s), followed by Phong (M = 13.21 s) and illustrative visualization (M = 14.04 s). Particularly, the FN condition seems to be difficult and delays decisions (M = 13.95 s), while for all other conditions subjects needed approximately the same amount of time. The significant triple interaction seems to be caused by conditions FN

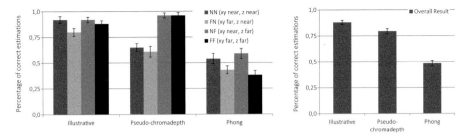

Fig. 5. Results for the distance estimation on a scale from 0 (false) to 1 (right). The errors bars represent the standard error.

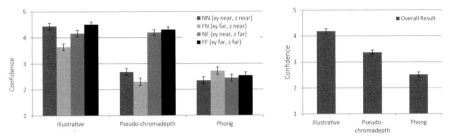

Fig. 6. Confidence rated on a 5-point Likert scale (5 = very confident, 1 = very unconfident). The errors bars represent the standard error.

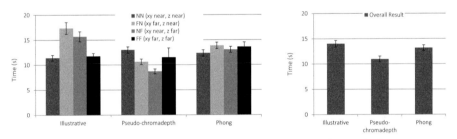

Fig. 7. Time for task completion. The errors bars represent the standard error.

and NF which are the best for pseudo-chromadepth and worst for illustrative, while NN and FF are approximately equal for all visualization techniques.

4   Discussion

Illustrative visualization has a high potential to improve the spatial perception of complex vascular models. The proposed visualization method provides strong monocular depth cues without the requirement of a medium able to display color and intensity gradients. However, color coding can be used to encode additional information. Especially if relative distances between vascular structures are small, supporting lines and illustrative shadows are a great help to perceive the depth.

According to the results of the qualitative study, the depth-dependent contour was rarely used, as differences in contour width were hard to perceive. The contour might not be the main depth cue when illustrative shadows and supporting lines are available. One idea was to use the contour to encode additional information, e.g., instead of using a white contour, color-coding can be applied to encode distances. However, contours can yield a false assessment of vessel diameters which might be critical in some cases.

Regarding our qualitative study, we made minor alterations and conducted a web-based quantitative evaluation with 50 subjects. The results prove that our new technique enhances depth assessment of vascular models for static 2D representations. Our approach leads to more correct depth assessments compared to pseudo-chromadepth rendering which was rated best in previous studies [4, 9]. Moreover, the subjects were even more confident in their decision. As a drawback, the subjects needed more time to assess the depth of the illustrative technique. This is because the supporting lines and the shadows need more cognitive effort to map from the 3D scene to the plane. Therefore, it is a tradeoff between a fast depth assessment and a correct estimation.

Acknowledgements. We thank Fraunhofer MEVIS for providing vascular models, the participants of our studies, and our medical experts: A. Diallo, J. Meyer, K. Oldhafer, E. Poloski, U. Preim, S. Rudolph and especially D. Komm. This work was partially funded by the BMBF (STIMULATE-OVGU: 13GW0095A).

References

1. Bruckner, S., Gröller, E.: Enhancing depth-perception with flexible volumetric halos. IEEE Trans. Vis. Comput. Graph. 13(6), 1344–1351 (2007)
2. Glueck, M., Crane, K., Anderson, S., Rutnik, A., Khan, A.: Multiscale 3D reference visualization. In: Proc. of Interactive 3D Graphics and Games, pp. 225–232 (2009)
3. Hahn, H.K., Preim, B., Selle, D., Peitgen, H.O.: Visualization and interaction techniques for the exploration of vascular structures. In: IEEE Visualization, pp. 395–402 (2001)
4. Kersten-Oertel, M., Chen, S.J.S., Collins, D.L.: An evaluation of depth enhancing perceptual cues for vascular volume visualization in neurosurgery. IEEE Trans. Vis. Graph. 20(3), 391–403 (2013)
5. Lawonn, K., Mönch, T., Preim, B.: Streamlines for Illustrative Real-time Rendering. Comp. Graph. Forum 32(3), 321–330 (2013)
6. Phong, B.T.: Illumination for computer generated pictures. Commun. ACM 18(6), 311–317 (1975)
7. Ritter, F., Hansen, C., Preim, B., Dicken, V., Konrad-Verse, O., Peitgen, H.O.: Real-Time Illustration of Vascular Structures for Surgery. IEEE Trans. Vis. Graph. 12, 877–884 (2006)
8. Ritter, F., Sonnet, H., Hartmann, K., Strothotte, T.: Illustrative shadows: Integrating 3D and 2D information displays. In: Proc. of Intelligent User Interfaces, pp. 166–173 (2003)
9. Ropinski, T., Steinicke, F., Hinrichs, K.H.: Visually supporting depth perception in angiography imaging. In: Butz, A., Fisher, B., Krüger, A., Olivier, P. (eds.) SG 2006. LNCS, vol. 4073, pp. 93–104. Springer, Heidelberg (2006)
10. Wang, X., Zu Berge, C.S., Demirci, S., Fallavollita, P., Navab, N.: Improved interventional x-ray appearance. In: IEEE International Symposium on Mixed and Augmented Reality, pp. 237–242 (2014)

Perfusion Paths: Inference of Voxelwise Blood Flow Trajectories in CT Perfusion

David Robben[1,*], Stefan Sunaert[2], Vincent Thijs[3], Guy Wilms[2],
Frederik Maes[1], and Paul Suetens[1]

[1] iMinds - Medical Image Computing (ESAT/PSI), KU Leuven, Belgium
[2] Department of Radiology, University Hospitals Leuven, KU Leuven, Belgium
[3] Department of Neurology, University Hospitals Leuven, KU Leuven, Belgium

Abstract. In CT perfusion imaging (CTP) multiple, consecutive 3D CT scans of an organ are made during the administration of contrast agent. This results in a 3D movie of the contrast agent entering and subsequently leaving the organ. Currently, this modality is mainly used for voxelwise analysis of perfusion parameters such as blood flow, blood volume, transit time etc. In this work, we propose to analyze these images in a more global fashion and introduce a method to infer the connectivity of the vascular structure underlying the perfusion – even if the vasculature itself is on a subvoxel scale. This novel approach enables several new applications for CTP. The feasibility of the method is illustrated on clinical data.

1 Introduction

The vascular system plays a crucial function in our body, permitting blood to circulate from the heart, through arteries and arterioles to the capillary bed, and through venules and veins back to the heart. In the capillary bed, perfusion takes places: the process of exchanging nutrients, oxygen, waste, etc. with the surrounding cells. Perfusion is essential for the function and survival of living tissue and hence there is vasculature virtually everywhere in the body. Traditional vascular imaging modalities, such as CT angiography (CTA) and MR angiography (MRA), have a limited imaging resolution. In the resulting image, the vascular structure is sparse and most voxels will be considered non-vessel, while in reality they do contain (micro)vasculature.

In CT perfusion imaging (CTP) multiple, consecutive 3D CT scans of an organ are made during the intravenous administration of a iodine contrast agent bolus. Each scan is a volumetric image, showing for every voxel the X-ray attenuation coefficient in Hounsfield units (HU). The result is a 3D movie of the contrast agent entering and subsequently leaving the organ. Alternatively, it can be considered as a 3D image with in every voxel a time series of the HU variation due to the local contrast passage. Subtracting the first image, which is made

---

* David Robben is supported by a Ph.D. fellowship of the Research Foundation - Flanders (FWO).

N. Navab et al. (Eds.): MICCAI 2015, Part II, LNCS 9350, pp. 407–414, 2015.
DOI: 10.1007/978-3-319-24571-3_49

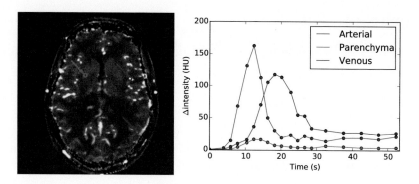

Fig. 1. Illustration of a cerebral CT perfusion. Left: axial slice of a cerebral CTP during the late arterial phase. The red, blue and green markers are located in respectively an artery, a vein and the grey matter. Right: time series in the markers.

before the contrast agent enters the organ, from the subsequent ones results in difference images that show the increase in HU due to the contrast agent. An illustration of a cerebral CTP image is given in Fig. 1.

This modality is very information rich and useful in clinical practice. First, each image of the movie can be considered a traditional CT angiography (CTA), thus allowing assessment of the vasculature in both arterial and venous phase images. More important, however, is the voxelwise calculation of clinically relevant parameters such as time to peak, mean transit time, blood flow and blood volume [8]. These voxelwise parameter maps are used for the diagnosis of stroke – a.o. for the assessment of the tissue at risk – and help making therapeutic decisions. Organs of interest include liver, lungs and brain, with the latter being the most important and also the focus of this work.

Although these voxelwise summary measures prove to be very useful in clinical practice, additional information may be deduced from CTP, especially regarding the vascular structure underlying the perfusion and the trajectories the blood follows throughout the organ. In this work, we propose a method to deduct the vascular connectivity throughout the organ – even if the vasculature itself is on a subvoxel scale. To the best of our knowledge, there is no other modality or image analysis technique that can infer this information, which has a wide range of potential applications. In clinical practice, it is relevant to determine the perfusion territories of arteries (i.e. the regions supplied by those arteries). There are atlases that describe the perfusion territories of the major arteries, but as there is considerable inter-subject variability, it is beneficial to measure them in vivo for each patient specifically [7]. With knowledge of the complete vascular connectivity, calculation of the perfusion territory of an arbitrary artery becomes possible. In research, one might want to investigate the inter-subject variability in vascular connectivity, how this changes during a stroke or whether there is correlation with incidence and outcome of vascular pathology.

In the following sections we first discuss related works, then present our method, and finally illustrate the feasibility of the method on clinical data.

2   Related Work

Currently, we can distinguish five techniques to image the perfusion territories.

In *catheter-based angiography*, an artery is selectively injected with contrast agent through a catheter and subsequently the region of interest perfused by this artery is imaged. Although this method gives excellent image quality, it is also very invasive and time consuming.

Regional arterial spin labeling is an MRI technique where arterial blood is selectively magnetized (labeled) and the magnetic disturbance of this labeled blood is imaged in the region of interest. This technique has several advantages, such as the ability to detect overlapping perfusion territories, the use of non-ionizing radiation and its non-invasive nature. On the other hand, there is very weak signal inside the gray matter, acquisition is time consuming and every additional artery for which the perfusion territory needs to be measured, demands more time.

Then, there is *CT and MR perfusion*. To the best of our knowledge, the only existing works regarding perfusion territory determination in those modalities are those of Christensen et al. The first work [3] describes a bolus tracking method for perfusion MRI. First, the arrival time of the bolus is calculated for every voxel in the image. The authors reason that the arrival times are monotonically rising from the point where the blood enters the image, along the vascular trajectories and towards the periphery. Hence, for every voxel, the least descending path is calculated, i.e. the path that visits each time the neighboring voxel with the highest arrival time that is lower than the arrival time of the current voxel. Such a path always ends in a local minimum of the arrival time, which they assume to be an arterial source along which blood enters the imaged region. They demonstrate the method on a single axial slice. In a second work [1,2], a method is presented for perfusion CT. The authors argue that, while the assumption of monotonically rising arrival times is true in theory, the high blood velocity in big arteries ($50\,\mathrm{cm/s}$), the relatively low sampling frequency ($1\,\mathrm{image/s}$) and the small voxel size (less than $1\,\mathrm{mm}^3$) make their estimation of the arrival time too noisy for the previous method to work: the many local minima in the arrival time will result in as many incorrect arterial sources. Instead they propose using competitive region growing on the arrival time image: starting from several anatomically labeled seed regions, region growing with a low threshold is applied, the selected voxels are added to their respective seed regions, the threshold is increased and the process is repeated. This is demonstrated on cerebral CTP images, where manual segmentations of the anterior, middle and posterior arterial trees are used as seeds and their method subsequently finds the associated perfusion territories.

Finally, there is the possibility of *extrapolation of the vascular image*. Selle et al. [6] predict the vascular territories of the liver by segmenting the hepatic arteries, anatomically labeling them and assigning each non-vessel voxel to its closest artery.

3   Mathematical Model

With a perfect, unlimited resolution scanner, modeling vascular connectivity would boil down to modeling the organ's microvasculature. But since our scanner's resolution is two magnitudes larger (a capillary has a diameter of $5\,\mu m$), this is impossible. Instead we propose to model the connectivity of the underlying vasculature as the connectivity of the voxels in the PCT image I.

This (now unknown) connectivity can be represented as a directed graph G=(V,E). Every voxel v_i in the image I is a vertex: $v_i \in V$. If there is blood flow between neighbouring voxels v_i and v_j ($v_j \in \mathcal{N}(v_i)$, using 26-connectivity), there is an edge $e_{ij} = (v_i, v_j) \in E$. We propose to model the arterial and venous connections separately. In this work, we further only consider the arterial case, but as discussed later, the same approach could be used for the veins.

Now, finding the vascular connectivity of an image, boils down to finding this unknown set of edges E. We want to find the most probable set:

$$E^* = argmax_{E \in \mathbb{E}} \log P(E|I), \tag{1}$$

where $\mathbb{E} = \{E\}$ is the set of acceptable edge sets. Let $V_s \subset V$ be the set of arterial voxels on the image border; these are the sources of blood in the imaged region. An edge set E is acceptable if every perfused voxel is reachable from a source $v_s \in V_s$ and the only perfused voxels without an incoming edge are those in V_s.

Finally, we do not consider vascular anastomoses: these are connections between two vascular trees, such as present in the Circle of Willis. If there is an anastomosis, only one connection will be modeled. This approximation reduces the problem complexity greatly: G contains now only tree-like structures. Or equivalently, every voxel v_i has a single path from a source $v_s \in V_s$, where a path is a tuple of neighboring voxels: $path(v_i) = (v_s, ..., v_j, ..., v_i)$. Additionally, for every other voxel v_j on that path it holds that $path(v_j) \subset path(v_i)$. We propose to call them *perfusion paths*: the voxel paths the blood appears to follow from the arterial sources towards each perfusion site. If those perfusion paths are known, the edges are also known: $E = \{(path(v_i)_j, path(v_i)_{j+1}) | v_i \in V, 1 \leq j \leq (|path(v_i)| - 1)\}$. Also, it is now easy to determine for every voxel v_i its perfusion territory $PT(v_i)$, the set of voxels that is perfused through this voxel: $PT(v_i) = \{v_j | v_i \in path(v_j)\}$.

We propose to find those perfusion paths by tracking the contrast bolus throughout the imaged volume. We can find those perfusion paths by minimizing for every voxel the cost of its path to a source independently. For a wide range of cost functions, this can be done efficiently with dynamic programming:

$$path(v_i) = \begin{cases} (v_i), & \text{if } v_i \in V_s \\ \arg\min_{p \in \mathcal{P}_i} (cost(p)), & \text{otherwise} \end{cases} \tag{2}$$

$$\mathcal{P}_i = \{path(v_j) + (v_i) \mid v_j \in \mathcal{N}(v_i)\} \tag{3}$$

Following the idea that the bolus arrival times should be monotonically rising from the arterial source towards the peripheral regions, we use:

$$cost(p) = \max_{v_j \in p} arrival(v_j), \tag{4}$$

with *arrival* giving the arrival time of the contrast bolus in that voxel. In Eq. 2, if a voxel is reached by several paths with the same cost, the path p whose second last vertex $p_{|p|-1}$ has the lowest cost $cost(path(p_{|p|-1}))$ will be taken.

The approach of Selle et al. [6] can also be described in our model and will be used for evaluation purposes. Its cost function is:

$$cost(p) = \sum_{2 \leq j \leq |p|} dist(p_{j-1}, p_j)(1 - A(p_j)), \tag{5}$$

with A a binary arterial segmentation and *dist* giving the Euclidean distance between a pair of voxels.

Arrival Time Estimation. Our method requires a very accurate estimation of the arrival time. Christensen et al. [3] describe several methods to estimate the arrival time and conclude after simulations that the first moment of the time series is the best metric. However, due to recirculation of the contrast agent, this metric will be heavily influenced by the tail of the timeseries (see Fig. 1) and overestimate the arrival time by a variable factor depending on the length of the tail. We propose to use the time to half max (THM), whose determination is better conditioned than the frequently used time to peak (TTP). Intuitively: the time series is much flatter at the maximum than at its half maximum, making determination of the exact time when the maximum is reached much more susceptible to noise. A formal proof is given in the supplementary material [1].

4   Experiments

There is no ground truth method for measuring the blood flow trajectories in vivo. Instead, we qualitatively evaluate our method by comparison with medical literature, demonstrate its feasibility and compare it with alternatives. We use four clinical cerebral CTP datasets from one healthy, one tumor and two stroke patients. Each dataset is acquired on a Toshiba Acquilion One, has 19 time points and has a voxel size of $0.443 \times 0.443 \times 0.5 mm^3$, resampled to $0.886 \times 0.886 \times 1.0 mm^3$ to speed up calculation and reduce noise. First, motion correction is performed: every image I_t with $t > 0$ is rigidly aligned to the first image I_0 using the Elastix Toolbox [4]. Noise is suppressed through both spatial and temporal filtering. Spatial filtering is done by bilateral Gaussian smoothing on the time series, called TIPS [5], with a σ of 4 mm. Temporal smoothing is done with a σ of 1 image. Finally, the images are processed with the proposed method.

---

[1] See www.medicalimagingcenter.be/public/MIC/publications/DR_MICCAI2015

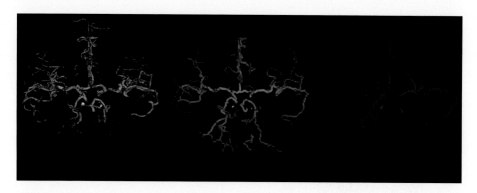

Fig. 2. Relation between the contrast enhancement during the arterial phase and perfusion territory volume (PTV). Three dimensional renderings of a subtraction image during the arterial phase (in grey) and of the logarithm of the PTV calculated using the proposed THM (in blue) and TTP (in red).

Perfusion Territory Volume. Intuitively, one would expect that voxels in the big arteries have large perfusion territories and vice versa. Hereto, we compare for the cerebral voxels their contrast enhancement during the arterial phase with their perfusion territory volume (PTV), the volume that is perfused through this voxel: $|PT(v_i)|$. Fig. 2 contains results obtained by our method using either THM or TTP for arrival estimation, showing that the proposed metric outperforms the latter. Even though the perfusion paths are calculated without knowledge of the amount of contrast enhancement, the results show that this relation indeed holds, suggesting that the perfusion paths are realistic and indeed follow the arteries. Nevertheless, there are places where the perfusion paths take 'shortcuts': it is for example impossible to distinguish the left and right anterior cerebral artery. For the four datasets, the correlations between the intensity and the logarithm of the PTV using TTP are: 0.15, 0.12, 0.13 and 0.14; using THM yields: 0.27, 0.20, 0.26 and 0.27. Visualizations can be found in the supplementary material.

Perfusion Territories of MCA, ACA and PCA. We manually place markers on the M1-segments, the A2-segments and P2-segments and visualize their perfusion territories using the proposed method and the method of Selle et al. [6]. Results for the healthy subject are shown in Fig. 3. Even though the boundaries produced by the proposed method are more crotchety, the results are more in concordance with the medical literature: the posterior inferior part of the brain is supplied by the PCAs, there is symmetry between the left and right PCA, and the superior posterior part of the brain is supplied by the ACA [7]. Furthermore, we speculate that in case of vascular pathology, such as stenosis, prediction of the territories based on the vasculature becomes even more unreliable. More examples and movies can be found in the supplementary material.

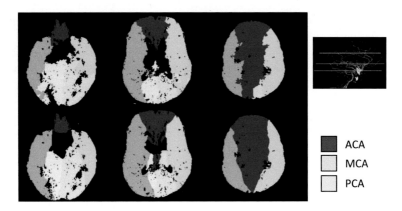

Fig. 3. The perfusion territories of the anterior cerebral arteries (ACAs), the left and right middle cerebral arteries (MCAs) and the left and right posterior cerebral arteries (PCAs). Three axial slices are shown in a healthy subject, the top row calculated by the proposed method, the bottom row by method of Selle et al. [6]. Note that, even though the boundaries produced by the proposed method are more crotchety, they are more in concordance with the medical literature (see text).

Perfusion Territory of the Lenticulostriate Performators. It is described that the lenticulostriate perforators, which branch off from the A1 and M1 segment, provide blood to the putamen [7]. To validate our method, we segment the putamen and calculate the volumetric fraction that is indeed perfused from the M1 and A1 segment. We find that the fraction of putamen volume perfused by the lenticulostriate perforators is in the four datasets: 0.70, 0.80, 0.57 and 0.93. In comparison, the method of Selle et al. [6] finds 0.31, 0.49, 0.38 and 0.56, which is significantly lower.

5   Discussion and Conclusion

We presented a method to infer the arterial perfusion paths. We showed the plausibility of the achieved results and demonstrated its advantage over existing methods.

From a methodological point of view, our formulation is a generalization of the works of Christensen et al. We follow the contrast flow like in [3], but due to the improved formulation and careful estimation of the arrival times, we did what they deemed impossible: trace the blood flow trajectories back to the arterial sources. The main advantage of our method over the competitive region growing approach of [1], is the ability to determine the territory of any single artery or even voxel, without prior segmentation of all 'competing' arteries or voxels.

The same formulation could be applied to infer the venous trajectories. Hereto, one should invert the modeling: the venous trees are rooted in the contrast sinks i.e. the venous voxels on the image border and there is a directed edge e_{ij} if voxel v_i receives venous blood from voxel v_j. The cost function is now in terms of the contrast departure time, which is in theory monotonically decreasing from the contrast sinks. As such, $cost(p) = \max_{v_j \in p} -departure(v_j)$.

The proposed cost function bears close resemblance to doing a watershed segmentation on the arrival time image, with the extension that the flow path of the water is stored. Currently, we only use the arrival time for inferring the vascular trajectories. It is however possible to include extra information, e.g. the maximum increase in intensity or even the full time series. Additionally, anatomical knowledge about the vascular connectivity can be included: e.g. there is no arterial connectivity between the two hemispheres. This can be enforced by excluding edges (v_i, v_j) with v_i and v_j in different hemispheres from the acceptable edge sets. Dynamic programming can naturally handle such constraints.

In future work, we will investigate more elaborate cost functions including intensity information and anatomical knowledge. Additionally, the method will be compared with regional arterial spin labeling to assess its accuracy in determining the perfusion territories.

Acknowledgement. We would like to thank Walter Coudyzer for the collection of the images.

References

1. Christensen, S.: Identification of vascular territories (WO 2013/159147A1) (2012)
2. Christensen, S., Brien, B.O., Menon, B., Bivard, A., Campbell, B.: Mapping of cerebral vascular territories using whole brain perfusion CT imaging : A new method. In: International Stroke Conference, vol. Acute Neur, p. Abstract 54 (2012)
3. Christensen, S., Calamante, F., Hjort, N., Wu, O., Blankholm, A.D., Desmond, P., Davis, S., Østergaard, L.: Inferring origin of vascular supply from tracer arrival timing patterns using bolus tracking MRI. Journal of Magnetic Resonance Imaging 27, 1371–1381 (2008)
4. Klein, S., Staring, M., Murphy, K., Viergever, M.A., Pluim, J.P.W.: Elastix: A toolbox for intensity-based medical image registration. IEEE Transactions on Medical Imaging 29(1), 196–205 (2010)
5. Mendrik, A.M., Vonken, E.J., van Ginneken, B., de Jong, H.W., Riordan, A., van Seeters, T., Smit, E.J., Viergever, M.A., Prokop, M.: TIPS bilateral noise reduction in 4D CT perfusion scans produces high-quality cerebral blood flow maps. Physics in Medicine and Biology 56, 3857–3872 (2011)
6. Selle, D., Preim, B., Schenk, A., Peitgen, H.O.: Analysis of vasculature for liver surgical planning. IEEE Transactions on Medical Imaging 21(11), 1344–1357 (2002)
7. Tatu, L., Moulin, T., Bogousslavsky, J., Duvernoy, H.: Arterial territories of the human brain. Neurology 50(6), 1699–1708 (1998)
8. Wintermark, M., Maeder, P., Thiran, J.P., Schnyder, P., Meuli, R.: Quantitative assessment of regional cerebral blood flows by perfusion CT studies at low injection rates: a critical review of the underlying theoretical models. European Radiology 11(7), 1220–1230 (2001)

Automatic Prostate Brachytherapy Preplanning Using Joint Sparse Analysis

Saman Nouranian[1], Mahdi Ramezani[1], Ingrid Spadinger[2], William J. Morris[2], Septimiu E. Salcudean[1], and Purang Abolmaesumi[1]

[1] Department of Electrical and Computer Engineering,
University of British Columbia, Vancouver, Canada
[2] Vancouver Cancer Centre, British Columbia Cancer Agency, Vancouver, Canada

Abstract. Prostate brachytherapy preplanning is the process of determining treatment target volume and arrangement of radioactive seeds w.r.t. the target volume prior to the implantation. Although preplanning is typically performed by a trained expert using a strict set of guidelines, the process remains highly subjective, resulting in significant user-dependent variability in the plans. In this work, we aim to reduce the preplanning variability by automating the seed arrangement process. We propose a novel framework which uses a retrospective treatment dataset to extract common radioactive seed patterns. The framework captures the inter-relation between the treatment volume delineation and seed arrangements through a joint sparse representation of retrospective data. This representation is used to estimate an initial seed arrangement for a new treatment volume, followed by a novel optimization process which captures the clinical guidelines, to fine-tune the seed arrangement. The proposed framework is evaluated on a dataset of 590 brachytherapy treatment cases by 5-fold cross validation. It achieves 86% success rate, when compared to the clinical guidelines and the actual plans.

1 Introduction

Low-dose-rate (LDR) prostate brachytherapy is an effective treatment option for localized prostate cancer. It is associated with a good long-term survival rate [1,2], requires less patient hospitalization when compared to radical prostatectomy, and is delivered in one session as opposed to alternative methods such as external beam therapy that need to be administered over a period of multiple sessions. In LDR brachytherapy, several small radioactive seeds, loaded into several needles in predefined patterns, are permanently implanted inside the prostate and its adjacent tissue to deliver a prescribed amount of radiation dose to the target anatomy. Arrangement of the seeds offers the advantage of controlling dose distribution inside the anatomy to minimize the risk of toxicity for organs such as urethra, rectal wall and crossing nerves.

Seed arrangements can be planned either prior to, right before or during implantation procedure. Prostate brachytherapy *preplanning* is a treatment approach, which requires pre-operative planning of seed arrangements, usually days

© Springer International Publishing Switzerland 2015
N. Navab et al. (Eds.): MICCAI 2015, Part II, LNCS 9350, pp. 415–423, 2015.
DOI: 10.1007/978-3-319-24571-3_50

before the implantation procedure. Seed planning takes place in an anisotropically dilated volume around the prostate boundary, known as Planning Target Volume (PTV). Standard-of-care for prostate brachytherapy preplanning and delivery is to use a standard brachytherapy grid template. This template is used for intra-operative delivery of the treatment, where needles are inserted according to the preplan, and confines needle placements to the grid points. Although clinical guidelines may vary somewhat between institutions, the preplanning treatment approach has shown excellent outcomes in the past decade [2].

Currently the standard-of-care in the majority of clinics is to create the plan manually, which is subject to a certain degree of observer variability. Treatment variability also stems from large set of possible solutions that all meet the clinical guidelines. However, a trained expert selects the recommended plan from this large set based on his/her expertise. Preplanning automation according to clinical guidelines and based on previous successful plans, can mitigate this problem. Over the last two decades, several solutions have been proposed for this automation [3,4,5,6,7]. A common approach to automating the seed placement is to define an inverse problem based on dose constraints applied to parameters that characterize features such as target coverage, dose uniformity, and dose to organs at risk. In this regard, various optimization techniques are employed including simulated annealing [4], genetic algorithms [7] and branch-and-bound solution for mixed-integer model [5]. The initialization for these techniques is normally with a random seed arrangement. Considering the very large size of the search space for optimal seed configuration, these solutions are highly subject to local minima and sensitive to initial seed configurations.

In this work, we propose a new framework to automate the prostate brachytherapy preplanning. It consists of two components: 1) a plan estimator that represents sparse joint patterns between PTV and seed plans, and 2) a stochastic optimizer that encodes clinical standards to fine-tune the outcome of the plan estimator. We show that the estimator aids the optimizer to converge to a solution that meets the clinical standards. We build the plan estimator by employing a sparse dictionary learning algorithm which encodes the joint patterns between PTV and seed plans in a large retrospective dataset, by a set of sparse joint dictionary elements. The estimated plan is used as an initial seed configuration for the optimizer. The stochastic optimizer is designed based on simulated annealing, while enforcing clinical requirements through a novel cost function that captures those requirements. The proposed pipeline is evaluated on a dataset of 590 patients who underwent brachytherapy treatment at the Vancouver Cancer Centre. We demonstrate an accuracy of 86%, defined on the basis of the clinical standards and previous treatment plans.

2   Methods

Fig. 1 shows the proposed framework which consists of two parts: 1) a one-time offline process of generating a model, based on the joint information between PTV and seed configurations in retrospective patient data. We use a joint Sparse

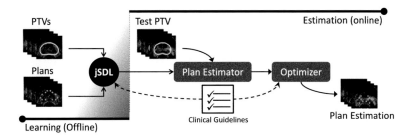

Fig. 1. Block diagram of the proposed framework. Initial estimation of a plan is optimized, based on a novel cost function, to ensure that clinical guidelines are met.

Dictionary Learning (jSDL) approach for training the model; and, 2) an online process of plan estimation and optimization. The optimizer rearranges the seed configuration in the neighborhood of the initial plan estimation.

2.1 Joint Sparse Dictionary Learning

We represent all patients' volumetric information, consisting of the PTV and seed coordinates, in a unique discrete Cartesian space of $\Omega \subset \mathbb{R}^3$, and a brachytherapy grid template space of $\Psi \subset \Omega$ with equal spatial spacing (e.g. 5 mm). We assume that this information is coregistered in the template space for further analysis. We define two information modalities as observation of two sets of labels assigned to each point in the discrete space of Ψ, i.e. labels w.r.t. the PTV volume and labels w.r.t. the seed distribution in Ψ. Specifically, for each patient $i \in \{1, 2, ..., N\}$ in a dataset of N patient treatment records, we use a unique spatial pattern in the space Ψ to generate $\mathbf{l}^{(i)} \in \mathbb{R}^{d \times 1}$ and $\mathbf{s}^{(i)} \in \{0, 1\}^{d \times 1}$, corresponding to PTV labels and seed placement labels in brachytherapy grid space, where d is the number of discrete coordinates in Ψ. We introduce joint observation vector $\mathbf{x}^{(i)} = [\mathbf{l}^{(i)T}, \mathbf{s}^{(i)T}]^T$ to train a dictionary of sparse joint patterns.

Our main objective is to introduce $\mathbf{D} \in \mathbb{R}^{2d \times K}$ as a dictionary of K atoms that satisfies $\mathbf{x}^{(i)} = \mathbf{D}\mathbf{c}^{(i)}$, where $\mathbf{c}^{(i)} \in \mathbb{R}^{K \times 1}$ is a vector of coefficients obtained for observation vector $i \in 1, 2, ..., N$.

We reformulate the dictionary training process by stacking the joint observation vectors $\mathbf{x}^{(i)}$ into a matrix of joint observations $\mathbf{X} \in \mathbb{R}^{2d \times N}$ expressing the joint dictionary learning as $\mathbf{X} = \mathbf{D}\mathbf{C}$, where $\mathbf{C} \in \mathbb{R}^{K \times N}$ refers to the coefficient matrix, and $\mathbf{D}$ contains atoms that jointly represent the observations in two parts, i.e. $\mathbf{D} = [\mathbf{D}^{lT}, \mathbf{D}^{sT}]^T$. Hence, atom coefficients are constrained to be equal for both modalities while satisfying the sparsity and efficient reconstruction conditions throughout the learning process. We use K-singular value decomposition (K-SVD) method [8] to train the model and generate $\mathbf{D}$. K-SVD is a generalization of the K-means clustering algorithm for vector quantization. This is an iterative approach that consists of two steps, 1) updating the atoms and their weights sequentially for the columns of $\mathbf{D}$ using singular value decomposition, and 2) to approximate sparsity using orthogonal mapping pursuit [9].

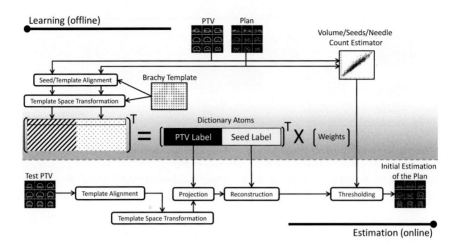

Fig. 2. Initial plan estimation using the joint sparse dictionary learning algorithm.

2.2   Seed Plan Estimation

We perform joint sparse dictionary learning on observation vectors which are defined on the brachytherapy grid space, i.e. $\Psi \subset \Omega$. Coordinates of the planning grid are obtained individually for each patient according to the clinical guidelines. Subsequently a randomly chosen case is used as reference to align all other planning grids. After transformation of PTVs and seed plans in space Ψ, we obtain aligned observation vectors of $\hat{\mathbf{l}}$ and $\hat{\mathbf{s}}$ for PTV and seed plan, respectively. We generate the observation matrix $\hat{\mathbf{x}}^{(i)} = [\hat{\mathbf{l}}^{(i)}, \hat{\mathbf{s}}^{(i)}]$ from the actual plan and the PTV to generate the joint sparse dictionary of $\mathbf{D}$, where $\hat{\mathbf{X}} = \mathbf{D}\mathbf{C}$ and $\mathbf{D} = [\mathbf{D}^{l^T}, \mathbf{D}^{s^T}]$. The dictionary $\mathbf{D}$ forms the model that captures the joint relationship between PTV labels and the corresponding seed arrangement.

An online *estimation* process includes an aligned PTV of a new case to form the observation vector $\mathbf{l}^t \in \{0,1\}^{d \times 1}$. Partial projection coefficients are obtained by solving a least squares problem $\tilde{\mathbf{c}}^t = \mathrm{argmin}_{\mathbf{c}^t} \|\hat{\mathbf{l}}^{\mathbf{t}} - \mathbf{D}^{\mathbf{l}}\mathbf{c}^t\|_2^2$, where $\|.\|_2^2$ denotes the Euclidean norm. Subsequently, a probability map of seed arrangement is calculated by linear weighted combination of the joint atoms, $P(\mathbf{s}^t) = \mathbf{D}^s \mathbf{c}^t$.

We propose to use a dynamic threshold value to convert the reconstructed $P(\mathbf{s}^t)$ into an initial estimation of the seed arrangement, $\tilde{\mathbf{s}}^t$. We take advantage of the high correlation between number of seeds and the size of the PTV, and generate a polynomial regression model from the training dataset. This model is then used to estimate the number of required seeds (according to a confidence interval), for a test case based on its PTV size.

Since the initial estimation is based on a learned model derived from retrospective data, it may not be optimal for a specific patient. We further propose an optimization step to fine-tune the initial estimation and to ensure compatibility with clinical guidelines.

2.3   Plan Optimization

We propose an optimization process to rearrange the estimated seed configuration towards maximizing adaptation of the plan to the clinical guidelines for a given patient. We follow the formalism proposed by Task Group #43 [10] to calculate the dose distribution map in the discrete space of Ω. Our main goal is to use simulated annealing (SA) architecture as a stochastic optimizer for a PTV volume, $l_{ptv} \subset \Omega$ and the corresponding estimated seed arrangement $s \subset \Psi$, which we hereafter refer to as a 2-tuple $\mathbf{y} =< l_{ptv}, s >$. We define plan quality indicators as: 1) $V_p(\mathbf{y})$, % of the PTV volume that is reached by at least $p\%$ of the prescribed dose; and 2) $D_p(\mathbf{y})$, the minimum dose that is reached by $p\%$ of the PTV volume. The objective function is defined as

$$J(\mathbf{y}) = \alpha J_{V_{100}}(\mathbf{y}) + \beta J_{V_{150}}(\mathbf{y}) + \gamma J_{V_{200}}(\mathbf{y}) + \delta J_{needles}(\mathbf{y}) + \Gamma(\mathbf{s}), \qquad (1)$$

where α, β, γ and δ are relative importance weights assigned to different terms of the objective function. Each term represents clinical quality indicators. Function $\Gamma(\mathbf{y})$ is defined to account for contiguity of the 150% isodose by counting the non-contiguous planes and penalizing the cost function. $J_{V_{100}}$, $J_{V_{150}}$ and $J_{V_{200}}$ are introduced to calculate deviation of the dose map from the boundary conditions:

$$J_{V_{100}}(\mathbf{y}) = 1 - V_{100}(\mathbf{y}), \qquad (2)$$

$$J_{V_{150}}(\mathbf{y}) = u(V_{150}(\mathbf{y})-0.6)(V_{150}(\mathbf{y})-0.6)+u(0.5-V_{150}(\mathbf{y}))(0.5-V_{150}(\mathbf{y})), \quad (3)$$

$$J_{V_{200}}(\mathbf{y}) = u(V_{200}(\mathbf{y}) - 0.21)(V_{200}(\mathbf{y}) - 0.21), \qquad (4)$$

$$J_{needles}(\mathbf{y}) = u(\mathcal{N}(\mathbf{s}) - R(\mathbf{y}))\frac{(\mathcal{N}(\mathbf{s}) - R(\mathbf{y}))}{R(\mathbf{y})} + \zeta(\mathbf{s}), \qquad (5)$$

where $u(x)$ is a Heaviside step function that returns zero for $x < 0$ and one for $x >= 0$. $\mathcal{N}(\mathbf{s})$ represents number of needles required for the seed configuration $\mathbf{s}$, and $R(\mathbf{y})$ is an estimation of the total needles expected for the seed configuration in $\mathbf{y}$. We use a high order polynomial regression model to provide priors for needle count and PTV size relationship. $\zeta(\mathbf{s})$ penalizes the cost function by returning 1, if there are more than two adjacent needles in a row or three in a column.

The SA algorithm iteratively anneals the seed arrangement $\mathbf{s}$. Number of seeds k and range of movement r are linearly modified in each iteration based on the temperature cool down function. In each iteration, seeds are ranked by assigning a movement probability value P_M, which is calculated by alternating between observations of two random variables: 1) ratio of locally non-overlapping volume between isodose volume and PTV, and 2) ratio of seed density over total number of seeds. Calculation of P_M is obtained in a neighborhood of size L which is also a linear function of the SA temperature. We propose the alternating approach for calculating P_M to push the annealing towards filling the uncovered areas, while making the seed arrangement more evenly distributed inside the PTV. Eventually, top k number of candidate seeds are chosen based on P_M.

Annealing procedure is followed by a seed arrangement correction procedure. Seed locations, rearranged in the annealing process, are marked in accordance to their adherence to the clinical guidelines, including seed spacing, brachytherapy grid mask and smaller number of needles. Those seeds that do not satisfy the clinical guidelines are moved in a neighborhood of size r until all seeds comply with the clinical guidelines.

3   Experiments and Results

A cohort of 590 patients who underwent prostate brachytherapy at the Vancouver Cancer Centre, is used to evaluate the proposed automatic preplanning framework. For each patient, PTV contours and actual seed arrangement used for the procedure are collected. All patients were treated with a plan based on the standard monotherapy dose prescription of 144 Gy mPD.

We performed our experiments by dividing the cohort of patients into 80% training and 20% test cases. A 5-fold cross validation approach was implemented to measure performance of the proposed framework. Objective function coefficients were heuristically chosen as $\alpha = 0.6$, $\beta = 0.7$, $\gamma = 1.0$ and $\delta = 0.1$.

The performance analysis consists of two parts: 1) plan estimation followed by optimization, and 2) optimization of randomly generated plans. We use the same parameters for the optimizer in the two experiments. Total number of required seeds, σ, is determined from the PTV size as indicated in Sec. 2.2.

We repeat our experiments for 95% confidence interval extremes, σ_- and σ_+, to determine the number of required seeds in both analyses; hence, we report performance of the plans for all three runs (i.e., with σ, σ_- and σ_+) for each test case. To tune the hyper-parameters of the proposed joint sparse dictionary model, we randomly partitioned the cohort into 80% training and 20% validation datasets. An exhaustive grid search on dictionary size and level of sparsity resulted in optimal number of 20 atoms with 5 sparse coefficients.

Fig. 3 shows general statistics of the plan quality indicators V_{100}, V_{150} and V_{200} obtained from the optimization process using estimated plan and randomly generated plan. Hatched area shows the recommended zone for each parameter according to clinical guidelines. Results tabulated in Table 1 further show performance of the proposed optimization algorithm in terms of dosimetry parameters and total number of needles. It is seen that the optimizer can further fine-tune the actual plans towards an improved set of quality indicators.

A successful plan needs to meet all or most clinical standards; therefore, we compare the percentage of successful preplans in terms of recommended clinical guidelines and actual delivered plans. Our observation shows 47% and 14% success rate for the optimizer initialized by estimated plan and random plan, respectively. These rates rise up to 86% and 65% when best of the optimization result is chosen for σ, σ_- and σ_+.

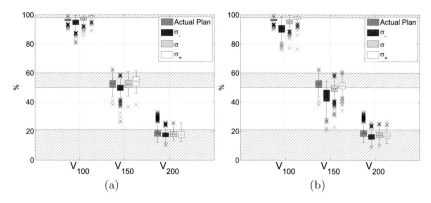

Fig. 3. Comparison between statistics of plan quality metrics for a) estimated plan followed by optimization, and b) randomly generated plan followed by optimization. Number of seeds used in both methods are obtained from polynomial regression model.

Table 1. Mean and standard deviation of the plan quality metrics calculated for actual, estimated and random plans with and without optimization.

	$V_{100}(\%)$	$V_{150}(\%)$	$V_{200}(\%)$	$D_{90}(Gy)$	#Needles
No Optimization:					
Actual	96.39±1.22	52.60±3.78	19.35±4.40	167.99±3.14	25±3
Proposed Estimator	91.71±5.56	54.99±7.57	25.48±5.85	156.27±14.89	26±4
Randomly Initialized	48.50±15.78	16.00±6.76	7.78±3.03	91.45±18.75	59±5
With Optimization:					
Actual	97.13±1.35	52.15±2.91	17.80±2.25	168.39±3.82	26±3
Proposed Estimator	97.12±1.95	52.32±3.48	18.03±2.54	167.79±6.62	28±4
Randomly Initialized	95.04±2.60	48.94±4.45	17.46±2.76	159.93±7.12	31±5

A paired t-test shows a statically significant difference between obtained quality indices ($p < 0.001$) comparing the optimization results for experiments with estimated plan and random plan.

4   Discussion and Conclusion

In this work, an automatic prostate brachytherapy treatment planning framework is introduced that incorporates previous successful treatment knowledge in a model by capturing joint sparse patterns between PTV and seed configuration. Results of the model, i.e. plan estimator, is further optimized by a stochastic optimizer that uses simulated annealing architecture and a novel cost function to apply clinical guidelines and improve the plan quality indicators. Initialization of the optimizer from the estimated plan reduces the very large search space for all possible plans to a neighborhood of the initially estimated plan.

The proposed system is evaluated on a retrospective dataset of treatment records at the Vancouver Cancer Centre. We evaluate performance of the system by reporting the statistics of the plan quality indicators against the actual delivered plan, and show a very high success rate to converge to acceptable plans in terms of clinical guidelines. We show that the automatically generated plans require same range of needles to deliver the plan when compared with the actual plans used for treatment.

Our proposed method can potentially aid the clinicians in training, decision support or suggesting plans which can be further modified. The optimization algorithm can also be used to reduce the number of needles used. The framework is computationally efficient, currently running on a commodity personal computer with an unoptimized MATLAB code within 2 minutes. Hence, it can be further optimized for intra-operative applications. The framework can also adapt to different institutions, requirements or datasets, and is capable of predicting a clinically acceptable plan that captures an implicit knowledge of a clinician or a group of clinicians, so that clinician-specific planning can be performed.

Acknowledgements. This work was funded by the Natural Sciences and Engineering Research Council of Canada (NSERC) and the Canadian Institutes of Health Research (CIHR).

References

1. Hinnen, K.A., Battermann, J.J., van Roermund, J.G.H., Moerland, M.A., Jürgenliemk-Schulz, I.M., Frank, S.J., van Vulpen, M.: Long-term biochemical and survival outcome of 921 patients treated with I-125 permanent prostate brachytherapy. Int. J. Radiat. Oncol. Biol. Phys. 76(5), 1433–1438 (2010)
2. Morris, W.J., Keyes, M., Spadinger, I., Kwan, W., Liu, M., McKenzie, M., Pai, H., Pickles, T., Tyldesley, S.: Population-based 10-year oncologic outcomes after low-dose-rate brachytherapy for low-risk and intermediate-risk prostate cancer. Cancer 119(8), 1537–1546 (2013)
3. Ferrari, G., Kazareski, Y., Laca, F., Testuri, C.E.: A model for prostate brachytherapy planning with sources and needles position optimization. Oper. Res. Heal. Care 3(1), 31–39 (2014)
4. Pouliot, J., Tremblay, D., Roy, J., Filice, S.: Optimization of permanent 125I prostate implants using fast simulated annealing. Int. J. Radiat. Oncol. Biol. Phys. 36(3), 711–720 (1996)
5. Meyer, R.R., D'Souza, W.D., Ferris, M.C., Thomadsen, B.R.: MIP Models and BB Strategies in Brachytherapy Treatment Optimization. J. Glob. Optim. 25(1), 23–42 (2003)
6. Lessard, E., Kwa, S.L.S., Pickett, B., Roach, M., Pouliot, J.: Class solution for inversely planned permanent prostate implants to mimic an experienced dosimetrist. Med. Phys. 33(8), 2773 (2006)
7. Yu, Y., Zhang, J.B., Brasacchio, R.A., Okunieff, P.G., Rubens, D.J., Strang, J.G., Soni, A., Messing, E.M.: Automated treatment planning engine for prostate seed implant brachytherapy. Int. J. Radiat. Oncol. Biol. Phys. 43(3), 647–652 (1999)

8. Aharon, M., Elad, M., Bruckstein, A.: K -SVD: An Algorithm for Designing Overcomplete Dictionaries for Sparse Representation. IEEE Trans. Signal Process. 54(11), 4311–4322 (2006)
9. Tropp, J.A.: Greed is Good: Algorithmic Results for Sparse Approximation. IEEE Trans. Inf. Theory 50(10), 2231–2242 (2004)
10. Rivard, M.J., Coursey, B.M., DeWerd, L.A., Hanson, W.F., Huq, M.S., Ibbott, G.S., Mitch, M.G., Nath, R., Williamson, J.F.: Update of AAPM Task Group No. 43 Report: A revised AAPM protocol for brachytherapy dose calculations. Med. Phys. 31(3), 633–674 (2004)

Bayesian Personalization of Brain Tumor Growth Model

Matthieu Lê[1], Hervé Delingette[1], Jayashree Kalpathy-Cramer[2],
Elizabeth R. Gerstner[3], Tracy Batchelor[3],
Jan Unkelbach[4], and Nicholas Ayache[1]

[1] Asclepios Project, INRIA Sophia Antipolis, France
[2] Martinos Center for Biomedical Imaging, Harvard–MIT Division of Health Sciences
and Technology, Charlestown, MA, USA
[3] Department of Neurology, Massachusetts General Hospital,
Boston, Massachusetts, USA
[4] Department of Radiation Oncology, Massachusetts General Hospital and Harvard
Medical School, Boston, MA, USA

Abstract. Recent work on brain tumor growth modeling for glioblastoma using reaction-diffusion equations suggests that the diffusion coefficient and the proliferation rate can be related to clinically relevant
information. However, estimating these parameters is difficult due to the
lack of identifiability of the parameters, the uncertainty in the tumor
segmentations, and the model approximation, which cannot perfectly
capture the dynamics of the tumor. Therefore, we propose a method
for conducting the Bayesian personalization of the tumor growth model
parameters. Our approach estimates the posterior probability of the parameters, and allows the analysis of the parameters correlations and uncertainty. Moreover, this method provides a way to compute the evidence
of a model, which is a mathematically sound way of assessing the validity
of different model hypotheses. Our approach is based on a highly parallelized implementation of the reaction-diffusion equation, and the Gaussian Process Hamiltonian Monte Carlo (GPHMC), a high acceptance
rate Monte Carlo technique. We demonstrate our method on synthetic
data, and four glioblastoma patients. This promising approach shows
that the infiltration is better captured by the model compared to the
speed of growth.

1 Introduction

Glioblastomas (GBM) are one of the most common types of primary brain tumors. In addition to being infiltrative by nature, they are also the most aggressive
of brain tumors. Reaction-diffusion equations have been widely used to model
the GBM growth, using a diffusion and a logistic proliferation term,

$$\frac{\partial u}{\partial t} = \underbrace{\nabla(D.\nabla u)}_{\text{Diffusion}} + \underbrace{\rho u(1 - u)}_{\text{Logistic Proliferation}} \tag{1}$$

$$D\nabla u.\overrightarrow{n}_{\partial\Omega} = 0 \tag{2}$$

© Springer International Publishing Switzerland 2015
N. Navab et al. (Eds.): MICCAI 2015, Part II, LNCS 9350, pp. 424–432, 2015.
DOI: 10.1007/978-3-319-24571-3_51

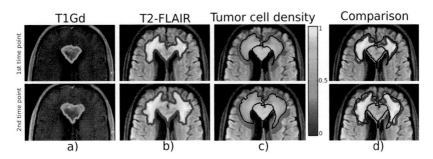

Fig. 1. For the two time points: a) T1Gd with the abnormality segmented in orange. b) T2-FLAIR with the abnormality segmented in red. c) Tumor cell density using the maximum a posteriori parameters with the 80% and 16% threshold outlined in black. d) Comparison between the clinician segmentations and the model segmentations.

Equation (1) describes the spatio-temporal evolution of the tumor cell density u, which infiltrates neighboring tissues with a diffusion coefficient D, and proliferates with a net proliferation rate ρ. Equation (2) enforces Neumann boundary conditions on the brain domain Ω. Equation (1) admits solutions which asymptotically behave like traveling waves with speed $v = 2\sqrt{D\rho}$ and infiltration length $\lambda = \sqrt{D/\rho}$ [1]. The infiltration length is related to the spatial rate of decay of the density u. Preliminary works suggest that D and ρ can help in assessing the response to therapy [2].

The personalization of D and ρ is based on serial acquisitions of Magnetic Resonance Images (MRIs). The tumor causes abnormalities on T1 post Gadolinium (T1Gd) and T2-FLAIR MRIs, which can be monitored over time. To relate the tumor cell density u to those images, it is usually assumed that the visible borders of these abnormalities correspond to a threshold of the tumor cell density [1]. Since the T2-FLAIR abnormality is larger than the T1Gd abnormality, the T2-FLAIR abnormality borders correspond to a lower threshold of tumor cell density (Fig. 1). Therefore, given MRIs of a patient at 2 time points, it is possible to extract the segmentations of the 4 visible abnormalities. Those can be used to personalize a tumor growth model, i.e. to find the set of parameters $\boldsymbol{\theta} = (D, \rho)$ which best fits those segmentations.

This problem was studied by Harpold *et al.* [1] who described a heuristic to relate the volumes of the four available segmentations to the speed $v = 2\sqrt{D\rho}$ and infiltration length $\lambda = \sqrt{D/\rho}$, based on the asymptotic behavior of the solutions of equation (1), hence allowing for the personalization of D and ρ. Konukoglu *et al.* [3] also elaborated a personalization strategy based on BOBYQA, a state-of-the-art derivative-free optimization algorithm. However, this latter method only considers one MRI modality per time point, and fails to simultaneously identify D and ρ. These estimation procedures provide single-solutions which are sensitive to the initialization, and do not provide any understanding about potential correlation between parameters.

To circumvent these drawbacks, we propose a method to estimate the posterior probability of $\boldsymbol{\theta} = (D, \rho)$ from the T1Gd and T2-FLAIR abnormalities at 2 time

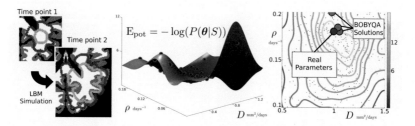

Fig. 2. a) Two synthetic time points with the simulated T1Gd and T2-FLAIR abnormalities (orange and red resp.). b) Gaussian process interpolation of E_{pot} using the evaluation of the posterior at well chosen points (in red). c) Kernel density estimate of the posterior using 1000 samples. Results of the BOBYQA optimization with multiple initializations in blue, true parameters in red.

points. We show how this method provides information on the confidence in the estimation, and provides a global understanding of the correlation between the parameters. We further demonstrate how the knowledge of the posterior distribution can be used to compare different model hypotheses. The method is based on the computation of the statistical evidence: the probability of observing the data given the model. The Bayes factor, defined as the ratio of the evidence of two different models, allows one to compare the models and select which better explains the data. This idea is applied to determine which tumor cell density threshold is the most adequate for the T2-FLAIR abnormality.

Naive Monte Carlo would be impractical due to computational overload. Some strategies rely on approximations of the posterior probability with sparse grids [4], approximations of the forward model based on reduced order models [5,6], or on expensive grid methods [7]. We present here a method based on the highly parallelized implementation of the reaction-diffusion equation using the Lattice Boltzmann Method (LBM), and the Gaussian Process Hamiltonian Monte Carlo (GPHMC), a high acceptance rate Monte Carlo technique.

2   Method

2.1   Tumor Growth Model

We consider the model defined in equations (1,2). Following previous work [1], the diffusion tensor is defined as $D = d_w \, \mathbb{I}$ in the white matter and $D = d_w/10 \, \mathbb{I}$ in the gray matter, where $\mathbb{I}$ is the 3x3 identity matrix. We further identify the parameter D with d_w. As such, the diffusion is heterogeneous and locally isotropic. This model reproduces the infiltrative nature of the GBM, takes into account anatomical barriers (ventricles, sulci, falx cerebri), and the tumor's preferential progression along white matter tracts such as the corpus callosum. The reaction-diffusion equation is implemented using the Lattice Boltzmann Method (LBM) [8]. The LBM are parallelized such that simulating 30 days of growth, with a time step of 0.1 day, takes approximately 80 seconds on a 60 core machine for a 1mm isotropic brain MRI. The initialization of the tumor cell density $u(t = t_1, \mathbf{x})$ at the time of the first acquisition is of particular importance, as it impacts the rest of the simulation. In this work, the tumor tail extrapolation algorithm described in [9] is used. The tumor cell density is computed outward (and inward) of the T1Gd abnormality borders as a static approximation of the wave-like solution of equation (1) with parameter $\boldsymbol{\theta}$. Consequently, the T1Gd abnormality falls exactly on the threshold of the tumor cell density at the first time point.

2.2   GPHMC

Given parameter $\boldsymbol{\theta}$, the model is initialized by extrapolating the tumor cell density from the T1Gd segmentation at time t_1. Its dynamics is then simulated using the LBM until time t_2. The thresholded tumor cell density is then compared to the segmentations S of the T1Gd at time t_2 and the T2-FLAIR at time t_1 and t_2 (Fig. 1). To cast the problem in a probabilistic framework, we follow Bayes rule: $P(\boldsymbol{\theta}|S) \propto P(S|\boldsymbol{\theta}) P(\boldsymbol{\theta})$. The likelihood is modeled as $P(S|\boldsymbol{\theta}) \propto \exp(-d(S, u)^2/\sigma^2)$, where the distance $d(S, u)$ is the mean symmetric Hausdorff distance between the border of the segmentations S and the isolines of the simulated tumor cell density u. The noise level is quantified through σ. Samples are drawn from the posterior probability using the Gaussian Process Hamiltonian Monte Carlo [10].

Hamiltonian Monte Carlo (HMC). HMC is a Markov Chain Monte Carlo algorithm which uses a refined proposal density function based on the Hamiltonian dynamics [10]. The problem is augmented with a momentum variable $\mathbf{p} \sim \mathcal{N}(\mathbf{0}, \mathbb{I})$. By randomly sampling $\mathbf{p}$, we define the current state $(\boldsymbol{\theta}, \mathbf{p})$. HMC is designed to propose a new state $(\boldsymbol{\theta}^*, \mathbf{p}^*)$ with constant energy $H = E_{\text{pot}} + E_{\text{kin}}$, with potential energy $E_{\text{pot}} = -\log(P(S|\boldsymbol{\theta})P(\boldsymbol{\theta}))$, and kinetic energy $E_{\text{kin}} = 1/2 \|\mathbf{p}\|_2^2$. The new state is the result of the Hamiltonian dynamics: $d\boldsymbol{\theta}_i/dt = \partial H/\partial \mathbf{p}_i$ and $d\mathbf{p}_i/dt = -\partial H/\partial \boldsymbol{\theta}_i$. The new state $(\boldsymbol{\theta}^*, \mathbf{p}^*)$ is accepted with probability $\mathcal{A} = \min[1, \exp(-H(\boldsymbol{\theta}^*, \mathbf{p}^*) + H(\boldsymbol{\theta}, \mathbf{p}))]$. The conservation of the energy during the Hamiltonian dynamics, up to the numerical discretization approximation, insures a high acceptance rate $\mathcal{A}$.

Gaussian Process Hamiltonian Monte Carlo (GPHMC). In the HMC, computing the Hamiltonian dynamics requires a significant amount of model evalutations. To circumvent this difficulty, E_{pot} is approximated with a Gaussian process [10] (Fig. 2). During an initialization phase, E_{pot} is evaluated by running the forward model at random locations. Those evaluation points are used to define the Gaussian process approximating E_{pot} - details in [10]. HMC is then run using the Gaussian process interpolation of E_{pot} to compute the Hamiltonian dynamics. Given that the Gaussian process well captures E_{pot}, the GPHMC benefits from the high acceptance rate of the HMC.

Posterior Density. $P(\boldsymbol{\theta}|S, \mathcal{M})$ is computed using a kernel density estimation on the drawn samples $\{\boldsymbol{\theta}_i\}_{i=1}^{N}$. A bounce-back boundary condition is applied to ensure the density integrates to 1 on the bounded parameter space.

2.3   Bayes Factor: Extension of the Chib's Method

The evidence of the model $\mathcal{M}$ can be expressed using Chib's method [11]

$$P(S|\mathcal{M}) = \frac{P(S|\boldsymbol{\theta}, \mathcal{M})P(\boldsymbol{\theta}|\mathcal{M})}{P(\boldsymbol{\theta}|S, \mathcal{M})} \propto \exp(-\frac{d(S, Y_{\boldsymbol{\theta}})^2}{\sigma^2})\frac{P(\boldsymbol{\theta}|\mathcal{M})}{P(\boldsymbol{\theta}|S, \mathcal{M})} \qquad (3)$$

In other words, the probability of observing the segmentation given the model (evidence) is equal to the likelihood times the prior, normalized by the posterior. The Chib's method evaluates this equation on a sample $\boldsymbol{\theta}$ of high posterior probability, like its mode. We propose instead a more robust estimation of the evidence, as an extension of the Chib's method, by averaging it over the samples $\{\boldsymbol{\theta}_i\}_{i=1}^{N}$ drawn from the posterior distribution,

$$P(S|\mathcal{M}) = \mathbb{E}_{\boldsymbol{\theta}|S, \mathcal{M}}\left[P(S|\mathcal{M})\right] \propto \frac{1}{N}\sum_{i=1}^{N}\exp(-\frac{d(S, Y_{\boldsymbol{\theta}_i})^2}{\sigma^2})\frac{P(\boldsymbol{\theta}_i|\mathcal{M})}{P(\boldsymbol{\theta}_i|S, \mathcal{M})} \qquad (4)$$

This estimator is less prone to errors when the kernel density estimation of the posterior approximately captures the real density at the modes. In order to compare two models $\mathcal{M}_1$ and $\mathcal{M}_2$, we can compute the Bayes factor $B = (P(S|\mathcal{M}_1)P(\mathcal{M}_1))/(P(S|\mathcal{M}_2)P(\mathcal{M}_2))$. If B is substantially larger than 1, it is evidence that $\mathcal{M}_1$ is better suited to explain the data than $\mathcal{M}_2$. This is a Bayesian alternative to the frequentist hypotheses testing approach.

3   Experiments and Results

We present results on synthetic and real data. The tumor cell density visibility thresholds are assumed to be 80% for the T1Gd abnormality and 16% for the T2-FLAIR abnormality [12]. The parameters are constrained such that $D \in [0.02, 1.5]$ mm^2/days, and $\rho \in [0.002, 0.2]$ days^{-1} [1]. The prior $P(\boldsymbol{\theta})$ is assumed uniform within this bounded box. After trials, the noise level has been manually tuned to $\sigma = 10$ mm. Our results are compared to the direct minimization of $d(S, Y)$ using BOBYQA. BOBYQA is run 9 times with 9 different initializations in the parameter space - around 20 iterations per BOBYQA were observed. Finally, we compare two models using two different tumor cell density visibility thresholds for the T2-FLAIR abnormality frontier: 16% for the first model $\mathcal{M}_1$, and 2% for the second model $\mathcal{M}_2$, following different studies [1]. The Bayes factor between $\mathcal{M}_1$ and $\mathcal{M}_2$ is computed to compare the models.

Synthetic Data. Starting from a manually drawn T1Gd abnormality segmentation, the growth of a tumor is simulated on an atlas of white and gray matter during 30 days with $D = 1.0$ mm^2.days^{-1} and $\rho = 0.18$ days^{-1}. The first and last images are thresholded in order to define the 4 segmentations (Fig. 2 left). 1000 samples are drawn with the GPHMC, using a GP interpolation of E$_{\text{pot}}$ with

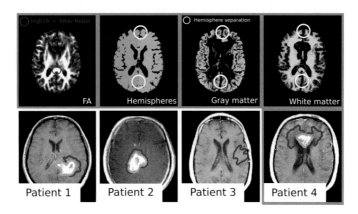

Fig. 3. Top: Data processing using the Fractional Anisotropy (FA) and the hemisphere segmentation to ensure the separation of the hemispheres in the white and gray matter. Bottom: T1Gd of the 4 real cases for the first time point. The T1Gd (resp. T2-FLAIR) abnormality is outlined in orange (resp. red).

35 points (Fig. 2 middle). The acceptance rate is 90%, demonstrating that the Gaussian process successfully captured E_{pot}. The best BOBYQA solutions are in very good agreement with the real parameters (Fig. 2 right). The existence of BOBYQA solutions somewhat distant from the true solution, demonstrates the need for multiple initializations of the algorithm. The true parameter is outlined by high posterior density isocontour, and the posterior reflects little correlation between the parameters (unimodal and somewhat peaked posterior). Finally, with equation (4), we computed a Bayes factor $B = P(S|\mathcal{M}_1)/P(S|\mathcal{M}_2) = 3$, indicating that $\mathcal{M}_1$ is better suited than $\mathcal{M}_2$ in the synthetic case.

GBM Cases. The method is applied to the 4 GBM patients shown in Fig. 3 (bottom panel). The T1Gd and T2-FLAIR abnormalities are segmented by a clinician. For each time point, the T2-FLAIR is rigidly registered to the T1Gd. The rigidly registered T2-FLAIR at time t_2 is then non-linearly registered to the T2-FLAIR at time t_1. All the segmentations are then mapped to the T1Gd image space at time t_1 where the white matter, gray matter and cerebrospinal fluid (CSF) are segmented (Fig. 3 top panel). Close attention is paid to the separation of the hemispheres to prevent tumor cells from invading the contralateral hemisphere. Voxels at the boundary of the hemispheres that show low Fractional Anisotropy value are tagged as CSF to ensure the separation of the hemispheres, while keeping the corpus calosum as white matter (Fig. 3).

The mean acceptance rate for the 4 patients is 74% (Fig. 1) which shows that the Gaussian process successfully interpolate E_{pot}. The BOBYQA solutions, although reasonable, fail to describe the spatial dynamics of the posterior (Fig. 4). This emphasizes the need for a global understanding of the posterior's behavior. We see that the model can capture the infiltration length of the tumor growth: the posterior is elongated along the line of constant infiltration $\lambda = \sqrt{D/\rho}$, es-

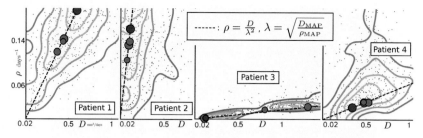

Fig. 4. Posterior estimation for the 4 real cases. The blue dots are the three best BOBYQA solutions. The red dot is the maximum a posteriori of the drawn samples $\boldsymbol{\theta}_{\mathrm{MAP}}$. The dashed black line is the line of constant infiltration $\rho = D/\lambda^2$.

Table 1. Presentation of the patients.

	$t_2 - t_1$ (days)	Acc. rate (%)	Bayes factor
Patient 1	105	90	2.8
Patient 2	29	80	1.8
Patient 3	26	51	0.49
Patient 4	29	75	1.2

pecially for patients 1, 2 and 3 (see the black dashed line on Fig. 4). A small infiltration λ corresponds to a T2-FLAIR abnormality close to the T1Gd abnormality (patient 1 Fig. 3) while a larger infiltration corresponds to more distant abnormalities (patient 4 Fig. 3). However, the model less successfully captures the speed of the growth, as the posterior does not present a clear mode on the constant infiltration line. For patient 3, the presence of two modes suggests that the speed of growth might be explained by two sets of parameters. Moreover, the presence of two modes is responsible for the relatively low acceptance rate of 51%. The posterior distribution is more complex and therefore harder to interpolate with the Gaussian process. For patient 4, the posterior is more peaked and suggests that both the infiltration and speed can be explained by the model. The simulation corresponding to the sample $\boldsymbol{\theta}$ of lowest potential energy $\mathrm{E}_{\mathrm{pot}}$ is presented on Fig. 1 (right). We note $\boldsymbol{\theta}_{\mathrm{MAP}} = (D_{\mathrm{MAP}}, \rho_{\mathrm{MAP}})$ the drawn sample corresponding to the lowest potential energy $\mathrm{E}_{\mathrm{pot}}$. It is interesting to note that $\boldsymbol{\theta}_{\mathrm{MAP}}$ can be slightly skewed on the edge of high posterior isocontour (patient 3 or 4 on Fig. 1). This is caused by the very high sensitivity of the output to the parameters' value, as well as the likelihood model which allows for a certain noise level σ. The Bayes factor between $\mathcal{M}_1$ and $\mathcal{M}_2$ was computed for the different patients (Fig. 1). We can see that for patients 1, 2, and 4, the Bayes factor leans toward validating the model $\mathcal{M}_1$ with a mean of 1.9. Patient 3 presents a lower Bayes factor supporting model $\mathcal{M}_2$, but this patient presents an odd posterior, which might indicate that the reaction-diffusion model less successfully captures the dynamics of the growth.

4   Conclusion

We presented a Bayesian personalization of the parameters of a tumor growth model on 4 patients. The computation of the posterior provides far more information than the direct optimization, and takes only five times longer. Our method provides a global understanding of the correlation between the parameters, and we showed that the model captures the infiltration way better than the speed of growth of the tumor. Furthermore, it provides a way to compute the Bayes factor and compare the validity of different model hypotheses, which showed that a threshold of 16% was probably better suited for the data. In the future, we want to apply this methodology to larger dimensional problems. Namely, the noise level σ could be included as an unknown, and depend on the image modality. Finally, we believe that such a method could be applied to personalized treatment planning.

Acknowledgments. Part of this work was funded by the European Research Council through the ERC Advanced Grant MedYMA 2011-291080.

References

1. Harpold, H.L., Alvord Jr., E.C., Swanson, K.R.: The evolution of mathematical modeling of glioma proliferation and invasion. J. of Neurop. & Exp. Neurol. (2007)
2. Neal, M.L., Trister, A.D., Ahn, S., Baldock, A., et al.: Response classification based on a minimal model of GBM growth is prognostic for clinical outcomes and distinguishes progression from pseudoprogression. Cancer research (2013)
3. Konukoglu, E., Clatz, O., Menze, B.H., Stieltjes, B., Weber, M.A., Mandonnet, E., et al.: Image guided personalization of reaction-diffusion type tumor growth models using modified anisotropic eikonal equations. MedIA 29(1), 77–95 (2010)
4. Menze, B.H., Van Leemput, K., Honkela, A., Konukoglu, E., Weber, M.-A., Ayache, N., Golland, P.: A generative approach for image-based modeling of tumor growth. In: Székely, G., Hahn, H.K. (eds.) IPMI 2011. LNCS, vol. 6801, pp. 735–747. Springer, Heidelberg (2011)
5. Konukoglu, E., Relan, J., Cilingir, U., Menze, B.H., Chinchapatnam, P., Jadidi, A., et al.: Efficient probabilistic model personalization integrating uncertainty on data and parameters: Application to eikonal-diffusion models in cardiac electrophysiology. Progress in Biophysics and Molecular Biology 107(1), 134–146 (2011)
6. Neumann, D., et al.: Robust image-based estimation of cardiac tissue parameters and their uncertainty from noisy data. In: Golland, P., Hata, N., Barillot, C., Hornegger, J., Howe, R. (eds.) MICCAI 2014, Part II. LNCS, vol. 8674, pp. 9–16. Springer, Heidelberg (2014)
7. Wallman, M., Smith, N.P., Rodriguez, B.: Computational methods to reduce uncertainty in the estimation of cardiac conduction properties from electroanatomical recordings. MedIA 18(1), 228–240 (2014)
8. Yoshida, H., Nagaoka, M.: Multiple-Relaxation-Time LBM for the convection and anisotropic diffusion equation. Journal of Computational Physics 229(20) (2010)

9. Konukoglu, E., Clatz, O., Bondiau, P.Y., Delingette, H., Ayache, N.: Extrapolating glioma invasion margin in brain magnetic resonance images: Suggesting new irradiation margins. MedIA 14(2), 111–125 (2010)

10. Rasmussen, C.E.: Gaussian processes to speed up hybrid monte carlo for expensive bayesian integrals. In: Bayesian Statistics, vol. 7 (2003)

11. Chib, S.: Marginal likelihood from the Gibbs output. Journal of the American Statistical Association 90(432), 1313–1321 (1995)

12. Swanson, K., Rostomily, R., Alvord, E.: A mathematical modelling tool for predicting survival of individual patients following resection of glioblastoma: a proof of principle. British Journal of Cancer 98(1), 113–119 (2008)

Learning Patient-Specific Lumped Models for Interactive Coronary Blood Flow Simulations

Hannes Nickisch[1], Yechiel Lamash[2], Sven Prevrhal[1], Moti Freiman[2],
Mani Vembar[3], Liran Goshen[2], and Holger Schmitt[1]

[1] Philips Research, Hamburg, Germany
[2] GRAD, CT, Philips Healthcare, Haifa, Israel
[3] Clinical Science, CT, Philips Healthcare, Cleveland, Ohio, USA

Abstract. We propose a parametric lumped model (LM) for fast patient-specific computational fluid dynamic simulations of blood flow in elongated vessel networks to alleviate the computational burden of 3D finite element (FE) simulations. We learn the coefficients balancing the local nonlinear hydraulic effects from a training set of precomputed FE simulations. Our LM yields pressure predictions accurate up to 2.76mmHg on 35 coronary trees obtained from 32 coronary computed tomography angiograms. We also observe a very good predictive performance on a validation set of 59 physiological measurements suggesting that FE simulations can be replaced by our LM. As LM predictions can be computed extremely fast, our approach paves the way to use a personalised interactive biophysical model with realtime feedback in clinical practice.

Keywords: CCTA, coronary blood flow, lumped parameter biophysical simulation, patient specific model.

1 Introduction

Fractional flow reserve (FFR) based on invasive coronary angiography is the gold-standard for the assessment of the functional impact of a lesion, thus helping

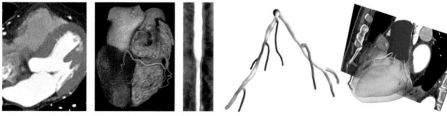

(a) Coronary CTA Scan   (b) Heart Segmentation   (c) Coronaries   (d) Centerlines + Cross Sections   (e) Blood Flow Simulation

Fig. 1. From image to simulation. The heart and its coronary arteries are (automatically) segmented from a CTA scan yielding a tree representation of centerline points and polygonal cross-sections (area encoded as color) used to conduct a patient-specific blood flow simulation (FFR encoded as color).

© Springer International Publishing Switzerland 2015
N. Navab et al. (Eds.): MICCAI 2015, Part II, LNCS 9350, pp. 433–441, 2015.
DOI: 10.1007/978-3-319-24571-3_52

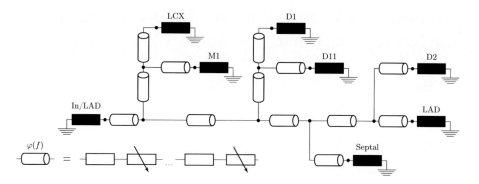

Fig. 2. Parametric nonlinear lumped model with $n = 21$ elements and $m = 15$ nodes including ground. Based on the centerline representation, we set up a lumped model with nonlinear resistances. The black boxes indicate inflow and outflow boundary conditions. The white tubes representing tree segment transfer functions $\varphi(f)$ are composed of a series of linear and nonlinear resistance elements reflecting both the local vessel geometry and hydraulic effects.

with clinical decisions for revascularization [14]. More recently, patient-specific simulations of physiologic information from the anatomic CCTA data have been proposed [7,16]. These computational fluid dynamics models are based on 3D finite element (FE) Navier-Stokes simulations, and are challenging both in terms of *computation* and *complexity*. Computation alone can be accelerated by performing them on GPUs, and complexity can be cut down by reduced order models e.g. [3,6,5], reuse of precomputations or lattice Boltzmann [10] methods. Operating a simulation pipeline from image to prediction (see Figure 1) in a failproof way is challenging as FE computations are sensitive to the quality of the underlying mesh. Besides complexity reduction, simpler and more robust models could be more appropriate for statistical reasons as many patient-specific parameters are unknown in practice. Lumped models (LM) were first used as systemic tree circulation model over 50 years ago [12] and later applied to the coronary circulation [9]. While machine learning techniques already assessed the sensitivity of a blood flow simulation to the segmentation [15], our goal is to use a data driven approach to approximate the FE simulation with a parametric LM that can be simulated extremely quickly. We determine the circumstances under which such an approximation is appropriate and accurate and use the LM for FFR predictions (Figure 1). The FFR value is defined as $FFR = P_d/P_a \in [0,1]$ where P_d and P_a are the pressures distal and proximal to the stenosis averaged over the cardiac cycle. Values above 0.8 are regarded as insignificant [17], and repeated measurements have a standard deviation of $\sigma = 0.025$ [13] suggesting a grey zone of $0.8 \pm 2\sigma$ where clinical decisions require additional information.

2   Methodology

Most FE models use lumped boundary conditions such as Windkessels [20]; and their coupling is not always simple. As we are seeking a fast, simple and

Hydraulic Effect	Geometry weights w_e, coefficients α_e and degrees d_e		Pictogram
1) Poiseuille friction	$w_P = 8\pi\mu\frac{\ell}{A^2}$	$d_P = 1$	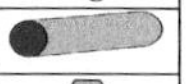
2) Expansion friction [18]	$w_E = \frac{\rho}{2}\max^2(0, \frac{1}{A_{in}} - \frac{1}{A_{out}})$	$d_E = 2$	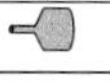
3) Ovality friction [11]	$w_O = w_P \cdot \left(\frac{P^2}{4\pi A}\right)^2$	$d_O = 1$	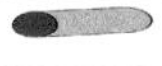
4) Curvature friction [1]	$w_C = w_P \cdot \max\left(0, \frac{19}{8}(r\kappa)^{\frac{1}{25}} - 1\right)$	$d_C = 1$	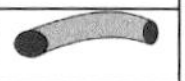
5) Bernoulli's principle	$w_B = \frac{\rho}{2}\left(\frac{1}{A_{in}^2} - \frac{1}{A_{out}^2}\right)$	$d_B = 2$	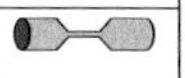
6) Bifurcation friction [19]	$w_{B_0} = \frac{\rho}{2A_{in}^2}, w_{B_1} = \frac{\rho}{2A_{out,1}^2}, w_{B_2} = \frac{\rho}{2A_{out,2}^2}$	$d_{B_0} = d_{B_1} = d_{B_2} = 2$	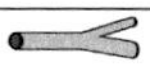
Local effect superposition	$\varphi^c(f) = \sum_{e=1}^{E} \alpha_e \varphi_e^c(f)$	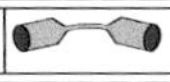 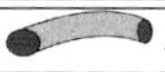 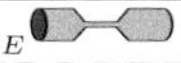	
Tree segment compression	$\varphi(f) = \sum_{c=1}^{C} \varphi^c(f)$	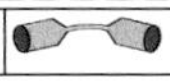	

Fig. 3. Transfer functions and hydraulic effects. The geometry weights are obtained from the vessel's local cross-sectional area A, perimeter P, length ℓ, radius r and curvature κ. Blood density is denoted by ρ and viscosity by μ. Note that our cross-sections are not circular. Local effect-specific transfer functions $\varphi_e^c(f)$ are linearly combined to yield local transfer functions $\varphi^c(f)$. The local transfer functions $\varphi^c(f)$ are summed along the centerline $c = 1..C$ to yield the tree segment transfer function $\varphi(f)$.

parametrisable FE alternative, a lumped model is a natural choice. Using the hydraulic analogy, we can identify volumetric flow rate f with electrical current and pressure p with voltage allowing the interpretation of the coronary hydraulic network as an electrical circuit. Resistors translate into (constricted) pipes, current and voltage sources correspond to dynamic pumps. Starting from the tree representation shown in Figure 1(a), we set up a circuit with two macroscopic component types: nonlinear vessel segment resistors (white tubes) and boundary conditions (black boxes). The boundary condition may be a pressure or flow source driving the network; but any (lumped) boundary condition driving a conventional FE model can be used here. The challenge is to translate the local geometry of the vessel (radius, perimeter, cross-sectional area) into parameters of the nonlinear resistor. In the following, we detail our translation process.

2.1 Transfer Functions and Hydraulic Effects

The hydraulic analogon to Ohm's law is Poiseuille's law stating that pressure drop p and flow f through a thin elongated pipe are linearly related by the linear transfer function p_F so that $p = \varphi_P(f) = w_P f$, where the resistance constant w_P depends on the length of the pipe and its cross-sectional area. Poiseuille friction is only one *hydraulic effect* causing a pressure drop (or energy loss) in hydraulic networks. Friction between blood and the vessel wall is caused by changes of cross-sectional area, bifurcations as well as ovality and curvature of the vessel.

In our framework (see Figure 3), we use piecewise polynomial (invertable and point symmetric) *effect transfer functions* $\varphi_e^c(f) = w_e^c \mathrm{sign}(f)|f|^{d_e}$ to model hydraulic effects with degree d_e and geometry-specific weights w_e^c depending solely on the local vessel geometry and material constants such as blood density ρ and viscosity μ. If $d_e = 1$, we recover *resistors* and if $d_e \neq 1$, we talk about *varistors*. The functional form of the effect transfer functions were taken from the fluid-mechanic literature [18,11,1,19] where the individual hydraulic effects had been experimentally and analytically studied in isolation. To combine multiple interdependent effects $e = 1..E$, we assume *local-effect superposition* $\varphi^c(f) = \sum_{e=1}^{E} \alpha_e \varphi_e^c(f)$ with *effect-specific coefficients* α_e. An illustration of local-effect superposition and tree segment compression is given at the bottom of Figure 3. In total, we include 6 different hydraulic effects, where the first 5 have a single coefficient each and the last one has three coefficients, yielding a total of 8 coefficients. To *compress* the size of the hydraulic network, we can sum up the transfer functions $\varphi^c(f)$ along a tree segment's centerline $c = 1..C$ into a single tree segment transfer function $\varphi(f) = \sum_{c=1}^{C} \varphi^c(f)$. This is possible because the flow through a tree segment is constant within the segment, as shown at the bottom of Figure 2. The compression operation can be inverted by *expansion*, once the simulation is done and the value of f is known. The hydraulic effects are also location specific in the sense that the first 5 effects are active everywhere except at bifurcations and the last one is active only at bifurcations. This representation of the hydraulic network as an assembly of transfer functions encoding hydraulic effects is now used to simulate blood flow.

2.2   Simulation

We make use of modified nodal analysis (MNA) [2] as employed in the popular circuit simulator SPICE[1]. A circuit graph is composed of $i = 1..m$ *nodes* and $j = 1..n$ *elements*. Note that $m < n$ since the circuit is connected. We wish to know the pressures p_j and flows f_j through all elements, a problem with $2n$ unknowns. In matrix-vector notation, we compute $\mathbf{p}, \mathbf{f} \in \mathbb{R}^n$ using *circuit topology* and *element properties* using the Newton-Raphson method. Typically, a handful of iterations are sufficient to solve the system up to machine precision which is due to two stepsize control mechanisms: damping and line search updates.

Topology. To impose Kirchhoff's laws (KL) on $\mathbf{p}$ and $\mathbf{f}$, MNA uses the (sparse) *node-to-element incidence matrix* $\mathbf{A}_0 = [a_{ij}]_{ij} \in \{\pm 1, 0\}^{m \times n}$ with $a_{ij} = 1$ if node i is input to element j, $a_{ij} = -1$ if node i is output to element j and $a_{ij} = 0$ otherwise. Selecting a ground node and removing the corresponding row yields the *reduced incidence matrix* $\mathbf{A} \in \{\pm 1, 0\}^{(m-1) \times n}$ allowing to express the KLs as $\mathbf{A}\mathbf{f} = \mathbf{0}$ (conservation law) and $\mathbf{p} = \mathbf{A}^\top \mathbf{q}$ (uniqueness law) where $\mathbf{q} \in \mathbb{R}^{m-1}$ contains the *absolute pressures relative to the ground node*. Hence, we are left with $n + m - 1$ free variables in $[\mathbf{f}; \mathbf{q}]$ instead of $2n$ variables in $[\mathbf{f}; \mathbf{p}]$ and have $m - 1$ additional constraints (one per node except ground) through $\mathbf{A}\mathbf{f} = \mathbf{0}$ so that the remaining number of degrees of freedom is n.

Element Properties. As a next step, we deal with the n remaining degrees of freedom by using the properties of the $n_R + n_P + n_F + n_V = n$ elements. We decompose $\mathbf{0} = \mathbf{A}\mathbf{f} = \mathbf{A}_R \mathbf{f}_R + \mathbf{A}_P \mathbf{f}_P + \mathbf{A}_F \mathbf{f}_F + \mathbf{A}_V \mathbf{f}_V$ into its constituents (resistors, pressure sources, flow sources, varistors). Using $\mathbf{f}_R = \mathbf{R}^{-1}\mathbf{p}_R$, $\mathbf{f}_F = \hat{\mathbf{f}}_F$,

---

[1] See http://www.eecs.berkeley.edu/Pubs/TechRpts/1973/22871.html.

$\mathbf{p}_P = \hat{\mathbf{p}}_P$, $\mathbf{f}_V = \boldsymbol{\varphi}^{-1}(\mathbf{p}_V)$, where $\mathbf{R}$ is the diagonal resistance matrix and $\hat{\mathbf{f}}_F, \hat{\mathbf{p}}_P$ are vectors containing the pressure/flow source parameters and $\boldsymbol{\varphi}^{-1}$ denotes the n_V inverse varistor transfer functions stacked into a vector, we obtain a system of $n_x = m - 1 + n_P$ nonlinear equations in the variables $\mathbf{x} = [\mathbf{q}; \mathbf{f}_P] \in \mathbb{R}^{n_x}$

$$\begin{bmatrix} \mathbf{A}_R \mathbf{R}^{-1} \mathbf{A}_R^\top \ \mathbf{A}_P \\ \mathbf{A}_P^\top \qquad \mathbf{0} \end{bmatrix} \begin{bmatrix} \mathbf{q} \\ \mathbf{f}_P \end{bmatrix} = \begin{bmatrix} -\mathbf{A}_F \hat{\mathbf{f}}_F \\ \hat{\mathbf{p}}_P \end{bmatrix} + \begin{bmatrix} -\mathbf{A}_V \boldsymbol{\varphi}^{-1}(\mathbf{A}_V^\top \mathbf{q}) \\ \mathbf{0} \end{bmatrix}. \tag{1}$$

2.3 Parameter Learning

In the following, we detail how we adapt the effect coefficient vector $\boldsymbol{\alpha}$ to minimise the quadratic distance between lumped model (LM) simulation results and a training set of precomputed 3D finite element (FE) simulations. The training set consists of flows $\mathbf{f}_i^{FE} \in \mathbb{R}^n$ through each of the n elements of the circuit and absolute pressures $\mathbf{q}_i^{FE} \in \mathbb{R}^M$ at every cross-section of the coronary tree. Note that $m < M$ since the former refers to the number of nodes in the compressed circuit as shown in Figure 2 and the latter to the number of nodes in the expanded circuit. We use the flow from the FE simulation $\mathbf{f}_i^{FE}$ to compute the lumped model pressure drop $\hat{\mathbf{p}}_i^{LM}$ as a sum over the contributions from the effects $e = 1..E$ and set the coefficients $\boldsymbol{\alpha}$ to make the absolute pressure of the FE simulation $\mathbf{q}_i^{FE}$ and the absolute pressure $\hat{\mathbf{q}}_i^{LM} = \mathbf{C}\hat{\mathbf{p}}_i^{LM}$ as predicted by the lumped model as similar as possible via nonnegative least squares [8]

$$\boldsymbol{\alpha}_* = \arg\min_{\boldsymbol{\alpha} \succeq 0} \sum_{i=1}^n \left\| \mathbf{q}_i^{FE} - \mathbf{C}\hat{\mathbf{p}}_i^{LM} \right\|^2, \quad \hat{\mathbf{p}}_i^{LM} = \sum_{e=1}^E \alpha_e \boldsymbol{\varphi}_e(\mathbf{f}_i^{FE}). \tag{2}$$

Here, the matrix $\mathbf{C}$ implements cumulative summation along the tree starting from the root to convert relative pressures $\mathbf{p}$ into absolute pressures $\mathbf{q}$. We use the nonnegativity constraint on the coefficients to discourage non-physical model behavior. Note that learning avoids running lumped simulations; we only employ transfer functions.

3 Experiments

In the following, we describe two cascaded evaluation experiments; the first reporting on how well finite element (FE) simulations can be predicted by lumped model (LM) simulations and the second explaining how well the LM approach is suited for the prediction of physiological FFR measurements.

We trained a model with $E = 8$ coefficients $\boldsymbol{\alpha}$ (see Figure 3) on a data set collected from 32 patients and containing 35 coronary trees (either left or right) using a 20-fold resampled equal split into training and test set to avoid overfitting and obtain sensitivities (runtime ~2min). We performed a total of 350 FE simulations (runtime ~20min each) on these datasets with 10 different biologically plausible inflows[2] per coronary tree and mapped the simulated pressure

---

[2] The 10 equispacedly sampled flow rates were automatically adjusted to yield physically valid pressure drops ranging from a few mmH to 100mmHg for the dataset.

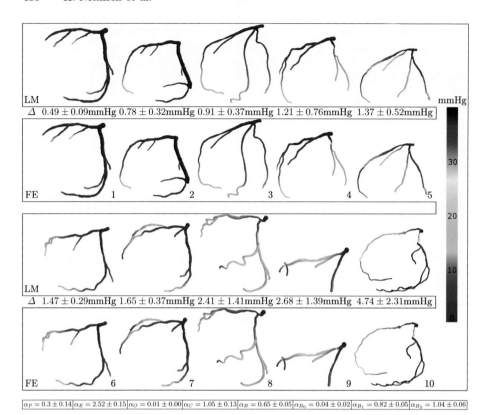

Fig. 4. Lumped model versus finite element simulations. We show LM simulated pressure drop $\mathbf{q}_{aorta} - \hat{\mathbf{q}}_i^{LM}$ and FE simulated pressure drop $\mathbf{q}_{aorta} - \mathbf{q}_i^{FE}$ for 10 exemplary coronary trees and measure their deviation Δ by the mean absolute error and its standard deviation averaged over the tree, 10 different flow rates and over the 20-fold resampling. We also report values for the coefficients $\boldsymbol{\alpha}$ along with standard error.

field and the velocity vector field on the centerline by averaging to generate the FE training data set consisting of volumetric flow rate $\mathbf{f}_i^{FE}$ and absolute pressure $\mathbf{q}_i^{FE}$ for every cross-section for the $i = 1..350$ runs. We used our own code for surface meshing and relied on Netgen[3] for volume meshing and OpenFOAM[4] to perform the calculations. From this dataset, leading to 10^5 terms in Equation 2, we computed the coefficient values as reported at the bottom of Figure 4 whose physical interpretation is hard. The predicted pressures in the 10 coronary trees of Figure 4 show a very good visual agreement and yield an average absolute deviation of 2.76mmHg±0.56mmHg.

We used another 41 patient data sets collected from multiple clinics with 59 FFR invasive measurements to benchmark our LM with the FE simulation on a clinical prediction task. As boundary conditions, for both models and left/right

---

[3] http://sourceforge.net/projects/netgen-mesher/

[4] We use the FV solver simpleFoam from http://www.openfoam.com/.

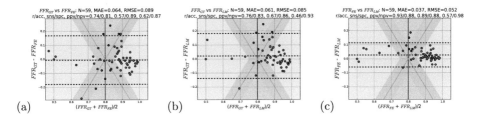

Fig. 5. Comparison of lumped model (LM, runtime <1s) and finite element (FE, runtime 20min) FFR prediction with invasive ground truth (GT) measurements: We show using a Bland-Altman plot for all pairs (a) GT/FE, (b) GT/LM and (c) FE/LM to underpin the equivalence of LM and FE for this prediction task. The green and red color correspond to correctly or incorrectly classified datapoints according to the clinical threshold of 0.8. Gray is the intrinsic error margin. RMSE is the root mean squared error and MAE denotes the mean absolute error. Further, we report the correlation coefficient (r), the accuracy (acc), the sensitivity (sns) and specificity (spc) as well as positive and negative predictive values (ppv,npv) for all pairs.

coronary trees independently, we employed an ostial pressure of $\hat{p} = 100$mmHg and outlet resistances R_i scaling with the outlet diameter d_i according to $R_i \propto d_i^{-1/3}$[4]. The result is summarised in Figure 5 showing similar performance for both FE (a) and LM (b) and a very good agreement between the two methods (c). The intrinsic error of $2\sigma = 0.05$ for a repeated FFR measurement [13] puts the dashed 2σ bands in Figures 5 (a)-(c) in perspective. The LM's accuracy and the deviation from the FE model are about the same.

4   Discussion and Conclusion

We have presented a steady-state parametric lumped model (LM) framework simulating FFR values with accuracy comparable to finite element (FE) simulations in a fraction of a second. The framework is extensible in at least three ways: 1) It is possible to envisage transient simulations by including capacitors or inductors. 2) Following this, one can directly use physiological measurements as training data instead of precomputed FE simulations. 3) Finally, derivatives w.r.t. transfer function parameters can be computed analytically by the implicit function theorem which sets the stage for learning boundary conditions directly from data. We have left open the question about the physical significance of the learned coefficients because the underlying hydraulic effects are not independent of each other. Instead, we prefer to regard the transfer functions of the hydraulic effects merely as *features* in a linear machine learning model. Our computations were based on CT images but other modalities such as interventional Xray can be targeted. We demonstrated comparable accuracy for both LM and FE models with deviations in the order of the ground truth variability; but even if LMs were not accurate enough for some cases, their simplicity and speed makes them a valuable interactive tool for segmentation guidance and quick estimation.

References

1. Ali, S.: Pressure drop correlations for flow through regular helical coil tubes. Fluid Dynamics Research 28(4), 295–310 (2001)
2. Ho, C.-W., Ruehli, A.E., Brennan, P.A.: The modified nodal approach to network analysis. IEEE Transactions on Circuits and Systems 22(6), 504–509 (1975)
3. van der Horst, A., Boogaard, F.L., Rutten, M.C.M., van de Vosse, F.N.: A 1D wave propagation model of coronary flow in a beating heart. In: ASME Summer Bioengineering Conference (2011)
4. Huo, Y., Kassab, G.S.: Intraspecific scaling laws of vascular trees. Journal of the Royal So 9, 190–200 (2012)
5. Huo, Y., Svendsen, M., Choy, J.S., Zhang, Z.D., Kassab, G.S.: A validated predictive model of coronary fractional flow reserve. Journal of the Royal Society Interface 9(71), 1325–1338 (2012)
6. Itu, L., Sharma, P., Mihalef, V., Kamen, A., Suciu, C., Comaniciu, D.: A patient-specific reduced order model for coronary circulation. In: ISBI (2012)
7. Kim, H.J., Vignon-Clementel, E., Coogan, J.S., Figueroa, C.A., Jansen, K.E., Taylor, C.A.: Patient-specific modeling of blood flow and pressure in human coronary arteries. Annals of Biomedical Engineering 38(10), 3195–3209 (2010)
8. Lawson, C.L., Hanson, R.J.: Solving Least Squares Problems. SIAM (1987)
9. Maasrani, M., Abouliatim, I., Ruggieri, V., Corbineau, H., Verhoye, J.P., Drochon, A.: Simulations of fluxes in diseased coronary network using an electrical model. In: International Conference on Electrical Machines (ICEM) (2010)
10. Melchionna, S., Bernaschi, M., Succi, S., Rybicki, E.K.F.J., Mitsouras, D., Coskun, A.U., Feldman, C.L.: Hydrokinetic approach to large-scale cardiovascular blood flow. Computer Physics Communications 181(3), 462–472 (2010)
11. Muzychka, Y., Yovanovich, M.: Pressure drop in laminar developing flow in non-circular ducts: a scaling and modeling approach. J. of Fluids Engin. 131(11) (2009)
12. Noordergraaf, A., Verdouw, P.D., Boom, H.B.K.: The use of an analog computer in a circulation model. Progress in Cardiovascular Diseases 5(5), 419–439 (1963)
13. Petraco, R., Sen, S., Nijjer, S., Echavarria-Pinto, M., Escaned, J., Francis, D.P., Davies, J.E.: Fractional flow reserve–guided revascularization: practical implications of a diagnostic gray zone and measurement variability on clinical decisions. JACC: Cardiovascular Interventions 6(3), 222–225 (2013)
14. Pijls, N., van Son, J., Kirkeeide, R., Bruyne, B.D., Gould, K.L.: Experimental basis of determining maximum coronary, myocardial, and collateral blood flow by pressure measurements for assessing functional stenosis severity before and after percutaneous transluminal coronary angioplasty. Circulation 87, 1354–1367 (1993)
15. Sankaran, S., Grady, L.J., Taylor, C.A.: Real-time sensitivity analysis of blood flow simulations to lumen segmentation uncertainty. In: Golland, P., Hata, N., Barillot, C., Hornegger, J., Howe, R. (eds.) MICCAI 2014, Part II. LNCS, vol. 8674, pp. 1–8. Springer, Heidelberg (2014)
16. Taylor, C.A., Fonte, T.A., Min, J.K.: Computational fluid dynamics applied to cardiac computed tomography for noninvasive quantification of fractional flow reserve. Journal of the American College of Cardiology 61(22), 2233–2241 (2013)

17. Tonino, P., Bruyne, B.D., Pijls, N., Siebert, U., Ikeno, F., van't Veer, M., Klauss, V., Manoharan, G., Engstrøm, T., Oldroyd, K., Lee, P.V., MacCarthy, P., Fearon, W.: Fractional flow reserve versus angiography for guiding percutaneous coronary intervention. The New England Journal of Medicine 360(3), 213–224 (2009)
18. Truckenbrodt, E.: Fluidmechanik. Springer (1980)
19. Ward-Smith, A.J.: Internal Fluid Flow. Clarendon Press (1980)
20. Westerhof, N., Lankhaar, J.W., Westerhof, B.E.: The arterial windkessel. Medical and Biological Engineering and Computing 47, 131–141 (2009)

Vito – A Generic Agent for Multi-physics Model Personalization: Application to Heart Modeling

Dominik Neumann[1,2], Tommaso Mansi[1], Lucian Itu[3], Bogdan Georgescu[1],
Elham Kayvanpour[4], Farbod Sedaghat-Hamedani[4], Jan Haas[4], Hugo Katus[4],
Benjamin Meder[4], Stefan Steidl[2], Joachim Hornegger[2], and Dorin Comaniciu[1]

[1] Imaging and Computer Vision, Siemens Corporate Technology, Princeton, NJ
[2] Pattern Recognition Lab, FAU Erlangen-Nürnberg, Germany
[3] Imaging and Computer Vision, Siemens Corporate Technology, Romania
[4] Department of Internal Medicine III, University Hospital Heidelberg, Germany

Abstract. Precise estimation of computational physiological model parameters from patient data is one of the main hurdles towards their clinical applicability. Designing robust estimation algorithms is often a tedious and model-specific process. We propose to use, for the first time to our knowledge, artificial intelligence (AI) concepts to learn how to personalize a computational model, inspired by how an expert manually personalizes. We reformulate the parameter estimation problem in terms of Markov decision process and reinforcement learning. In an off-line phase, the artificial agent, called Vito, automatically learns a representative state-action-state model through data-driven exploration of the computational model under consideration. In other words, Vito learns how the model behaves under change of parameters and how to personalize it. Vito then controls the on-line personalization by exploiting its automatically derived action policy. Because the algorithm is model-independent, personalizing a completely new model would require only adjusting some simple parameters of the agent and defining the observations to match, without the full knowledge of the model itself. Vito was evaluated on two challenging problems: the inverse problem of cardiac electrophysiology and the personalization of a lumped-parameter whole-body circulation model. Obtained results suggested that Vito could achieve equivalent goodness of fit than standard methods, while being more robust (up to 25% higher success rates) and with faster (up to three times) convergence rate. Our AI approach could thus make model personalization algorithms generalizable and self-adaptable to any patient, like a human operator.

1 Introduction

For the past decade, computational models of heart function have been explored to improve clinical management of patients with cardiomyopathies, from stratification to therapy planning [1,2]. Yet, the high model complexity and the often noisy and sparse clinical data still hinder their personalization; i.e. the estimation of their parameters such that they capture the observed physiology (e.g. cardiac motion, electrocardiogram, etc.) and can predict outcome. A wide variety of parameter estimation approaches have been explored to personalize cardiac models

© Springer International Publishing Switzerland 2015
N. Navab et al. (Eds.): MICCAI 2015, Part II, LNCS 9350, pp. 442–449, 2015.
DOI: 10.1007/978-3-319-24571-3_53

from clinical data [3,4]. They all aim to iteratively reduce the misfit between model output and measurements using automatic optimization algorithms (e.g. variational or filtering approaches). Applied blindly, those techniques could easily fail on unseen data, if not supervised, due to parameter ambiguity. Therefore, complex algorithms have been designed combining cascades of optimizers in a very specific way to achieve the required robustness [5]. However, such methods are not generic and their generalization to varying data quality cannot be guaranteed. Reversely, an experienced human can almost always succeed in manually personalizing a model for any subject. One reason is that an expert is likely to have an intuition of model behavior from his prior knowledge on physiology and model design, and past personalization experience. This intuition definitely helps to solve the personalization task more effectively, even on unseen data.

Instead, we propose to address personalization from a learning perspective, inspired by the "human expert". Based on neuroscience theories of animal learning, reinforcement learning (RL) encompasses a set of approaches to make a virtual agent learn by interacting with the environment [6]. RL was first applied to game or simple control tasks. However, the past few years saw tremendous breakthroughs in RL for more complex, real-world problems [7]. In [8], the authors combine RL with deep learning to train an agent to play with 49 Atari games, yielding better performance than an expert in the majority of them thanks to an outstanding generalization property of the RL algorithm.

Motivated by these recent successes, we propose a novel RL-based personalization approach, henceforth called *Vito*, with the goal of designing a framework that can, for the first time to our knowledge, learn by itself how to estimate model parameters from clinical data while being model-independent. First, like an expert, Vito assimilates the behavior of the model in an off-line, one-time only data-driven exploration phase. From this knowledge, Vito learns the optimal strategy encoded by the MDP state-action-state tuples using RL [6]. The goal of Vito is to choose an action that maximizes future rewards, and therefore bring it to the state representing the solution of the personalization problem. To setup the algorithm, the user just needs to define what observations need to be matched and the agent state space discretization. Then everything is learned automatically. The algorithm does not depend on the underlying model. Vito is evaluated on two different tasks: the inverse problem of cardiac electrophysiology and the personalization of a lumped-parameter model of whole-body circulation. Obtained results suggest that Vito can achieve equivalent goodness of fit as standard optimization methods, is more robust and has faster convergence rate.

2 Method

2.1 Markov Decision Processes for Modeling Agent Behavior

An MDP (Fig. 1) is a tuple $\mathcal{M} = (\mathcal{S}, \mathcal{A}, \mathcal{T}, \mathcal{R}, \gamma)$, where $\mathcal{S} = \{s_1, \ldots, s_{|\mathcal{S}|}\}$ is a set of states that describe the agent, $\mathcal{A} = \{a_1, \ldots, a_{|\mathcal{A}|}\}$ is the set of actions, $\mathcal{T} : \mathcal{S} \times \mathcal{A} \times \mathcal{S} \to [0; 1]$ and $\mathcal{R} : \mathcal{S} \times \mathcal{A} \times \mathcal{S} \to \mathbb{R}$ describe the probability of transitioning from one state to another upon action a_t; and the immediate reward after doing

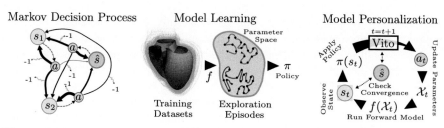

Fig. 1. Left: Simplified MDP (3 states, 1 action). Line width signifies $\mathcal{T}$. Negative rewards are given for all transitions, except when reaching state $\hat{s}$ (model personalized). **Mid**: Off-line model learning from training datasets. **Right**: On-line personalization.

so, respectively. γ is the discount factor that controls the importance of future versus immediate rewards [6]. The solution of an MDP is a policy $\pi : \mathcal{S} \to \mathcal{A}$ that maximizes the discounted expected reward $\sum_{t=0}^{\infty} \gamma^t \mathcal{R}(s_t, a_t, s_{t+1})$.

2.2   Reformulation of the Model Personalization Problem into RL

Any computational model f is governed by a set of parameters $\mathcal{X} = \{x_1, \ldots, x_{|\mathcal{X}|}\}$ and characterized by state variables, some of them, $\mathcal{Y} = \{y_1^c, \ldots, y_{|\mathcal{Y}|}^c\}$, are observable and can be used to estimate $\mathcal{X}$. The goal is to minimize a set of objectives $\mathcal{C} = \{c_1, \ldots, c_{|\mathcal{C}|}\}$, where $c_i = d(y_i^c, y_i^m)$, y_i^m is the measured data and d a distance function. Personalization is mapped to an MDP as follows. First, we define the MDP **states** $\mathcal{S}$ as $|\mathcal{C}|$-dimensional vectors with components $s_{t,i} = c_i$, encoding a combination of objective values. Hence, a state is characterized by its "distance" to the solution, which is patient-invariant. Continuous objective values are discretized into K_i bins, yielding K_i states per dimension i. The problem is therefore characterized by $\prod_i^{|\mathcal{C}|} K_i$ states. Next, mimicking a human operator, Vito will learn how to change the parameters $\mathcal{X}$ to fulfill the objectives $\mathcal{C}$. As such, the **actions** $\mathcal{A}$ modify the parameters, and consist in either in- or decrementing a parameter $x \in \mathcal{X}$ by $1\times$ or $10\times$ a user-specified reference value Δx. Inspired by the Mountain Car benchmark [6], we define the **reward** as always being equal to $\mathcal{R}(s_t, a_t, s_{t+1}) = -1$ (i.e. punishment) except when the agent performs an action that reaches the solution, i.e. when s_{t+1} is the state representing the smallest error $\hat{s}$. In that case, $\mathcal{R}(s_t, a_t, s_{t+1} = \hat{s}) = 0$. The **discount factor** $\gamma = 0.99$ encourages finding a policy that favors future over immediate rewards, as the latter could prefer finding local over global optima. Finally, the stochastic **transition function** $\mathcal{T}$ is learned automatically from f as described below.

2.3   Transition Function as Probabilistic Model Representation

The MDP transition probabilities $\mathcal{T}$ encode the agent's knowledge about the computational model f. Like a human operator, the agent first learns how the model "behaves" through self-guided "sensitivity analyses" (Fig. 1). First, we collect a batch of sample transitions from model exploration episodes $\mathcal{E} = \{e_1, \ldots, e_{|\mathcal{E}|}\}$, i.e. sequences of state-action-state transitions, where each episode contains a fixed number of m (=100 in this work) consecutive transitions. An episode e is initiated by generating random model parameters $\mathcal{X}_0^e$ within physiologically plausible ranges. From the output of a forward model run $f(\mathcal{X}_0^e)$, we derive the initial state s_0^e as described in Sec. 2.2. Next, we employ a random exploration policy π_{rand} that randomly selects an action $a_0^e = \pi_{\mathrm{rand}}(s_0^e)$ (uniform distribution) and applies a_0^e to $\mathcal{X}_0^e$, yielding $\mathcal{X}_1^e$. From $f(\mathcal{X}_1^e)$ the next state s_1^e is determined. We then select the next action $a_1^e = \pi_{\mathrm{rand}}(s_1^e)$ and repeat this process $m-1$ times. Hence, each episode can be seen as a set of state-action-state tuples: $e = \{(s_t^e, a_t^e, s_{t+1}^e), t = 0 \ldots m-1\}$. Transition probabilities $\mathcal{T}$ are made patient-independent by exploring the model using different patients and combining the episodes computed on all of them in one big episode set $\mathcal{E}$. Finally, the transition probabilities $\mathcal{T}$ for each possible state-action-state transition are estimated. To this end, for each action $a \in \mathcal{A}$ and state $s \in \mathcal{S}$, we compute the relative frequency of (s, a, s') tuples in $\mathcal{E}$ among all $(s, a, \cdot)$ in $\mathcal{E}$, for all $s' \in \mathcal{S}$.

2.4   Learning How to Personalize a Model

Now that all components of $\mathcal{M}$ are defined, we compute a policy π that Vito will later use to decide which action to take given any possible state of a model personalization. To this end, value-iteration, a traditional MDP solving technique based on dynamic programming [6] is used. Value-iteration iteratively refines the state-value function V, which represents the expected sum of accumulated discounted rewards for any given state in the MDP: $V(s) = \sum_{s' \in \mathcal{S}} \mathcal{T}(s, \pi(s), s') [\mathcal{R}(s, \pi(s), s') + \gamma V(s')]$. The algorithm is guaranteed to converge to the optimal value function V^* for the given MDP. The optimal policy is given by $\pi(s) = \arg\max_{a \in \mathcal{A}} \sum_{s'} \mathcal{T}(s, a, s') [\mathcal{R}(s, a, s') + \gamma V^*(s')]$.

2.5   On-line Model Personalization

Once trained, Vito personalizes the computational model as follows. Starting from a default parameter set (e.g. normal values), Vito decides from the learned optimal policy π the first action to take, and walks through state-action-state sequences, guided by π, to personalize the computational model f. As observed in previous RL works [7], Vito could start oscillating between states. Since π is deterministic, oscillations can be automatically detected and Vito restarts the personalization from a randomly-selected state (attained by randomly sampling the model parameters). The personalization terminates when either Vito reaches the optimum $\hat{s}$, or when a maximum number of iterations N=100 is reached.

3   Experiments and Results

Two experiments were conducted to evaluate Vito: personalization of a cardiac electrophysiology (EP) model from ECG-derived parameters and personalization of a lumped whole-body circulation (WBC) model from volume and pressure measurements. For both experiments, the same set of 28 consecutive patients

Image Segmentation   Fiber Architecture   Depolarization Map   Torso
                                                                Mapping   ECG

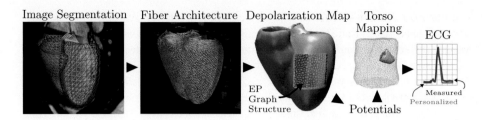

                                                   EP
                                                   Graph   Measured
                                                   Structure   Personalized
                                                              Potentials

Fig. 2. EP simulation pipeline illustrated on a typical case (see text for details). The rightmost plot shows a personalization result provided by Vito against the ground-truth. As one can see, Vito was able to perfectly match the observed QRS signal.

with no severe cardiac arrhythmias (QRS duration $\leq 120\,$ms) was used. For each patient, the bi-ventricular anatomy was segmented (Fig. 2) and tracked from short-axis MRI stacks using shape-constraints, learned motion models and diffeomorphic registration [5], from which ventricular volume curves were derived. At end-diastole, a tetrahedral anatomical model including myofibers was estimated and a torso atlas affinely registered to the patient based on MRI scout images [9]. We then randomly selected eight cases to determine Vito's hyper-parameters. More precisely, various state space discretization settings (K and the bin sizes) were manually tested, and the set yielding the best personalization was selected. It should be noted that this procedure could be easily automatized. Once the hyper-parameters were set, Vito was evaluated on the remaining 20 cases using a leave-one-out strategy: the off-line estimation of the transition probabilities $\mathcal{T}$ was carried out excluding the patient that was being personal-ized during the on-line phase. For fair comparison, just like Vito, the parameter estimation algorithms of reference terminated once all convergence criteria were met, and the maximum number of forward model runs was set to 100.

3.1   Personalization of Cardiac Electrophysiology Model

Forward Model Description: The depolarization time at each node of the tetrahedral anatomical model was computed using a shortest-path graph-based algorithm [10] (Fig. 2). Tissue anisotropy was modeled by modifying the edge costs to take into account fiber orientation. A time-varying voltage map was then derived according to the depolarization time: at a given time t, mesh nodes whose depolarization time was higher than t were assigned a trans-membrane potential of $-70\,$mV, $30\,$mV otherwise. The time-varying potentials were then propagated to a torso model and QRS duration (QRSd) and electrical axis (EA) were computed [11]. The model was controlled by the conduction velocities (in m/s) of myocardial tissue, left and right Purkinje network ($\mathcal{X}_{\mathrm{EP}} = \{v_{\mathrm{Myo}}, v_{\mathrm{LV}}, v_{\mathrm{RV}}\}$), the latter two domains modeled as fast endocardial conducting tissue. The goal of EP personalization was to estimate $\mathcal{X}_{\mathrm{EP}}$ from the measured QRSd and EA. Accounting for uncertainty in the measurements, the model was considered per-sonalized if QRSd and EA misfits were below $5\,$ms and $10°$ respectively.

States and Actions: During hyper-parameters selection, large variations in the number of states (9 to 121) were tested. Yet, the observed variability in personalization outcomes was relatively low (standard deviation of ≈ 1 ms and $4°$ for mean QRSd and EA errors, respectively), suggesting that Vito's performance could be robust w.r.t. state discretization settings. The best results on eight datasets were obtained with $|\mathcal{S}|=49$ ($K=7$), with bin borders at $\{\pm 45, \pm 15, \pm 5\}$ ms for QRSd and $\{\pm 60, \pm 30, \pm 10\}$ degrees for EA. Reference increment values (Sec. 2.2) to build the action set of size $|\mathcal{A}|=12$ were set to $\Delta x = 5$ m/s for all three $x \in \mathcal{X}_{EP}$.

Evaluation: $|\mathcal{E}|=100$ exploration episodes were generated per patient. Vito's personalization results were compared to BOBYQA, a standard, gradient-free optimization method where the objective function is the sum of absolute QRSd and EA errors. Vito achieved mean errors of 3.0 ± 2.0 ms and $9.0 \pm 10.5°$. The average goodness of fit yielded by BOBYQA was slightly better in terms of QRSd (1.4 ± 2.6 ms) and slightly worse in terms of EA ($9.9 \pm 14.7°$). It required less forward model evaluations until convergence (31 ± 7 versus 37 ± 33 for Vito), however, this came at the cost of poor robustness: the personalization criteria could not be met in $7/20$ cases. In comparison, Vito produced 70% less fail-cases. Despite the inherent ambiguity of states (several conduction velocity combinations could yield the same state), Vito was still able to personalize $18/20$ cases.

3.2   Personalization of Whole-Body Circulation Model

Forward Model Description: The WBC model to personalize (Fig. 3) contained a heart model (left ventricle (LV) and atrium, right ventricle (RV) and atrium, valves), the systemic circulation (arteries, capillaries, veins) and the pulmonary circulation (arteries, capillaries, veins) [12]. Time-varying elastance models were used for all four chambers of the heart. The valves were modeled through a resistance and an inertance. A three-element Windkessel model was used for the systemic and pulmonary arterial circulation, while a two-element Windkessel model was used for the systemic and pulmonary venous circulation. The inputs of the model were the MRI-derived end-diastolic (ED) and end-systolic (ES) LV volumes, the heart rate and the systolic, diastolic, and average aortic pressures, as measured during catheterization. In this experiment, Vito learned how to personalize the systemic circulation to match five objectives: ED and ES LV volumes and the systolic, diastolic and average aortic pressures. To that end, we asked Vito to estimate five parameters $\mathcal{X}_{WBC}$: the initial LV volume, LV maximum elastance, LV dead volume, total arterial resistance and arterial compliance. To account for measurement noise, a personalization was considered successful if the final misfit was below $\approx 10\%$ of average measured values in our population: 10 mmHg for pressure-, and 20 mL for volume-based objectives.

States and Actions: Like for EP, Vito appeared to be robust with respect to tested discretization settings, as quantified by the standard deviations of the mean errors after personalization (on average < 2.3 mmHg (or mL) for the five objectives). The best results were achieved with $|\mathcal{S}|=675$ ($K=3$ for pressures and $K=5$ for volumes), with bin borders at $\{\pm 10\}$ mmHg and $\{\pm 40, \pm 20\}$ mL. Based

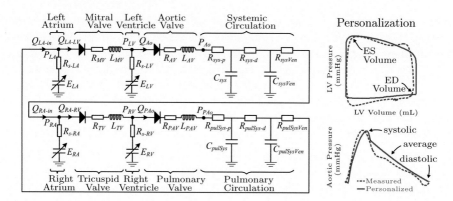

Fig. 3. Left: Whole-body lumped-parameter closed loop model of the cardiovascular system. P, Q, R, E, C and L represent pressures, flow, resistance, elastance, compliance and inertance, respectively. **Right**: Personalization objectives and results.

on the physiological ranges of parameter values, the reference increment values to build the action set of size $|\mathcal{A}|=20$ were set to $\Delta x=\{6\,\mathrm{mL}, 10^{-2}\,\mathrm{mmHg/mL}, 4\,\mathrm{mL}, 8\,\mathrm{g\,cm^{-4}\,s^{-1}}, 1.5\cdot 10^{7}\mathrm{cm^4\,s^2\,g^{-1}}\}$ for the five parameters in $\mathcal{X}_{\mathrm{WBC}}$ (see above).

Evaluation: As one patient had no pressure data, evaluation was performed on the remaining 19 cases, for which $|\mathcal{E}|=300$ exploration episodes each were generated. Vito was compared to a standard optimization using the dogleg trust-region method [12]. Average errors over all pressure-based and all volume-based objectives after personalization were equivalent: $5\pm5\,\mathrm{mmHg}$ and $9\pm7\,\mathrm{mL}$ for Vito, and $5\pm5\,\mathrm{mmHg}$ and $9\pm6\,\mathrm{mL}$ for the comparison method. Vito was however more robust (2 versus 3 failed cases), and at the same time converged three times faster (16 ± 30 versus 48 ± 30 forward model runs), despite the large complexity of the model. Furthermore, preliminary experiments on ten randomly selected sets of initial parameter values suggested that Vito is robust w.r.t. initializations.

4   Discussion and Conclusion

This paper presented a novel personalization approach, Vito, based, for the first time, on AI concepts. We successfully applied it to two challenging personalization tasks in cardiac computational modeling. Inspired by the human approach, Vito first learns the underlying characteristics of the model under consideration using a data-driven approach. This knowledge is then utilized for automatically building a model-specific MDP. Vito is generic in the sense that beyond minimal user input (parameter ranges and authorized updates, discretization bins), it is able to learn by itself how to personalize a model. Setting up Vito thus does not require strong model knowledge. We showed that Vito can be faster and more robust than standard personalization methods, the same we would have expected from a human operator. As such, Vito could become a unified framework for personalization of any physiological model, potentially eliminating the need for an expert operator with in-depth knowledge to design complex optimization procedures. Important challenges still remain, like the definition of states and their discretization. In this work we rely on manually defined bins, which could be seen as ordinal evaluation of the goodness of fit (e.g. "good", "satisfactory" and "bad" states). However, advanced approaches for continuous RL with value function approximators [6] could be integrated to fully circumvent discretization issues. At the same time, such methods could improve Vito's scalability towards higher-dimensional estimation tasks. Experience replay [8] or similar techniques could be employed to increase training data efficiency, which becomes important when computationally expensive models are considered. In the future, a thorough evaluation of convergence properties for both training and personalization will be carried out. Beyond these challenges, Vito showed promising performance and versatility, making it a first step towards an automated, self-taught model personalization agent.

References

1. Trayanova, N.A.: Whole-heart modeling applications to cardiac electrophysiology and electromechanics. Circulation Research 108(1), 113–128 (2011)
2. Nordsletten, D., Niederer, S., Nash, M., Hunter, P., Smith, N.: Coupling multi-physics models to cardiac mechanics. PBMB 104(1), 77–88 (2011)
3. Wallman, M., Smith, N.P., Rodriguez, B.: Computational methods to reduce uncertainty in the estimation of cardiac conduction properties from electroanatomical recordings. Med. Image Anal. 18(1), 228–240 (2014)
4. Wong, K.C., Sermesant, M., Rhode, K., Ginks, M., Rinaldi, C.A., Razavi, R., Delingette, H., Ayache, N.: Velocity-based cardiac contractility personalization from images using derivative-free optimization. J. Mech. Behav. Biomed. 43 (2015)
5. Seegerer, P., et al.: Estimation of regional electrical properties of the heart from 12-lead ECG and images. In: Camara, O., Mansi, T., Pop, M., Rhode, K., Sermesant, M., Young, A. (eds.) STACOM 2014. LNCS, vol. 8896, pp. 204–212. Springer, Heidelberg (2015)
6. Sutton, R., Barto, A.: Reinforcement Learning: An Introduction. MIT Press (1998)
7. Kveton, B., Theocharous, G.: Kernel-based reinforcement learning on representative states. In: Association for the Advancement of Artificial Intelligence (2012)
8. Mnih, V., Kavukcuoglu, K., Silver, D., Rusu, A.A., Veness, J., Bellemare, M.G., Graves, A., Riedmiller, M., Fidjeland, A.K., Ostrovski, G., et al.: Human-level control through deep reinforcement learning. Nature 518(7540), 529–533 (2015)
9. Neumann, D., et al.: Robust image-based estimation of cardiac tissue parameters and their uncertainty from noisy data. In: Golland, P., Hata, N., Barillot, C., Hornegger, J., Howe, R. (eds.) MICCAI 2014, Part II. LNCS, vol. 8674, pp. 9–16. Springer, Heidelberg (2014)
10. Wallman, M., Smith, N.P., Rodriguez, B.: A comparative study of graph-based, eikonal, and monodomain simulations for the estimation of cardiac activation times. IEEE Transactions on Biomedical Engineering 59(6), 1739–1748 (2012)
11. Zettinig, O., Mansi, T., Neumann, D., Georgescu, B., Rapaka, S., Seegerer, P., Kayvanpour, E., Sedaghat-Hamedani, F., Amr, A., Haas, J., Steen, H., Meder, B., Navab, N., Kamen, A., Comaniciu, D.: Data-driven estimation of cardiac electrical diffusivity from 12-lead ECG signals. Med. Image Anal. 18(8), 1361–1376 (2014)
12. Itu, L., Sharma, P., Georgescu, B., Kamen, A., Suciu, C., Comaniciu, D.: Model based non-invasive estimation of PV loop from echocardiography. In: Engineering in Medicine and Biology Society (EMBC), pp. 6774–6777 (2014)

Database-Based Estimation of Liver Deformation under Pneumoperitoneum for Surgical Image-Guidance and Simulation

S.F. Johnsen[1,2], S. Thompson[1], M.J. Clarkson[1], M. Modat[1,2], Y. Song[1],
J. Totz[1], K. Gurusamy[3], B. Davidson[3], Z.A. Taylor[4], D.J. Hawkes[1],
and S. Ourselin[1,2]

[1] University College London, Centre for Medical Image Computing, London, UK
[2] University College London, Translational Imaging Group, CMIC, London, UK
[3] University Dept Surgery, Royal Free Campus, UCL, London UK
[4] University of Sheffield, CISTIB, Insigneo, Sheffield, UK

Abstract. The insufflation of the abdomen in laparoscopic liver surgery leads to significant deformation of the liver. The estimation of the shape and position of the liver after insufflation has many important applications, such as providing surface-based registration algorithms used in image guidance with an initial guess and realistic patient-specific surgical simulation.

Our proposed algorithm computes a deformation estimate for a patient subject from a database of known insufflation deformations, as a weighted average. The database is built from pre-operative and intra-operative 3D image segmentations. The estimation pipeline also comprises a biomechanical simulation to incorporate patient-specific boundary conditions (BCs) and eliminate any non-physical deformation arising from the computation of the deformation as a weighted average.

We have evaluated the accuracy of our intra-subject registration, used for the computation of the displacements stored in the database, and our liver deformation predictions based on segmented, in-vivo porcine CT image data from 5 animals and manually selected vascular landmarks. We found root mean squared (RMS) target registration errors (TREs) of 2.96-11.31mm after intra-subject registration. For our estimated deformation, we found an RMS TRE of 5.82-11.47mm for four of the subjects, on one outlier subject the method failed.

1 Introduction

Many of the algorithms currently being proposed for the registration of the pre-operative segmentation to intra-operative surface reconstructions [10] in image-guided laparoscopic liver surgery (e.g. Iterative Closest Points method) suffer from a tendency to converge to local cost-function minima when not well initialised. The main application for our pneumoperitoneum-deformation estimates is the initialisation of such registrations and thus avoid a manual initialisation

© Springer International Publishing Switzerland 2015
N. Navab et al. (Eds.): MICCAI 2015, Part II, LNCS 9350, pp. 450–458, 2015.
DOI: 10.1007/978-3-319-24571-3_54

step, which is desirable for both workflow and accuracy reasons. They could also help produce better patient-specific surgical simulations for the planning of a laparoscopic procedure.

Few algorithms have been proposed for this particular purpose: Work conducted by Bano et al. [1], investigated the possibility of simulating pneumoperitoneum to guide port placement. Their method was based on a finite element simulation of the patient abdomen which modelled the effects of the gas pressure and gravity. While it was not their primary objective, they also evaluated their method's ability to predict the position of the abdominal viscera in a pig model, and found errors in terms of mesh vertex distances of 5.7 ± 4.9mm with the larger errors being concentrated near the liver. A complete pipeline, from image segmentation through to visual output to the surgeon, for the same purpose was presented by Kitasaka et al. [5]. The tissue biomechanical model they employed was a mass-spring one to which they directly applied gas-pressure forces. However, none of the simulation parameters were given and no registration error evaluation was performed. Bosman et al. [2] looked at different ways of incorporating ligaments in surgical simulations, with pneumoperitoneum being one application. While their experiments were purely synthetic, the work does illustrate how difficult it is to generate a model that correctly takes into account all the effects of surrounding anatomy on the liver configuration under pneumoperitoneum.

Atlas-based methods have been proposed for a number of related tasks. Clements et al. [3] presented a method for the compensation of liver deformation in open hepatic surgery. Their deformation estimates were computed as a weighted average of solutions obtained with a computational model of the patient liver. Their results, while good, were obtained with only simple deformations being applied to a physical liver phantom. Plantefeve et al. [9] developed an atlas-based transfer of FEM BCs. The atlas BCs were computed with Principal Component Analysis performed on a large number of input segmentations of ligaments, blood vessels, and similar structures. Their method yielded good results, but it was limited to the mapping of easily identifiable anatomy, and no validation involving the multitude of interactions determining the liver deformation in real surgery was performed.

In this submission we propose a novel algorithm that extrapolates for a patient liver a likely deformation based on a database containing known insufflation deformations. It is more akin to the aforementioned atlas-based methods, and motivated by the assumption that accurately modelling the interactions occurring during insufflation between the liver and the surrounding tissues is too challenging, since the latter largely consist of tissues that due to their softness and mobility cannot be reliably segmented, meshed and modelled. The data required to build the database have to be acquired with dense intra-operative 3D imaging, but once the database is built it can be used at other sites where such modalities are not available.

2 Methods

2.1 Algorithm Overview

The proposed algorithm computes for a subject with an unknown liver configuration under pneumoperitoneum (unseen subject) an estimate for the displacement of its liver due to pneumoperitoneum. The estimate is computed as a weighted average of displacements observed in other subjects (training subjects) by means of intra-operative imaging and stored in a database. In the simplest case, the database only has to store for the training subjects the original pre-operative liver mesh, an augmented spectral embedding of that mesh, the displacements, and the insufflation pressure. The spectral embedding is used for registration with unseen-subject livers. The original liver mesh and the gas pressure are used in the computation of the weights used in the averaging process.

The algorithm comprises two processing pipelines (Fig. 1): 1) A pipeline processing training data given by CT images of the pre-operative and the intra-operative configuration of the abdomen, and corresponding anatomical segmentations. 2) A pipeline for the estimation of the deformation due to pneumoperitoneum for unseen subjects. This pipeline only requires a pre-operative segmentation as input.

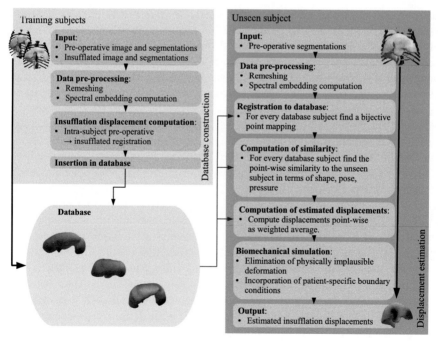

Fig. 1. Flowchart overview over the proposed deformation estimation pipeline. Left: processing of training data. Right: processing of an unseen subject for displacement estimation.

2.2   Image Data and Segmentations

For this work we had segmented, contrast-enhanced CT images of the pre-operative and insufflated anatomy of 5 pigs (subsequently referred to as P1, P2, P3, P4, and P5). The pigs were anaesthetised with isoflurane. They were insufflated with CO_2 at a pressure of approx. 12mmHg, in one case (P1) we assumed a pressure of 16mmHg due to an approx. 50% higher mean displacement compared to other 12mmHg subjects, and in one case the pressure had to be lowered to 8mmHg (P5). A total of 4-5 ports were put in place (1 umbilical, 1 epigastric, 1 left upper quadrant, and 1 or 2 right upper quadrant ports). The CT images were acquired at full exhale, with a resolution of $0.85 \times 0.85 \times 2.5$mm. All pigs were scanned with the same scanner (GE LightSpeed16). The segmentations were done by Visible Patient (http://www.visiblepatient.com/en/service/), and all included the liver, the hepatic artery, the hepatic and portal vein tree, the gall bladder, and the rib cage.

2.3   Registration

Both the intra-subject registration, required to determine the displacements in training subjects, and the inter-subject registration of unseen subjects to the database rely on a mesh registration using spectral point correspondences.

Spectral Embeddings.   The spectral method establishes correspondences based on the shape topology rather than spatial configurations. This is highly advantageous for this application, since the relative size of pig liver lobes can vary considerably. The livers are also highly deformable and their lobes are very mobile. The basic form of our spectral embeddings is based on ref. [4] and is derived from bending and scale invariate geodesic distances of the different parts of the liver surface. The affinity matrix A, whose dominant eigenmodes form the spectral embedding, is computed as follows, with D denoting the matrix of the mutual geodesic distances of the liver-mesh surface nodes:

$$A_{ij} = \exp(-\alpha D_{ij}^2), \ \alpha = 4/ \max_{k,l} D_{kl}^2 \tag{1}$$

To guide the registration algorithm, the following structures are projected onto the liver: the centreline of the trunks of the hepatic and portal veins and the hepatic artery, and the gall bladder. The projection attributes are defined on all liver-mesh nodes and consist of values inversely proportional to the node's shortest distance to the projected structure. For a projected feature mesh Y, they are of the following type:

$$^Y a(\boldsymbol{x_i}) = \exp\left(-\beta ||\boldsymbol{x_i} - \arg \min_{\boldsymbol{y_j} \in Y} ||\boldsymbol{y_j} - \boldsymbol{x_i}||||^2 \right), \ \beta > 0, \ \boldsymbol{x_i} \in \{\text{Liver-mesh nodes}\} \tag{2}$$

This results in an augmented spectral embedding $\hat{\boldsymbol{X}}$ consisting of the first six eigenmodes of (1) and four projection components defined by (2).

Spectral Point Correspondences. Point correspondences are established by non-rigidly registering the augmented spectral embeddings [4]. The registration is done with the Coherent Point Drift (CPD) algorithm [8]. This is mathematically consistent with applications to 4+ dimensional data. For mapping attributes from one subject onto another after establishment of correspondences, a Gaussian interpolation in spectral space is employed, as done by Lombaert et al. [6].

Intra-subject Registration. To make the most use of the available data an intensity-based registration of the CT images corresponding to the segmentations used for building the database is performed with the velocity-field algorithm of NiftyReg [7]. The image registration is initialised with the result of the spectral mesh registration and augmentations are applied to the images by blending the CT images with the segmentation masks corresponding to the hepatic vein, portal vein, gall bladder, and hepatic artery.

2.4   Displacement Computation

The displacement computation for an unseen subject requires a registration and known point-wise correspondences to every liver in the database. With these mutual point correspondences in place, the displacement field is computed nodewise as a weighted average of the corresponding point displacements found in the database. The following three similarity metrics are employed as weights:

Embedding similarity: s_S is given by the similarity of the *unwarped*, augmented spectral embeddings of the unseen mesh u and the training mesh t. For the purpose of the metric's evaluation the spectral embedding is treated like any multivariate node attribute that can be mapped from one subject onto another.

$$^{ut}s_S = -||\hat{x}(x_u) - \hat{x}(\phi_{u2t}(x_u))||/||\hat{x}(x_u)|| \qquad (3)$$

where $\phi_{u2t}(x_u)$ is the coordinate mapping from u to t, and thus $\hat{x}(\phi_{u2t}(x_u))$ the spectral embedding value of the point on t corresponding to x_u.

Transform similarity: s_X is computed from local 3×3 affine transforms P_{t2u}, in turn computed from the spectral point correspondences, by penalising departures from the identity transform (I):

$$^{ut}s_X = -\sum_{i,j} |(P_{t2u})_{ij} - \mathrm{I}_{ij}| \qquad (4)$$

Gas-pressure similarity: s_G is computed from the relative difference in insufflation gas pressure (p):

$$^{ut}s_G = -|p_u - p_t|/p_u \qquad (5)$$

The computation of the similarity for all nodes of the unseen mesh and all training meshes results in three $N \times M$ similarity matrices S, where N is the number of nodes and M is the number of training subjects. These are then normalised via

$$\tilde{S} = (S - \min S)/(\max S - \min S) \qquad (6)$$

Finally, the predicted displacements $\boldsymbol{u_p}$ are computed at every node of the output mesh from the following weighted average:

$$\boldsymbol{u}(\boldsymbol{x_u}) = \frac{1}{\sum_{\tau \in \{\text{database}\}} {}^{u\tau}\tilde{s}_S \, {}^{u\tau}\tilde{s}_X \, {}^{u\tau}\tilde{s}_G} \sum_{t \in \{\text{database}\}} {}^{ut}\tilde{s}_S \, {}^{ut}\tilde{s}_X \, {}^{ut}\tilde{s}_G \, \boldsymbol{u}(\boldsymbol{\phi_{u2t}}(\boldsymbol{x_u})) \frac{p_u}{p_t} \tag{7}$$

The factor p_u/p_t provides a first-order approximation for the displacement magnitude as a function of pressure.

After a first displacement field is computed with (7) one has the option to impose this surface displacement field as a boundary condition on a biomechanical simulation to obtain a displacement solution for the liver parenchyma. If the boundary conditions are formulated as penalty forces one further has the means to eliminate any physically implausible deformation from the solution, e.g. excessive volume change. This solution can also easily be combined with patient-specific boundary conditions extracted from the patient CT, such as zero-displacement constraints at attachment points of major vasculature. The settings of these simulations can be optimised on the training data.

If the database is large, by introducing a reference liver geometry to which the unseen liver and all training livers are registered, one can evaluate (7) with one inter-subject registration per unseen subject.

3   Experiments

3.1   Intra-subject Registration

The validation of the intra-subject registration pipeline is based on easily identifiable vascular landmarks evenly distributed throughout the liver parenchyma. Per subject we used 6–8 landmarks. The RMS TREs are listed in Table 1(a). The first row shows the RMS errors after an alignment of the centre of gravity of the segmentation masks. The last row of Table 1(a) shows the max, mean, and min surface displacement computed with the full pipeline. An example of the images produced in the various stages of the pipeline can be seen in Fig. 2(a).

The TREs in Table 1(a) indicate that the surface registration handles large deformations well - this is especially evident in the case of P1, but to achieve the best possible registration error in most cases an intensity-based image registration step is required. In all cases but P3, whose images are severely degraded by breathing motion artefacts, the RMS error obtained after the image registration is below 5mm.

3.2   Displacement Estimation

Table 1(b) lists the RMS TREs obtained with a leave-one-out analysis of the predicted displacements on the same landmarks as used for validation of the intra-subject registration pipeline. The first data column in Table 1(b) contains the

Table 1. RMS registration errors. All values in mm.

(a) Intra-subject registration errors (RMS TRE):

	P1	P2	P3	P4	P5
Rigid alignment	13.83	13.61	16.27	12.53	9.69
Mesh registration	8.00	7.65	11.31	9.54	4.29
Mesh + image registration	3.88	3.52	12.04	3.80	2.96
Surface displacement (max/mean/min)	65.8/41.4/6.3	51.6/19.4/1.34	33.4/15.1/0.2	57.2/19/1.3	28.4/13.6/1.0

(b) RMS TREs arising from application of the displacement predicted with (7)

Subject	Weighted-average displacement	Weighted-average displacement and biomechanical simulation
P1	37.57	34.98
P2	7.73	8.89
P3	13.89	11.47
P4	8.61	10.53
P5	6.03	5.82

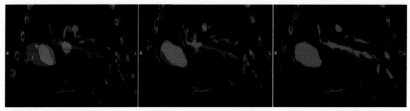

(a) The CT images corresponding to the different stages of the intra-subject registration pipeline with target image overlaid (red): coronal slices through images of P2; Left to right: enhanced source image; surface-registration result; result of intensity-based registration.

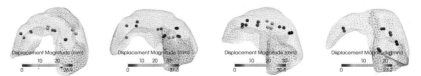

(b) Displacement-estimation pipeline final results with landmarks (left to right): P2, P3, P4, P5; displacement magnitude colour mapped; corresponding landmarks (source, target) shown as spheres with same colour.

Fig. 2. Result configurations of the intra-subject registration pipeline and the displacement estimation pipeline

RMS TREs obtained with the weighted-average database displacements given by (7); the second column lists the errors obtained when additionally running a biomechanical simulation as described towards the end of Sect. 2.4.

The full pipeline results in Table 1(b) show: on all subjects except P1 the RMS TRE is comparable to the registration error after the intra-subject surface registration and significantly better than what is obtained with a rigid alignment of the pre- and post-insufflation meshes (Table 1(a)). P1 is an outlier not only in terms of its displacement magnitude but also due to segmentation errors leading to lobes being fused together in two places and the liver being slightly rotated about the ventro-dorsal axis. Since there is no match in the database for such a liver, the method can only fail. The biomechanical simulation seems to be most beneficial where the weighted average displacement computed with (7) works poorly, in particular on subject P1.

4 Conclusions

We have presented a new method that can approximate the effects on the liver of the complex mechanical interactions of the abdominal viscera occurring during gas insufflation in laparoscopic surgery. The displacements are computed node-wise as the weighted average of displacements observed in training subjects where the insufflated configuration was captured with CT imaging. The weights are provided by custom similarity metrics comparing unseen and training data.

The proposed method achieves an error that is comparable to what has been reported for methods relying on sophisticated biomechanical modelling with a 5.82-11.47mm RMS TRE on subsurface landmarks. While it has some disadvantages handling outliers, it achieves so without using any intra-operatively acquired data for the unseen subject whatsoever and with a very small database of training subjects. Further, considering that the biomechanical simulation currently only acts as a rudimentary safeguard against non-physical deformation and the method can be easily combined with more advanced biomechanical modelling, the current implementation likely only hints at its true potential. This is also true when considering applications to human livers where the inter-patient variability is not as pronounced as in pigs and consistent segmentation is simpler. It was also shown that the intra-subject registration component when used on its own can provide sub-surface accuracy in the range 3-4mm, which is more than adequate for the intended application.

Acknowledgements. The authors were supported by the following funding bodies and grants: EPSRC EP/H046410/1, NIHR BRC UCLH/UCL High Impact Initiative BW.mn.BRC10269, UCL Leonard Wolfson Experimental Neurology Centre, EU-FP7 FP7-ICT-2011-9-601055. The data was supplied by the Wellcome/DoH HICF project T4-317.

References

1. Bano, J., et al.: Simulation of the abdominal wall and its arteries after pneumoperi-toneum for guidance of port positioning in laparoscopic surgery. In: Bebis, G., et al. (eds.) ISVC 2012, Part I. LNCS, vol. 7431, pp. 1–11. Springer, Heidelberg (2012)
2. Bosman, J., Haouchine, N., Dequidt, J., Peterlik, I., Cotin, S., Duriez, C.: The role of ligaments: patient-specific or scenario-specific? In: Bello, F., Cotin, S. (eds.) ISBMS 2014. LNCS, vol. 8789, pp. 228–232. Springer, Heidelberg (2014)
3. Clements, L.W., Dumpuri, P., Chapman, W.C., Galloway, R.L., Miga, M.I.: Atlas-based method for model updating in image-guided liver surgery. In: Proceedings of SPIE, vol. 6509, pp. 650917–650917–12. SPIE (2007)
4. Jain, V., Zhang, H., Van Kaick, O.: Non-rigid spectral correspondence of triangle meshes. International Journal of Shape Modeling 13(01), 101–124 (2007)
5. Kitasaka, T., Mori, K., Hayashi, Y., Suenaga, Y., Hashizume, M., Toriwaki, J.-I.: Virtual pneumoperitoneum for generating virtual laparoscopic views based on volumetric deformation. In: Barillot, C., Haynor, D.R., Hellier, P. (eds.) MICCAI 2004. LNCS, vol. 3217, pp. 559–567. Springer, Heidelberg (2004)
6. Lombaert, H., Sporring, J., Siddiqi, K.: Diffeomorphic spectral matching of cortical surfaces. In: Gee, J.C., Joshi, S., Pohl, K.M., Wells, W.M., Zöllei, L. (eds.) IPMI 2013. LNCS, vol. 7917, pp. 376–389. Springer, Heidelberg (2013)
7. Modat, M., Daga, P., Cardoso, M.J., Ourselin, S., Ridgway, G.R., Ashburner, J.: Parametric non-rigid registration using a stationary velocity field. In: Proceedings of the Workshop on Mathematical Methods in Biomedical Image Analysis, pp. 145–150 (2012)
8. Myronenko, A., Song, X.: Point set registration: coherent point drift. IEEE Transactions on Pattern Analysis and Machine Intelligence 32(12), 2262–2275 (2010)
9. Plantefève, R., Peterlik, I., Courtecuisse, H., Trivisonne, R., Radoux, J.-P., Cotin, S.: Atlas-based transfer of boundary conditions for biomechanical simulation. In: Golland, P., Hata, N., Barillot, C., Hornegger, J., Howe, R. (eds.) MICCAI 2014, Part II. LNCS, vol. 8674, pp. 33–40. Springer, Heidelberg (2014)
10. Totz, J., Thompson, S., Stoyanov, D., Gurusamy, K., Davidson, B.R., Hawkes, D.J., Clarkson, M.J.: Fast semi-dense surface reconstruction from stereoscopic video in laparoscopic surgery. In: Stoyanov, D., Collins, D.L., Sakuma, I., Abolmaesumi, P., Jannin, P. (eds.) IPCAI 2014. LNCS, vol. 8498, pp. 206–215. Springer, Heidelberg (2014)

Computational Sonography

Christoph Hennersperger[1], Maximilian Baust[1],
Diana Mateus[1], and Nassir Navab[1,2]

[1] Computer Aided Medical Procedures, Technische Universität München, Germany
[2] Computer Aided Medical Procedures, Johns Hopkins University, USA
christoph.hennersperger@tum.de

Abstract. 3D ultrasound imaging has high potential for various clinical applications, but often suffers from high operator-dependency and the directionality of the acquired data. State-of-the-art systems mostly perform compounding of the image data prior to further processing and visualization, resulting in 3D volumes of scalar intensities. This work presents computational sonography as a novel concept to represent 3D ultrasound as tensor instead of scalar fields, mapping a full and arbitrary 3D acquisition to the reconstructed data. The proposed representation compactly preserves significantly more information about the anatomy-specific and direction-depend acquisition, facilitating both targeted data processing and improved visualization. We show the potential of this paradigm on ultrasound phantom data as well as on clinically acquired data for acquisitions of the femoral, brachial and antebrachial bone.

1 Introduction

Tracked freehand 3D ultrasound (US) yields 3D information of the scanned anatomy by acquiring 1D scanlines or 2D images, respectively, along with their position and orientation in space. For further processing and visualization, the data is then often interpolated with respect to a regular grid. This procedure is commonly referred to as 3D reconstruction or *compounding* [10] and can be performed in different ways, *e.g.* forward, backward or functional interpolation. All these approaches reconstruct scalar intensity values per voxel,however, such conventional compounding techniques suffer from two inconveniences.

First, they imply a significant loss of information and neglect the directionality-dependent nature of ultrasound. Second, in order to avoid artifacts, they impose acquisition protocols (*e.g.* straight probe motion) modifying the physician's common practice (acquisition guided by interactive motion of the probe).

In this work we propose a novel paradigm for 3D US representation, called *Computational Sonography* (CS), based on the the reconstruction of tensor fields instead of the traditional intensity volumes, *cf.* Fig. 1. In our approach, at every 3D location a 2nd order tensor is optimized to compactly encode the amount of reflected signal expected from each direction. In this way, both the anatomy- and the acquisition-specific directionalities are preserved.

N. Navab et al. (Eds.): MICCAI 2015, Part II, LNCS 9350, pp. 459–466, 2015.
DOI: 10.1007/978-3-319-24571-3_55

The advantages of this novel reconstruction paradigm are as follows:

1. It preserves directional information while allowing for the retrieval of scalar intensity volumes for arbitrary directions. This calls for novel (interactive) visualization techniques which better reflect the directional nature of US.
2. The proposed reconstruction paradigm can be applied to arbitrary scanning trajectories. Thus, the clinician is not subjected to strict scanning protocols.
3. The presented method is fast in terms of reconstruction time (easily parallelizable), while leading to a compact representation (constant storage/voxel).
4. Beyond visualization, the preserved information in CS provides additional value for tasks where 3D ultrasound is used for further processing, *e.g.* registration, segmentation or tracking [6,3,13]. Furthermore, CS also enables using post-processing techniques specialized to tensor-valued data, *e.g.* [12].

The proposed method is inspired by *computational photography*, where light fields instead of just intensities are stored and available to subsequent processing steps [8]. Our vision is that tensor fields become the standard format for freehand 3D US acquisitions, enabling a plenitude of novel computational techniques. We demonstrate the potential of this new paradigm for both phantom and in-vivo data and compare it to state-of-the-art compounding methods.

Related Work: A popular and successful example of tensor fields is Diffusion Tensor Imaging (DTI), for which a vast literature addressing tensor fitting,

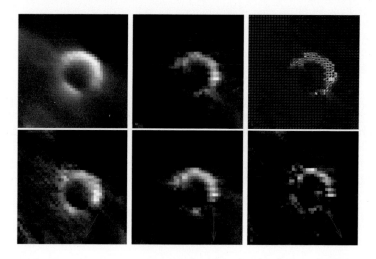

Fig. 1. Top: Reconstruction Comparison. (left) Conventional reconstruction from arbitrarily sampled vascular ultrasound data obtained by backward-interpolation using median compounding. **(middle)** Absolute value of the trace of the reconstructed tensors. **(right)** Tensors visualized as colored ellipses. Note that the trace image nicely resembles the high intensities of the boundary and that tensors align with the global orientation of the imaged structures. **Bottom: Directionality of Tensors.** Reconstructed tensors allow for a reconstruction of directional B-Mode ultrasound information in arbitrary directions, as indicated by red arrows.

visualization, *etc.* [7] exists. In contrast to DTI, compounding of freehand 3D US data is today only considered in terms of reconstructing scalar intensity volumes [10], which neglects most of the directional information acquired along the trajectory of the scan. Recently, a method for incorporating directionality of ultrasound acquisitions was proposed, clustering data from different directions for 3D compounding [1]. While this method utilizes information from different directions for a combined reconstruction, it still reconstructs only scalar values per voxel, and thus directional information is not available for further processing. In [9], the spatial coherence of ultrasound information observed for different orientations and focal regions has been used for tensor reconstructions. While the method is promising, it requires both a specialized hardware setup and a fixed scanning protocol. In contrast, our approach can be seamlessly integrated into the clinical workflow and applied directly to clinical 3D ultrasound acquisitions. Furthermore, the reconstructed tensor fields result in a compact representation of the directional information observed during the acquisition, which remains available for subsequent processing tasks.

2   Computational Sonography for 3D Ultrasound

The basis for any 3D ultrasound reconstruction is a set of ultrasound samples $S = \{s_i\}_i^N$. The samples typically lie on rays (scanlines) that are more or less arbitrarily distributed in 3D space based on the acquisition trajectory. Each sample, denoted here by s_i, is given by a tuple $s_i = \{I_i, p_i, v_i\}$ consisting of the ultrasound intensity I_i, the sample position $p_i = (p_{i,x}, p_{i,y}, p_{i,z})^\top$ and the corresponding ray direction $v_i = (v_{i,x}, v_{i,y}, v_{i,z})^\top$. Current 3D ultrasound techniques use only intensities I_i and positions p_i to reconstruct 3D intensity volumes. Because the content of ultrasound images is direction-dependent, we argue that preserving the directionality is both important and beneficial, which calls for a paradigm change in US data representation. We propose here to rely on tensors to encode such complex behavior, as this resembles the anisotropic nature of ultrasound waves best, with varying visibility of structures and a change penetration depth using different scanning trajectories. The key idea of Computational Sonography is thereby to reconstruct a 3D tensor field from the collection of samples S, where each tensor will compactly and optimally encode the local intensity for each viewing direction. In practice, to reconstruct tensor data from the samples, a two-step approach is proposed, comprising of a selection of US samples in proximity to the respective voxel, followed by the tensor reconstruction through least-squares minimization, *cf.* Fig. 2.

2.1   Sample Selection

At first, we select the subset of the ultrasound samples $s_i \in S$ which contribute to the tensor estimation at a specific volume point $p = (p_x, p_y, p_z)^\top \in P$. Here $P \in \mathbb{Z}^3$ denotes the lattice (set of positions) at which the tensors shall be reconstructed. A proper selection of the respective subset of samples is important,

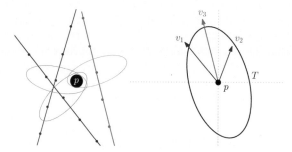

Fig. 2. Reconstruction Process: (left) Ultrasound sample selection from a set of samples close to the target volume position. **(right)** Reconstruction of a 2nd order tensor from measurements originating from different ultrasound rays.

because (i) the selected samples should contain complementary information, i.e., the corresponding measurements should be independent, and ii) potential outliers should be removed in order to avoid a distortion of the subsequent tensor estimation. In this regard and inspired by [2], all input samples S are traversed and a sample s_i is selected if p_i lies within an ellipsoid defined around the ultrasound sample, *cf.* left panel in Fig. 2:

$$\left(\frac{p_x - p_{i,x}}{a}\right)^2 + \left(\frac{p_y - p_{i,y}}{b}\right)^2 + \left(\frac{p_z - p_{i,z}}{c}\right)^2 \leq 1, \tag{1}$$

where a, b, c represent the maximum distances in the native sampling space in x-, y-, and z-direction, respectively. This sample selection w.r.t. the coordinate systems of the original ultrasound rays (in a backward fashion) is of special interest if physical parameters of an acquisition, such as frequency, probe element width, height, pitch, or focus, are incorporated into the reconstruction approach. Based on Eq. (1), multiple samples of each scan line would be selected depending on the proximity of a ray to the target position p. As better tensor reconstructions can be obtained from complementary information, only the nearest sample of each ray is selected instead of all samples fulfilling (1), thus restricting the set to contain only one sample per scanline.

2.2   Tensor Reconstruction

As a result of the sample selection, every voxel position p has an assigned set of samples $s_1, \ldots, s_n \subset S$, which can be used for the reconstruction of a tensor $T \in \mathbb{R}^{3\times3}$. In our CS conception, the 3D reconstruction should be able to reproduce as faithfully as possible the directionality dependence of the acquisition. To this end, we assume that for each sample s_i, ideally the following relationship holds:

$$v_i^\top T v_i = I_i, \quad \text{where} \quad T = \begin{bmatrix} T_{xx} & T_{xy} & T_{xz} \\ T_{xy} & T_{yy} & T_{yz} \\ T_{xz} & T_{yz} & T_{zz} \end{bmatrix}. \tag{2}$$

This results in the recovery of the tensor that preserves the intensities for each orientation best, given the sample subset assigned to the voxel. If estimated properly, it will then be possible to retrieve an intensity volume for an arbitrary viewing direction $v \in \mathbb{R}^3$ by evaluating the tensor w.r.t. this direction, i.e., by computing $v^\top T v$ at all voxel positions.

As T shall be symmetric, it is possible to rewrite (2) as follows:

$$[\, v_{i,x}^2, \, v_{i,y}^2, \, v_{i,z}^2, \, 2v_{i,x}v_{i,y}, \, 2v_{i,x}v_{i,z}, \, 2v_{i,y}v_{i,z}\,]\,\big[\,T_{xx}\ T_{yy}\ T_{zz}\ T_{xy}\ T_{xz}\ T_{yz}\,\big]^\top = I_i. \tag{3}$$

This means that we need at least six sampling points in order to compute the six coefficients T_{xx}, T_{yy}, T_{zz}, T_{xy}, T_{xz}, and T_{yz}. In practice, however, we use more than six samples, typically between 12 and 500 samples. As a consequence, we end up with a least squares problem

$$\|Ax - b\|_2^2, \tag{4}$$

where the i-th entry of $b \in \mathbb{R}^n$ is given by I_i, the i-th row of $A \in \mathbb{R}^{n \times 6}$ is given by $(v_{i,x}^2, v_{i,y}^2, v_{i,z}^2, 2v_{i,x}v_{i,y}, 2v_{i,x}v_{i,z}, 2v_{i,y}v_{i,z})^\top$, and $x \in \mathbb{R}^6$ denotes the solution vector. We solve this least squares problem for all volume points simultaneously using Cholesky decompositions implemented on a GPU.

At this point it is important to note that the symmetry of T is ensured by the used parametrization (3). However, as intensities are expected to be positive, T should be positive definite ($v^\top T v > 0$), which is not yet enforced in our scheme. This can partially result in erroneous tensor estimates, especially in areas with severe shadows or almost no meaningful information. We suggest to detect these areas by means of other approaches, e.g. by computing confidence values as suggested by [4], and exclude them from further processing.

3   Experimental Evaluation

For evaluating the potential of computational sonography as a new paradigm for 3D ultrasound reconstruction, we performed experiments on both phantom and in-vivo data. All 3D freehand image acquisitions were performed with an Ultrasonix RP system and a linear transducer (L14-5/38) tracked with an Ascension EM system. For the relevant sample selection, we chose $a = b = c = 1.5\ mm$. Volumetric spacing can be chosen freely as a balance between reconstruction quality (finer spacing) and speed (coarser); here all datasets were reconstructed with a spacing of 0.5mm in accordance with previous work. One advantage of computational sonography is the possibility to directly reconstruct information w.r.t. any viewing direction v by evaluating all the tensors according to $v^\top T v$, yielding an intensity volume corresponding to the direction v. Storing an acquired US sweep as a tensor volume thus facilitates the optimal resembling of the directional nature of ultrasound in any kind of interactive visualization for instance. As this possibility is conceptually similar to computational photography and particularly light field imaging, where the focus plane can be chosen

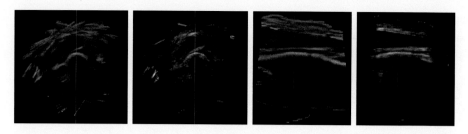

Fig. 3. Comparison of 3D Reconstructions - Real Data: Transverse **(column 1)** and longitudinal **(column 3)** slices for median compounding and similarly for the absolute value of the tensor trace of our reconstruction **(columns 2,4)** from a rotational scan of the Brachial bone. Note that conventional compounding depicts mainly the bone structure, while our reconstruction better resembles the overall structures in the volume.

and modified after the image acquisition process, we chose the term *computational sonography*. It can be observed in Fig. 3 and Fig. 4 that this procedure yields high quality reconstructions. Considering the directional information thus results in the possibility to retrieve texture information as it would be observed from arbitrarily chosen directions, in comparison to conventional reconstruction approaches which do not take directional information into account. In particular for Fig. 3, the median-reconstructed frame does not show anatomical information except for the shadowing/bone. Moreover, it is also distorted due to components from different views. In contrast to this, *computational sonography* allows for a reconstruction of directional information, preserving the original image information. It should be noted that the lack of speckle patterns in both images is mainly due to the large cell size (0.5mm with ∼500samples/voxel).

In order to demonstrate this effect also quantitatively, we reconstructed volumes for different acquisitions using the orientations of the corresponding original images. For evaluation, we compared the reconstructed intensity values with the original ultrasound samples, where we used the Mean Absolute Distance (MAD) to the original US image as well as the Peak Signal to Noise Ratio (PSNR) as evaluation metrics. As a baseline method, we employed the median compounding strategy, which is often recommended due to its preservation of the original US image appearance [11]. We performed this evaluation on two different sets of data: i) Five freehand scans of an in vitro silicone vessel phantom immersed in gelatin (2% gelatin, 1% agar, 1% flour) in order to allow for a scanning of realistic anatomies in a static environment, and ii) Ten freehand scans of the Femoral bone as well as the Antebrachial and Brachial bones using varying trajectories to evaluate the feasibility in a realistic setup. For both sets, we performed acquisitions using rotationally and overlapping trajectories, where a target volume position is imaged several times from different directions as this scenario well resembles the daily routine for US diagnostics. We perform a quantitative evaluation on 5 datasets (avg. 167 ± 103 slices) for the silicone phantom and 10 in-vivo datasets (avg. 243 ± 84 slices). Table 1 shows that CS provides on average higher peak SNR values as well as slightly lower absolute

Table 1. Quantitative results

Method	Phantom		In-vivo	
	MAD	PSNR	MAD	PSNR
Median Compounding	17.70 ± 1.81	20.31 ± 0.91	20.79 ± 2.27	18.67 ± 0.97
Computational Sonography	17.46 ± 2.47	57.67 ± 8.79	19.64 ± 2.89	66.35 ± 9.43

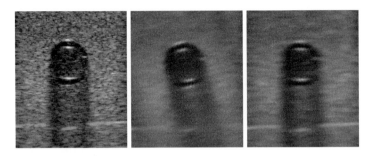

Fig. 4. Consistency with Original Acquisitions - Phantom Data: (left) Original B-mode image from a scan of the vessel phantom. **(middle)** Conventional reconstruction using median compounding. **(right)** Result computed from the proposed tensor representation using the direction v corresponding to the original image. Note the significant loss of original information in case of the regular compounding.

distances, while being partially susceptible to varying imaging conditions, as indicated by increased PSNR variability for CS. Observed high PSNR values show the potential of computational sonography as a new paradigm in 3D ultrasound imaging. Our future work includes enforcing the positive definiteness of T [5] to improve the results and developing a more efficient implementation (for a spacing of 0.5mm, the computational time is about 4 minutes per volume).

4   Conclusion

In this work we presented *computational sonography* as new paradigm for 3D ultrasound, reconstructing tensor fields from the acquired data instead of scalar intensities being used in today's practice. For tensor retrieval, we propose a two-step approach with a sample selection performed first, followed by a tensor reconstruction through least-squares solution. Our results show that the approach preserves the original (B-mode) ultrasound data better compared to state-of-art methods and yields a high potential for utilization of tensor information in further processing and visualization steps. With improved reconstruction schemes such as tensor fitting with direct regularization, as used frequently in DTI, computational sonography will hopefully evolve as a standard for reconstruction of 3D ultrasound data in the future. Applications that could benefit from our new representation are: multi-modal registration, segmentation, tracking, free viewpoint approximation (e.g. for educational simulation), online guidance of the acquisition to optimize the 3D reconstruction as well as analysis and comparison of different acquisitions. The additional information can be further used online to guide the current acquisition, e.g. acoustic window optimization, or offline, enabling targeted image analysis by allowing different users to extract different relevant information based on their technical or clinical objectives.

References

1. zu Berge, C.S., Kapoor, A., Navab, N.: Orientation-driven ultrasound compounding using uncertainty information. In: Stoyanov, D., Collins, D.L., Sakuma, I., Abolmaesumi, P., Jannin, P. (eds.) IPCAI 2014. LNCS, vol. 8498, pp. 236–245. Springer, Heidelberg (2014)
2. Hennersperger, C., Karamalis, A., Navab, N.: Vascular 3D+T freehand ultrasound using correlation of doppler and pulse-oximetry data. In: Stoyanov, D., Collins, D.L., Sakuma, I., Abolmaesumi, P., Jannin, P. (eds.) IPCAI 2014. LNCS, vol. 8498, pp. 68–77. Springer, Heidelberg (2014)
3. Hu, N., Downey, D.B., Fenster, A., Ladak, H.M.: Prostate boundary segmentation from 3D ultrasound images. Medical Physics 30(7), 1648–1659 (2003)
4. Karamalis, A., Wein, W., Klein, T., Navab, N.: Ultrasound confidence maps using random walks. Medical Image Analysis 16(6), 1101–1112 (2012)
5. Koay, C.G., Chang, L.-C., Carew, J.D., Pierpaoli, C., Basser, P.J.: A unifying theoretical and algorithmic framework for least squares methods of estimation in diffusion tensor imaging. Journal of Magnetic Resonance 182(1), 115 (2006)
6. Lang, A., Mousavi, P., Gill, S., Fichtinger, G., Abolmaesumi, P.: Multi-modal registration of speckle-tracked freehand 3D ultrasound to ct in the lumbar spine. Medical Image Analysis 16(3), 675–686 (2011)
7. Le Bihan, D., Mangin, J.F., Poupon, C., Clark, C.A., Pappata, S., Molko, N., Chabriat, H.: Diffusion tensor imaging: concepts and applications. Journal of Magnetic Resonance Imaging 13(4), 534–546 (2001)
8. Ng, R., Levoy, M., Brédif, M., Duval, G., Horowitz, M., Hanrahan, P.: Light field photography with a hand-held plenoptic camera. Computer Science Technical Report CSTR 2(11) (2005)
9. Papadacci, C., Tanter, M., Pernot, M., Fink, M.: Ultrasound backscatter tensor imaging (BTI): analysis of the spatial coherence of ultrasonic speckle in anisotropic soft tissues. IEEE Transactions on Ultrasonics, Ferroelectrics and Frequency Control 61(6), 986–996 (2014)
10. Solberg, O.V., Lindseth, F., Torp, H., Blake, R.E., Nagelhus Hernes, T.A.: Freehand 3D ultrasound reconstruction algorithms - a review. Ultrasound in Medicine and Biology 33, 991–1009 (2007)
11. Wein, W., Pache, F., Röper, B., Navab, N.: Backward-warping ultrasound reconstruction for improving diagnostic value and registration. In: Larsen, R., Nielsen, M., Sporring, J. (eds.) MICCAI 2006. LNCS, vol. 4191, pp. 750–757. Springer, Heidelberg (2006)
12. Weinmann, A., Demaret, L., Storath, M.: Total Variation Regularization for Manifold-Valued Data. SIAM Journal on Imaging Sciences 7(4), 2226–2257 (2014)
13. Yang, L., Georgescu, B., Zheng, Y., Meer, P., Comaniciu, D.: 3D ultrasound tracking of the left ventricle using one-step forward prediction and data fusion of collaborative trackers. In: IEEE Conf. on Comp. Vision and Pattern Recognition (2008)

Hierarchical Shape Distributions for Automatic Identification of 3D Diastolic Vortex Rings from 4D Flow MRI

Mohammed S.M. Elbaz[1], Boudewijn P.F. Lelieveldt[1,2], and Rob J. van der Geest[1]

[1] Division of Image Processing, Department of Radiology,
Leiden University Medical Center, Leiden, The Netherlands
[2] Department of Intelligent Systems, Delft University of Technology, Delft, The Netherlands
mohammed.elbaz@lumc.nl

Abstract. Vortex ring formation within the cardiac left ventricular (LV) blood flow has recently gained much interest as an efficient blood transportation mechanism and a potential early predictor of the chamber remodeling. In this work we propose a new method for automatic identification of vortex rings in the LV by means of 4D Flow MRI. The proposed method consists of three elements: 1) the 4D Flow MRI flow field is transformed into a 3D vortical scalar field using a well-established fluid dynamics-based vortex detection technique. 2) a shape signature of the cardiac vortex ring isosurface is derived from the probability distribution function of pairwise distances of randomly sampled points over the isosurface 3) a hierarchical clustering is then proposed to simultaneously identify the best isovalue that defines a vortex ring as well as the isosurface that corresponds to a vortex ring in the given vortical scalar field. The proposed method was evaluated in a datasets of 24 healthy controls as well as a dataset of 23 congenital heart disease patients. Results show great promise not only for vortex ring identification but also for allowing an objective quantification of vortex ring formation in the LV.

1   Introduction

A growing body of evidence [1-6] suggests a critical role of vortex ring formation within cardiac left ventricular blood flow during diastole as a significant contributor to efficient blood transportation [2] and as a potential clinical biomarker for early prediction of cardiac remodeling and diastolic dysfunction [4,5]. A vortex is generally characterized by a swirling motion of a group of fluid elements around a common axis. Among different types of vortical flow structures, vortex rings are most abundant in nature due their stability [6]. In the LV, the asymmetrical redirection of blood flow through the LV results in the development of a vortex ring distal to the mitral valve (Fig.1) [1].

In fluid dynamics, different methods exist to define a vortex structure [7]. Most of these methods are based on a function of the velocity gradient tensor of the flow field. 4D Flow MRI enables non-invasive acquisition of the blood flow velocity field

© Springer International Publishing Switzerland 2015
N. Navab et al. (Eds.): MICCAI 2015, Part II, LNCS 9350, pp. 467–475, 2015.
DOI: 10.1007/978-3-319-24571-3_56

providing all three velocity components (in-plane and through-plane) over the three spatial dimensions and over the cardiac cycle [1]. Therefore, 4D Flow MRI provides all the flow field information needed for 3D vortex analysis [3].

A typical 3D vortex ring identification problem consists of three steps 1) convert the 3D velocity flow field into some 3D vortical scalar field in which a vortex is defined given some criteria; 2) manually (empirically) select an isovalue threshold that can define a vortex ring structure from the 3D vortical field. Given that different vortex structures may be present in the same flow field, the selected isovalue may result in multiple co-existing isosurfaces of other vortex structures in addition to the target vortex ring. 3) Manually identify the isosurface that corresponds to a vortex ring. It is obvious that manual isovalue selection and vortex ring selection can be time consuming and subjective. This may limit the applicability of a 3D vortex ring analysis in a clinical setup in which objective and reproducible analysis is crucial.

To our knowledge, there have been no studies on fully automatic identification of a vortex ring (i.e. both steps 2 and 3) from 4D Flow MRI. In our previous work [8], only the automatic identification of a vortex ring (step 3) was addressed using a spectral shape analysis [9]. However, this was based on the assumption that an isovalue was already predefined; therefore the problem of automatic isovalue selection has not been addressed. In addition, spectral shape analysis can be computationally intensive, hence may not be suitable for a multi-level search.

In this work, we propose a new method that simultaneously and automatically identifies the isovalue and the vortex ring isosurface. The proposed method has three elements: First, the flow field from peak inflow phase of 4D Flow MRI is converted into a 3D vortical scalar field using a well-established fluid-dynamics-based vortex identification method called the Lambda2 method [10]. Second, a reference shape signature defining the vortex ring isosurface is computed from a training set using D2 shape distributions [11]. Finally, simultaneous identification of isovalue and vortex ring is achieved using hierarchical clustering that allows for an iterative search for the best D2 shape distribution match with the reference signature. To evaluate the objectivity and generalizability of the proposed method in a clinical setup, the defined vortex ring was quantified using the method introduced in [3] in a dataset of 24 healthy controls as well as in a challenging dataset of 23 congenital heart disease patients who were previously reported to have abnormal diastolic inflow [12].

2   Methodology

2.1   3D Vortical Scalar Field from 4D Flow MRI Using the Lambda2 Method

Among different fluid dynamics based vortex identification methods [7], the lambda2 (λ_2) method is considered the most accepted definition of a vortex [6]. The lambda2 method extracts vortex structures from the flow field by means of vortex-cores. The input for the Lambda2 method is the three velocity components of the velocity vector field and the output is a 3D scalar field in which each voxel is assigned a scalar value (λ_2). This scalar value can then be used to determine whether or not a voxel belongs to a vortex. For more formal definition, if U, V and F denote the three velocity components of the flow field acquired using 4D Flow and X, Y, Z denote the three spatial dimensions each of size $I \times J \times W$ with I as 4D Flow MRI's slice width, J as its height and W as the number of slices. Then the λ_2 method can be applied as follows. First, the velocity gradient tensor $\mathbf{J}$ is computed. Second, the tensor $\mathbf{J}$ is decomposed into its symmetric part, the strain deformation tensor $\mathbf{S} = \frac{\mathbf{J}+\mathbf{J}^T}{2}$ and the antisymmetric part, the spin sor $\mathbf{\Omega} = \frac{\mathbf{J}-\mathbf{J}^T}{2}$, where T is the transpose operation. Then, eigenvalue analysis is applied only on $\mathbf{S}^2 + \mathbf{\Omega}^2$. Finally, a voxel is labeled as part of a vortex only if it has two negative eigenvalues i.e. if $\lambda_1, \lambda_2, \lambda_3$ are the eigenvalues whereas $\lambda_1 \geq \lambda_2 \geq \lambda_3$ then a voxel is labeled as vortex if its $\lambda_2 < 0$. Isosurfaces of a λ_2 isovalue threshold (T_{λ_2}) <0 can be used to visualize different vortex structures in the flow field. A single T_{λ_2} isovalue can result in multi isosurfaces of different vortex structures among which a vortex ring may or may not be present. Different T_{λ_2} isovalues can be used to reveal different levels of details of vortices in the flow.

There are two outputs of this step. 1) A 3D volume denoted by $L_{i,j,w}$ where

$$L_{i,j,w} = \begin{cases} 0, & if\ \lambda_2(i,j,w) \geq 0 \\ \lambda_2(i,j,w) & if\ \lambda_2(i,j,w) < 0 \end{cases}, i = 1, \dots I. j = 1, \dots J. \ w = 1, \dots W.$$

2) A 1D feature vector Q_d, $d = 1, \dots P$ that stores all scalar values $L_{i,j,w} \neq 0$ (i.e. all possible T_{λ_2} thresholds). Q_d represents the isovalue feature vector. P represents the total number of scalar values $L_{i,j,w} \neq 0$.

Throughout the rest of the paper, the term vortex refers to a vortex core under the λ_2 definition explained above.

3   D2 Signature of Shape Distributions

The signature of shape distributions was first introduced in [11] for shape retrieval in computer vision tasks. The idea behind shape distributions' signature is to statistically encode a 3D model using a probability distribution of some parametric function that measures geometric properties of the given 3D model. This reduces the shape matching/retrieval problem into a simple distribution comparison [11]. D2 signature (Fig.1) is a shape distribution signature where the parametric function is defined by the Euclidean distances between randomly sampled pairs of points over the 3D surface. The D2 distribution can globally define the surface of interest (in our case, the vortex ring isosurface). Compared to other global shape signatures e.g. spectral signatures [9], the major advantage of the D2 distribution signature is its simplicity, essentially the shape matching problem is reduced to random sampling of points, histogram construction and finally histogram comparison using a dissimilarity metric.

Being a distribution, the D2-signature is invariant to rotation, translation and scaling (after normalization), therefore allowing matching of different shapes without the need for pre-registration or alignment. In addition, it is robust to small shape perturbations or deformations (e.g. due to noise) [11] which makes it sufficient for tasks that require multi shape comparisons as in our case.

In this work, the D2 signature is constructed following a similar procedure to that proposed in [11]: 1) Represent the 3D shape of interest as an isosurface. 2) Randomly sample N point pairs over the vortex-ring isosurface. $N=512^2$ pair of samples was used in this work. 3) Compute Euclidean distances between the N samples using L2-norm. 4) Construct a histogram of B bins of the pairwise distances. B =100 equally space bins was used in this work. 5) Normalize the resulting histogram using root mean square deviation. This step makes the signature scale invariant. 6) Define a dissimilarity metric to be used for histogram matching with a new given 3D model. In this work we used the normalized L1-norm (normalized by L1 norm of the reference signature) as dissimilarity metric. Though similar, cardiac vortex rings differ between subjects. To account for this, we derive an average reference signature from a cohort of healthy subjects for matching purposes. Of note, increasing N and B more than the specified numbers did not yield significant improvement.

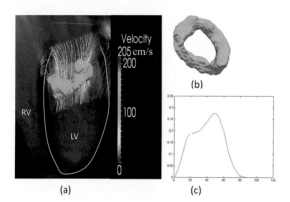

Fig. 1. (a) A four chamber view showing the 3D vortex ring isosurface (in green) with super-imposed streamlines in the LV at peak inflow phase in a sample healthy subject. (b) Separate view of the 3D vortex ring isosurface shown in (a). (c) The reference (average) D2 shape distributions' signature determined from the 24 healthy controls in this study.

4   Hierarchical Shape Distributions for Vortex Ring Identification

In principle, the vortex ring isosurface may be defined by any isovalue in the Q_d feature vector. This can result in a large search space as multiple shape matching tasks are needed per each value to find the target isosurface. To reduce the search space, we propose to compress the isovalue feature vector into a subset of representative isovalues using the vector quantization technique [13]. Given a vector of features, the vector quantization process involves compression of the input set of points into a smaller set. This works by dividing the input vector into groups, each group is then defined by one value given some criteria [13]. The well-known K-means clustering algorithm is a vector quantization method [13] in which a long input feature vector can be compressed into a vector of K cluster centroids that minimize the within-cluster sum of square distances.

In this work, we use an iterative hierarchical K-means scheme in which there is no need to predefine the number of centroids K. This allows avoiding the possible bias when K is predefined. The proposed scheme is as follows: Given the isovalue feature vector Q_d, initialize with K=1 and apply the K-means clustering algorithm (i.e. Q_d feature vector is reduced to a single candidate isovalue). Then, K is iteratively incremented by one until convergence or a predefined stopping criterion is satisfied. This results in a hierarchical multi-level vector $V^{r,k}$, in which each level $k = 1, ... P$ carries $r = 1, ... k$ candidate isovalues.

Given an isovalue level k, each isovalue $V^{r,k}$ can define $U_t^{r,k}, t = 1, ... E$ isosurfaces of different vortex structures from among them a vortex ring may or may not be present. Therefore, to identify the vortex ring isosurface we need to solve two problems. 1) Find the isovalue $V^{r,k}$ in which a vortex ring is one of its E resulting isosurfaces. 2) Find the isosurface $U_t^{r,k}$ that corresponds to a vortex ring.

Using the proposed hierarchical vector quantization scheme and the reference D2 shape distribution signature, we are able to simultaneously solve these two problems by minimizing the shape distribution distances as follows: for each isovalue $V^{r,k}$ at level k, extract the corresponding $U_t^{r,k}$ vortex isosurfaces. Then, for each isosurface $U_t^{r,k}$, construct the D2 shape distribution following the procedure explained above. Compute the dissimilarity distance $d_t^{r,k}$ with the reference signature using the normalized L1 norm (i.e. normalized by the L1-norm of the reference signature). Repeat this for every isovalue level until convergence ($d_t^{r,k}< \epsilon$) or stopping criteria is satisfied. We wish to identify the best surface match by finding the indices $\hat{r}, \hat{k}$ and $\hat{t}$ such that

$$\{\hat{r}, \hat{k}, \hat{t}\} = arg\min_{r,k,t} d$$

As a result the target two problems are simultaneously solved by defining the isosurface $U_{\hat{t}}^{\hat{r},\hat{k}}$ as the target vortex ring isosurface and corresponding isovalue $V^{\hat{r},\hat{k}}$ as the target isovalue. To avoid local minima, for each iteration, the K-means algorithm was replicated T times (T =10 was used in this work) using different initial centroids. Then, the centroids with minimum within-cluster sums of point-to-centroid distances were chosen. Two stop criteria were defined 1) reaching a maximum number of predefined iterations (set to 50 in this work). In all our experiments, less than 15 iterations were enough to find $\{\hat{r}, \hat{k}, \hat{t}\}$, and 2) The dissimilarity distance was increasing for three consecutive iterations. This decreases the possibility of stopping at local minima when only a single diverging iteration is used instead.

5   Quantitative Characterization of the Identified Vortex Ring in the LV

After the identification of the vortex ring isosurface, it was quantified using the parameters proposed in [3]. These parameters are the vortex ring orientation and normalized cylindrical (Circumferential (C), Longitudinal (L) and Radial(R)) 3D position of the vortex ring center relative to the LV. L and R were normalized relative to the LV long-axis length and the radius of the LV endocardial cavity, respectively. Vortex orientation is defined as the angle between the LV long axis and the fitting plane of the vortex isosurface.

6   Dataset, Preprocessing and Validation

We evaluated the proposed method on two datasets: one dataset of 24 healthy controls (mean age: 21±10 years) as previously described in [3] and a dataset of 23 patients (27±11) after atrioventricular septal defect correction. All subjects underwent retrospectively-gated 4D Flow MRI at 3.0 T (Philips) with spatial resolution of 3-4 mm^3 and a temporal resolution of ~30 ms covering all 4 chambers of the heart. This data was then linearly interpolated spatially to result in a 1mm^3 spatial resolution. More details on the acquisition parameters can be found in [3].

To localize the LV ROI, the LV was manually segmented from only the peak-inflow diastolic phase in the 4D Flow volume as explained in [3]. As the vortex ring is a connected region of voxels within the LV, accurate segmentation is not required for the purpose of vortex ring identification. Only rough over-segmentation of the LV (to ensure the LV is covered) was enough to roughly define the LV ROI. In this work, an over-segmentation of about 0.5 cm around LV border was used to define LV ROI.

To generate the ground truth for the vortex ring isosurface in the two included datasets, for the healthy control dataset, we used the vortex ring isosurfaces interactively generated with low inter and intra observer variability in a previously validated workflow [3]. Same procedure in [3] was used to blindly generate the ground truth for patient dataset. To quantitatively evaluate the performance of the proposed method in the first dataset of healthy controls, leave-one-out cross-validation was used to avoid bias in the selection of the reference averaged D2 signature.

To test the generalization performance in a clinical setting, the dataset of 23 patients was evaluated using a reference signature derived only from the 24 healthy control subjects. To evaluate the identification performance relative to the ground truth, we performed two sets of evaluations. The accuracy of the identified isosurface object was assessed using the Hausdorff distance and dice coefficient for surface overlap. In addition, a paired student's t-test comparison of the automatically defined isovalues and the one used to generate the ground truth isosurfaces was performed. Second, paired student's t-test was used to statistically compare the quantitative vortex ring parameters of the automatically identified vortex-ring isosurfaces to those of the ground truth. For all statistical tests a p-value <0.05 was considered significant.

7   Results

In all subjects of both datasets, a vortex ring isosurface was successfully identified from the Lambda2 scalar field with qualitatively similar shape to that of the ground truth (Fig. 2). Detailed results of the quantitative evaluation over the two datasets is given in Table 1 where a Hausdorff distance of 8.36±7.55 mm in healthy control dataset and 11.73±6.57 mm in the patients dataset were found. The surface overlap (dice coefficient) was 0.81±0.09 in controls and 0.77±0.14 in patients. The identified isovalues using the proposed method were highly comparable to those of the ground truth and not statistically different (p=0.86). Quantitative parameters of the automatically identified vortex rings were in good agreement with the ground truth.

8   Discussion and Conclusion

This paper presents a framework for objective identification and quantification of 3D vortex ring in the LV from 4D PC MRI by means of isosurfaces. The problem of vortex ring identification from the 3D vortical scalar field was reduced to histogram comparison and hierarchical K-means vector quantization. The reported results on healthy controls as well as patients show great promise of the proposed method. The generalizability of the proposed method was evaluated with abnormal vortex rings being identified from 23 patients with a signature trained solely on normal vortex ring isosurfaces from healthy controls. The proposed method provided high performance and agreement with the blindly generated ground truth. It is important to emphasize that the exact size/volume of a vortex ring is generally undefined as it is isovalue dependent. Therefore, volumetric measurements like Hausdorff distance or dice overlap may not sufficiently capture the validity of the identified vortex rings. Instead, the evaluated quantitative characterization parameters (C, L, R and orientation) may provide more objective evaluation of the method and its potential clinical value. In this work, the vortex ring identification was limited to the phase of peak LV inflow which is considered the moment around full vortex development [3,6], however vortex formation in the LV is a dynamic process over the entire diastole involving vortex evolution and dissipation with corresponding shape deformations. Future work will address the method's performance in other diastolic phases. The proposed method allows for objective quantitative characterization of the peak-inflow vortex ring formation in the LV with results comparable to those previously validated [3]. With the increasing interest in vortex ring formation as a potential biomarker for LV (dys)function [2,4,6], the proposed method can play an important role in providing objective 3D vortex analysis for assessment of vortex ring formation in the LV from 4D Flow MRI.

Table 1. Qunatitative evaluation results

Parameter	24 Controls			23 Patients		
	Ground truth	Proposed method	p-value (paired t-test)	Ground truth	Proposed method	p-value (paired t-test)
C	87±20	85±24	0.12	67±19	63±23	0.07
L	0.19±0.04	0.19±0.04	0.92	0.22±0.06	0.22±0.05	0.74
R	0.27±0.07	0.27±0.07	0.91	0.33±0.09	0.33±0.1	0.61
Vortex Orientation	70±55	65±54	0.65	57±25	57±40	0.87
Lambda2 Isovalue*	-7.2±-3.43	-7.3±-3.2	0.82	-7.27±-11.24	-7.7±-5.45	0.86
Surface Overlap (Dice Coeffecient)	0.81±0.09			0.77±0.14		
Hausdorff distance (mm)	8.36±7.55			11.73±6.57		

*The absolute lambda2 isovalue doesn't have direct interpretation here and was provided only to give impression on how similar were they in test cases compared to ground truth

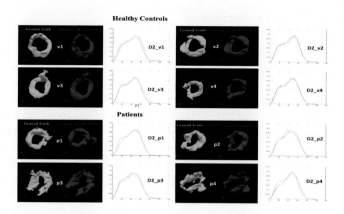

Fig. 1. Sample results of the proposed method on 4 healthy controls (top two rows: v1 to v4) and 4 patients (bottom two rows: p1 to p4). For every subject, the ground truth is presented on left (green) and the automatically identified peak-inflow vortex ring isosurface on right (red). D2_v1 to D2_v4 and D2_p1 to D2_p4 show the best matched D2 distributions corresponded to the automatically identified vortex ring isosurface (red curve) overlaid on the reference signature (average over healthy controls) in blue.

Acknowledgement. This work is supported by Dutch Technology Foundation (STW): project number 11626.

References

1. Kilner, P.J., et al.: Asymmetric redirection of flow through the heart. Nature 404(6779), 759–761 (2000)
2. Martinez-Legazpi, P., et al.: Contribution of the diastolic vortex ring to left ventricular filling. J. Am. Coll. Cardiol. 64, 1711–1721 (2014)
3. Elbaz, M.S.M., et al.: Vortex flow during early and late left ventricular filling in normal subjects: quantitative characterization using retrospectively-gated 4D flow cardiovascular magnetic resonance and three-dimensional vortex core analysis. J. Cardiovasc. Magn. Reson. 16(1), 78 (2014)
4. Pedrizzetti, G., et al.: The vortex–an early predictor of cardiovascular outcome? Nat. Rev. Cardiol. 11, 545–553 (2014)
5. Gharib, M., et al.: Optimal vortex formation as an index of cardiac health. Proc. Natl. Acad. Sci. U.S.A 103, 6305–6308 (2006)
6. Kheradvar, A., Pedrizzetti, G.: Vortex formation in the cardiovascular system. Springer Science & Business Media (2012)
7. Jiang, M. et al.: Detection and visualization of vortices. In: Visualization Handbook (2004)
8. ElBaz, M.S.M., Lelieveldt, B.P.F., Westenberg, J.J.M., van der Geest, R.J.: Automatic extraction of the 3D left ventricular diastolic transmitral vortex ring from 3D whole-heart phase contrast MRI using laplace-beltrami signatures. In: Camara, O., Mansi, T., Pop, M., Rhode, K., Sermesant, M., Young, A. (eds.) STACOM 2013. LNCS, vol. 8330, pp. 204–211. Springer, Heidelberg (2014)

9. Reuter, M., et al.: Laplace–Beltrami spectra as 'Shape-DNA' of surfaces and solids. Computer-Aided Design 38(4), 342–366 (2006)

10. Jeong, J., Hussain, F.: On the identification of a vortex. J. Fluid Mech. 285, 69–94 (1995)

11. Osada, R., et al.: Shape distributions. ACM Trans. Graph. 21(4), 807–832 (2002)

12. Calkoen, E.E., et al.: Characterization and improved quantification of left ventricular inflow using streamline visualization with 4DFlow MRI in healthy controls and patients after atrioventricular septal defect correction. J. Magn. Reson. Imaging (2014)

13. Gersho, A., Gray, R.M.: Vector quantization and signal compression. Springer Science & Business Media (1992)

Robust CT Synthesis for Radiotherapy Planning: Application to the Head and Neck Region

Ninon Burgos[1], M. Jorge Cardoso[1,2], Filipa Guerreiro[3], Catarina Veiga[4],
Marc Modat[1,2], Jamie McClelland[5], Antje-Christin Knopf[3],
Shonit Punwani[6,7], David Atkinson[6], Simon R. Arridge[5], Brian F. Hutton[8,9],
and Sébastien Ourselin[1,2]

[1] Translational Imaging Group, CMIC, University College London, London, UK
[2] Dementia Research Centre, Institute of Neurology, UCL, London, UK
[3] The Institute of Cancer Research, Radiotherapy Imaging Department, London, UK
[4] Radiation Physics Group, UCL Medical Physics and Bioengineering, London, UK
[5] Centre for Medical Image Computing, UCL, London, UK
[6] Centre for Medical Imaging, UCL, London, UK
[7] Department of Radiology, University College London Hospitals, London, UK
[8] Institute of Nuclear Medicine, UCL, London, UK
[9] Centre for Medical Radiation Physics, University of Wollongong, NSW, Australia

Abstract. In this work, we propose to tackle the problem of magnetic resonance (MR)-based radiotherapy treatment planning in the head & neck area by synthesising computed tomography (CT) from MR images using an iterative multi-atlas approach. The proposed method relies on pre-acquired pairs of non-rigidly aligned T2-weighted MRI and CT images of the neck. To synthesise a pseudo CT, all the MRIs in the database are first registered to the target MRI using a robust affine followed by a deformable registration. An initial pseudo CT is obtained by fusing the mapped atlases according to their morphological similarity to the target. This initial pseudo CT is then combined with the target MR image in order to improve both the registration and fusion stages and refine the synthesis in the bone region.

Results showed that the proposed iterative CT synthesis algorithm is able to generate pseudo CT images in a challenging region for registration algorithms. We demonstrate that the robust affine decreases the overall absolute error compared to a single affine transformation, mainly in images with small axial field-of-view, whilst the bone refinement process further reduces the error in the bone region, increasing image sharpness.

1 Introduction

Magnetic resonance imaging (MRI) is often preferred over computed tomography (CT) as a structural imaging modality, mainly for its excellent soft-tissue contrast. However, MRI does not provide photon density information, which is essential for several applications such as performing dosimetry for MR-based radiotherapy treatment planning (RTP) or attenuation correction in the context of Positron Emission Tomography (PET)/MR scanners. To overcome this limitation, a solution is to recreate a CT image from the available MR images.

© Springer International Publishing Switzerland 2015
N. Navab et al. (Eds.): MICCAI 2015, Part II, LNCS 9350, pp. 476–484, 2015.
DOI: 10.1007/978-3-319-24571-3_57

Several methods exist to obtain synthetic CT images and many have been applied to RTP. Results presented in [1] are obtained from a Gaussian mixture regression model linking the MRI intensity values to the CT Hounsfield units (HU). In [2], bones are manually segmented and the MRI intensity values are converted to HU using a dual model, within and outside of the bone class. Other approaches, called registration- or atlas-based methods, rely on a single [3] or a database [4–6] of MRI and CT image pairs and consist of registering each atlas MR image to the target MRI, applying the same transformation to the associated CT image and finally, for multi-atlas methods, fusing the registered CT images. The fusion can be obtained by computing the voxelwise median [4], using a probabilistic Bayesian framework [5], an arithmetic mean process or pattern recognition with Gaussian process [6]. Atlas-based methods have also been applied to MR-based attenuation correction. In [7], the fusion is obtained via a voxelwise weighting scheme where the weights are defined according to the morphological similarity between the deformed atlas and target images.

Most of these methods address the problem in the brain [1,4–6], some in the pelvic area [2,3], but none in the neck. CT synthesis in the neck is challenging for three main reasons. First, the mixture of bone and air present in this area makes the conversion of MRI intensity values to HU difficult as both bone and air have usually low intensities in MR images. A second challenge comes from the wide range of target image fields of view (FOV). Images with large axial FOV can cover an area starting from the top of the lungs to the middle of the head (Fig 1, bottom), while images with small axial FOV (Fig 1, top) only focus on a target area, such as a tumour. These disparities are a problem when aligning the atlas images to the target. The last challenge arises from the large-scale postural changes, such as flexion or extension of the neck, or the position of the jawbone, which reduces the performances of registration methods.

We propose to redesign the synthesis process and present an iterative multi-atlas algorithm to synthesise CT images in the neck region. The contribution of this paper, compared to the current atlas-based methods, consists of four points.

1. To form the database, the CT and MR images are non-rigidly aligned to account for the different positions between the two acquisitions. We also align all the MR-CT pairs to a common coordinate frame.
2. The first step to synthesise a pseudo CT is to register all the MRI atlases to the target MRI. Large differences in the FOV were observed between the subjects, which can hinder the inter-subject registration. To overcome this problem, we propose a robust alignment exploiting the fact that all the atlases are pre-aligned in the same coordinate frame.
3. Similarly to [7], the pseudo CT is obtained by fusing the mapped atlases according to their morphological similarity to the target. A similarity measure taking into account mismatches between FOVs is proposed.
4. The algorithm relies on the ability to accurately map T2 images from different subjects, a process that can be challenging, particularly in low-contrast areas. We propose to combine multiple modalities, an initial pseudo CT and the target MR image to improve the synthesis accuracy in the bone region.

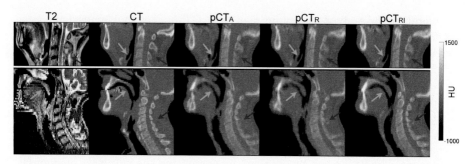

Fig. 1. Examples of T2-w MRI, CT, and pseudo CT images for a subject from dataset 1 (top) and dataset 2 (bottom). Note that the method is able to generate a pseudo CT even in the presence of motion and large-scale postural changes such as neck flexion.

2   Method

The proposed iterative multi-atlas algorithm aims at synthesising CT from MR images of the neck region using a database of non-rigidly aligned MRI and CT pairs. In this section, we apply a robust process to align the atlas images to the target image and propose an iterative process aiming at improving the synthesis in the bone region, critical for radiotherapy planning.

2.1   MR-CT Database Building

The CT synthesis method relies on pre-acquired pairs of T2-weighted MRI and CT images of the neck. For each subject, the MRI is mapped to the CT using a non-rigid deformation algorithm [8] to compensate for neck flexion. The MRI from the atlases are then mapped to a common coordinate frame via an affine groupwise registration [9]. The transformations are then applied to the MR-CT pairs by updating their image coordinate system, thus forming a database of MR and CT images aligned in a common space.

2.2   Inter-subject Mapping

The first step to synthesise a CT for a given MRI is to register all the MRIs in the atlas database to the target MRI. This inter-subject coordinate mapping can be obtained using a symmetric global registration followed by a non-rigid registration [7]. However, when the FOV of the target MRI is limited, which can occur when a tumour is the sole target of the imaging protocol, the affine alignment can be inaccurate. To overcome this weakness, we propose a robust affine which relies on the fact that the atlases are aligned to the same space.

Robust Affine. The robust affine alignment consists of three steps. Each atlas MR is first affinely mapped to the target. The average transformation, computed in the log space, is obtained from all the pairwise affine transformations. This average affine is then used to initialise a second affine registration step to refine the alignment. As all the atlases are aligned to the same space, applying the average affine transformation to all of them guarantees that each atlas is initially aligned with the target.

Non-rigid Registration. The robust affine alignment between atlas and target images is used to initialise a cubic B-spline parametrised non-rigid registration, using normalised mutual information as a measure of similarity [8]. These non-rigid transformations are also applied to all the CTs in the atlas database. Through this registration and resampling procedure, one obtains a series of MRI/CT pairs aligned to the target MRI.

2.3   CT Synthesis

Similarly to [7], the pseudo CT is obtained by fusing the mapped atlases according to their morphological similarity to the target. A local image similarity measure between the target MRI and the set of registered MRIs from the database is used as a surrogate of the underlying morphological similarity, under the assumption that if two MRIs are similar at a certain spatial location, the two CTs will also be similar at this location.

Image/Morphological Similarity. Due to different acquisition FOVs, the inter-subject mapping and resampling processes introduce areas where no information is available. Those areas have to be accounted for when the similarity measure is computed and during the intensity fusion process. We extend the convolution-based local normalised correlation coefficient (LNCC) method by Cachier *et al.* [10] to irregular regions-of-interest (ROI-LNCC).

Let the target subject's MRI be denoted by I^{MRI} and, for each of the N atlases in the database, let the mapped MR image of atlas n be denoted by J_n^{MRI}. The ROI-LNCC between I^{MRI} and J_n^{MRI} at voxel x is then given by

$$\text{ROI-LNCC}_n(x) = \frac{\langle I^{MRI}(x), J_n^{MRI}(x) \rangle}{\sigma(I^{MRI}(x))\,\sigma(J_n^{MRI}(x))} \quad . \tag{1}$$

Let Ω be a density function equal to 1 where the fields of view overlap, and 0 otherwise. The standard deviation σ and the correlation $<,>$ are defined as in [7], but instead of a normal convolution process, a density normalised convolution is used, i.e. the mean will be estimated as $(G * I)/(G * \Omega)$, where G represents a Gaussian kernel, $*$ denotes the convolution operator, and $G * \Omega$ represents a density normalisation term that compensates for areas with missing information. The ROI-LNCC values outside the FOV are set to $-\infty$.

Intensity Fusion. The ROI-LNCCs at each voxel are ranked across all atlas images in the database and the ranks, noted as $r_n(x)$, are converted to weights by applying an exponential decay function $w_n(x) = e^{-\beta r_n(x)}$ with $w_n(x)$ being the weight associated with the nth mapped atlas image at voxel x and $\beta = 0.5$ [7].

As in [7], the final pseudo CT (I^{pCT}) is obtained by applying a spatially varying weighted averaging

$$I^{pCT}(x) = \frac{\sum_{n=1}^{N} w_n(x) \cdot J_n^{CT}(x)}{\sum_{n=1}^{N} w_n(x)} \quad . \tag{2}$$

2.4   Iterative Bone Refinement Process

In contrast to CT images, T2-weighted MR images do not provide a good estimate of the bone location. We propose to combine multiple modalities to regularise the registration in low-contrast areas, providing more realistic mappings.

An initial pseudo CT (pCT) is synthesised following the method described previously. This pCT is then combined with the MR image to form a MRI-pCT pair. The MRI-pCT pair is registered to all the MRI-CT pairs from the database. The inter-subject coordinate mapping is obtained using the robust affine followed by a multichannel non-rigid registration. Normalised mutual information is used as a similarity measure for the T2-weighted MR channel while the sum of squared differences is computed for the second channel, exploiting the quantitative property of the CT intensities. A refined pseudo CT is obtained by fusing the mapped MRI-CT pairs according to their morphological similarity to the target MRI-pCT pair, which is assessed using a multivariate LNCC (MV ROI-LNCC) defined as MV-ROI-LNCC$_n$ = ROI-LNCC $\left(I^{MRI}, J_n^{MRI} \right)$ + ROI-LNCC $\left(I^{pCT}, J_n^{CT} \right)$.

3   Validation and Results

Data Images from two retrospective studies were used to build the MR-CT database and validate the proposed method.

Dataset 1: Small axial FOV. Six subjects with a small axial FOV were used to assess the robustness of the method. They have both T2-weighted MRI (voxel size $1 \times 1 \times 2$ mm^3, matrix size $192 \times 192 \times 40$) and CT (voxel size $1 \times 1 \times 2$ mm^3, matrix size $512 \times 512 \times 200$) images.

Dataset 2: Large axial FOV. Seventeen subjects with a large axial FOV were used to build the database and validate the method. They have both T2-weighted MRI (voxel size $0.7 \times 0.7 \times 3.3$ mm^3, matrix size $256 \times 256 \times 60$) and CT (voxel size $1 \times 1 \times 2.5$ mm^3, matrix size $512 \times 512 \times 160$) images.

3.1   Algorithmic Comparison

Subjects from dataset 2 were used to build the database. Using the proposed technique, we first synthesised pseudo CTs for all subjects in dataset 1 to study the benefits of the robust affine compared with a single affine. We then performed a leave-one-out cross validation using all the subjects from dataset 2 to study the impact of the bone refinement process on the pseudo CT images. For each subject in both datasets, three pseudo CTs were synthesised:

- pCT$_A$, obtained using a single affine between the atlases and target;

Table 1. Average ± SD of the MAE and SAE computed between the reference CT and the pseudo CTs, and of the FDE computed for each pseudo CT.

		Dataset 1			Dataset 2		
		pCT_A	pCT_R	pCT_{RI}	pCT_A	pCT_R	pCT_{RI}
MAE	Bone	204.5 ± 19.2	193.6 ± 23.2	196.8 ± 16.0	208.0 ± 19.6	205.2 ± 18.2	192.1 ± 13.4
(HU)	Soft	41.2 ± 1.7	40.2 ± 2.2	39.1 ± 1.9	41.1 ± 5.3	40.6 ± 5.1	40.4 ± 4.6
	Air	63.4 ± 8.4	55.6 ± 8.4	56.6 ± 10.3	133.8 ± 29.4	133.0 ± 23.0	126.7 ± 25.4
SAE	Bone	201.8 ± 40.0	189.5 ± 45.1	186.9 ± 34.9	184.4 ± 14.8	182.0 ± 14.1	169.7 ± 10.9
(HU)	Soft	45.8 ± 1.6	44.5 ± 2.1	43.4 ± 2.0	46.5 ± 3.7	46.1 ± 3.7	46.0 ± 3.4
	Air	114.7 ± 11.4	106.0 ± 11.1	108.6 ± 13.7	145.4 ± 18.5	143.8 ± 13.1	150.2 ± 20.6
FDE	All	18.40 ± 0.12	18.11 ± 0.13	17.77 ± 0.13	19.73 ± 0.32	19.69 ± 0.32	19.44 ± 0.34

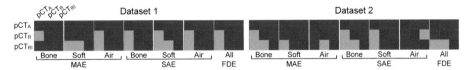

Fig. 2. Results of the one-tailed Wilcoxon signed-rank test at the 5% significance level for the MAE, SAE and FDE metrics. The colour green indicates a significant decrease for the row method when compared to the column method, while the red indicates that the difference is not significant.

– pCT_R, obtained using the robust affine;
– pCT_{RI}, obtained after the robust affine and the iterative bone refinement.
The mean absolute error (MAE) and the standard deviation of the absolute error (SAE) were calculated for every subject between the reference CT non-rigidly aligned to the MR (R^{CT}) and each of the pseudo CTs (I^{CT}), in a region of interest comprising V voxels: $\text{MAE} = \frac{1}{V}\sum_x |I^{CT}(x) - R^{CT}(x)|$, $\text{SAE} = \frac{1}{V-1}\sqrt{\sum_x (|I^{CT}(x) - R^{CT}(x)| - \text{MAE})^2}$. The MAE gives information on the amount of error while the SAE gives information on the amount of dispersion of the error. We focus the validation on three regions: air (< -100 HU), soft-tissue (between -100 and 300 HU), and bone (>300 HU). As inaccuracies exist in the registration between the real CT and T2-weighted images, we also provide a reference-free metric using the entropy of the pseudo CT images in the frequency domain as a measure of sharpness: $\text{FDE} = -\sum (f \log_2 (f))$ where f is the normalised absolute amplitudes of frequencies of the pseudo CT image [11].

3.2   Robust Affine: Validation with Small Axial FOV

The average and standard deviation (SD) of the MAE, SAE and FDE metrics are presented in Table 1. Using the robust instead of a single affine transform decreases the MAE, SAE and FDE in all the regions. Colour coded statistical test results are presented in Fig 2. These results show significant improvements when comparing synthesis using the robust affine to synthesis using a single affine. An example of MR, CT and pCT images are displayed in Fig 1 (top).

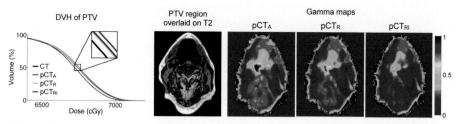

Fig. 3. Results of the dose calculations performed for a test subject from dataset 1.

3.3   Iterative Bone Refinement: Validation with Large Axial FOV

After one iteration of the bone refinement process, the MAE and SAE in the bone region and the FDE are significantly decreased (Table 1 & Fig 2). An example of MR, CT and pCT images are displayed in Fig 1 (bottom).

3.4   Case Study: Dosimetry Calculations

To test the impact of the proposed improvements in RTP, dose calculations were performed for a test subject from dataset 1. We compared the cumulative dose volume histogram (DVH) obtained for the pseudo CTs to the DVH obtained for the reference CT image in the planning target volume (PTV). The DVHs displayed in Fig 3 show a close agreement between the pseudo CTs and the CT. A 2D gamma analysis [12], evaluated at 2%/2 mm dose difference/distance to agreement, was used to compare axial dose distributions. A gamma index greater than 1 means that the calculation does not meet the acceptance criteria. The gamma maps displayed in Fig 3 show that the robust affine improves the results compared with a single affine and that the bone refinement process further reduces the error to an acceptable range ($\gamma < 1$).

4   Discussion and Conclusion

This paper presents a CT synthesis algorithm based on a multi-atlas information propagation scheme and iterative process able to generate pseudo CT images in the neck, a region challenging for registration algorithms. The results displayed in Table 1 demonstrate that the robust affine decreases the absolute error compared to the single affine, particularly when the axial FOV of the target image is limited, and that the bone refinement process further reduces the error in the bone region, producing sharper images. Most of the errors observed when comparing with results obtained in the brain [7] can be explained by inaccuracies in the inter-subject registrations due to a complex mixture of tissues present in the neck area, and by large epiglottis/tongue mismatch between MR and CT data.

Note that while the main focus of the proposed technique is to estimate dose deposition in the context of MR-based RTP, the proposed method could also be used for attenuation correction in PET/MR imaging studies of the neck. As a proof of concept, dose calculations were performed for a test subject (Fig 3), showing close agreement between the proposed pseudo CT and the reference CT, within acceptable error margins ($\gamma < 1$). Further experiments are required to verify the suitability of this proposed framework for dose calculation and to study the effect of anatomical abnormalities, such as tumours, on the results. We will also explore the effect of the number of iterations on the synthesis accuracy.

Acknowledgements. This work was supported by an IMPACT studentship funded by Siemens and the UCL FES. Funding was received from the EPSRC (EP/H046410/1, EP/J020990/1, EP/K005278), the MRC (MR/J01107X/1), the EU-FP7 project VPH-DARE@IT (FP7-ICT-2011-9-601055), Alzheimer's Research UK, the Brain Research Trust, the NIHR BRU (Dementia), the UCL Leonard Wolfson Experimental Neurology Centre (PR/ylr/18575), the Fundação para a Ciência e a Tecnologia (SFRH/BD/76169/2011), and by researchers at the NIHR UCLH BRC (including the High Impact Initiative).

References

1. Jonsson, J., Akhtari, M., Karlsson, M., Johansson, A., Asklund, T., Nyholm, T.: Accuracy of inverse treatment planning on substitute CT images derived from MR data for brain lesions. Radiation Oncology 10(1) (2015)
2. Korhonen, J., Kapanen, M., Keyriläinen, J., Seppälä, T., Tenhunen, M.: A dual model HU conversion from MRI intensity values within and outside of bone segment for MRI-based radiotherapy treatment planning of prostate cancer. Medical Physics 41(1), 011704 (2014)
3. Dowling, J.A., Lambert, J., Parker, J., Salvado, O., Fripp, J., Capp, A., Wratten, C., Denham, J.W., Greer, P.B.: An atlas-based electron density mapping method for magnetic resonance imaging (MRI)-alone treatment planning and adaptive MRI-based prostate radiation therapy. International Journal of Radiation Oncology · Biology · Physics 83(1), e5–e11 (2012)
4. Sjölund, J., Forsberg, D., Andersson, M., Knutsson, H.: Generating patient specific pseudo-CT of the head from MR using atlas-based regression. Physics in Medicine and Biology 60(2), 825 (2015)
5. Gudur, M.S.R., Hara, W., Le, Q.-T., Wang, L., Xing, L., Li, R.: A unifying probabilistic Bayesian approach to derive electron density from MRI for radiation therapy treatment planning. Physics in Medicine and Biology 59(21), 6595 (2014)
6. Uh, J., Merchant, T.E., Li, Y., Li, X., Hua, C.: MRI-based treatment planning with pseudo CT generated through atlas registration. Med. Phys. 41(5) (2014)
7. Burgos, N., Cardoso, M.J., Thielemans, K., Modat, M., Pedemonte, S., Dickson, J., Barnes, A., Ahmed, R., Mahoney, C.J., Schott, J.M., Duncan, J.S., Atkinson, D., Arridge, S.R., Hutton, B.F., Ourselin, S.: Attenuation Correction Synthesis for Hybrid PET-MR Scanners: Application to Brain Studies. IEEE Transactions on Medical Imaging 33(12), 2332–2341 (2014)
8. Modat, M., Ridgway, G.R., Taylor, Z.A., Lehmann, M., Barnes, J., Hawkes, D.J., Fox, N.C., Ourselin, S.: Fast free-form deformation using graphics processing units. Computer Methods and Programs in Biomedicine 98(3), 278–284 (2010)

9. Modat, M., Cash, D.M., Daga, P., Winston, G.P., Duncan, J.S., Ourselin, S.: Global image registration using a symmetric block-matching approach. Journal of Medical Imaging 1(2), 024003 (2014)

10. Cachier, P., Bardinet, E., Dormont, D., Pennec, X., Ayache, N.: Iconic feature based nonrigid registration: the PASHA algorithm. Computer Vision and Image Understanding 89(2-3), 272–298 (2003)

11. Kristan, M., Pernus, F.: Entropy based measure of camera focus. In: Proc. ERK 2004, pp. 179–182 (2004)

12. Low, D.A., Harms, W.B., Mutic, S., Purdy, J.A.: A technique for the quantitative evaluation of dose distributions. Medical Physics 25(5), 656–661 (1998)

Mean Aneurysm Flow Amplitude Ratio Comparison between DSA and CFD

Fred van Nijnatten[1,*], Odile Bonnefous[2,*], Hernan G. Morales[2], Thijs Grünhagen[1], Roel Hermans[1], Olivier Brina[3], Vitor Mendes Pereira[3,4], Daniel Ruijters[1]

[1] interventional X-Ray, Philips Healthcare, Best, The Netherlands
{fred.van.nijnatten,thijs.grunhagen,roel.hermans,
danny.ruijters}@philips.com
[2] Medisys - Philips Research, Paris, France
{odile.bonnefous,hernan.morales}@philips.com
[3] Division of Neuroradiology, Department of Medical Imaging,
University Hospitals of Geneva, Switzerland
olivier.brina@hcuge.ch
[4] Division of Neuroradiology, Department of Medical Imaging and Division of Neurosurgery,
Department of Surgery, Toronto Western Hospital,
University Health Network, Toronto, Ontario, Canada
vitormpbr@hotmail.com

Abstract. The Mean Aneurysm Flow Amplitude ratio (MAFA-ratio) has been proposed to evaluate the efficacy of flow diverting stents during minimally invasive intracranial aneurysm treatment. A method has been described for calculating the MAFA-ratio on high frame-rate digital subtraction angiography (DSA) acquisitions using an optical flow algorithm. In this article we have generated computational fluid dynamics (CFD) simulations using six distinct aneurysms and computed the MAFA-ratios based on these data. Furthermore, the simulations have been used to create virtual angiograms, in order to calculate the MAFA-ratios using the DSA approach. An analysis of the MAFA-ratios generated by both methods shows that there is a monotone increasing relation between the DSA and CFD based ratios, albeit without a slope being identity. Overall, it can be concluded that the DSA-based ratio is a predictor for the magnitude of aneurysm flow reduction, i.e., for the efficacy of flow diverting stents.

Keywords: Mean aneurysm flow amplitude, Flow diversion, Digital subtraction angiography, Computational fluid dynamics.

1 Introduction

Digital subtraction angiography (DSA) and three-dimensional rotational angiography (3DRA) are currently the gold standard for imaging and navigation of intravascular

---

* Fred van Nijnatten and Odile Bonnefous are joint first authors.

© Springer International Publishing Switzerland 2015
N. Navab et al. (Eds.): MICCAI 2015, Part II, LNCS 9350, pp. 485–492, 2015.
DOI: 10.1007/978-3-319-24571-3_58

devices during minimally invasive intracranial aneurysm treatment. While traditional DSA and 3DRA are unrivalled regarding imaging the vascular morphology, they lack functional information. Recently, aneurysm treatment by flow diverting stents has been gaining popularity. These devices reduce the inflow of blood into the aneurysm with the objective to cause the blood in the aneurysm to thrombose in the months following the intervention. The reduction of blood inflow causes flow alterations in both amplitude and patterns in the aneurysm sac, which are considered to predict rupture and clotting [1,2,3,4].

A linear dependency between the amplitude of the aneurysm flow and the arterial flow rate in the feeding vessel has been shown in [5]. Therefore, the possible variation of arterial flow conditions should be taken into account when evaluating the aneurysm flow reduction induced by a flow diverter. This can be achieved by normalization of aneurysm flow measurements with their corresponding arterial flow measurements.

The normalized mean aneurysm flow amplitude ratio (MAFA-ratio) has been introduced as a parameter that can be used to measure the efficacy of the flow diverting stent during the course of the intervention [6,7,8]. The MAFA-ratio R is defined as:

$$R = \frac{M_{post}}{M_{pre}} \cdot \frac{Q_{pre}}{Q_{post}} \tag{1}$$

Whereby the *pre* and *post* subscripts indicate measured quantities prior and after deploying the flow diverting stent. Q represents the time-averaged arterial flow of the feeding parent blood vessel, which is used to normalize the MAFA-ratio for overall flow changes [9]. The mean flow in the aneurysm sac M is calculated as follows:

$$M = \frac{\int_T \int_V |\vec{v}(\vec{x},t)| d\vec{x}dt}{\int_T \int_V d\vec{x}dt} \tag{2}$$

Whereby T is the time window, t represents time, V the aneurysm sac volume, $\vec{x}$ position, and $\vec{v}$ blood velocity.

The MAFA-ratio can be measured peri-interventionally using high frame-rate DSA sequences. During the acquisition of the DSA data, iodine contrast agent is injected intra-arterially at a very modest pace (1.5 ml/s). The contrast agent is consequently modulated by the flow pulsatility at the injection point, driven by the cardiac cycle. The contrast will be denser during the diastole phase and less dense during the systole phase. The modulated contrast agent pattern travels through the vessels and aneurysm sac, and is followed using an optical flow algorithm [10].

2   Methods

In this article, we compare the MAFA-ratios calculated from computational fluid dynamics (CFD) with high frame-rate DSA (60 fps) calculations. For this purpose, CFD simulations were performed, using 3DRA reconstructions of intracranial aneurysms acquired from six patients, see Figure 1. All aneurysms were located on the internal carotid artery. Aneurysm size ranged from small (5mm) to large (15mm), see Table 1.

Nine CFD input flow conditions were imposed for each 3DRA, with mean flow rates ranging from 1 ml/s to 5 ml/s in increments of 0.5 ml/s. The arterial flow curves were created by scaling a reference flow curve as described in [5,9]. Hexahedral meshes were generated from the vasculature segmented in the 3DRA data with the SnappyHexMesh utility from OpenFoam. The CFD simulations were performed with OpenFoam v2.2.1.

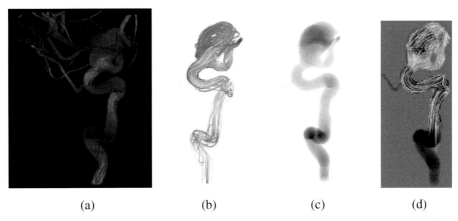

| (a) | (b) | (c) | (d) |

Fig. 1. (a) 3DRA reconstruction of an intracranial aneurysm. (b) Computational fluid simulation (CFD), whereby the stream lines illustrate the 3D vector field. (c) Virtual angiogram view generated from the CFD data. (d) 2D flow field obtained by the optical flow algorithm from the contrast motion in the time dependent virtual angiograms.

Table 1. Aneurysm dimensions.

Patient nr.	1	2	3	4	5	6
Largest diameter (mm)	8.3	15.0	5.3	5.1	8.0	7.6

The CFD simulations were performed without and with virtual stents placed, as described in [5,9]. The first stent had a porosity of 0.72, which is chosen to mimic the Silk flow diverter stent. Two additional CFD simulations were performed for three out of six aneurysms. One with a stent having a porosity of 0.92, and another one also with a porosity of 0.92, but this time the stent did not fully cover the aneurysm ostium to mimic an ill-positioned stent. The CFD simulations yielded a time-dependent 3D vector field representing the displacements of blood, which was used to calculate the space and time averaged CFD aneurysm flow.

The CFD simulations were also used to generate virtual angiograms from two different viewing angles [3], see Fig. 1. The virtual angiograms were loaded in the Aneurysm Flow software (Philips Healthcare, Best, the Netherlands) to compute the mean aneurysm flow and arterial flow based on high frame-rate DSA. The mean flow for the CFD data was calculated on the 3D flow vector field, whereas the flow for the DSA data was computed on the 2D projection images, using an optical flow algorithm [10].

The simulations allowed to perform a lot of experiments while varying selected parameters while keeping others the same, which would not have been possible in-vivo. The following conditions were varied in the experiments:

- Six 3DRA geometries of different aneurysms.
- Nine flow rates: ranging from 1 ml/s to 5 ml/s in increments of 0.5 ml/s.
- CFD simulations: without stent, with stent 1 with porosity 0.72, with stent 2 with porosity 0.92 (for three aneurysms), with ill-positioned stent 3 with porosity 0.92 (for three aneurysms).
- Two projection angles for the virtual angiograms.

In total 9*4=36 CFD simulations were performed for the first three aneurysms and 9*2=18 simulations for the second three aneurysms, yielding a total of 36+18=54 CFD simulations. Per simulation two virtual angiograms were computed from different projection angles, delivering in total 108 virtual angiograms.

MAFA-ratios were computed from two angiograms for the same aneurysm and the same projection angle, one without stent and one with stent, whereby the difference in pre- and post-deployment arterial flow was ≤ 1.5 ml/s. This range was selected based on the analysis of arterial flow changes prior and after stenting in 61 clinical cases. This yielded 9+8+8+7+7+6+6=51 ratios for each aneurysm-stent-view combination.

3   Results

The MAFA-ratio computed on the virtual angiograms is plotted versus the MAFA-ratio computed on the CFD data for each aneurysm. Figure 2 presents an example of such a graph. From this data, available for every aneurysm, the average and standard deviation of the MAFA-ratios are calculated for each aneurysm-stent combination, see Fig. 3. A regression line fitted through these points delivers: $y = 0.68 \cdot x + 0.34$, with the coefficient of determination r^2 being 0.96.

Furthermore, the pooled standard deviation σ_p is computed from the standard deviations that are calculated for each aneurysm-stent combination as follows:

$$\sigma_p = \sqrt{\frac{\sum (n_i - 1) \cdot \sigma_i^2}{\sum (n_i - 1)}} \tag{3}$$

Whereby n_i is the size of a stent group of aneurysm i and σ_i the standard deviation of a stent group of aneurysm i. The average MAFA-ratios for the stents are presented in Table 2, while the results of the pooled standard are provided in Table 3.

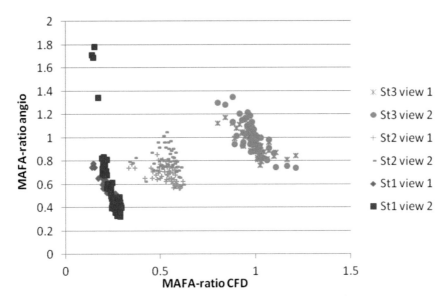

Fig. 2. For a particular aneurysm geometry (patient 2) the MAFA-ratio based on the virtual angiograms (vertical axis) is plotted versus the MAFA-ratio based on the CFD vector fields (horizontal axis). The MAFA-ratio was calculated for three simulated stents; stent 1 (St1) has a porosity of 0.72, stent 2 (St2) a porosity of 0.92 and stent 3 (St3) also a porosity of 0.92, but is ill-deployed. Each view number represents a distinct projection angle.

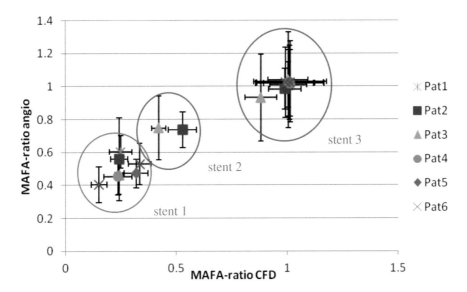

Fig. 3. Average MAFA-ratio based on the virtual angiograms (vertical axis) vs. average MAFA-ratio based on CFD (horizontal axis) for each aneurysm-stent combination. The averages are computed over both views combined. The error bars indicate the standard deviation.

Finally, the pooled standard deviation for the two combined DSA views is evaluated as a function of the absolute arterial flow difference $\Delta Q = |Q_{post} - Q_{pre}|$, as shown in Fig. 4.

Table 2. Average MAFA-ratio for the three different stents and without stent.

Average	CFD	View 1	View 2	View 1&2
Stent 1	0.24	0.49	0.50	0.49
Stent 2	0.43	0.70	0.64	0.67
Stent 3	0.95	0.98	0.98	0.98
Without stent	1.01	1.02	1.02	1.02

Table 3. Pooled standard deviation of the three different stents and without stent.

Pooled stddev. σ_p	CFD	View 1	View 2	View 1&2
Stent 1	0.05	0.11	0.16	0.14
Stent 2	0.05	0.15	0.11	0.15
Stent 3	0.09	0.21	0.21	0.21
Without stent	0.13	0.23	0.22	0.22

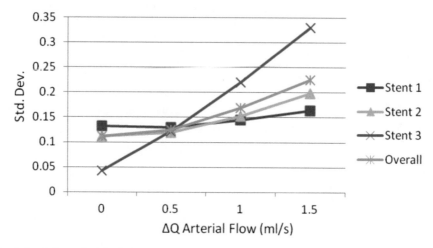

Fig. 4. Pooled standard deviation (vertical axis) from the combined views 1 & 2 for each stent, and overall (combined data of view 1 and 2) for all stents together, as a function of the ΔQ absolute arterial flow difference (horizontal axis).

4   Discussion

In the ideal case, the six stent-view combinations would show up as three points in Fig. 2 without any spread. This would mean that there is no difference in the MAFA-ratio if you would choose a different viewing angle, and that the MAFA-ratio is invariant to changes in arterial flow. Each stent, however, yields a distinct cloud of points in the plot that compares the MAFA-ratios computed from the virtual angiograms and from the CFD data, as can be seen in Fig. 2. The point clouds produced by the two different projection angles map very well on each other. This trend is also observed for the other five aneurysms.

The data for all aneurysms are represented in a single graph (Fig. 3), whereby each data point represents the mean and standard deviation for each aneurysm-stent combination. The data points appear to represent a linear relation nearly passing through coordinate (1,1), which indicates that when the CFD MAFA-ratio indicates no flow reduction (R=1), the DSA MAFA-ratio indicates the same (R=1), independently of the projection angle. For the stents we expect lower MAFA-ratios for lower porosity values, as can be observed in Table 2 and Fig. 3. A flow reduction ($R < 1$) also is confirmed in both measurements, and a stronger reduction ($R_1 < R_2$) is also consistently found in both CFD and DSA measurements, due to their monotone increasing relation.

In the ideal case, the MAFA-ratios of the angiograms would be exactly equal to the MAFA-ratios of the CFD. However, the slope of the relation is not 1, which might be caused by the differences between the dimensionality of the two methods; The CFD MAFA-ratio is calculated in 3D space, whereas the DSA MAFA-ratio is obtained in a projective 2D space, which suffers from phenomena like foreshortening, overlapping structures, laminar flow effects, etc. This means that threshold analysis performed on one technique (e.g., CFD) cannot be applied to the other one (e.g., DSA).

The standard deviation of the aneurysm-stent combinations is presented in Fig. 3 as horizontal bars for the CFD and vertical bars for the DSA. While the averages of the various stents for a clear trend, there is overlap of the standard deviations on the vertical axis, which has implications on the predictive power of a single DSA-based MAFA measurement, and should be taken into account when determining safety margins around clinically relevant thresholds.

The fact that also the CFD simulations possess a standard deviation > 0 implies that the normalization by the arterial flow in Equation 1 is not perfect. This is confirmed in Figure 4, where a larger difference between pre- and post-deployment arterial flow tends to increase the standard deviation. This effect is stronger when the MAFA-ratio R is close to 1, as is the case with stent 3 (see also Table 3). This phenomenon might be caused by phenomena like the development of vortices and unsteady flow features, and by a non-linear relation between the aneurysm flow magnitude and the arterial flow, due to the ratio of shear flow versus influx flow being dependent on the arterial flow magnitude. Furthermore, the normalized MAFA-ratio definition does not take any bias effects into account [5], which may have an impact on the standard deviation. Future research might investigate this effect further. In clinical practice this can be taken into account by applying a larger safety margin to a chosen threshold when the arterial flow differs more.

5   Conclusion

In this article we have examined the relation between the MAFA-ratios obtained directly from CFD simulations with the DSA based MAFA-ratios by generating virtual angiograms from the CFD data. We have found that while the slope of a regression line through the ratios is not 1, the ratios have a monotone increasing relation and correspond in predicting (practically) no flow reduction, as well as increasingly stronger reductions. Therefore, it can be concluded that the DSA-based MAFA-ratio can be used as a tool in interventional intracranial aneurysm treatment to evaluate the efficacy of a flow diverting stent. Since the slope of the DSA-based MAFA-ratios and the CFD-based ratios is not the identity, any threshold analysis to associate a MAFA-ratio range with certain clinical outcome is only valid for the respective technique used to acquire the input data of that analysis.

References

1. Augsburger, L., Reymond, P., Fonck, E., Kulcsar, Z., Farhat, M., Ohta, M., Stergiopulos, N., Rüfenacht, D.A.: Methodologies to assess blood flow in cerebral aneurysms: Current state of research and perspectives. J. Neuroradiol. 36, 270–277 (2009)
2. Sforza, D.M., Putman, C.M., Cebral, J.R.: Hemodynamics of cerebral aneurysms. Annu. Rev. Fluid Mech. 41, 91–107 (2009)
3. Sun, Q., Groth, A., Bertram, M., Waechter, I., Bruijns, T., Hermans, R., Aach, T.: Phantom-based experimental validation of computational fluid dynamics simulations on cerebral aneurysms. Med. Phys. 37, 5054–5065 (2010)
4. Groth, A., Waechter-Stehle, I., Brina, O., Perren, F., Mendes Pereira, V., Rüfenacht, D., Bruijns, T., Bertram, M., Weese, J.: Clinical study of model-based blood flow quantification on cerebrovascular data. In: Wong, K.H., Holmes III, D.R. (eds.) SPIE Medical Imaging: Visualization, Image-Guided Procedures, and Modeling, vol. 7964, pp. 79640X. SPIE Press (2011)
5. Morales, H.G., Bonnefous, O.: Unraveling the relationship between arterial flow and intra-aneurysmal hemodynamics. J. Biomech. 48, 585–591 (2015)
6. Mendes Pereira, V., Bonnefous, O., Ouared, R., Brina, O., Stawiaski, J., Aerts, H., Ruijters, D., Narata, A.P., Bijlenga, P., Schaller, K., Lovblad, K.-O.: A DSA-Based Method Using Contrast-Motion Estimation for the Assessment of the Intra-Aneurysmal Flow Changes Induced by Flow-Diverter Stents. AJNR Am. J. Neuroradiol. 34, 808–815 (2013)
7. Mendes Pereira, V., Ouared, R., Brina, O., Bonnefous, O., Stawiaski, J., Aerts, H., Ruijters, D., van Nijnatten, F., Perren, F., Bijlenga, P., Schaller, K., Lovblad, K.-O.: Quantification of Internal Carotid Artery Flow with Digital Subtraction Angiography: Validation of an Optical Flow Approach with Doppler Ultrasound. AJNR Am. J. Neuroradiol. 35, 156–163 (2014)
8. Brina, O., Ouared, R., Bonnefous, O., van Nijnatten, F., Bouillot, P., Bijlenga, P., Schaller, K., Lovblad, K.-O., Grünhagen, T., Ruijters, D., Mendes Pereira, V.: Intra-Aneurysmal Flow Patterns: Illustrative Comparison among Digital Subtraction Angiography, Optical Flow, and Computational Fluid Dynamics. AJNR Am. J. Neuroradiol. 35, 2348–2353 (2014)
9. Morales, H.G., Bonnefous, O.: Peak systolic or maximum intra-aneurysmal hemodynamic condition? Implications on normalized flow variables. J. Biomech. 47, 2362–2370 (2014)
10. Bonnefous, O., Mendes Pereira, V., Ouared, R., Brina, O., Aerts, H., Hermans, R., van Nijnatten, F., Stawiaski, J., Ruijters, D.: Quantification of arterial flow using digital subtraction angiography. Med. Phys. 39, 6264–6275 (2012)

Application of L0-Norm Regularization to Epicardial Potential Reconstruction

Liansheng Wang[1], Xinyue Li[1], Yiping Chen[1], and Jing Qin[2,3]

[1] Department of Computer Science, School of Information Science and Engineering,
Xiamen University, Xiamen, China
lswang@cse.cuhk.edu.hk
[2] School of Medicine, Shenzhen University, China
[3] Guangdong Key Laboratory for Biomedical Measurements and Ultrasound Imaging, China

Abstract. Inverse problem of electrocardiography (ECG) has been extensively investigated as the estimated epicardial potentials (EPs) reflecting underlying myocardial activities. Traditionally, L2-norm regularization methods have been proposed to solve this ill-posed problem. But L2-norm penalty function inherently leads to considerable smoothing of the solution, which reduces the accuracy of distinguishing abnormalities and locating diseased regions. Directly using L1-norm penalty function, however, may greatly increase the computational complexity due to its non-differentiability. In this study, we present a smoothed L0 norm technique in order to directly solve the L0 norm constrained problem. Our method employs a smoothing function to make the L0 norm continuous. Extensive experiments on various datasets, including normal human data, isolated canine data, and WPW syndrome data, were conducted to validate our method. Epicardial potentials mapped during pacing were also reconstructed and visualized on the heart surface. Experimental results show that the proposed method reconstructs more accurate epicardial potentials compared with L1 norm and L2 norm based methods, demonstrating that smoothed L0 norm is a promising method for the noninvasive estimation of epicardial potentials.

1 Introduction

Inverse ECG problem has been paid much attention recently as it is an efficient tool for the characterization of cardiac electrical events. In the study of ECG inverse problem, the electrical activity of the heart can be described by the reconstructed epicardial potentials [1]. In our study, supposing the torso surface potentials are given, we attempt to compute the potentials on the epicardial surface.

As it subjects to both the Dirichlet and Neumann boundary conditions, this problem is a boundary value problem. Assuming the human torso is homogeneous and isotropic, this boundary value problem can be solved by a boundary element method (BEM), which relates the potentials at the torso nodes (expressed as a m-dimensional vector Φ_T) to the potentials at the epicardial nodes (expressed as a n-dimensional vector Φ_E):

$$\Phi_T = A\Phi_E \qquad (1)$$

where A is the transfer coefficient matrix $(m * n)$ with $n < m$. The transfer coefficient matrix A is determined entirely by the geometric integrands and thus can be calculated analytically with a BEM solution.

© Springer International Publishing Switzerland 2015
N. Navab et al. (Eds.): MICCAI 2015, Part II, LNCS 9350, pp. 493–500, 2015.
DOI: 10.1007/978-3-319-24571-3_59

To find a practical solution, regularization is usually employed to tackle the ill-posedness and reduce the outliers of the inverse solution [2]. In these regularizations, Tikhonov regularizations with zeroth, first, and second orders impose constraints on the magnitude or derivatives of the epicardial potential Φ_E to overcome the ill-posed inverse problem [3] [4]. The truncated total least squares (TTLS) method is introduced to solve the inverse problem with adaptive BEM in [5]. TTLS can deal with the measurement errors and geometry errors at the same time, but it suffers from large reconstruction errors when the measurement errors and geometry errors increase. These regularizations are all in the L2 norm which will smooth the reconstructed results.

Except L2 norm regularization, total variation (TV) has been recently applied to the inverse problem of ECG and achieve good comparable results in terms of L_1-norm [6] [7]. However, the implementation of TV is complicated due to the non-differentiability of the penalty function with L_1-norm.

L0 norm is an efficient scheme for solving the inverse problem of ECG. However, due to the discontinuity of the penalty function, investigators had to develop L2 norm methods and L1 norm methods to approximate the L0 norm [8]. In this study, we present a smoothed L0 norm solution [9] to epicardial potential reconstruction which directly solves the inverse problem of ECG. Through a smooth measure approximating the L0 norm, a smoothed L0 norm solves the inverse problem in an iterative manner. The smoothed L0 norm is validated on various datasets, including isolated canine heart data, normal human data, and WPW syndrome data.

2   The Smoothed L0-Norm Method

The inverse problem of ECG can be carried out by solving the unconstrained minimization:

$$min\{\|A\Phi_E - \Phi_T\|_2 + \lambda\|\Phi_E\|_0\} \tag{2}$$

where λ is the regularization parameter. However, as discussed, the L0 norm faces two challenges. The first is the discontinuity which means that we have to perform a combinatorial search for its minimization. The second is its high noise sensitivity. We meet these two challenges by employing a smoothed L0-norm method.

The main idea of the smoothed L0 is to employ a smoothing function (continuously) for the L0 norm minimization. For the inverse problem of ECG, we approximate the L0 norm of the potential vector Φ_E by a smoothing function $F_\sigma(\Phi_E)$, where the value of σ controls the accuracy of the approximation.

Given the potential vector $\Phi_E = [\phi_1, ..., \phi_n]^T$, the L0 norm of Φ_E is valued as the number of the non-zero components in Φ_E. We define it as follows:

$$v(\phi) = \begin{cases} 1 & \phi \neq 0 \\ 0 & \phi = 0. \end{cases} \tag{3}$$

Thus, the L0 norm of Φ_E can be expressed as:

$$\|\Phi_E\|_0 = \sum_{i=1}^{n} v(\phi_i). \tag{4}$$

It is obvious that the L0 norm is discontinuous because of the discontinuities of the function v. If we can replace v with a continuous function, the L0 norm will be continuous. With the smoothed L0 norm, we apply the zero-mean Gaussian family of functions for the inverse problem of ECG. By defining:

$$f_\sigma(\phi) = \exp(-\phi^2/2\sigma^2), \tag{5}$$

we have:

$$\lim_{\sigma \to 0} f_\sigma(\phi) = \begin{cases} 1 & \phi = 0 \\ 0 & \phi \neq 0, \end{cases} \tag{6}$$

and thus we can obtain:

$$\lim_{\sigma \to 0} f_\sigma(\phi) = 1 - v(\phi). \tag{7}$$

Then, we define:

$$F_\sigma(\phi) = \sum_{i=1}^{n} f_\sigma(\phi_i), \tag{8}$$

and the L0 norm of Φ_E is approximated with $n - F_\sigma(\phi)$:

$$||\Phi_E||_0 = n - F_\sigma(\phi). \tag{9}$$

The σ determines the effect of the approximation. If the σ is too large, the approximation will be too smooth to accurately reflect the L0 norm of Φ_E. If the σ is too small, it is easily trapped in the local minima searching for σ. We employ the scheme proposed in the Graduated Non-Convexity (GNC) [10] method to control the value of σ for escaping from the local minima, where the value of σ is decreased gradually.

The final smoothed L0 norm for the inverse problem of ECG is summarized in the following algorithm:

Algorithm 1. Smoothed L0 norm method for inverse problem of ECG

1: **(Initialization)**:
   1. Given $\widehat{\phi}$ as an arbitrary solution to the inverse problem of ECG obtained from a pseudo-inverse of A.
   2. Choose a suitable decreasing sequence for σ, $[\sigma_1, ..., \sigma_K]$.
2: **(FOR Loop)**:k=1,...,K
   1. Let $\sigma = \sigma_j$;
   2. Maximize (approximately) the function F_σ on the feasible set of inverse problems of ECG using L iterations of the steepest ascent algorithm
   (1)Initialization: $\phi = \widehat{\phi}_j$.
   (2)for $j = 1, ..., L$ (loop L times):
   (a)$\delta \overset{\Delta}{=} [\phi_1 \exp(-\phi_1^2/2\sigma^2), ..., \phi_n \exp(-\phi_n^2/2\sigma^2)]^T$
   (b) Let $\phi \leftarrow \phi - \omega\delta$ (where ω is a small positive constant).
   (c) Project ϕ back onto the feasible set: $\phi \leftarrow \phi - A^T(AA^T)^{-1} - (A\phi - \Phi_T)$.
   3. Set $\widehat{\phi}_j = \phi$.
3: **(END FOR Loop)**
4: **(Results)**: $\widehat{\phi} = \widehat{\phi}_K$.

---

3   Experimental Data and Protocols

In order to evaluate the proposed smoothed L0 norm, L2 norm method TTLS (L2-TTLS) [5] and L1 norm method GPSR (L1-GPSR) [8] are compared with our presented method. In the experiments, the slowly decreasing sequences of σ are fixed to $[1, 0.5, 0.2, 0.1, 0.05, 0.02, 0.01]$ and δ is fixed to 2.5 based on our data.

3.1   Data

Three different types of data were used in our experiments.

Normal Human Data. Three normal male data were collected for the normal case study. The geometric heart model and torso model were built from MRI scanning images. The high-resolution 65-lead body surface potential mapping were collected for these normal cases.

Isolated Canine Heart Data. The normal canine data is obtained from the Center for Integrative Biomedical Computing (CIBC) at the University of Utah. The details of the data collection procedure are reported in [11]. The torso surface potentials are computed in a forward solution. A homogenous torso geometry including the epicardial sock electrodes (490 nodes and 976 triangles) and torso tank (771 nodes and 1254 triangles) is used in the forward solution. The forward solution used BEM from Matti Stenroos *et al.* [12]. To mimic the realistic conditions, $25dB$ signal-to-noise (SNR) Gaussian noise (independent, zero mean) are added to the computed torso surface potentials. The added noise is zero mean and unit standard variation distribution.

WPW Syndrome Data. The WPW syndrome data was collected from seven patients (3 female) with overt ventricular pre-excitation who underwent an electrophysiologic examination. The patients were as assessed through prior transthoracic echocardiography to make sure they had structurally normal hearts for this study. Patients in this study had not received antiarrhythmic drug therapy [13].

3.2   Evaluation Protocols

We quantitatively evaluate the accuracy of the ECG inverse problem by using two standard criteria: relative error (RE) and correlation coefficient (CC). The RE is defined as:

$$RE = \frac{||\Phi_H - \hat{\Phi}_H||_2}{||\hat{\Phi}_H||_2}, \tag{10}$$

and the CC is defined as:

$$CC = \frac{\sum\limits_{k=1}^{N_k} (\Phi_H(k) - \bar{\Phi}_H(k))(\hat{\Phi}_H(k) - \bar{\hat{\Phi}}_H(k))}{\sqrt{\sum\limits_{k=1}^{N_k} (\Phi_H(k) - \bar{\Phi}_H(k))^2 \sum\limits_{k=1}^{N_k} (\hat{\Phi}_H(k) - \bar{\hat{\Phi}}_H(k))^2}}, \tag{11}$$

where N_k is the total number of nodes on the heart geometry surface. The Φ_H is the potential value on the heart surface. The superscript '^' refers to the reference values and the superscript '‾' refers to the mean values.

4   Experiments and Results

In our experiments, all methods were implemented in MATLAB R2012a running on a Dell computer with Intel Core2 i3-2120 CPU 3.30GHz and 4.00GB RAM.

Figure 1 shows the epicardial potential maps of human data during pacing, 13ms after onset of QRS. Measured data is shown in figure 1(a) with the pacing site marked by an plus sign. Elliptic shapes of negative potential (in dark blue) spread out as a round shape into two sides of positive potentials areas (in red). Figure 1(b) shows reconstructed data by L2-TTLS. While L2-TTLS reconstructs the pattern of negative potentials (in dark blue) around the pacing site (plus sign) flanked by a broad area of positive potentials (in red), it overestimates the spatial gradients between the area of negative potentials and the area of positive potentials on the sides, which leads to significant errors in the reconstructions with high RE (RE=0.36) and low CC (CC=0.65). Figure 1(c) shows the reconstructed results by the L1-GPSR [8]. Although the reconstruction accuracy improves (RE=0.19, CC=0.88), the negative potentials around the pacing site are also overestimated, which is shown in a big parallel circle. The L0-norm solution ((RE=0.10, CC=0.97)) demonstrates high fidelity compared with the measured data shown in figure 1(d), in which the shape of the negative potentials is well preserved. More importantly, the spatial gradients (blue to red) around the pacing site are more accurately estimated. The values of the RE and CC also show the highest reconstruction accuracy and best spatial features compared to the L2-norm and L1-norm methods.

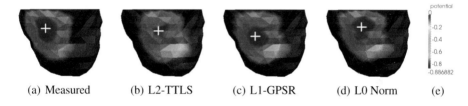

(a) Measured	(b) L2-TTLS	(c) L1-GPSR	(d) L0 Norm	(e)

Fig. 1. Reconstructed epicardial potential maps, 13ms after onset of QRS, for different methods. The plus sign shows the pacing site. The unit of potential is V.

Figure 2 shows the epicardial electrograms of the pre- and post-infarction. Two epicardial sites are chosen; marked on the surface of the heart. Site 1 is chosen within the infarct area and site 2 is chosen away from the infarct area. While the form of the electrograms at site 2 remains unchanged in the pre-infarct and post-infarct, electrograms at site 1 are reversed in negative and positive. The L0-norm solution preserves better form of the electrograms compared to L2-TTLS and L1-GPSR in terms of RE and CC.

QRST integral mapping has been shown to be a useful noninvasive method to assess the spatial distribution of primary ventricular recovery properties [14]. QRST integral maps were computed by using of the sum of all potentials from the QRS onset to the T-wave offset in each lead. The epicardial QRST integral maps of the canine data computed from measured and reconstructed data are shown in figure 3. The warm area of the LV with high QRST integral values is shown in red color while the cooler region with lower values is shown in dark blue. Although the reconstructed maps achieve the low and high QRST integral values, the L2-TTLS solution shows over-computed high integral values with larger RE (RE=0.78). Meanwhile, parts of the high integral values are missed in the result of the L1-GPSR solution with a lower CC (CC=0.57). Our L0-norm method achieved the best results.

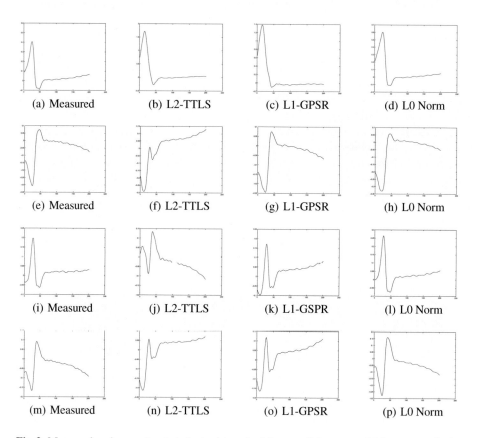

(a) Measured   (b) L2-TTLS   (c) L1-GPSR   (d) L0 Norm

(e) Measured   (f) L2-TTLS   (g) L1-GPSR   (h) L0 Norm

(i) Measured   (j) L2-TTLS   (k) L1-GSPR   (l) L0 Norm

(m) Measured   (n) L2-TTLS   (o) L1-GPSR   (p) L0 Norm

Fig. 2. Measured and reconstructed electrograms by L2-norm, L1-norm and L0-norm methods. The upper two rows are for site 1 and bottom two rows are for site2. For site 1 and site 2, the first row for pre-infarct and the second row for post-infarct.

Figure 4 shows the epicardial activation map in a male patient with WPW syndrome. The time step for this activation isochrones is 2ms. The L2-norm solution shows a large flat area of early activation (in pink color) while the L1-norm solution shows the one distinct early activation areas which means there is one diseased region. However, the L0-norm solution shows two distinct early activation areas of which one early activation area cannot be found in the L1-norm solution. These two distinct areas of early activation are very important for surgeons making a surgical plan. The reconstructed results demonstrate that the proposed L0-norm method achieves more accurate results than the L2-TTLS method and the L1-GPSR method.

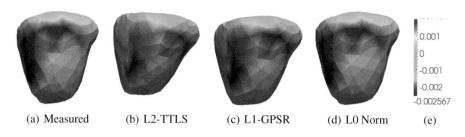

| (a) Measured | (b) L2-TTLS | (c) L1-GPSR | (d) L0 Norm | (e) |

Fig. 3. Epicardial QRST integral maps from measured and reconstructed data. The unit is $V - ms$.

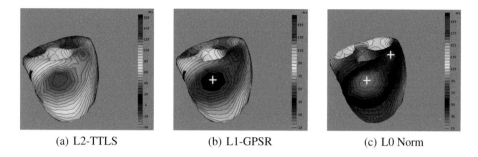

| (a) L2-TTLS | (b) L1-GPSR | (c) L0 Norm |

Fig. 4. Activation maps for Wolff Parkinson White (WPW) patient reconstructed by the L2 norm, L1 norm, and L0 norm. The plus sign indicates the distinct early activation area.

5   Conclusion

A L0-norm base regularization technique was applied to the inverse problem of ECG for epicardial potentials reconstruction in this study. In order to overcome the discontinuity of the L0 norm, a smooth measure is employed for direct reconstruction of epicardial potentials in an iterative manner. The experiments were conducted in different types data of isolated canine heart, normal human, and patients with WPW syndrome. The reconstructed results were compared to the L2-norm based method and the L1-norm based method. Experimental results showed that the proposed L0-norm base method is a promising method for the inverse problem of ECG which achieves more accurate results than L2-norm and L1-norm based methods.

Acknowledgement. This work was supported by National Natural Science Foundation of China (Grant No. 61301010), the Natural Science Foundation of Fujian Province (Grant No. 2014J05080), Research Fund for the Doctoral Program of Higher Education (20130121120045), by CCF-Tencent Open Research Fund and by the Fundamental Research Funds for the Central Universities (Grant No. 2013SH005, Grant No. 20720150110).

References

1. Wang, D., Kirby, R.M., Johnson, C.R.: Resolution Strategies for the Finite-Element-Based Solution of the ECG Inverse Problem. IEEE Transactions on Biomedical Engineering 57(2), 220–237 (2010)
2. Milanic, M., Jazbinsek, V., Wang, D., Sinstra, J., MacLeod, R.S., Brooks, D.H., Hren, R.: Evaluation of approaches to solving electrocardiographic imaging problem. In: IEEE Computers in Cardiology, pp. 177–180 (2010)
3. Dössel, O.: Inverse problem of electro-and magnetocardiography: Review and recent progress. International Journal of Bioelectromagnetism 2(2) (2000)
4. Rudy, Y., Messinger-Rapport, B.J.: The inverse problem in electrocardiography: Solutions in terms of epicardial potentials. Critical Reviews in Biomedical Engineering 16(3), 215–268 (1988)
5. Shou, G., Xia, L., Jiang, M., Wei, Q., Liu, F., Crozier, S.: Truncated total least squares: a new regularization method for the solution of ECG inverse problems. IEEE Transactions on Biomedical Engineering 55(4), 1327–1335 (2008)
6. Ghosh, S., Rudy, Y.: Application of L1-norm regularization to epicardial potential solution of the inverse electrocardiography problem. Annals of Biomedical Engineering 37(5), 902–912 (2009)
7. Shou, G., Xia, L., Liu, F., Jiang, M., Crozier, S.: On epicardial potential reconstruction using regularization schemes with the L1-norm data term. Physics in Medicine and Biology 56, 57–72 (2011)
8. Wang, L., Qin, J., Wong, T., Heng, P.: Application of l1-norm regularization to epicardial potential reconstruction based on gradient projection. Physics in Medicine and Biology 56, 6291 (2011)
9. Mohimani, H., Babaie-Zadeh, M., Jutten, C.: A fast approach for overcomplete sparse decomposition based on smoothed norm. IEEE Transactions on Signal Processing 57(1), 289–301 (2009)
10. Blake, A., Zisserman, A.: Visual reconstruction. MIT Press, Cambridge (1987)
11. MacLeod, R.S., Lux, R.L., Taccardi, B.: A possible mechanism for electrocardiographically silent changes in cardiac repolarization. Journal of Electrocardiology 30, 114–121 (1998)
12. Stenroos, M., Haueisen, J.: Boundary element computations in the forward and inverse problems of electrocardiography: comparison of collocation and Galerkin weightings. IEEE Transactions on Biomedical Engineering 55(9), 2124–2133 (2008)
13. Berger, T., Fischer, G., Pfeifer, B., Modre, R., Hanser, F., Trieb, T., Roithinger, F., Stuehlinger, M., Pachinger, O., Tilg, B., et al.: Single-beat noninvasive imaging of cardiac electrophysiology of ventricular pre-excitation. Journal of the American College of Cardiology 48(10), 2045–2052 (2006)
14. Wilson, F., Macleod, A., Barker, P., Johnston, F.: The determination and the significance of the areas of the ventricular deflections of the electrocardiogram. American Heart Journal 10(1), 46–61 (1934)

MRI-Based Lesion Profiling of Epileptogenic Cortical Malformations

Seok-Jun Hong, Boris C. Bernhardt, Dewi Schrader, Benoit Caldairou,
Neda Bernasconi, and Andrea Bernasconi

Neuroimaging of Epilepsy Laboratory, McConnell Brain Imaging Centre,
Montreal Neurological Institute and Hospital, McGill University, Montreal, Quebec, Canada
sjhong@bic.mni.mcgill.ca

Abstract. Focal cortical dysplasia (FCD), a malformation of cortical development, is a frequent cause of drug-resistant epilepsy. This lesion is histologically classified into Type-IIA (dyslamination, dysmorphic neurons) and Type-IIB (dyslamination, dysmorphic neurons, and balloon cells). Reliable *in-vivo* identification of lesional subtypes is important for preoperative decision-making and surgical prognostics. We propose a novel multi-modal MRI lesion profiling based on multiple surfaces that systematically sample intra- and subcortical tissue. We applied this framework to histologically-verified FCD. We aggregated features describing morphology, intensity, microstructure, and function from T1-weighted, FLAIR, diffusion, and resting-state functional MRI. We observed alterations across multiple features in FCD Type-IIB, while anomalies in IIA were subtle and mainly restricted to FLAIR intensity and regional functional homogeneity. Anomalies in Type-IIB were seen across all intra- and subcortical levels, whereas those in Type-IIA clustered at the cortico-subcortical interface. A supervised classifier predicted the FCD subtype with 91% accuracy, validating our profiling framework at the individual level.

Keywords: Intracortical, FCD, Multimodal MRI, Histopathological prediction.

1   Introduction

Focal cortical dysplasia (FCD), a highly epileptogenic malformation of cortical development, is a frequent cause of drug-resistant epilepsy in children and adults. Surgical resection of these lesions is the only effective treatment to arrest the seizures.

Histologically, FCD is characterized by cortical dyslamination associated with various intra-cortical cytological anomalies: large dysmorphic neurons typify FCD Type-IIA, while clusters of balloon cells and dysmorphic neurons are characteristic of Type-IIB [1]. In addition to cortical abnormalities, neuronal density is increased in the white matter immediately below the cortical interface. Radiological assessments suggest that these histological subtypes may have diverging morphological and intensity signatures, with Type-IIA being generally more subtle than IIB [1]. Moreover, difficulties to discern lesional boundaries from the surrounding normal cortex, together

N. Navab et al. (Eds.): MICCAI 2015, Part II, LNCS 9350, pp. 501–509, 2015.
DOI: 10.1007/978-3-319-24571-3_60

with a more extended epileptogenic network [2], explain less favorable surgical out-come prospects in FCD Type-IIA compared to type-IIB [3].

Given the irreversible nature of surgery, it is important to predict FCD subtypes *in vivo*. We propose a surface-based multivariate MRI framework that jointly assesses morphology, intensity, diffusion, and functional characteristics, taking advantage of their covariance for improved lesion profiling. To model FCD-related cortical dyslamination and white matter gliosis, we sampled imaging parameters on multiple surfaces at various cortical and subcortical depths. We used a supervised classifier to automatically predict the histological subtype from multiparametric MRI.

2   Methods

Figure 1 summarizes our approach. Each step is detailed in the text below.

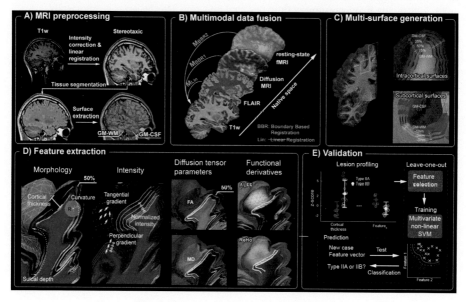

Fig. 1. Flowchart of the proposed method

2.1   MRI Acquisition

Acquisition. Multimodal MRI was acquired on a 3T Siemens TimTrio using a 32-channel head coil. Structural MRI included a 3D T1-weighted (T1w) MPRAGE (TR = 2300ms, TE=2.98ms, FA=9°, FOV=256mm^2, voxel size= 1×1×1mm^3) and fluid-attenuated inversion recovery (FLAIR; TR=5000ms, TE=389 ms, TI=1.8ms, FA=120°, FOV=230mm^2, voxel size=0.9×0.9×0.9mm^3). Diffusion-weighted MRI data were obtained using a 2D-EPI sequence (TR=8400ms, TE=90ms, FA=90°, FOV=256mm^2, voxel size=2×2×2mm^3, 64 directions, b=1000s/mm^2, 1 B0). Resting-state fMRI (rs-fMRI) was acquired using a 2D-BOLD-EPI sequence (TR=2020ms, TE=30ms, FA=90°, FOV=256mm^2, 34 slices, voxel size=4×4×4mm^3, 150 volumes).

2.2   MRI Preprocessing and Multimodal Data Fusion (Fig. 1A, B)

T1w underwent intensity inhomogeneity correction, intensity standardization, linear registration to MNI152 space, as well as classification into white matter (WM), gray matter (GM), and cerebro-spinal fluid (CSF) [4]. GM-WM and GM-CSF surface models were constructed using CLASP, an algorithm relying on intensity and geometric constraints [5]. Notably, as the GM-CSF surface is generated directly from the GM-WM surface, both surfaces have the same number of vertices. Moreover, corresponding vertices on both surfaces can be connected using straight line, a so-called *t-link*. A surface registration based on cortical folding improved inter-subject alignment. After intensity correction, FLAIR data were co-registered to native T1w. Diffusion-weighted data were corrected for motion, eddy currents, and geometric distortions; we obtained fractional anisotropy (FA) and mean diffusivity (MD) using FSL (v5.0; http://fsl.fmrib.ox.ac.uk/fsl/). The rs-fMRI data were corrected for slice-time, motion, geometric distortions, and nuisance signals of WM and CSF. Scrubbing corrected residual motion confounds [6]. Diffusion-weighted MRI and rs-fMRI were co-registered to T1w using boundary-based registration [7].

2.3   Multi-surface Generation (Fig. 1C)

We reconstructed three intracortical surfaces equidistantly positioned between GM-CSF and GM-WM boundaries along the t-link at 25, 50, and 75% thickness. Although these surfaces do not necessarily reflect exact cortical laminae, they capture relative differences along the axis perpendicular to the cortical mantle. A set of subcortical surfaces was constructed to probe intensity and diffusion parameters in the WM immediately below the cortex; for each individual, a Laplacian deformation field running from the GM-WM interface towards the ventricles guided subcortical surface placement. A Laplacian field represents a map of smoothly increasing equipotential surfaces between two boundaries S_0 and M and guarantees a similar triangular topology throughout the deformation. Let ψ denote the electrostatic potential at equilibrium of some quantity. Then, the net flux of ψ through the boundary S of a control volume V is defined as following:

$$\int \nabla\psi \bullet \mathbf{n} \, dS = 0 \tag{1}$$

where dS is the area of an infinitesimal surface element on the boundary and $\mathbf{n}$ is a surface normal vector. In Cartesian coordinates, Laplace's equation is expressed as:

$$\Delta\psi = \nabla^2\psi = \frac{\partial\psi}{\partial x^2} + \frac{\partial\psi}{\partial y^2} + \frac{\partial\psi}{\partial z^2} \tag{2}$$

Given boundary conditions as $\psi_1 = S_0$ (GM-WM interface) and $\psi_2 = M$ (ventricle), solving **Eq. (2)** results in a smooth transition of equipotentials within V. Intervals between subcortical surfaces were adapted to the native resolution of each modality (T1/FLAIR: 1/0.9mm and diffusion: 2mm). Please note that the use of more widely-spaced surfaces for the sampling of diffusion parameters minimized residual misregistration errors due to EPI-specific image distortions.

2.4   Surface-Based Feature Extraction

Features were extracted in the native space of the respective modalities to minimize interpolation. To control for regional feature variability after surface smoothing (FWHM=5mm), measures in a given patient were z-transformed at each vertex with respect to the corresponding distribution in controls (*see below*).

Intensity and Texture. To assess lesional intensity, we calculated the difference between the T1w (and FLAIR) intensity at a given voxel and averaged GM-WM boundary intensity, and normalized it by the mode of the intensity histogram. These *normalized intensity* values were mapped to surfaces using a linear interpolation. To model intracortical dyslamination, we computed intensity gradients in perpendicular and tangential direction with respect to cortical surface geometry. *Perpendicular gradient* was computed as the difference in intensity between corresponding vertices above and below a vertex v_i on neighboring surfaces, divided by their distance. *Tangential gradient* was computed along each surface, by averaging differences of intensity of the surface-neighbors of v_i, divided by the mean distance from neighboring vertices. We did not sample intensity at the outermost GM-CSF surface to avoid large CSF partial volume effects *(PVE_{CSF})*. At other surfaces, PVE_{CSF} was corrected similar to a previous approach [8]. In brief, we automatically estimated PVE_{GM} and PVE_{CSF} on T1w- and FLAIR-MRI [9] and mapped these values to intra-cortical surfaces. Observed intensity (I) at v_i was modeled as: $I=PVE_{GM}\times I_{GM}(v_i)+PVE_{CSF}(v_i)\times I_{CSF}(v_i)$, where I_{GM}/I_{CSF} are pure intensities of GM/CSF. $I_{CSF}(v_i)$ was computed by averaging intensity of neighboring voxels considered 'pure' CSF (voxels with $PVE_{CSF}=1$, within a radius of 10 mm around v_i). Solving the equation provides the remaining term RI_{GM} (*i.e.*, the hypothetical CSF–free GM intensity) at each vertex.

Morphology. Cortical thickness was calculated as the Euclidean distance between corresponding vertices on the GM-WM and GM-CSF surfaces [5]. As small FCD lesions are often located at the bottom of a sulcus [10], we computed sulcal depth by overlaying a brain hull on the GM-CSF boundary to detect gyral crowns; for a given vertex, sulcal depth was computed as the shortest geodesic distance from a crown.

Diffusion tensor parameters. FA and MD are proxies for fiber architecture and microstructure. Due to lower resolution, we sampled FA and MD at the 50% intra-cortical, the GM-WM boundary and subcortical surfaces lying at 2 and 4 mm depth.

Functional MRI metrics. We calculated two voxel-wise markers of local functional integrity: amplitude of low frequency fluctuations (ALFF) and regional homogeneity (ReHo) [11]. While ALFF is computed as the total time-series power in the 0.01-0.08 Hz band, ReHo quantifies local time-series variance within a 27-voxel-neighborhood. Functional features were sampled on the 50% intra-cortical surface.

3   Experiment and Results

3.1   Subjects

We studied 33 consecutive patients (17 males; mean±SD age=28±10 years) with histologically-proven FCD Type-II (9 IIA, 24 IIB) admitted to our Hospital for the investigation of focal epilepsy. The presurgical workup included a neurologic examination, assessment of seizure history, neuroimaging, and video-EEG telemetry. The FCD subgroups did not show statistical differences in age, sex, age at onset, disease duration, and focus lateralization. As control group, we studied 41 age- and sex-matched healthy individuals (21 males; mean±SD age=30±7 years).

3.2   Lesion Profiling

Manual Segmentation. Two trained raters independently segmented FCD lesions on co-registered T1w and FLAIR images; their consensus volume label was intersected with the surface models, thereby generating surface-based lesion labels.

Lesion Profiling. For each patient, z-scores of a given feature **(2.3)** were averaged across all intracortical/subcortical vertices within the consensus label to obtain a global lesion profile. Global profiling was complemented by systematic analysis of feature variations across individual intracortical and subcortical surfaces.

Statistical Analysis. Using two-sample Student's t-tests, we compared global and multi-surface profiles between each patient group (*i.e.*, FCD Type-IIA and IIB) to controls, and patient cohorts to each other. We utilized the Benjamini-Hochberg procedure to control the false discovery rate (FDR) to be below q=0.05 [12].

3.3   Machine-Learning Prediction of Histological Subtypes

A support vector machine (SVM) with a polynomial 3rd-order kernel was used to automatically predict the histological FCD subtype in individual patients. Using a leave-one-out cross-validation scheme, we performed a forward-sequential feature selection, trained the classifier, and evaluated prediction performance. The forward-sequential procedure added features to an empty set until classification rates were not further improved. We evaluated the *box-constraint* parameter C, a penalty for non-separable samples, across C=0.1-1000. As accuracies were stable across the entire range, C was set to the default of 1. We visualized classification results through multidimensional scaling. SVM performance was evaluated for three different feature categories: *i)* Global features from single modalities (*e.g.*, only features derived from FLAIR); *ii)* Global multi-modal features (*e.g.*, combinations of features derived from T1w, FLAIR, DWI, and rs-fMRI); *iii)* multimodal and multi-surface (intracortical and subcortical) features.

3.4   Results

Global Lesion Profiling (**Fig. 2**). Compared to controls, FCD Type-IIB was associated with a wide range of morphological and intensity anomalies (*increased* cortical thickness, sulcal depth, intracortical/subcortical FLAIR intensity, subcortical MD; *decreased* perpendicular T1w/FLAIR gradient, tangential T1w gradient), while anomalies in Type-IIA were restricted to increased FLAIR intensity (q_{FDR}=0.05). Directly comparing both FCD cohorts revealed increased FLAIR intensity, cortical thickness, sulcal depth, and decreased vertical T1w gradient in Type-IIB (q_{FDR}<0.05). Functional profiling revealed decreased ALFF and ReHo in Type-IIB compared to controls (q_{FDR} <0.03). Type-IIA, on the other hand, showed marginally increased ReHo compared to controls (q_{FDR}<0.07). Direct subtype comparisons confirmed significant decreases across both features in Type-IIB (q_{FDR} <0.01).

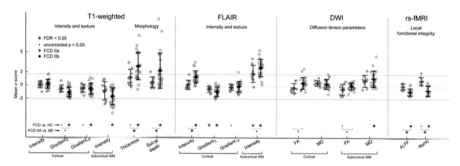

Fig. 2. Global lesion profiling. Graphs show feature z-scores *w.r.t.* controls in FCD Type-IIA (*red*) and IIB (*black*). Significant differences from controls and between patient groups are indicated by asterisks (q_{FDR}<0.05), trends are displayed as small circles (p<0.05).

Multi-Surface Profiling (**Fig. 3**). Multi-surface analysis revealed marked abnormalities across virtually all intracortical levels in Type-IIB (increased FLAIR intensity, decreased vertical T1w/FLAIR gradient), while alterations in IIA were proximal to the GM-WM interface (decreased T1w/FLAIR gradients). Likewise, WM alterations in Type-IIB were found across all subcortical surfaces (decreased T1w intensity, increased FLAIR intensity and MD; q_{FDR}<0.02). Type-IIA presented with FLAIR intensity increases in subcortical WM at 1 mm depth (q_{FDR}<0.02). Direct FCD cohort comparisons revealed increased FLAIR intensity in Type-IIB relative to IIA across all intracortical and the 1 mm deep subcortical WM surfaces (q_{FDR}=0.03). Conversely, FA was reduced in Type-IIA relative to IIB (q_{FDR}=0.05).

Prediction of Histological Subtypes (**Fig. 4**). An SVM trained on multi-surface features derived from structural and functional modalities accurately predicted the FCD subtype in 91% (21/23, missing one IIA and one IIB), outperforming SVMs trained on single modalities (52-70%) or classifiers using only global features (83%). We repeated the analysis with a 10-fold cross-validation (100 times) and addressed unbalanced group sizes by adding 'bagging' (100 times; randomly selecting equal numbers of training cases from each subtype). Using this scheme, we observed a slightly lower, but still excellent overall performance (87% accuracy, sensitivity: 89%, specificity: 85%). Permutation tests with 10,000 iterations confirmed that the achieved accuracy exceeded chance-level (p<0.001). A mean±SD=3±1 features were selected across leave-one-out iterations at optimal accuracy. In order of contribution, these were: ReHo, T1w-vertical gradient (75% depth), FLAIR intensity (25 and 50% depth), cortical thickness, subcortical FA (2mm depth), and ALFF.

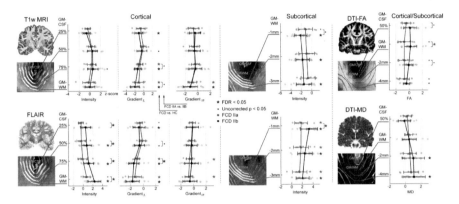

Fig. 3. Plots display multi-surface lesion profiles at various intra-/subcortical depths. Circles indicate FCD subtypes (*red/black* for Type IIA/IIB). For a given lesion, feature values are z-normalized relative to controls and averaged within the consensus label. Inter-surface spacing is based on the relative native imaging resolution.

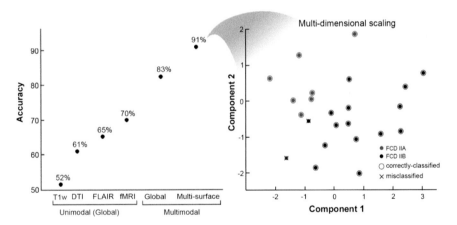

Fig. 4. MRI-based FCD subtype prediction across feature combinations *(left)*. For display purposes, the high dimensional feature space was projected to 2D using multi-dimensional scaling *(right)*. Circles indicate FCD subtypes (*red/black* for Type IIA/IIB). Correctly classified cases are surrounded by a *circle*, misclassified cases are marked by x.

4   Discussion

Global lesion profiling showed that cortical thickening, T1w hypointensity, FLAIR hyperintensity, and increased sulcal depth are associated with FCD Type-IIB lesions, while Type-IIA has a more subtle impact on neuroimaging markers. The subtype divergence was refined by the multi-surface analysis, revealing marked intensity and gradient abnormalities in IIB across all intracortical surfaces; conversely, anomalies in IIA were located proximal to the GM-WM interface. The selective alteration of upper cortical surfaces in IIB relate to the preferential location of immature progenitors, including balloon cells, in superficial laminae [13].

Subtypes also diverged with regards to functional metrics. Our finding of decreased ReHo in FCD Type-IIB may indicate abnormal intracortical signal integration that possibly results from the presence of balloon cell clusters acting as barriers to cortico-cortical connections [2]. Conversely, increased ReHo in Type-IIA may reflect enhanced functional synchronization due to excessive activation of dysmorphic neurons.

Few previous studies modeled FCD lesions, either using voxel- [14] or surface-based analysis [10, 15]. Feature modeling was generally limited to T1w features. Moreover, no work attempted to differentiate histological subtypes. The novelty of our work resides in: i) modeling cortical dyslamination via a multi-surface approach; ii) multicontrast MRI features targeting both the GM and the subcortical WM, iii) probing functional integrity; iv) predicting FCD subtypes through machine-learning. In the latter machine-learning experiment, we could validate our profiling approach by predicting histological subtypes with excellent (91%) accuracy. Our results emphasize the utility of integrating metrics of structure and function to dissociate neuroimaging signatures of surgically remediable epileptogenic malformations, with potential application to various neurological conditions in which disease staging is important, such as neurodegenerative disorders, multiple sclerosis, and tumors.

Reference

1. Blumcke, I., et al.: The clinicopathologic spectrum of focal cortical dysplasias: a consensus classification proposed by an ad hoc Task Force of the ILAE Diagnostic Methods Commission. Epilepsia 52(1), 158–174 (2011)
2. Boonyapisit, K., et al.: Epileptogenicity of focal malformations due to abnormal cortical development: Direct electrocorticographic histopathologic correlations. Epilepsia 44(1), 69–76 (2003)
3. Tassi, L., et al.: Electroclinical, MRI and neuropathological study of 10 patients with nodular heterotopia, with surgical outcomes. Brain 128(Pt. 2), 321–337 (2005)
4. Zijdenbos, A.P., Forghani, R., Evans, A.C.: Automatic "pipeline" analysis of 3-D MRI data for clinical trials: application to multiple sclerosis. IEEE Trans. Med. Imaging 21(10), 1280–1291 (2002)
5. Kim, J.S., et al.: Automated 3-D extraction and evaluation of the inner and outer cortical surfaces using a Laplacian map and partial volume effect classification. Neuroimage 27(1), 210–221 (2005)
6. Power, J.D., et al.: Spurious but systematic correlations in functional connectivity MRI networks arise from subject motion. Neuroimage 59(3), 2142–2154 (2012)
7. Greve, D.N., Fischl, B.: Accurate and robust brain image alignment using boundary-based registration. Neuroimage 48(1), 63–72 (2009)

8. Shafee, R., Buckner, R.L., Fischl, B.: Gray matter myelination of 1555 human brains using partial volume corrected MRI images. Neuroimage 105, 473–485 (2015)
9. Tohka, J., Zijdenbos, A., Evans, A.: Fast and robust parameter estimation for statistical partial volume models in brain MRI. Neuroimage 23(1), 84–97 (2004)
10. Besson, P., et al.: Small focal cortical dysplasia lesions are located at the bottom of a deep sulcus. Brain 131(Pt. 12), 3246–3255 (2008)
11. Yuan, R., et al.: Regional homogeneity of resting-state fMRI contributes to both neurovascular and task activation variations. Magn. Reson. Imaging 31(9), 1492–1500 (2013)
12. Benjamini, Y., Hochberg, Y.: Controlling the false discovery rate: a practical and powerful approach to multiple testing. Journal of the Royal Statistical Society. Series B (Methodological), 289–300 (1995)
13. Sakakibara, T., et al.: Delayed maturation and differentiation of neurons in focal cortical dysplasia with the transmantle sign: analysis of layer-specific marker expression. J. Neuropathol. Exp. Neurol. 71(8), 741–749 (2012)
14. Colliot, O., et al.: In vivo profiling of focal cortical dysplasia on high-resolution MRI with computational models. Epilepsia 47(1), 134–142 (2006)
15. Thesen, T., et al.: Detection of epileptogenic cortical malformations with surface-based MRI morphometry. PLoS One 6(2), e16430 (2011)

Patient-specific 3D Ultrasound Simulation Based on Convolutional Ray-tracing and Appearance Optimization

Mehrdad Salehi[1,3], Seyed-Ahmad Ahmadi[2], Raphael Prevost[1],
Nassir Navab[3,4], and Wolfgang Wein[1]

[1] ImFusion GmbH, München, Germany
[2] Department of Neurology, Klinikum der Universität München, LMU, Germany
mehrdad.salehi@tum.de
[3] Computer Aided Medical Procedures, Technische Universität München, Germany
[4] Computer Aided Medical Procedures, Johns Hopkins University, Baltimore, USA

Abstract. The simulation of medical ultrasound from patient-specific data may improve the planning and execution of interventions e.g. in the field of neurosurgery. However, both the long computation times and the limited realism due to lack of acoustic information from tomographic scans prevent a wide adoption of such a simulation. In this work, we address these problems by proposing a novel efficient ultrasound simulation method based on convolutional ray-tracing which directly takes volumetric image data as input. We show how the required acoustic simulation parameters can be derived from a segmented MRI scan of the patient. We also propose an automatic optimization of ultrasonic simulation parameters and tissue-specific acoustic properties from matching ultrasound and MRI scan data. Both qualitative and quantitative evaluation on a database of 14 neurosurgical patients demonstrate the potential of our approach for clinical use.

1 Introduction

A realistic simulation of medical ultrasound is an important tool, e.g. for transducer design, training of physicians or multi-modal image-registration through simulation. A further attractive application is pre-operative planning, in which a patient-specific ultrasound simulation of the operational situs could help the surgeon to anticipate tissue appearance or optimal transducer positioning. However, a wide adoption in this context has been prevented by two problems. First, computation times of realistic ultrasound simulation methods still prevent interactive frame rates. Second, deriving the required acoustic parameters of tissue from a CT or MRI scan of the same patient is difficult due to different physical imaging principles and limited resolution of the source modalities. In this work, we are addressing both problems by proposing an interactive and realistic simulation based on convolution and ray-tracing with simulation parameters that can be optimized to match the appearance of real ultrasound images.

© Springer International Publishing Switzerland 2015
N. Navab et al. (Eds.): MICCAI 2015, Part II, LNCS 9350, pp. 510–518, 2015.
DOI: 10.1007/978-3-319-24571-3_61

Ultrasound simulation approaches can be roughly categorized into wave-based, ray-based and convolution-based methods. Wave-based methods offer the highest realism and physical accuracy due to actual simulation of wave-front propagation in tissue. However, they are computationally expensive, requiring up to one hour for rendering of a single frame even on modern graphic card hardware [9]. Another approach is to simulate the spatial impulse response of the ultrasound system and convolve it with an artificial map of micro-scatters. A well-known software to employ this model is Field II, which takes up to one minute for simulation of a 2D image [8] and often serves as gold standard in validation of other methods. Another convolution-based approach was introduced by Bamber [1] and expanded by Meunier [11], in which the image is created by convolution of the imaging system's point-spread-function (PSF) with a map of points representing the position and reflectivity of scatterers. A comparison study in [5] shows that recently proposed convolution-based method, COLE [4], can provide similar image quality and statistics compared to Field II, while offering real-time simulation speeds. A problem in these methods, however, is the inability to mimic specific types of US imaging artifacts such as refractions, mirroring, range distortion, shadowing, and enhancement.

Ray-based simulation techniques focus on generating real-time images using ray optics. They cover acoustic brightness of tissue regions, reflections at tissue boundaries and shadowing artefacts, but they are lacking speckle noise or reflection- and refraction-induced artefacts.

In [2], a computer graphics ray-tracing scheme is adapted for fast convolution-based ultrasound simulation. The ray-tracing depends on exact surface models of brain regions, requiring extensive pre-processing of the data and post-processing to overcome simplifications of the ray-based approach. We adopt and extend this method to work directly on volume data, which can be derived from a patient's MRI or CT in a number of simple image processing steps. Moreover, our method interleaves convolution and ray-tracing, such that scattering properties of the tissue are propagated throughout the entire ultrasound beam formation process. Additionally, we demonstrate for the first time a method to directly optimize ultrasound simulation parameters and acoustic properties of the underlying tissue maps through image-based matching of patient-specific ultrasound and MRI data. An overview of the proposed system is shown in Fig. 1.

2 Methods

2.1 Patient-Specific Acoustic Data from MRI

Six acoustic parameters are defined for each medium. Speed of sound c, acoustic impedance Z, and attenuation coefficient α are used in the ray-tracing engine to compute the intensity and relative time of the rays at each point. Three other parameters, μ_0, μ_1, and σ_0 drive a generative model for the distribution and intensity of scatterer points in each medium (detailed description in [2]). The ray-tracing part is performed on a label volume containing the tissue indices corresponding to the parameters table. The pre-processing part thus consists of segmenting and labeling the source modality, in our case MRI data.

A well-established approach for multi-class segmentation of MRI is to cluster image intensities using a Gaussian Mixture model and optimizing the fitting using the Expectation-Maximization (EM) algorithm [14]. Instead of enforcing spatial regularization during EM, we pre-process the MRI with a guided filter [6] which acts as a very fast anisotropic diffusion step. The resulting label maps are sufficiently smooth and accurate to be used as input to our simulation algorithm. No further processing or meshing of the segmentation is required.

2.2   Ultrasound Simulation

A ray-tracing engine is at the core of this method and builds the data for each radio frequency (RF) scanline separately. The recorded echo for each scanline i at the distance l from the transducer is defined as a sum of two main terms:

$$E_i(l) = R_i(l) + B_i(l) \tag{1}$$

where $R_i(l)$ is the reflected energy from the tissue boundaries and $B_i(l)$ is the backscattered energy from the scattering points throughout the scan line.

Reflection and Attenuation: We use a model similar to [13] to approximate both specular and diffuse reflections. Let $H(l)$ be the PSF of the imaging system, and $G(x, y, z)$ be an indicator function that returns 1 for points on the surface boundaries and 0 otherwise. Then, the reflected energy can be written as:

$$R_i(l) = \left| I_i(l) * \cos\theta_i{}^n * \left(\frac{Z_1 - Z_2}{Z_1 + Z_2} \right)^2 \right| * H(l) \otimes G(x, y, z) \tag{2}$$

The term $\cos\theta_i$ comes from Lambert's cosine law and θ_i is the angle of incidence. The exponent n is a simple modification to describe the heterogeneity on the surface and $I_i(l)$ is the remaining ultrasound wave amplitude. Z_1 and Z_2 are the acoustic impedances of two adjacent tissues. The sound energy gets attenuated during tissue traversal, which causes artefacts like shadowing and enhancement. The remaining energy of the sound beam $I_i(l)$ is modeled using the Beer-Lambert Law as $I_i(l) = I_0\, e^{-\alpha l f}$, where I_0 is the initial energy, f is the sound frequency, and α is the attenuation coefficient of the medium.

Backscattering Term: The other term in the returned echo, the back-scattered energy $B_i(l)$, is the product of the remaining wave amplitude and the convolution of the PSF $H(l)$ with random scatterers:

$$B_i(l) = I_i(l) * H(l) \otimes T(x, y, z). \tag{3}$$

Similar to [2], we create the scatterers from a generative model. It is based on two random textures which are combined using the tissue-specific parameters μ_0, μ_1, and σ_0. For each tissue, the model generates scatterers of various spatial and acoustic density. We refer the reader to [2] for details. The spatial PSF $H(x, y, z)$ (or $H(l)$ along the ray) is modeled with a cosine function modulated by a 3D

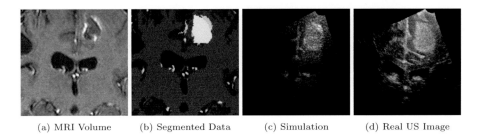

(a) MRI Volume   (b) Segmented Data   (c) Simulation   (d) Real US Image

Fig. 1. Simulation/optimization pipeline; (a) Input modality, (b) Label-map after segmentation, (c) Simulation result before parameter optimization, (d) real US image, which is used for optimization of simulation parameters.

Gaussian envelope, which is sufficient to approximate the far-field [11]. The convolution kernel can be separated [1] into three 1D components, i.e. $H(x, y, z) = H_x(x) \times H_y(y) \times H_z(z)$, with an axial pulse $H_x(x) = \exp(-0.5x^2/\sigma_x^2)\cos(2\pi f x)$, and lateral and elevational beam profiles $H_y(y) = \exp(-0.5y^2/\sigma_y^2)$ and $H_z(z) = \exp(-0.5z^2/\sigma_z^2)$. The beam profile can thus be spatially varying, which allows for simulation of a sharper, user-defined focus zone and blurrier out-of-focus regions by dispersal of the beam profile. The convolution between the PSF and the scatterers texture is calculated during the entire ray-tracing for each pixel on the RF scan-lines.

Ray-Tracing: A binary tree structure keeps the data for the ray-tracing engine, which is based on optical principles. Each crossing of a ray with a tissue interface generates a reflected and a refracted ray, which are further traced into the medium. The remaining intensity (according to Fresnel equation), direction (according to Snell's law) and the relative time to transducer are passed to the child rays. The final result for each RF scan-line is the sum of all child rays covering that scan-line. Each ray terminates if (i) it leaves the imaging frame, (ii) its remaining intensity decreases lower than a user-defined threshold or (iii) its relative time to transducer exceeds the image penetration depth and thus the maximum allowed run-time. The whole simulation pipeline and post-processing steps are parallelized on GPU using OpenCL and OpenGL libraries, which makes it independent of proprietary ray-tracing engines as in [2].

Post-processing: Post-processing is performed using a simple RF to B-mode conversion scheme. We first add (Gaussian) amplifier noise to the signal and proceed with time gain compensation (TGC), envelope detection and dynamic range limiting of the signal [7]. The RF data is log-compressed and 8-bit quantized. Finally, the fan geometry and ultrasound image are calculated through scan conversion.

2.3 Automatic Optimization

We use registered MRI and 3D freehand ultrasound data from all 14 patients of the BITE neurosurgical database [10]. The following cost function is used in a non-linear optimization of the simulation parameters with respect to the real ultrasound images as reference.

$$L(A, B) = \rho(A, B) + \lambda * \mathrm{SAD}(A, B) \tag{4}$$

$$\rho(A, B) = \frac{1}{N} \sum_{i}^{N} \sqrt{1 - \sum_{j}^{M} \sqrt{P_{ij} Q_{ij}}} \tag{5}$$

$\rho(A, B)$ is our proposed local Bhattacharyya distance between images A and B; P_i and Q_i are normalized distributions of patch number i of the images, M is the number of bins, and N is the number of patches. This is a modification of Bhattacharyya-based metric distribution distance proposed by Comaniciu *et al.* [3]. It caters to the fact that simulated speckle positions can not match with the real ultrasound, but their intensity distributions shall be similar. The localized version is required to prevent arbitrary configurations of tissue parameters which may nevertheless align the overall image histograms. We compute the average Bhattacharyya distance within local square image regions of width 5 mm. Through λ, it is weighted to the sum of absolute differences (SAD) of the image intensities. This assures the overall matching of large-scale structures, brightness and contrast. This measure, therefore, allows us to optimize (i) global post-processing parameters, which are typically unknown and different in every ultrasound acquisition and (ii) the acoustic parameters of each modeled tissue.

3   Evaluation

3.1   Acoustic Model

We demonstrate various US phenomena and artifacts of our simulation on a synthetic phantom. Obvious ones include shadowing or enhancement after high- or low-attenuation areas. Compared to purely ray-based or convolutional approaches, our hybrid algorithm can also simulate more subtle effects such as mirroring, reverberation or refraction at acoustic impedance interfaces, as well as geometric range distortions due to variations of speed of sound (Fig. 2).

3.2   Qualitative Results on Patient Data

We also illustrate the fidelity of our simulation using real-life, co-registered MRI and 3D US data from the BITE database. In Fig. 3, simulation results before and after optimization are shown alongside the real US image and MRI plane. Images are simulated using a pulse frequency of 5 MHz.

Direct comparison of this method to convolution-based approaches is challenging due to different scatterer map models. However, in future works our proposed similarity measure can be used for comparing different simulation approaches to real US data.

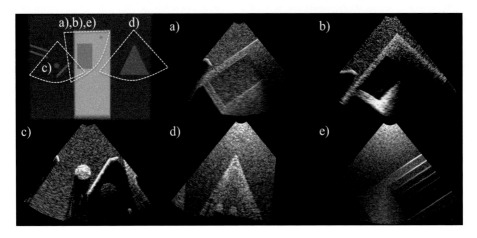

Fig. 2. Ultrasound artifacts exhibited in the artificial phantom (top left). a) Shadowing, b) Range distortion due to (exaggerated) speed of sound differences in tissue, c) mirroring, d) refraction and e) reverberation

3.3 Quantitative Evaluation and Optimization

For the evaluation of the statistical characteristics, the simulation was performed on a random scatterer volume with pixel dimension of 20 μm^3 and density of 1250 per mm^3 [11]. When using an unfocused beam-profile, intensity distribution for the produced analytic signal is known to follow Rayleigh statistics [12]. The result for the distribution fit is shown in Fig. 4. The sum of squares due to errors (SSE) was $3.14e$-05, which can be considered simlarly low as in literature [5], even though a direct comparison would require exactly identical source data. The goodness-of-fit between the measured histogram and its Rayleigh fit demonstrates that our simulation can produce accurate speckle characteristics despite the complex decomposition of the 3D convolution between separate rays. Please note that only envelope-detected, reflection/refraction-free data was used in this experiment, without post-processing.

Performance: Simulation performance is dependent on scatterers size, image depth, axial resolution, and depth of the rays binary tree. Simulation time including post-processing lies between 0.1-1s, which mainly depends on the number of scan-lines, depth of reflections, and axial resolution of the RF data (OpenCL implementation run on a laptop with NVIDIA GTX 850M). We also limited the binary trees depth to six since further reflections usually do not contribute significantly to the final image due to reduced ray intensities.

Optimization: Table 1 shows the parameters after optimization on 14 datasets; the visual appearance significantly improved in all cases. An exemplary result is shown in Fig. 3. The values for μ_0 and μ_1 are more consistent, while σ_0 and α vary for different patients. An explanation is that the latter two depend on log-compression and TGC parameters which are being simultaneously optimized.

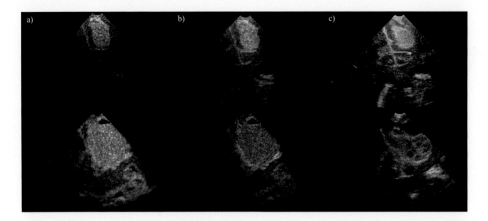

Fig. 3. Columns show (a): Simulation before optimization, (b): after optimization, (c): real US image. Both rows show a tumor next to the cerebral falx. Inaccuracies in b) are caused by segmentation errors (partly due to brain-shift) and the assumption of homogeneous scatterer properties per tissue type.

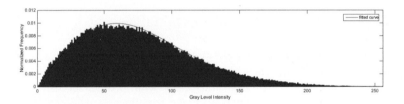

Fig. 4. Rayleigh Distribution Fit. $\sigma = 59.09$, SSE $= 3.14e\text{-}05$

Table 1. α, μ_0, σ_0, and μ_1 are brain white-matter's acoustic properties. μ and σ are mean and standard deviation of acoustic parameters after optimization.

AC Prop.	Initial Values	Optimized Parameters for each Patient														Statistics	
		1	2	3	4	5	6	7	8	9	10	11	12	13	14	μ	σ
α	0.54	0.59	0.71	0.43	0.59	0.28	0.31	0.57	0.93	0.20	0.44	0.24	0.25	0.39	0.34	0.452	0.207
μ_0	0.40	0.40	0.36	0.06	0.37	0.33	0.39	0.44	0.40	0.30	0.30	0.32	0.34	0.27	0.32	0.332	0.089
σ_0	0.15	0.16	0.05	0.31	0.38	0.07	0.07	0.26	0.24	0.01	0.07	0.01	0.23	0.13	0.23	0.163	0.119
μ_1	0.00	0.00	0.00	0.04	0.00	0.00	0.00	0.00	0.01	0.00	0.00	0.00	0.00	0.00	0.00	0.004	0.013

4   Conclusion

We have presented a patient-specific US simulation from MRI at interactive frame rates, using a hybrid, convolutional ray-tracing approach with limited data pre-processing. Furthermore, for the first time, we propose a similarity formulation for optimization of both US system and tissue acoustic parameters. This improves simulation realism and further closes the gap between underlying physics and information contents of both modalities. Possible applications go beyond typical usages of ultrasound simulation today. For example, pre-operative tissue appearance anticipation from MRI and planning of transducer positioning could help with tight time constraints in US-guided interventions. A shortcoming of our simulation is its high dependence on the segmentation accuracy. Future work could address this with a hybrid model for the scatterers texture, which combines the label map with original intensities of MRI/CT source data. The simulation and optimization accuracy should be also further evaluated, ideally in a controlled acquisition environment with known tissue parameters.

Acknowledgments. Bayerische Forschungsstiftung (BFS) grant RoBildOR and Deutsche Forschungsgesellschaft (DFG) grant BO 1895/4-1.

References

1. Bamber, J.C., Dickinson, R.J.: Ultrasonic B-scanning: a computer simulation. Physics in Medicine and Biology 25(3), 463–479 (1980)
2. Bürger, B., Bettinghausen, S., Rädle, M., Hesser, J.: Real-time GPU-based ultrasound simulation using deformable mesh models. IEEE Transactions on Medical Imaging 32(3), 609–618 (2013)
3. Comaniciu, D., Ramesh, V., Meer, P.: Kernel-based object tracking. IEEE Transactions on Pattern Analysis and Machine Intelligence 25, 564–577 (2003)
4. Gao, H., Choi, H.F., Claus, P., Boonen, S., Jaecques, S., Van Lenthe, G.H., Van der Perre, G., Lauriks, W., D'hooge, J.: A fast convolution-based methodology to simulate 2-D/3-D cardiac ultrasound images. IEEE Transactions on Ultrasonics, Ferroelectrics, and Frequency Control 56(2), 404–409 (2009)
5. Gao, H., Hergum, T.T.R., Torp, H., D'hooge, J.: Comparison of the performance of different tools for fast simulation of ultrasound data. Ultrasonics 52(5), 573–577 (2012)
6. He, K., Sun, J., Tang, X.: Guided image filtering. In: Daniilidis, K., Maragos, P., Paragios, N. (eds.) ECCV 2010, Part I. LNCS, vol. 6311, pp. 1–14. Springer, Heidelberg (2010)
7. Hedrick, W.R., Starchman, D.E., Hykes, D.L.: Ultrasound physics and instrumentation, 4th edn. Elsevier Mosby, St. Louis (2005)
8. Jensen, J.A.: A multi-threaded version of Field II. In: 2014 IEEE International Ultrasonics Symposium, pp. 2229–2232, September 2014
9. Karamalis, A., Wein, W., Navab, N.: Fast ultrasound image simulation using the Westervelt equation. In: Jiang, T., Navab, N., Pluim, J.P.W., Viergever, M.A. (eds.) MICCAI 2010, Part I. LNCS, vol. 6361, pp. 243–250. Springer, Heidelberg (2010)
10. Mercier, L., Del Maestro, R., Petrecca, K., Araujo, D., Haegelen, C., Collins, D.: Online Database of Clinical MR and Ultrasound Images of Brain Tumors. Medical Physics 39, 3253 (2012)
11. Meunier, J., Bertrand, M.: Ultrasonic texture motion analysis: theory and simulation. IEEE Transactions on Medical Imaging 14(2), 293–300 (1995)

12. Wagner, R.F., Insana, M.F., Brown, D.G.: Statistical properties of radio-frequency and envelope-detected signals with applications to medical ultrasound. Journal of the Optical Society of America. A, Optics and image Science 4, 910–922 (1987)
13. Wein, W., Brunke, S., Khamene, A., Callstrom, M., Navab, N.: Automatic CT-Ultrasound Registration for Diagnostic Imaging and Image-Guided Intervention. Medical Image Analysis 12(5), 577 (2008)
14. Zhang, Y., Brady, M., Smith, S.: Segmentation of brain mr images through a hidden markov random field model and the expectation-maximization algorithm. IEEE Transactions on Medical Imaging 20(1), 45–57 (2001)

Robust Transmural Electrophysiological Imaging: Integrating Sparse and Dynamic Physiological Models into ECG-Based Inference

Jingjia Xu[1], John L. Sapp[2], Azar Rahimi Dehaghani[1], Fei Gao[3], Milan Horacek[2], and Linwei Wang[1]

[1] Rochester Institute of Technology, Rochester, NY, 14623, USA
xujingjia.zju@gmail.com
[2] Dalhousie Unviersity,Halifax, NS, Canada
[3] Molecular Imaging Division, Siemens Medical Solutions, Knoxville, TN, 37932, USA

Abstract. Noninvasive inference of patient-specific intramural electrical activity from surface electrocardiograms (ECG) lacks a unique solution in the absence of prior assumptions. While 3D cardiac electrophysiological models emerged to be a viable vehicle for constraining this inference with knowledge about the spatiotemporal dynamics of cardiac excitation, it is important for the inference to be robust to errors in these high-dimensional model predictions given the limited ECG data. We present an innovative solution to this problem by exploiting the low-dimensional structure of the solution space – a powerful regularizer in overcoming the lack of measurements – *within* the dynamic inference guided by physiological models. We present the first Bayesian inference framework that allows the exploration of both the spatial sparsity of cardiac excitation and its complex nonlinear spatiotemporal dynamics for an improved inference of patient-specific intramural electrical activity. The benefit of this integration is verified in both synthetic and real-data experiments, where we present one of the first detailed, point-by-point comparison of the reconstructed electrical activity to *in-vivo* catheter mapping data.

1 Introduction

Despite significant advances in diagnostic imaging, a considered gap remains between the way to assess cardiac electrical and mechanical functions. To date, clinical assessment of cardiac electrophysiology remains at a gross view with several electrocardiogram (ECG) traces, while a more detailed image requires a invasive mapping using catheters. This gap has motivated the research in *noninvasive electrophysiological (EP) imaging* that, in analogy to computed tomography, collects ECG data external to the body and computationally reconstructs patient-specific electrical activity [1]. It underscores a notoriously ill-posed inverse problem: surface ECG is not only limited in number but, more importantly, different intramural electrical sources may produce identical ECG data [2].

To bypass the challenge of non-unique intramural solutions, a common approach has been to restrict the reconstruction to the surface of the heart [1].

© Springer International Publishing Switzerland 2015
N. Navab et al. (Eds.): MICCAI 2015, Part II, LNCS 9350, pp. 519–527, 2015.
DOI: 10.1007/978-3-319-24571-3_62

Therefore, to obtain a unique intramural solution, proper assumptions must be made. In the few existing approaches, 3D excitation models have emerged to be a useful constraint for ECG-based inference, containing rich physiological knowledge about the spatiotemporal electrical dynamics within the myocardium [3]. However, since the ECG data is limited relative to the high-dimensional model prediction, it becomes important for ECG-based inference to be robust to *priori* model errors. In dynamic inference, a common solution is to augment the unknown system state with auxiliary variables representing unknown model errors [4]. Although this allows the prior model to adapt to measurement data, it leads to an even higher-dimensional unknown space. Outside the traditional regime of dynamic inference, the low-dimensional structure of a signal (*i.e.*, its sparsity in a certain basis) has become a powerful regularizer to overcome the lack of measurements by focusing on the most important region of a high-dimensional solution space [5]. Its use in noninvasive EP imaging was recently reported [6,1], *e.g.*, by extracting the sparsity of action potential in the gradient domain using total-variation [6]. However, sparse reconstructions are mostly studied in a static context in separation from dynamic inference. In the few recent efforts toward dynamic sparse inference, a linear dynamic model is typically used to describe the slow-changing property of the sparse signal in time [7].

In this paper, we present a hierarchical Bayesian approach to integrate dynamic physiological knowledge with sparse constraint in ECG-based inference of transmural electrical activity. It allows the incorporation of: 1) complex physiological knowledge produced by quasi Monte Carlo simulation of 3D cardiac excitation models, which can be of arbitrary form and nonlinearity running as a blackbox behind the inference; and 2) sparsity structure of intramural action potential emphasizing its spatial gradient localized between active and inactive regions. These two models are mutually complementary: while the former provides inference with complex domain knowledge about nonlinear spatiotemporal dynamics, the latter addresses the inference robustness by emphasizing the low-dimensional structure in the high-dimensional model prediction. The benefit of this integration is first verified in synthetic experiments designed to test the robustness of the inference to errors in *a priori* physiological knowledge. Its capacity in complex pathological applications is then demonstrated in a pilot study on post-infarction ventricular tachycardia patients, where the reconstructed excitation maps are quantitatively verified with *in-vivo* catheter mapping data.

2   Methods

Cardiac electrical excitation produces voltage data on the body surface following the *quasi-static* electromagnetism [2]. With numerical discretization of the heart-torso anatomy of a given subject, a biophysical model $\phi_k = \mathbf{H}\mathbf{u}_k$ can be derived that relates transmural action potential $\mathbf{u}_k$ to surface ECG data ϕ_k at each time instant k. $\mathbf{H}$ is specific to each individual's anatomy and typically assumed time-invariant to simplify the inference problem. In the Bayesian setting, the likelihood $p(\phi_k|\mathbf{u}_k,\varepsilon)$ can be modeled as a normal distribution $\mathcal{N}(\mathbf{H}\mathbf{u}_k,\varepsilon\mathbf{I})$, where ε denotes the precision (inverse variance) of data error.

Prior decomposition: To exploit the sparse structure of $\mathbf{u}_k$ while utilizing physiological knowledge regarding its spatiotemporal dynamics, we introduce an extra layer into the Bayesian hierarchy to decompose $\mathbf{u}_k$ into two independent variables $\mathbf{s}_k$ and $\mathbf{t}_k$, each incorporating the corresponding signal structure of $\mathbf{u}_k$. We consider a simple decomposition model $\mathbf{u}_k = \mathbf{s}_k \cdot \mathbf{t}_k + \delta$, where $\cdot$ denotes dot product and δ is a zero-mean Gaussian residual with precision β. We obtain:

$$p(\mathbf{u}_k|\mathbf{s}_k, \mathbf{t}_k, \beta) = \mathcal{N}(\mathbf{s}_k \cdot \mathbf{t}_k, \beta\mathbf{I}) \tag{1}$$

Physiological dynamic prior: $\mathbf{t}_k$ in (1) is a dimension-less descriptor of the nonlinear temporal profile of action potential. Physiological knowledge regarding its spatiotemporal behavior can be incorporated through a 3D cardiac EP model. In general, the presented framework can incorporate models as a blackbox running behind the inference. Here, the monodomain *Aliev-Panfilov* model [8] will be used to balance physiological plausibility and computational complexity:

$$\begin{cases} \frac{\partial \mathbf{t}}{\partial t} = \nabla \cdot (\mathbf{D}\nabla\mathbf{t}) + k\mathbf{t} \cdot (\mathbf{t} - a) \cdot (1 - \mathbf{t}) - \mathbf{t} \cdot \mathbf{v} \\ \frac{\partial \mathbf{v}}{\partial t} = -e(\mathbf{v} + k\mathbf{t} \cdot (\mathbf{t} - a - 1)) \end{cases} \tag{2}$$

where $\mathbf{v}$ stands for recovery current and the diffusion tensor $\mathbf{D}$ is considered anisotropic. The 3D myocardial fiber structure is mapped from an *ex-vivo* ventricular fibrous model [9]. The rest of the parameters are adopted from literature [8],so that no patient-specific pathological knowledge is assumed *a priori*.

Given posterior distribution of $\mathbf{t}_{k-1}$, the prior distribution of $\mathbf{t}_k$ can be predicted according to (2). Due to the nonlinearity of this model, a close-form prediction is not possible. Instead, simulation-based approach is used where a set of samples is drawn from the posterior distribution of $\mathbf{t}_{k-1}$ and individually passed through the excitation model; deterministic sampling based on the *unscented transform* [10] is used to reduce the number of samples needed for the high-dimensional $\mathbf{t}$ $(\sim 10^3)$. The mean $\bar{\mathbf{t}}_k^-$ and covariance $\mathbf{P}_{\mathbf{t}_k}^-$ of the new samples are used to approximate the prior distribution of $\mathbf{t}_k$ as:

$$p(\mathbf{t}_k|\phi_{1:k-1}) \sim \mathcal{N}(\bar{\mathbf{t}}_k^-, \mathbf{P}_{\mathbf{t}_k}^- + \mathbf{Q}_k) \tag{3}$$

where $\mathbf{Q}_k$ is a pre-defined covariance matrix to account for errors in the prior excited model (2) caused by factors such as heart motion, fiber model, etc. Variable $\mathbf{v}$ is not modeled or inferred because it is not directly related to the measurement. Note that the sampling and model simulation runs as a blackbox behind the inference, allowing a flexible *plug-and-play* of different EP models.

Sparse prior: The error covariance $\mathbf{Q}_k$ is only able to account for errors in the prior excitation model (2) to an extent. Since the model prediction is much higher in dimension than ECG data, additional structure of the solution space should be explored to avoid the inference being dominated by model predictions. Recent studies show that the sparsity of action potential in its gradient domain (*i.e.*, localized gradient between active and inactive regions) is an effective regularizer for ECG-based inference [6]. Thus, we define a spatial profile $\mathbf{s}_k$ for action potential and approximate the continuous form of its total-variation with a numerical integration using $N_g \sim 10^5$ Gaussian quadrature points:

$$\text{TV}(\mathbf{s}_k) = \int_{\Omega_h} |\nabla s_k| d\Omega_h \approx \Sigma_{i=1}^{N_g} \sqrt{\mathbf{s}_k^T \nabla\varphi_i^T \nabla\varphi_i \mathbf{s}_k} \tag{4}$$

where ∇s_k on each Gauss point is approximated by a linear combination of its neighboring nodes in the discrete ventricular mesh using shape functions φ_i.

Accordingly, the sparsity prior can be written as:

$$p(\mathbf{s}_k|\alpha) = c\alpha^{2m} \exp(-\alpha \mathrm{TV}(\mathbf{s}_k)) = c\alpha^{2m} \exp[-\alpha \Sigma_{i=1}^{N_g} \sqrt{\mathbf{s}_k^T \nabla \varphi_i^T \nabla \varphi_i \mathbf{s}_k}] \quad (5)$$

where c is constant, m is the dimension of $\mathbf{s}_k$.

Hyperparameters: The precision parameters (α, β and ε) of the above distributions control their relative contributions to the inference. To reduce the reliance on an *ad-hoc* tuning of these parameters, we assume them to be unknown with Gamma distributions (the conjugate of Gaussian distributions) [11].

Hierarchical Bayesian model: Because the excitation model (2) involves a first-order derivative in time, it is reasonable to assume $\mathbf{t}_k$ to be a first-order Markov process. The prior for sparsity and all hyperparameters can be assumed to be not informed by the previous ECG data, *i.e.*, independent with $\phi_{1:k-1}$:

$$p(\mathbf{s}_k|\alpha, \phi_{1:k-1}) \equiv p(\mathbf{s}_k|\alpha), \quad p(\theta|\phi_{1:k-1}) \equiv p(\theta), \theta \in \{\alpha, \beta, \varepsilon\} \quad (6)$$

Therefore, given ECG data $\phi_{1:N}$ throughout N time instants in a cardiac cycle, we can recursively compute the joint posterior distribution of all the unknowns $\Theta_k = (\mathbf{u}_k, \mathbf{t}_k, \mathbf{s}_k, \alpha, \beta, \varepsilon)$ given the data available up to the time instant k:

$$\begin{aligned} p(\Theta_k|\phi_{1:k}) &\propto p(\phi_k|\Theta_k)p(\Theta_k|\phi_{1:k-1}) \\ &= p(\phi_k|\mathbf{u}_k, \varepsilon)p(\mathbf{u}_k|\mathbf{t}_k, \mathbf{s}_k, \beta)p(\mathbf{t}_k|\phi_{1:k-1})p(\mathbf{s}_k|\alpha)p(\alpha)p(\beta)p(\varepsilon) \end{aligned} \quad (7)$$

Fig. 1(a) outlines the hierarchical Bayesian model at one time instant.

Variational Bayesian inference: The posterior distribution in (7) is analytically intractable. We adopt the variational Bayesian method to seek a tractable distribution $q(\Theta_k)$ with minimal Kullback-Leibler (KL) divergence to (7):

$$\hat{q}(\Theta_k) = \arg\min_{q(\Theta_k)} C_{KL}(q(\Theta_k)\|p(\Theta_k|\Phi_{1:k})) = \int q(\Theta_k) \log(\frac{q(\Theta_k)}{p(\Theta_k|\Phi_{1:k})})d\Theta \quad (8)$$

The solution to the above optimization problem is given by:

$$q(\Theta_{k,i}) \propto \exp(E_{\Theta\backslash\Theta_{k,i}}[\ln p(\Theta_k, \Phi_{1:k})]) \quad (9)$$

where $E_{\Theta_k\backslash\Theta_{k,i}}[\cdot]$ denotes the expectation with respect to all variables in the set of Θ_k except the variable of interest $\Theta_{k,i}$. Because the total-variation prior (5) prevents us from solving equation (9) analytically, we introduce an auxiliary vector $\mathbf{w}$ and define $p(\mathbf{s}_k, \mathbf{w}|\alpha) = c\alpha^{\gamma m} \exp(-\frac{\alpha}{2} \sum_i^{N_g} \frac{\mathbf{s}_k^T \nabla \varphi_i^T \nabla \varphi_i \mathbf{s}_k + w_i}{\sqrt{w_i}})$. Because $p(\mathbf{s}_k, \mathbf{w}|\alpha) \leq p(\mathbf{s}_k|\alpha)$ given the geometric-arithmetic mean inequality, replacing $p(\mathbf{s}_k|\alpha)$ with $p(\mathbf{s}_k, \mathbf{w}|\alpha)$ in equation (8) gives us an upper bound of the KL divergence. We can thus recursively minimize and monotonically decrease this upper bound until convergence to the original solution to (8) [11]. We randomly initialize $\mathbf{u}^1$ and then enter an iterative procedure. In each iteration, we cycle through each variable in Θ_k to update its posterior distribution according to (9). The main algorithm flow is illustrated in Fig. 1(b).

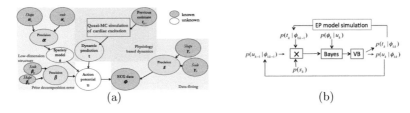

(a)   (b)

Fig. 1. Illustration of the hierarchical Bayesian model (a) and algorithm flow (b).

3 Experiments and Results

3.1 Simulation Study

Synthetic experiments are designed on pathological conditions to test the robustness of the inference to errors in *a priori* models. Experiments are conducted on 3 realistic human heart-torso models derived from CT scans (heart: ~ 2000 meshfree nodes; torso: 120 nodes). In all experiments, simulated time sequences of 120-lead ECGs are corrupted with 20-db white Gaussian noise. We compare the presented method with that constrained by 1) dynamic excitation model only [3] and 2) sparse total-variation model only [6]. The accuracy is measured by *correlation coefficient* (CC) between the reconstructed and simulated sequences of action potential.

Myocardial infarction: 10 cases of myocardial infarction are test, where ventricular action potential is simulated with the model(2) using parameters modified at the region of infarct scar [8]. It is noteworthy that the inference is guided by models with standard parameters, invoking *a priori* model parameter errors.

Fig. 2(a) top row shows snapshots of the simulated propagation of action potential during apical pacing with an infarct localized at the mid-basal lateral region of the LV (labeled by purple line). Before the excitation encounters (a1) or after it leaves the infarct region (a4), the *a priori* model error is minimal; therefore, result constrained by the excitation model shows high consistence with the ground truth (row 2 & 3). However, as the wavefront encounters and gets disrupted by the infarct region (a2), prior model errors start to have a visible impact on the solution accuracy (a2; row 3). In comparison, our method accurately reconstructs the abnormal excitation caused by the anatomical block, *demonstrating an improved robustness to model errors brought by simultaneously focusing on the sparse structure of the solution* (a2; row 2). During ECG ST-segment (a3), constrained by the dynamic model only, the inference is only able to overcome the model error and to reflect the inactive necrosis to a certain extent (a3; row 2); the exploit of sparse structure evidently improve this ability (a3; row 3): two additional examples from ECG ST-segments on different infarcted hearts are listed in Fig. 2(b). Inspection of the reconstructed temporal waveform of action potential tells a similar story (Fig. 2(2-3)): when strong prior dynamic knowledge is imposed, exploiting the low-dimensional structure of intramural action potential helps the inference to better combat the error in this knowledge.

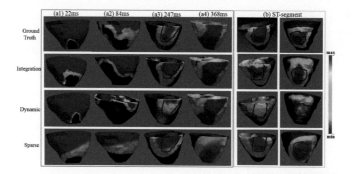

Fig. 2. Snapshots of intramural action potential propagation on infarcted hearts: simulated ground truth *vs.* inferences with physiological dynamic constraint only (Dynamic), sparsity constraint only (Sparse), and combined constraints (Integration).

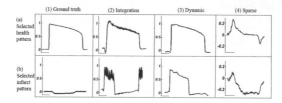

Fig. 3. Temporal morphology of simulated and reconstructed action potential.

Conversely, when only sparsity model is used, the inference is successful in capturing a gross division between active versus inactive regions. However, the excitation wavefront loses its intricate details (Fig. 2(a4)) and, more importantly, temporal morphology of action potential cannot be reproduced (Fig. 2(4)).

Premature ventricular contraction (PVC): In another 5 set of experiments, we consider abnormal ectopic foci that are not known *a priori* in the sinus-rhythm excitation model. Thus, the relevant model error primarily occurs in the early stage of ventricular excitation. As shown in Fig. 3.1(a), inference constrained by the dynamic model shows erroneous activation at standard sinus-rhythm sites. The integration with sparsity models is able to help correct this model error and produce PVC sites close to the simulated ground truth.

Statistical analysis: Quantitative analysis on CC are summarized in all cases across both settings. Fig. 3.1(b1) shows CC calculated on the complete temporal sequence of reconstructed action potential: in comparison to using sparsity models only, the use of prior excitation models can significantly improve CC by providing temporal morphology that is physiologically correct ($p < 0.01$, paired-t). Fig. 3.1(b2) shows CC calculated on the first half sequence within the cardiac cycle when less ECG data are available to the inference: in comparison to using dynamic models only, the exploitation of sparsity significantly improves CC by better overcoming model errors given limited data ($p < 0.01$, paired-t).

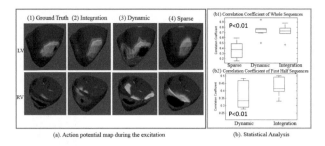

Fig. 4. Snapshots of intramural action potential resulting from ectopic foci (a) and correlation coefficients across n=15 synthetic cases (b).

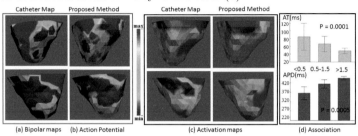

Fig. 5. Comparison with invasive catheter mapping on a post-infarction patient.

3.2 Real-Data Study

A case study is conducted on a patient who underwent catheter ablation of scar-related ventricular tachycardia. Transmural action potential is inferred from 120-lead ECG data on CT-derived anatomical model. *In-vivo* bipolar voltage map (Fig. 5(a1)) was collected during invasive EP study, where two low-voltage regions were revealed at lateral RV and lateral-basal LV (dense scar: blue, $\leq$ 0.5mV; scar border: green, 0.5-1.5mV). Action potential reconstructed by our method during ECG ST-segment exhibits low amplitude at the same regions (Fig. 5(a2)). Fig. 5(b1) shows the invasive activation map acquired on the same patient in stable rhythm: comparing activation (b1) and voltage maps (a1) side by side, we can appreciate the intrinsic native-rhythm activation within the low-voltage region. This is consistent with recent study that some critical isthmuses may exist within low-voltage areas, underscoring the importance of an accurate, high-resolution activation map in identifying culprit tissue for surgery planning [12]. Fig. 5(b2) illustrates the activation map obtained from our method, which exhibits similar pattern to the invasive map and is able to delineate intrinsic electrical activity around low-voltage regions.

Statistical analysis on 208 epicardial points (Fig. 5(c)) verified a negative association between the reconstructed activation time and bipolar voltage (p = 0.0002, Spearman's ρ), and a positive association between the reconstructed action potential duration and bipolar voltage (p = 0.0001, Spearman's ρ). With decreasing voltage, significant differences are also found in three action potential features: delay of activation (p = 0.001, ANOVA), reduction of duration (p = 0.005, ANOVA), and increase of repolarization heterogeneity (p < 0.05, F-test for standard deviation). These changes are consistent with documented action potential biomarkers associated with ischemic hearts [12].

3.3   Conclusion

This paper has two major contributions: 1) the improved robustness of transmural EP imaging will contribute to its reliable clinical use; this is also one of the first studies to associate noninvasive solutions with *in-vivo* catheter maps on human subjects; and 2) bridging the gap between dynamic inference and sparse regularization, this is to our knowledge the first theoretical framework for statistical inference that supports the use of the low-dimensional structure in concurrence with its domain knowledge yielded by complex nonlinear dynamic models. It provides a novel solution to the general challenge regarding the robustness of dynamic inference to *a priori* model errors. Future work will study the robustness of this framework to additional model errors, *i.e.* cardiac motion, cardiac fiber model and the setting of algorithm parameters. Note that, due to the difficulty of invasive mapping, its discrepancy with noninvasive solutions should be interpreted with caution.

Acknowledgement. This work is supported by the National Science Foundation under CAREER Award ACI-1350374 and the National Institute of Heart, Lung, and Blood of the National Institutes of Health under Award R21Hl125998.

References

1. Ghosh, S., Rudy, Y.: Application of l1-norm regularization to epicardial potential solutions of the inverse electrocardiography problem. Annals of Biomedical Engineering 37, 902–912 (2009)
2. Plonsey, R.: Bioelectric phenomena. Wiley Online Library (1999)
3. Wang, L., Dawoud, F., Yeung, S.K., Shi, P., Wong, K.C., Liu, H., Lardo, A.C.: Transmural imaging of ventricular action potentials and post-infarction scars in swine hearts. IEEE Transactions on Medical Imaging 32, 731–747 (2013)
4. Haykin, S.: Adaptive Filter Theory. Prentice Hall (1996)
5. Candes, E.J., Romberg, J., Tao, T.: Robust uncertainty principles: Exact signal reconstructions from highly incomplete frequency information. IEEE Transactions on Information Theory 52, 489–509 (2006)
6. Xu, J., Dehaghani, A., Gao, F., Wang, L.: Noninvasive transmural electrophysiological imaging based on minimization of total-variation functional. IEEE Transactions on Medical Imaging 33, 1860–1874 (2014)
7. Carmi, A., Gurfil, P., Kanevsky, D.: Methods for sparse signal recovery using kalman filtering with embedded pseudo-measurement norms and qausi-norms. IEEE Transactions on Signal Processing 58, 2405–2409 (2010)
8. Aliev, R.R., Panfilov, A.V.: A simple two-variable model of cardiac excitation. Chaos, Solitons & Fractals 7, 293–301 (1996)

9. Nash, M.: Mechanics and Material Properties of the Heart using an Anatomically Accurate Mathematical Model. PhD thesis, Univ. of Auckland (1998)
10. Julier, S.: The scaled unscented transform. International Journal for Numerical Methods in Engineering 47, 1445–1462 (2000)
11. Smídl, V., Quinn, A.: The variational Bayes method in signal processing. Springer (2006)
12. Jamil-Copley, S., Vergara, P., Carbucicchio, C., et al.: Application of ripple mapping to visualise slow conduction channels within the infarct-related left ventricular scar. Circulation Arrhythmia and Electrophysiology (2014). Epub ahead of print

Estimating Biophysical Parameters from BOLD Signals through Evolutionary-Based Optimization

Pablo Mesejo[1], Sandrine Saillet[2,5], Olivier David[2,5], Christian Bénar[3,4],
Jan M. Warnking[2,5], and Florence Forbes[1]

[1] INRIA, Univ. Grenoble Alpes, LJK, F-38000, Grenoble, France
pablo.mesejo-santiago@inria.fr
[2] INSERM, U836, F-38000, Grenoble, France
[3] INSERM, UMR1106, Marseille, France
[4] Aix-Marseille Université, Institut de Neurosciences des Systèmes, Marseille, France
[5] Univ. Grenoble Alpes, GIN, F-38000, Grenoble, France

Abstract. Physiological and biophysical models have been proposed to link neural activity to the Blood Oxygen Level-Dependent (BOLD) signal in functional MRI (fMRI). They rely on a set of parameter values that cannot always be extracted from the literature. Their estimation is challenging because there are more than 10 potentially interesting parameters involved in non-linear equations and whose interactions may result in identifiability issues. However, the availability of statistical prior knowledge on these parameters can greatly simplify the estimation task. In this work we focus on the extended Balloon model and propose the estimation of 15 parameters using an Evolutionary Computation (EC) global search method. To combine both the ability to escape local optima and to incorporate prior knowledge, we derive the EC objective function from Bayesian modeling. This novel method provides promising results on a challenging real fMRI data set involving rats with epileptic activity and compares favorably with the conventional Expectation Maximization Gauss-Newton approach.

Keywords: Functional MRI, BOLD signal, Biophysical parameters, Evolutionary Computation, Differential Evolution, Expectation Maximization.

1 Introduction

In the past decade, physiological models have been proposed to describe the processes that link the neural and the hemodynamic activity in the brain. Different variations of the widely used *"Balloon model"*[2] have been introduced that provide a complete description of the physiological processes underlying hemodynamic activity, from neural activation to the Blood-Oxygen-Level-Dependent (BOLD) effect measurement [1,10]. These models all depend on physiological parameters for which different competing values have been proposed in the literature, e.g. [10,11]. Most approaches that focus on such models currently use one of these empirical sets of values with no real justification, e.g. [8,14], although it has been shown in [8], and to a lesser extent in [14], that the selection of these parameters had a more critical impact than the choice of the Balloon model variant itself, via their influence on the system dynamics. Estimating these physiological parameters from observed data may therefore be of interest in a number of fMRI

© Springer International Publishing Switzerland 2015
N. Navab et al. (Eds.): MICCAI 2015, Part II, LNCS 9350, pp. 528–535, 2015.
DOI: 10.1007/978-3-319-24571-3_63

studies. A general method for estimating parameters involved in a dynamic system has been proposed [9] based on a Bayesian approach which allows the incorporation of prior knowledge. Such *a priori* knowledge is typically summarized by a Gaussian distribution for each physiological parameter and provides a generally accepted consensus avoiding the commitment to arbitrarily fixed values. The method in [9] has then been widely used as the method of reference to estimate the hemodynamic response in dynamical causal modelling (DCM). It is based on an Expectation-Maximization Gauss-Newton search (EM/GN) which requires the linearization of the original system and approximation such as the Laplace approximation for tractability. The EM algorithm is also more generally known to be sensitive to initialization and prone to get stuck in local optima. Alternative approaches include sampling, e.g. Monte Carlo Markov Chain (MCMC), or other stochastic techniques, e.g. Metaheuristics (MHs). Sampling techniques offer a number of attractive features such as robust and reliable performance and ability to escape local optima. MHs are in addition general purpose procedures that do not even require the availability of the objective function in analytic form. In the DCM context, the need for the Laplace approximation is relaxed by [3] which uses a MCMC implementation of the Bayesian inversion scheme of [9] and shows that the Laplace approximation actually yields sensible inferences under a large set of conditions. However, MCMC needs thousands of iterations to converge, constraints are not easy to introduce and it does not provide mechanisms to control the trade-off exploration-exploitation. Also, [3] focuses on DCM and neuronal parameter estimation while nothing is reported on the impact on the non-neuronal physiological parameters. In contrast, in [16] the authors consider the Balloon model in a non-Bayesian setting using standard MHs with an objective, or so-called *fitness* function which does not include prior information. Without such valuable prior knowledge, it is quite challenging to put all parameters into the proposed optimization scheme due to potential identifiability issues. It results that the approach in [16] is limited to the estimation of three of the physiological parameters out of the 15 considered in this paper.

In this work, our goal is to combine both the benefits from a Bayesian approach which allows incorporation of prior knowledge and from MHs which are general-purpose global optimization techniques able to avoid local optima. Following the Bayesian inversion scheme of [9], we derive a fitness function that is directly comparable to EM/GN search DCM standard. It follows an estimation procedure able to estimate all physiological parameters of interest while being less likely to get trapped in local minima. This novel method is assessed on a challenging real EEG/fMRI data set involving rats with epileptic activity. A qualitative comparison with the EM/GN approach shows the ability of our method to provide more physiologically sensible parameter values.

2   The Extended Balloon Model

The Balloon model was first proposed in [2] to link neuronal and vascular processes by considering the venous vascular compartment as a balloon that inflates under the effect of blood flow variations. More specifically, the model describes how, after some stimulation, the local blood flow $f_{in}(t)$ increases and leads to the subsequent augmentation of the local deoxygenated blood volume $v(t)$. The incoming blood is strongly oxygenated, and since the relative blood flow increase exceeds the increase in oxygen consumption, local deoxyhemoglobin concentration $q(t)$ decreases and induces a BOLD signal increase. The Balloon model was subsequently extended [10] to include the effect of the neuronal activity on the variation of some auto-regulated flow inducing signal $s(t)$ so as to eventually link neuronal to hemodynamic activity. Variable $n_e(t)$ represents the activity of the excitatory neuron population and $n_i(t)$ the inhibitory neuron population [12]. The experimentally controlled input function (stimulus) is represented by $u(t)$. In the following, the explicit time dependence '(t)' of the state variables will be omitted for compactness. The global physiological model corresponds then to a non-linear system with six state variables $x = \{n_e, n_i, s, f_{in}, v, q\}$ related to the excitatory and inhibitory neuronal activity, normalized flow inducing signal, local blood flow, local deoxygenated blood volume, and deoxyhemoglobin concentration. Their interactions over time are described by the following non-linear differential equations:

$$\frac{dn_e}{dt} = -En_e - \exp\left(A + Bu^{se} + D^T \begin{pmatrix} n_e \\ s \\ f_{in} - 1 \end{pmatrix} \right) n_i + Cu^{se}$$

$$\frac{dn_i}{dt} = n_e - 2En_i \ , \quad \frac{ds}{dt} = n_e - sd\,s - ar\,(f_{in} - 1) \ , \quad \frac{d\,ln(f_{in})}{dt} = \frac{s}{f_{in}} \quad (1)$$

$$\frac{d\,ln(v)}{dt} = \frac{1}{tt}\frac{f_{in} - v^{\frac{1}{\alpha}}}{v} \ , \quad \frac{d\,ln(q)}{dt} = \frac{1}{tt}\left(\frac{1 - (1 - E_0)^{\frac{1}{f_{in}}}}{E_0}\frac{f_{in}}{q} - v^{\frac{1}{\alpha} - 1} \right)$$

From these state variables, the observed BOLD signal y is derived using an observation equation that includes intra- and extravascular BOLD signal components [1]:

$$y = V_0 \left[k_1\,(1 - q) + k_2 \left(1 - \frac{q}{v} \right) + k_3\,(1 - v) \right] \quad (2)$$

where k_1, k_2, k_3 are physiology- and scanner-dependent constants $k_1 = 4.3\,\theta_0 E_0 TE$, $k_2 = \varepsilon\,r_0 E_0\,TE$ and $k_3 = 1 - \varepsilon$.

The value θ_0 is the frequency offset at the outer surface of the magnetized vessel for fully deoxygenated blood, it is equal to $40.3\,\text{Hz} \cdot b_0/1.5\,\text{T}$, where b_0 is the magnetic field strength. TE is the echo time and r_0 is the slope of the relation between the intravascular relaxation rate and oxygen saturation, which is set to 300 Hz [13]. E_0 is the oxygen extraction fraction at rest and is considered as a free parameter as well as ε, the ratio of intra to extravascular signal.

The remaining parameters are the following: A, B, C, D and E are parameters as in non-linear Dynamic Causal Models [15], $D = (D_1, D_2, D_3)^T$ being the new component in the non-linear state equation above. Parameter se is the spike exponent introduced for the present dataset to control the scaling of the synaptic activity with respect to the spike amplitude derived from local field potentials (LFPs), sd is the vasodilatory signal decay, ar is the rate constant for autoregulatory feedback by blood flow, and tt represents the transit time of blood from the arteriolar to the venous compartment. The Grubb's vessel stiffness exponent corresponds to α, while V_0 is the resting venous cerebral blood volume fraction. The whole model depends on 15 different scalar parameters to optimize $\theta = \{A, B, C, D, E, se, sd, ar, tt, \alpha, E_0, V_0, \varepsilon\}$.

3   Bayesian Estimation of Dynamical Systems

MHs require the definition of a fitness function to measure the goodness of the parameters found. We use the Bayesian inversion scheme of [9] to derive an appropriate fitness function. In the Balloon model, the first part describes the transitional dynamics of the state vector $\boldsymbol{x} = \{n_e, n_i, s, f_{in}, v, q\}$. The system is defined as $\frac{d\boldsymbol{x}}{dt} = f(\boldsymbol{x}, \boldsymbol{u}, \boldsymbol{\psi})$, with $\boldsymbol{\psi} = \{A, B, C, \boldsymbol{D}, E, se, sd, ar, tt, \alpha, E_0\}$. The second part of the model is the observational equation for the BOLD signal $\boldsymbol{y}$ which is assumed to be observed with some additive Gaussian noise (in this context of BOLD data sampled at discrete time points, we represent both data and state variables as vectors of discrete samples), $\boldsymbol{y} = g(\boldsymbol{x}, \boldsymbol{\phi}) + \boldsymbol{\eta}$, with $\boldsymbol{\phi} = \{V_0, E_0, \varepsilon\}$ and $\boldsymbol{\eta}$ is a random error vector distributed according to the Gaussian distribution $\mathcal{N}(0, \sigma_\eta^2 \mathbf{I})$ assuming unstructured noise. Under additional distributional assumptions about the model parameters $\boldsymbol{\theta} = \{\boldsymbol{\psi}, \boldsymbol{\phi}\}$ and noise variance σ_η^2, we can apply Bayesian inference. In [9], Gaussian priors are chosen for all parameters. As explained in [14] for ε, it is more natural to use log-normal priors for parameters that are positive. A simple way to account for positivity while remaining in a Gaussian setting is to change the model parameterization. We consider equivalently $\tilde{\boldsymbol{\theta}} = \{\tilde{A}, \tilde{B}, \tilde{C}, \tilde{\boldsymbol{D}}, \tilde{E}, \tilde{se}, \tilde{sd}, \tilde{ar}, \tilde{tt}, \tilde{\alpha}, \tilde{E_0}, \tilde{V_0}, \tilde{\varepsilon}\}$, where $\{\tilde{A}, \tilde{B}, \tilde{C}, \tilde{\boldsymbol{D}}\} = \{A, B, C, \boldsymbol{D}\}$ remain unchanged while the other parameters take the form $\tilde{\theta} = \log(\theta/\mu_\theta)$ where the specific μ_θ values may depend on the experiment (see section 5). An exception is E_0 for which we set $E_0 = \arctan(\tilde{E_0} + \tan(\pi(\mu_{E_0} - 0.5)))/\pi + 0.5$ in order to ensure $E_0 \in [0, 1]$. Gaussian priors can then be assumed for $\tilde{\boldsymbol{\theta}}$ and the state and observational equations above lead to, $\boldsymbol{y} = h(\tilde{\boldsymbol{\theta}}, \boldsymbol{u}) + \boldsymbol{\eta}$, with $\boldsymbol{\eta} \sim \mathcal{N}(0, \sigma_\eta^2 \mathbf{I})$, $\tilde{\boldsymbol{\theta}} \sim \mathcal{N}(\bar{\boldsymbol{\theta}}, \boldsymbol{\Sigma}_{\tilde{\theta}})$ and $\sigma_\eta^2 \sim p(\sigma_\eta^2)$. As another difference with [9,14], we use a semi-conjugate prior for the unknown parameters $(\tilde{\boldsymbol{\theta}}, \sigma_\eta^2)$ in which $\tilde{\boldsymbol{\theta}} \sim \mathcal{N}(\bar{\boldsymbol{\theta}}, \boldsymbol{\Sigma}_{\tilde{\theta}})$ independently of σ_η^2 and a non-informative prior is used for σ_η^2, i.e. $p(\sigma_\eta^2) \propto (\sigma_\eta^2)^{-1}$. Bayesian inference is then based on the posterior distribution $p(\tilde{\boldsymbol{\theta}}, \sigma_\eta^2 | \boldsymbol{y}) \propto p(\boldsymbol{y} | \tilde{\boldsymbol{\theta}}, \sigma_\eta^2) \, p(\tilde{\boldsymbol{\theta}}) \, p(\sigma_\eta^2)$ whose mode provides the maximum a posteriori (MAP) estimate:

$$(\tilde{\boldsymbol{\theta}}, \sigma_\eta^2)_{MAP} = \arg\max_{\tilde{\boldsymbol{\theta}}, \sigma_\eta^2} \{\log p(\boldsymbol{y} | \tilde{\boldsymbol{\theta}}, \sigma_\eta^2) + \log p(\tilde{\boldsymbol{\theta}}) + \log p(\sigma_\eta^2)\} \qquad (3)$$

$$= \arg\min_{\tilde{\boldsymbol{\theta}}, \sigma_\eta^2} \{(N+2)\log\sigma_\eta^2 + \frac{||\boldsymbol{y} - h(\tilde{\boldsymbol{\theta}}, \boldsymbol{u})||^2}{\sigma_\eta^2} + (\tilde{\boldsymbol{\theta}} - \bar{\boldsymbol{\theta}})^T \boldsymbol{\Sigma}_{\tilde{\theta}}^{-1}(\tilde{\boldsymbol{\theta}} - \bar{\boldsymbol{\theta}})\} \ .$$

where N is the $\boldsymbol{y}$ signal length. Setting to zero the gradient with respect to σ_η^2 yields $(\sigma_\eta^2)_{MAP} = \frac{||\boldsymbol{y} - h(\tilde{\boldsymbol{\theta}}_{MAP}, \boldsymbol{u})||^2}{N+2}$. Plugin in $(\sigma_\eta^2)_{MAP}$ into expression (3) leads to

$$\tilde{\boldsymbol{\theta}}_{MAP} = \arg\min_{\tilde{\boldsymbol{\theta}}} \{(N+2)\log||\boldsymbol{y} - h(\tilde{\boldsymbol{\theta}}, \boldsymbol{u})||^2 + (\tilde{\boldsymbol{\theta}} - \bar{\boldsymbol{\theta}})^T \boldsymbol{\Sigma}_{\tilde{\theta}}^{-1}(\tilde{\boldsymbol{\theta}} - \bar{\boldsymbol{\theta}})\} \ . \qquad (4)$$

The left-hand side above corresponds to our fitness function to be used in the EC framework described in the next section. In contrast to the conventional Laplace approximation and EM estimation algorithm, EC does not require the linearization or approximation of $h(\tilde{\boldsymbol{\theta}}, \boldsymbol{u})$. It does not require an analytic form of the likelihood and $h(\tilde{\boldsymbol{\theta}}, \boldsymbol{u})$ can typically be used as a numerical function. Another advantage of EC is its flexibility in particular as regards hard constraints often imposed for stability of the differential equations (1). The hyperparameters $\bar{\boldsymbol{\theta}}$ and $\boldsymbol{\Sigma}_\theta$ are specified in section 5.

4   Evolutionary Computation

Evolutionary Computation (EC) methods are population-based MH algorithms [7]. They include several computational models that reproduce natural evolution processes to reach a target which is generally represented as a fitness function to optimize. In practice, they implement an iterative process (artificial evolution) in which solutions improve over generations until they converge to an optimum, starting from an initial pool of randomly generated solutions. EC procedures are based on achieving a trade-off between intensification (exploitation of the best solutions, usually through selection operators and replacement strategies) and diversification (exploration of the search space thanks to crossover and mutation operators).

In this work, we choose to use Differential Evolution (DE) [5], which has recently been shown to be one of the most successful EC methods for global continuous optimization. DE perturbs individuals in the current generation by the scaled differences of other randomly selected and distinct individuals. In DE, each individual acts as a parent vector, and for each of them a new solution, called donor vector, is created. In the basic version of DE, the donor vector for the ith parent ($\tilde{\boldsymbol{\theta}}_i$) is generated by combining three random and distinct elements $\tilde{\boldsymbol{\theta}}_{r1}$, $\tilde{\boldsymbol{\theta}}_{r2}$ and $\tilde{\boldsymbol{\theta}}_{r3}$. The donor vector V_i is computed as $V_i = \tilde{\boldsymbol{\theta}}_{r1} + F \cdot (\tilde{\boldsymbol{\theta}}_{r2} - \tilde{\boldsymbol{\theta}}_{r3})$, where F (scale factor) is a parameter that strongly influences DE's performance and typically lies in the interval $[0.4, 1]$. The original method described above is called DE/rand/1, which means that the first element of the donor vector equation $\tilde{\boldsymbol{\theta}}_{r1}$ is randomly chosen and only one difference vector (in this case $\tilde{\boldsymbol{\theta}}_{r2} - \tilde{\boldsymbol{\theta}}_{r3}$) is added. After mutation, every parent-donor pair generates a child (called trial vector) by means of a crossover operation. The crossover is applied with a certain probability, defined by a parameter Cr (crossover rate) that, like F, is one of the control parameters of DE. Then, the trial vector is evaluated and its fitness is compared to the parent's. The best, in terms of fitness, survives and will be part of the next generation.

5   Experimental Results

The BOLD data used in the experiments was recorded with the goal of testing biophysical models in the context of epileptic activity in rats. An intracortical silica capillary was surgically implanted in the right primary somatosensory cortex of male Wistar rats ($\sim$400 g) and subdural carbon EEG electrodes were placed close to the injection site and over the cerebellum. Epileptic activity was elicited using bicuculline methochloride (2.5 mM, 1 µl/5 min) injected intra-cortically during the MRI session. Simultaneous EEG and BOLD-fMRI data were acquired under <2% isoflurane anesthesia.

The EEG/fMRI data were acquired on a 4.7 T Advance III Bruker Biospec.In each scan, 300 volumes of five slices ($0.25 \times 0.25 \times 0.8$ mm^3 voxel size) were acquired using single-shot GE EPI with TE/TR of 20/600 ms. A total of 3-12 scans were performed for each of 12 rats (27 min of EEG/fMRI data per animal on average). The data from 3 animals were unexploitable and thus excluded from the analysis. Epileptic discharges (EDs) were automatically identified from the EEG data and ED amplitudes and onsets were recorded. For each rat, a single average fMRI signal concatenating all scans was extracted from the largest cluster of significantly active voxels identified in a linear analysis with a FIR hemodynamic response model. The fMRI signal size N ranged from 894 to 3576 with a median value of 2684. The EDs were entered in the biophysical model via the input function u as a series of short (8 ms) events.

To palliate the absence of ground truth (GT) in real data, a synthetic dataset is created to study the methods behavior under controlled conditions. Rat 5, whose physiological conditions are amongst the most stable ones, is selected as a reference to create this dataset, and the parameter estimates found by EM/GN are defined as the GT. BOLD signals are generated from either a full set of measured spikes or a subset (25%) to simulate more sparse events, adding $AR(1)$ noise with three target SNRs (0.10, 0.46 and 2.15). The average distance to GT using 25% subsampling and the full set of spikes are 0.56 and 2.8 in EM/GN, and 0.28 ± 0.09 and 0.15 ± 0.01 in DE, respectively.

Then, for each rat, physiological parameters θ are estimated using DE with fitness function (4) and transforming back the resulting $\tilde{\theta}$ into θ. Each of the positive parameters in $\tilde{\theta}$ is specified using $\tilde{\theta} = \log(\theta/\mu_\theta)$ with μ_θ defined respectively by $\{\mu_E, \mu_{se}, \ldots, \mu_\varepsilon\} = \{1, 1, 0.64, 0.41, 0.98, 0.32, 0.55, 0.4, 1\}$ [6]. The prior means are then set to $\tilde{\theta} = 0$ and the prior covariance $\Sigma_{\tilde{\theta}}$ is a diagonal matrix containing the prior variances set to $\{0.25, 0.25, 54.6, 0.05, 0.05, 0.05, 0.05, 0.14, 0.14, 0.05, 0.05, 0.007, 0.007, 0.05, 0.14\}$ for each parameter in $\tilde{\theta}$. The DE parameters used are among the most common ones in the state of the art [5]: $F = 0.85$, $Cr = 1$, with a DE/local-to-best/1 strategy that attempts a balance between robustness and fast convergence, and a population size of 150. The EM/GN algorithm [9] starts from physiologically reasonable parameter values (the prior means), which facilitates its convergence to a good solution. Since DE is a stochastic approach several runs need to be executed to evaluate its average performance. In this study, the number of runs per rat and the number of iterations per run are empirically set to 15 and 300, respectively. DE shows a very stable behavior with a standard deviation of the mean fitness values between 0.001% and 0.042%.

The θ parameter estimations from DE and EM/GN are shown in Table 1. The experimental conditions for all animals were controlled as closely as possible. It is therefore expected that the physiologically meaningful parameters show limited variability across animals. However, the parameters related to the scaling of the stimulus and the neuronal signals (notably, A, B, C, D, E and se) may vary significantly, since the amplitudes of the elicited EEG responses varied between sessions. Estimates for 4 of the parameters that are expected to be among the most stable ones are shown in Figure 1. The ratio between intra- and extravascular signals, ε, depends on field strength, blood T_2, and vascular geometry, but little on physiology. The values estimated by DE are markedly more stable between animals than the values obtained with EM/GN. Quantitatively, both methods yield plausible results. Blood transit times from arterioles to the deoxygenated vascular compartment estimated with DE are generally longer, and closer to the expected value, than those obtained with EM/GN, which are rather too short. For comparison, mean transit times across the entire vascular tree in a cortical voxel observed using DSC MRI in anesthetized rats are on the order of 1.6 s [4]. Inversely, resting venous blood volumes estimated with DE are lower than those obtained with EM/GN. The prior estimate used here for this parameter, 4%, corresponds to the total cortical resting blood volume in isoflurane anesthetized male Wistar rats [4]. In hindsight, the value that should actually be considered in the model is however only the

Table 1. EM estimates and DE medians for each of the 9 rats and each parameter in θ.

	A	B	C	D_1	D_2	D_3	E	se	sd	ar	tt	α	V_0	E_0	ε
RAT1 DE	0.56	0.02	0.10	0.01	0.02	0.05	0.84	1.44	0.89	0.53	0.83	0.32	0.38	0.55	0.90
EM/GN	0.14	-0.01	0.02	0.01	0.01	0.01	0.86	1.11	0.61	0.44	0.65	0.31	0.53	0.55	1.77
RAT2 DE	0.48	0.03	3.00	-0.14	-0.10	0.46	0.73	0.40	2.02	0.25	0.91	0.35	0.20	0.53	0.35
EM/GN	0.03	-0.00	0.02	0.01	0.01	0.01	0.96	0.60	0.73	0.36	0.44	0.30	0.58	0.54	2.13
RAT3 DE	-0.66	-0.01	3.00	-0.14	-0.09	0.58	0.73	0.96	1.00	0.26	0.85	0.33	0.15	0.52	0.42
EM/GN	1.35	0.02	0.26	0.07	-0.01	0.18	0.72	0.83	1.12	0.59	0.65	0.32	0.34	0.54	0.94
RAT4 DE	-0.14	0.01	2.18	0.31	-0.43	0.05	0.40	0.50	1.95	0.36	0.72	0.33	0.15	0.54	0.41
EM/GN	-0.14	0.01	2.10	0.33	-0.42	0.07	0.41	0.50	1.86	0.35	0.71	0.33	0.16	0.54	0.41
RAT5 DE	1.11	0.03	1.60	-0.08	-0.11	0.17	0.57	0.82	2.05	0.46	0.67	0.35	0.23	0.54	0.36
EM/GN	1.07	0.03	1.21	-0.09	-0.12	0.19	0.56	0.78	2.07	0.46	0.65	0.34	0.26	0.55	0.39
RAT6 DE	-0.85	0.01	3.00	0.23	0.24	0.18	0.44	0.33	1.15	0.25	0.97	0.33	0.22	0.52	0.49
EM/GN	0.21	-0.01	0.03	0.03	0.04	0.03	0.71	1.13	1.04	0.39	0.38	0.30	0.62	0.55	2.38
RAT7 DE	1.75	-0.03	0.09	-0.00	0.00	0.01	0.65	1.23	1.30	0.47	0.65	0.32	0.40	0.55	1.16
EM/GN	1.70	-0.03	0.07	-0.00	0.00	0.01	0.65	1.23	1.25	0.47	0.64	0.31	0.42	0.55	1.30
RAT8 DE	0.10	0.07	2.99	-0.43	-0.47	-0.02	0.39	0.19	1.92	0.14	0.60	0.31	0.22	0.53	0.49
EM/GN	-0.67	0.08	0.30	-0.08	-0.10	0.11	0.50	0.14	1.40	0.57	0.51	0.31	0.32	0.54	1.14
RAT9 DE	0.74	0.03	0.55	0.02	-0.01	0.06	0.45	0.68	2.74	0.38	0.58	0.32	0.36	0.55	0.60
EM/GN	0.74	0.03	0.52	0.01	-0.01	0.07	0.45	0.68	2.71	0.38	0.57	0.32	0.37	0.55	0.62

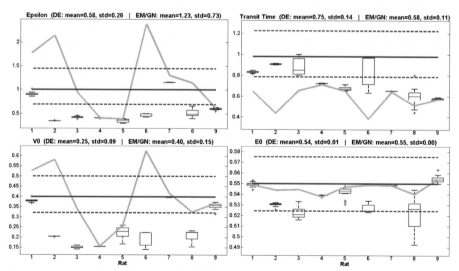

Fig. 1. Boxplots of the DE runs and EM/GN results (green line) for ε, transit time (tt), V_0 and E_0. The parameter prior mean (resp. standard deviation) is indicated by the red (resp. blue) line.

venous (deoxygenated) fraction of that, such that a value of 2% actually seems much more realistic than the higher values of up to 6% estimated using EM/GN. Finally, both methods yield similar values for the resting oxygen extraction fraction. In summary, the estimates obtained from DE for these values seem both more realistic and more stable or at least as stable across sessions as the estimates from EM/GN.

6 Conclusion and Future Work

A novel method to infer physiological parameters from observed BOLD signals has been described, showing the robustness and flexibility of global search optimization methods while being able to incorporate prior information in a principled Bayesian way. This has not been proposed before and could have a strong impact on a number of fMRI studies. Traditionally, these parameters are manually set or, only few of them, are determined by using conventional but potentially suboptimal local search methods like EM. Preliminary results on synthetic and real data showed promising results providing sensible and more stable parameter estimates. Possible future research includes testing on multimodal fMRI data, since information from cerebral blood flow and volume dynamics may help to further improve the reliability of the parameter estimates.

References

1. Buxton, R.B., Uludağ, K., Dubowitz, D.J., Liu, T.T.: Modeling the hemodynamic response to brain activation. Neuroimage 23, S220–S233 (2004)
2. Buxton, R.B., Wong, E.C., Frank, L.R.: Dynamics of blood flow and oxygenation changes during Brain activation: the balloon model. Magn. Reson. Med. 39, 855–864 (1998)
3. Chumbley, J.R., Friston, K.J., Fearn, T., Kiebel, S.J.: A Metropolis-Hastings algorithm for dynamic causal models. Neuroimage 38(3), 478–487 (2007)
4. Coquery, N., Francois, O., Lemasson, B., Debacker, C., Farion, R., Rémy, C., Barbier, E.L.: Microvascular MRI and unsupervised clustering yields histology-resembling images in two rat models of glioma. J. Cereb. Blood Flow Metab. 34(8), 1354–1362 (2014)
5. Das, S., Suganthan, P.: Differential Evolution: A Survey of the State-of-the-Art. IEEE T. Evolut. Comput. 15, 4–31 (2011)
6. David, O., Guillemain, I., Saillet, S., Reyt, S., Deransart, C., Segebarth, C., Depaulis, A.: Identifying neural drivers with functional MRI: an electrophysiological validation. PLoS Biol. 6(12), 2683–2697 (2008)
7. Eiben, A.E., Smith, J.E.: Introduction to Evolutionary Computing. Springer (2003)
8. Frau-Pascual, A., Ciuciu, P., Forbes, F.: Physiological models comparison for the analysis of ASL fMRI data. In: EEE International Symposium on Biomedical Imaging (ISBI) (2015)
9. Friston, K.J.: Bayesian estimation of dynamical systems: an application to fMRI. Neuroimage 16, 513–530 (2002)
10. Friston, K.J., Mechelli, A., Turner, R., Price, C.J.: Nonlinear responses in fMRI: the balloon model, Volterra kernels, and other hemodynamics. Neuroimage 12, 466–477 (2000)
11. Khalidov, I., Fadili, J., Lazeyras, F., Van De Ville, D., Unser, M.: Activelets: Wavelets for sparse representation of hemodynamic responses. Signal Process 91(12), 2810–2821 (2011)
12. Marreiros, A., Kiebel, S., Friston, K.: Dynamic causal modelling for fMRI: A two-state model. NeuroImage 39, 269–278 (2008)
13. Silvennoinen, M., Clingman, C., Golay, X., Kauppinen, R., van Zijl, P.: Comparison of the dependence of blood R2 and R* on oxygen saturation at 1.5 and 4.7 Tesla. Magn. Reson. Med. 49(1), 47–60 (2003)
14. Stephan, K.E., Weiskopf, N., Drysdale, P.M., Robinson, P.A., Friston, K.J.: Comparing hemodynamic models with DCM. Neuroimage 38(3), 387–401 (2007)
15. Stephan, K., Kasper, L., Harrison, L., Daunizeau, J., den Ouden, H., Breakspear, M., Friston, K.: Nonlinear dynamic causal models for fMRI. NeuroImage 42(2), 649–662 (2008)
16. Vakorin, V.A., Krakovska, O.O., Borowsky, R., Sarty, G.E.: Inferring neural activity from BOLD signals through nonlinear optimization. Neuroimage 38(2), 248–260 (2007)

Radiopositive Tissue Displacement Compensation for SPECT-guided Surgery

Francisco Pinto[1,2]*, Bernhard Fuerst[1,2]*, Benjamin Frisch[2],
and Nassir Navab[1,2]

[1] Computer Aided Medical Procedures,
Johns Hopkins University, Baltimore, MD, USA
[2] Computer Aided Medical Procedures,
Technical University of Munich, Germany

Abstract. We present a new technique to overcome a major disadvantage of SPECT-guided surgery, where a 3D image of the distribution of a radiotracer augments the live view of the surgical situs in order to identify radiopositive tissue for resection and subsequent histological analysis. In current systems, the reconstructed SPECT volume is outdated as soon as the situs is modified by further surgical actions, due to tissue displacement. Our technique intraoperatively estimates the displacement of radiopositive tissue, which enables the update of the SPECT image augmentation. After the initial SPECT reconstruction is complete, we deploy a 2D γ-camera along with a technique to optimize its placement. We automatically establish a correspondence between regions of interest in the reconstructed volume and the near real-time 2D γ images. The 3D displacement of the radiopositive nodules is then continuously estimated based on the processing of the aforementioned γ-camera's output. Initial results show that we can estimate displacements with ± 1 mm accuracy.

1 Introduction

The Sentinel Lymph Node Biopsy (SLNB) is part of the standard of care for the treatment of melanoma [14], breast cancers [5,6] and vulvar cancers [12,15]. It further has demonstrated clinical value in the staging of head and neck [3], gastric [8], prostate [10], and cervical [4] cancers. In an SLNB, a radioactive tracer (usually a ^{99m}Tc nanocolloid) or a colored dye is injected close to a tumor, under the assumption that it primarily drains to the sentinel lymph nodes. Lymph nodes identified that way are resected and sent for subsequent histological analysis. In this paper, we focus on radioguided SLNB, which relies on either pre-interventional whole-body Single Photon Emission Computerized Tomography (SPECT) imaging or the use of a γ-detector for the live intraoperative identification of radiopositive tissue. Types of γ-detectors are 1D γ-probes and 2D γ-cameras that provide the surgeon with a planar view of the radioactivity

---

* F. Pinto and B. Fuerst are joint first authors.

© Springer International Publishing Switzerland 2015
N. Navab et al. (Eds.): MICCAI 2015, Part II, LNCS 9350, pp. 536–543, 2015.
DOI: 10.1007/978-3-319-24571-3_64

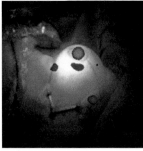 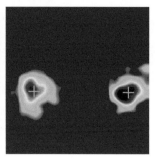 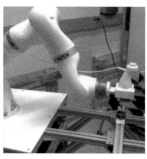

(a) SPECT system showing several SLNs via Augmented Reality. Courtesy SurgicEye GmbH.

(b) Interpolated γ-camera output for two sources, showing the auto-marked centers.

(c) γ-camera mounted on a KUKA iiwa industrial lightweight robot. An off-screen PC collects data.

Fig. 1. γ-detectors and respective outputs.

distribution in the area (see Fig. 1b). Brouwer et al. combine SPECT/CT with the intraoperative use of a laparoscopic γ-probe and γ-camera in their dual detector approach, improving SLN detection by 20% as compared to the sole use of pre-interventional information [2].

The intraoperative acquisition of several thousand γ-activity recordings over a region of interest with a spatially tracked detector allows for the 3D reconstruction of the nuclear information and its display via Augmented Reality (AR) overlays, a technique called freehand SPECT [9,13]. The latter is applied in open and laparoscopic surgeries, such as SLNB for head and neck [7] or breast [1] cancer.

The AR visualization of SPECT information becomes outdated as soon as the tissue is manipulated, such as during any incision, when the radioactively marked tissue gets displaced. The acquisition of a new intraoperative SPECT volume to replace the previously augmented one is problematic as it requires prolonged handling of a γ-detector, delaying the procedure. Another solution is the use of a 1D or a 2D detector to acquire additional information about the γ distribution, losing the benefit of AR and disrupting the workflow. An alternate solution proposed in [11] is the registration of a pre-acquired 3D SPECT volume to an intraoperative 1D γ-probe signal, which requires a γ-probe, a model of its behavior (sensitivity, collimator aperture, etc.) and several hundred tracked γ-activity recordings. In a clinical scenario where lymph nodes can have a diameter of less than 1 cm, their demonstrated accuracy of 8 mm may prove insufficient.

Proposed Solution: Displacement Compensation. We propose a new method for continuous SLN displacement compensation. We utilize a 2D γ-camera rather than a 1D detector, and focus on minimally invasive SLN biopsies. The solution provides an update of the intraoperative SPECT image, by placing the γ-camera relative to the SLNs and estimating their displacement. Results are presented based on displacements in ex-vivo experiments and show an average accuracy of under 1 mm.

2   Materials and Methods

The proposed displacement compensation technique requires a SPECT volume, acquired by preoperative SPECT/CT [2] or intraoperative freehand SPECT [13], and a tracked γ-camera.

2.1   SPECT Imaging and Technical Background

The system we propose is based on a two step intraoperative workflow (see Fig. 2). The first step is the acquisition of a SPECT volume. In the case of preoperative SPECT/CT, the volume has to be registered to the patient e.g. by using fiducials. In the case of freehand SPECT, registration is unnecessary as the reconstruction is done relative to an optically tracked reference target fixed to the patient's body. The SPECT volume is then visualized intraoperatively using an AR overlay, as in Fig. 1a. To display the SPECT AR overlay and its continuous updates, we employ the commercially available declipse®SPECT (SurgicEye GmbH, Munich, Bavaria, Germany). The second step is to use the tracked γ-camera to calculate the displacement of each of the segmented lymph nodes.

2.2   2D γ-camera

The CrystalCam (Crystal Photonics GmbH, Berlin, Germany) is a handheld, miniaturized γ-camera capable of producing images with a resolution of 16×16 pixels. The selected collimator, the Tungsten-based LEHS (Crystal Photonics GmbH, Berlin, Germany), has dimensions of $44 \times 44 \times 11.5$ mm, with each square pixel having 2.16 mm long sides. This is a parallel collimator; The produced images can be compared to a parallel projection of the radioactivity in the observed area. Based on a single image, a 0.925 MBq (25 Ci) ^{57}Co source is identifiable within distances up to 15 cm.

We use an infrared tracking system (henceforth designated as *IR*) to track the γ-camera and patient. The system we chose, due to the convenience of it being perfectly integrated into the declipse®SPECT system, is the Polaris Vicra (Northern Digital Inc., Waterloo, Ontario, Canada).

2.3   Displacement Compensation

Positioning of γ-camera: With the $^{\gamma\text{-camera}}\mathbf{T}_{\text{patient}}$ transformation computed as in (1), and given that the SPECT volume is reconstructed relative to the IR patient target (in the case of freehand SPECT) or registered to the patient (in the case of preoperative SPECT/CT), we can keep the γ-camera focused on the

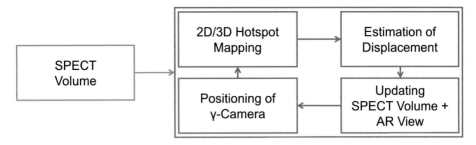

Fig. 2. The workflow of the proposed solution

global centroid of the lymph nodes. A possible robotic-assisted solution to the γ-camera positioning problem is described in Sec. 4.

$$^{\gamma\text{-camera}}\mathbf{T}_{\text{patient}} = {}^{\gamma\text{-camera}}\mathbf{T}_{\text{IR}} \cdot {}^{\text{IR}}\mathbf{T}_{\text{patient}} \tag{1}$$

2D/3D Hotspot Mapping: We segment the 3D image, via thresholding, into several 'hotspots' each corresponding to a different lymph node. The end objective is to translate these hotspots according to their displacement and update the AR overlay. The tissue displacement has translational and rotation components. However, since each nodule is well approximated as an anatomical structure with spherical geometry, we are interested in its 3D position. Our 2D sensor can estimate well its movement parallel to the sensor plate. We also estimate the motion orthogonal to the sensor using γ-camera's Lookup Tables. As described within the discussion section, we also propose to guide the motion of the γ-camera based on the tracked motion of the surgical tool as the tissue displacement mostly occurs due to the tool tissue interaction. In this way, we propose a system which intelligently positions the sensor in order to dynamically optimize the estimation of radiopositive tissue displacement taking the surgical action into account.

We post process the 2D image produced by the γ-camera (see Fig. 1b for an example) by first segmenting regions of interest where the reported radioactivity is both a local and one of few global maxima. The distribution of radioactivity in the hotspot can be approximated using a Gaussian distribution. Therefore, we employ Gaussian fitting, which provides us with an estimated center for the resulting 2D blob.

Knowing both the γ-camera's pose and the location of each lymph node computed before, we can compare the 3D SPECT hotspot centroids and 2D blob centers. This can be done by backprojecting the 3D hotspots onto the γ-camera's collimator view plane. The same Gaussian fitting method can be applied to the backprojection and we can then establish a 3D hotspot to 2D blob mapping by comparing the distance between centers.

Estimation of Displacement: With continuous γ-camera acquisitions, we update the SPECT volume accordingly, albeit with translations solely parallel to the

γ-camera's collimator view plane. Z-direction translations are recovered with a lesser degree of accuracy by referring to the γ-camera's Lookup Tables (LUT), which allows the user to estimate relative, but not absolute, depth changes.

Updating SPECT Volume: After quantification of displacement is achieved as explained above, we feed back the corrections into the SPECT system, where the AR overlay (see Fig. 1a) is duly adjusted to reflect the SLNs' translations. These are applied independently of the underlying SPECT volume's voxel grid, thereby allowing for translations of virtually arbitrary magnitude.

3   Experiments & Results

Experimental Setup: To validate our workflow and algorithm, we perform free-hand SPECT reconstruction of a pair of sealed point-like 0.925 MBq ^{57}Co sources, which were chosen due to their similarity to ^{99m}Tc, the radioactive element usually present in the injectable nanocolloid for SPECT. ^{57}Co's longer half-life and safer handling makes it more suitable for laboratory use. The sources are placed on a specially designed mount so that we know their relative position with high certainty. After the reconstruction is complete, we translate the sources by several defined amounts and calculate the displacement as described in Sec. 2.3. We estimate the translations applied to each lymph node and compare them to the ground truth.

Evaluation: For our first ex-vivo experiment (Table 1), the γ-camera was kept static and placed so that the collimator's plane was parallel to the direction of source movement. The source was moved to 5 different points ($p\{0-4\}$), which are colinear and 5 mm apart from each neighbor.

Table 1. Results for displacement estimation when $p\{0-4\}$ interdistance is 5 mm.

$\vec{r}$	$p1 = 5$ mm	$p2 = 10$ mm	$p3 = 15$ mm	$p4 = 20$ mm
$p0$	5.44 mm	10.92 mm	16.31 mm	21.54 mm
$p1$		5.49 mm	10.87 mm	16.11 mm
$p2$			5.39 mm	10.62 mm
$p3$				5.24 mm
$\bar{\epsilon} \approx 0.79$ mm, $\sigma \approx 0.43$ mm				

Our second ex-vivo experiment (Table 2) was done under the same circumstances, with the sole difference being that the γ-camera was angled at 45° relative to the direction of source motion.

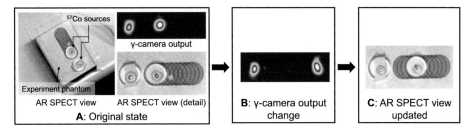

Fig. 3. Workflow for updating the SPECT AR overlay based on 2D γ-camera acquisitions. We start with original state **A**. When the tracked γ-camera's (off-screen) output changes as in **B**, the overlay is updated as in **C**.

Table 2. Results for displacement estimation when $p\{0-4\}$ interdistance is 5 mm $*$ $\sin(45°) \cong 3.54$ mm.

$\vec{r}$	$p1 = 3.54$ mm	$p2 = 7.07$ mm	$p3 = 10.61$ mm	$p4 = 14.14$ mm
$p0$	3.40 mm	7.06 mm	11.25 mm	14.46 mm
$p1$		3.66 mm	7.85 mm	11.07 mm
$p2$			4.19 mm	7.41 mm
$p3$				3.21 mm
$\bar{\epsilon} \cong 0.38$ mm, $\sigma \cong 0.25$ mm				

Multiple sources in view are accurately handled, as in Fig. 1b.

Performance: The algorithm operates at a frequency of 2 Hz. γ-camera output is computed using compound exposures on a sliding-window basis. The window's width is configurable and varies, but is usually between 1 to 5 seconds. Assuming 2 seconds of exposure, the end result is that displacements are presented to the user with a 2.5 second delay in the worst case, which is acceptable for an intraoperative scenario.

4 Discussion and Conclusion

Stable 2D-3D Matching: In our 2D-3D matching algorithm described in Sec. 2.3, we focus on deriving a 2D blob to 3D hotspot correspondence. This correspondence is not guaranteed to be stable in practice, i.e., a 2D blob may not always correspond to the *same* 3D hotspot. One example of this behavior occurring is if the lymph nodes move into close proximity with each other, and then apart again. However, this does not represent a major clinical problem as all radiopositive lymph nodes are treated as equivalent and the end result is their resection.

Robotic Platform for Automated Tool Tracking: Our ideal operating room setup is composed of one of the scenarios described in Sec. 2 and an additional lightweight industrial robot such as the KUKA LBR iiwa (KUKA Roboter GmbH, Augsburg, Bavaria, Germany) that would be programmed to automatically track either the tip of a Minimally Invasive Surgery (MIS) robot's tool (as displacement is most likely to occur in its vicinity) or the centroid of the SPECT-identified lymph nodes, depending on the scenario. An example of the proposed setup is depicted in Fig. 1c.

Wide Field-of-View γ-cameras: One of the upper bounds for the quality of displacement estimation presented in this paper is the area covered by our current γ-camera. Wide field-of-view collimators would allow for improved results requiring smaller displacement of the γ-camera. Alternatively, the robotically controlled γ-camera could follow displacement of SLNs, resulting in radioguided visual servoing.

Conclusion: In this paper, we introduced a novel technique for radiopositive tissue displacement compensation. Our initial ex-vivo experiments show that estimation accuracy is in the sub-millimeter range, which motivates full integration of our approach into existing intra-operative freehand SPECT acquisition systems system and further feasibility studies.

Acknowledgements. The authors would like to thank Anton Deguet for robotics hardware support; and Intuitive Surgical Inc. for loaning the daVinci® surgical system used for testing.

References

1. Bluemel, C., Schnelzer, A., Ehlerding, A., Scheidhauer, K., Kiechle, M.: Changing the Intraoperative Nodal Status of a Breast Cancer Patient Using Freehand SPECT for Sentinel Lymph Node Biopsy. Clinical Nuclear Medicine 39(5), e313–e314 (2014)
2. Brouwer, O.R., Valdes Olmos, R.A., Vermeeren, L., Hoefnagel, C.A., Nieweg, O.E., Horenblas, S.: SPECT/CT and a portable gamma-camera for image-guided laparoscopic sentinel node biopsy in testicular cancer. Journal of Nuclear Medicine 52(4), 551–554 (2011)
3. Hellingman, D., de Wit–van der Veen, L.J., Klop, W.M.C., Olmos, R.A.V.: Detecting Near-the-Injection-Site Sentinel Nodes in Head and Neck Melanomas With a High-Resolution Portable Gamma Camera. Clinical Nuclear Medicine 40(1), e11–e16 (2015)
4. Holman, L.L., Levenback, C.F., Frumovitz, M.: Sentinel Lymph Node Evaluation in Women with Cervical Cancer. Journal of Minimally Invasive Gynecology 21(4), 540–545 (2014)
5. Krag, D.N., Anderson, S.J., Julian, T.B., Brown, A.M., Harlow, S.P., Costantino, J.P., Ashikaga, T., Weaver, D.L., Mamounas, E.P., Jalovec, L.M., Frazier, T.G., Noyes, R.D., Robidoux, A., Scarth, H.M., Wolmark, N.: Sentinel-lymph-node Resection Compared with Conventional Axillary-lymph-node Dissection in Clinically Node-negative Patients with Breast Cancer: Overall Survival Findings from the NSABP B-32 Randomised Phase 3 Trial. The Lancet Oncology 11(10), 927–933 (2010)

6. Lyman, G.H., Giuliano, A.E., Somerfield, M.R., Benson, A.B., Bodurka, D.C., Burstein, H.J., Cochran, A.J., Cody, H.S., Edge, S.B., Galper, S., Hayman, J.A., Kim, T.Y., Perkins, C.L., Podoloff, D.A., Sivasubramaniam, V.H., Turner, R.R., Wahl, R., Weaver, D.L., Wolff, A.C., Winer, E.P.: American Society of Clinical Oncology guideline recommendations for sentinel lymph node biopsy in early-stage breast cancer. Journal of Clinical Oncology 23(30), 7703–7720 (2005)

7. Mandapathil, M., Teymoortash, A., Heinis, J., Wiegand, S., Güldner, C., Hoch, S., Roeßler, M., Werner, J.A.: Freehand SPECT for Sentinel Lymph Node Detection in Patients with Head and Neck Cancer: First Experiences. Acta Oto-Laryngologica 134(1), 100–104 (2014)

8. Miyashiro, I., Kishi, K., Yano, M., Tanaka, K., Motoori, M., Ohue, M., Ohigashi, H., Takenaka, A., Tomita, Y., Ishikawa, O.: Laparoscopic Detection of Sentinel Node in Gastric Cancer Surgery by Indocyanine Green Fluorescence Imaging. Surgical Endoscopy 25(5), 1672–1676 (2010)

9. Navab, N., Blum, T., Wang, L., Okur, A., Wendler, T.: First deployments of augmented reality in operating rooms. Computer 99, 48–55 (2012)

10. Vermeeren, L., Olmos, R.A.V., Meinhardt, W., Bex, A., van der Poel, H.G., Vogel, W.V., Sivro, F., Hoefnagel, C.A., Horenblas, S.: Value of SPECT/CT for Detection and Anatomic Localization of Sentinel Lymph Nodes Before Laparoscopic Sentinel Node Lymphadenectomy in Prostate Carcinoma. Journal of Nuclear Medicine 50(6), 865–870 (2009)

11. Vetter, C., Lasser, T., Okur, A., Navab, N.: 1D-3D Registration for Intra-Operative Nuclear Imaging in Radio-Guided Surgery. IEEE Transactions on Medical Imaging 34(2), 608–617 (2015)

12. Vidal-Sicart, S., Doménech, B., Luján, B., Pahisa, J., Torné, A., Martínez-Román, S., Lejárcegui, J.A., Fusté, P., Ordi, J., Paredes, P., Pons, F.: Sentinel Node in Gynaecological Cancers. Our Experience. Revista Española de Medicina Nuclear (English Edition) 28(5), 221–228 (2009)

13. Wendler, T., Hartl, A., Lasser, T., Traub, J., Daghighian, F., Ziegler, S.I., Navab, N.: Towards Intra-operative 3D Nuclear Imaging: Reconstruction of 3D Radioactive Distributions Using Tracked Gamma Probes. In: Ayache, N., Ourselin, S., Maeder, A. (eds.) MICCAI 2007, Part II. LNCS, vol. 4792, pp. 909–917. Springer, Heidelberg (2007)

14. Wong, S.L., Balch, C.M., Hurley, P., Agarwala, S.S., Akhurst, T.J., Cochran, A., Cormier, J.N., Gorman, M., Kim, T.Y., McMasters, K.M., et al.: Sentinel lymph node biopsy for melanoma: American Society of Clinical Oncology and Society of Surgical Oncology joint clinical practice guideline. Journal of Clinical Oncology 30(23), 2912–2918 (2012)

15. Van der Zee, A.G., Oonk, M.H., De Hullu, J.A., Ansink, A.C., Vergote, I., Verheijen, R.H., Maggioni, A., Gaarenstroom, K.N., Baldwin, P.J., Van Dorst, E.B., Van der Velden, J., Hermans, R.H., van der Putten, H., Drouin, P., Schneider, A., Sluiter, W.J.: Sentinel node dissection is safe in the treatment of early-stage vulvar cancer. Journal of Clinical Oncology 26(6), 884–889 (2008)

A Partial Domain Approach to Enable Aortic Flow Simulation Without Turbulent Modeling

Taha S. Koltukluoglu[1,*], Christian Binter[3], Christine Tanner[1], Sven Hirsch[2], Sebastian Kozerke[3], Gábor Székely[1], and Aymen Laadhari[1]

[1] Computer Vision Lab., Swiss Federal Institute of Technology, Zürich, Switzerland
ktaha@vision.ee.ethz.ch
[2] Inst. of Applied Simulation, Zurich University of Applied Sciences, Wädenswil, Switzerland
[3] Inst. for Biomed. Eng., Swiss Federal Institute of Technology, Zürich, Switzerland

Abstract. Analysis of hemodynamics shows great potential to provide indications for the risk of cardiac malformations and is essential for diagnostic purposes in clinical applications. Computational fluid dynamics (CFD) has been established as a valuable tool for the detailed characterization of volumetric blood flow and its effects on the arterial wall. However, studies concentrating on the aortic root have to take the turbulent nature of the flow into account while no satisfactory solution for such simulations exists today. In this paper we propose to combine magnetic resonance imaging (MRI) flow acquisitions, providing excellent data in the turbulent regions while showing only limited reliability in the boundary layer, with CFD simulations which can be used to extrapolate the measured data towards the vessel wall. The solution relies on a partial domain approach, restricting the simulations to the laminar flow domain while using MRI measurements as additional boundary conditions to drive the numerical simulation. In this preliminary work we demonstrate the feasibility of the method on flow phantom measurements while comparing actually measured and simulated flow fields under straight and spiral flow regimes.

1 Introduction

A wide range of flow problems can be approximated using computer assisted numerical methods. The physics of the flow field is described by the Navier-Stokes equations in terms of non-linear partial differential equations. Usually an analytical solution does not exist (except for simple geometries). Therefore, the governing equations are discretized resulting in an algebraic system of equations. Simplifications can be applied depending on, e.g., the compressibility and/or viscosity of the fluid. In biomechanical studies, the blood flow is usually approximated with a divergence-free assumption in large arteries.

---

* This work was supported by the Swiss National Science Foundation grant 320030-149567.

N. Navab et al. (Eds.): MICCAI 2015, Part II, LNCS 9350, pp. 544–551, 2015.
DOI: 10.1007/978-3-319-24571-3_65

Analysis of hemodynamics shows great potential to provide indications for the risk of cardiac malformations and is essential for diagnostic purposes in clinical applications [4]. In the last decade, combined studies based on computational fluid dynamics and magnetic resonance imaging have been under extensive research. Recent advances in three-directional velocity encoded phase contrast MRI [2] enable to capture complex flow patterns within the arteries including the aortic root. Some major drawbacks of MRI are the limitations with respect to signal-to-noise ratio, resolution and partial volume effects, which restrict the analysis of hemodynamic parameters [3].

Inflow velocity data are frequently determined by 2-D flow MRI and used in CFD as boundary conditions (BCs) [5]. Morbiducci et al. [6] recently demonstrated the importance of realistic inflow conditions and its substantial impact on the flow field. In [8], flow rates were applied as BCs. In [7], Boutsianis implemented a Schwarz-Christoffel technique to map measured MRI data for setting BCs at an inflow surface.

All of these studies apply the flow conditions at the inlet and perform flow simulations on the entire domain. However, due to the complex geometry of the aortic root and high flow velocities at positions near the valves, turbulent flow can be observed in a core region of the ascending aorta. In the surrounding the flow is transitional i.e., depending on the heart phase, it usually oscillates between laminar and turbulent [10]. Still in all cases, the velocities are zero at the vessel wall due to adhesion forces. Since blood is a viscid fluid, a parabolic profile is developed very near the vascular wall, which is lined by a laminar boundary layer. These regions are illustrated in Fig. 1b.

Numerical simulation of turbulent flows is a notoriously complex problem and no satisfactory solution for turbulent blood flow simulation exists today. Under these circumstances it is mandatory to search for alternative approaches when investigating the physiology of the aortic root. While MRI phase contrast flow measurements provide excellent data in the turbulent region, no reliable measurements can be expected in the boundary layer due to very poor signal-to-noise ratio at low velocities.

In this paper we propose a new method which explores this complementarity between CFD simulations and MRI measurements by restricting the simulation to a partial domain covering regions with laminar flow, while using MRI measurements at positions with sufficiently high velocities as additional BCs to drive the numerical simulations. The approach has been tested by comparing MRI measurements on a rigid vessel phantom with preliminary simulation results using both classical CFD and partial domain simulations.

2   The Partial Domain Approach

Let us define a set of manifolds $\Gamma_i, \Gamma_p, \Gamma_o, \Gamma_w \subset \mathbb{R}^3$. The subscripts stand for inlet, partial layer, outlet and wall, respectively. We define a domain $\Omega \subset \mathbb{R}^3$ with the boundary $\partial\Omega = \Gamma_i \cup \Gamma_p \cup \Gamma_o \cup \Gamma_w$ (see Fig. 1a and 1b). The flow is modeled as homogeneous, incompressible and Newtonian fluid governed by the

546   T.S. Koltukluoglu

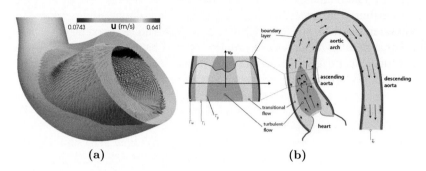

(a)   (b)

Fig. 1. (a): Partial domain, (b): Illustration of laminar boundary layer, transitional region and turbulent region.

Navier Stokes equations (2.1) and (2.2). Let $u = u(t, x) : [0, T] \times \Omega \to \mathbb{R}^3$ be the velocity and $p = p(t, x) : [0, T] \times \Omega \to \mathbb{R}$ stands for the pressure, $t \in [0, T]$ being the time and $x \in \Omega$. Suitable initial and BCs of both types (Dirichlet and Neumann) are required to ensure the well-posedness of the problem, which reads: $\forall t \in [0, T]$, find u and p such that

$$\rho \left(\partial_t u + u \cdot \nabla u \right) - \mu \Delta u + \nabla p = f \qquad \text{in } [0, T] \times \Omega \qquad (2.1)$$

$$\nabla \cdot u = 0 \qquad \text{in } [0, T] \times \Omega \qquad (2.2)$$

$$u(0, \cdot) = \tilde{u}^\star(\cdot) \qquad \text{in } \{0\} \times \Omega \qquad (2.3)$$

$$u = 0 \quad \text{and} \quad \nabla p \cdot n = 0 \qquad \text{on } [0, T] \times \Gamma_w \qquad (2.4)$$

$$u = s \quad \text{and} \quad \nabla p \cdot n = 0 \qquad \text{on } [0, T] \times (\Gamma_i \cup \Gamma_p) \qquad (2.5)$$

$$p = 0 \quad \text{and} \quad \nabla u \cdot n = 0 \qquad \text{on } [0, T] \times \Gamma_o \qquad (2.6)$$

where ρ is the density, μ is the viscosity, n is the outward normal of the corresponding boundary and $\tilde{u}^\star$ is some observation (see Section 4). The body forces are neglected in this work. The equations (2.1) and (2.2) are the momentum and conservation equations, respectively. Non-homogeneous BCs are applied on the inlet and the partial layer for u (2.5). The rest of the applied BCs are homogeneous. By restricting the simulations to the aortic volume between the surface Γ_p and the wall, we have to account only for regions with laminar flow and rely on standard numerical methods for solving the Navier-Stokes equations. The price we have to pay for it is, that additional BCs have to be defined on the surface Γ_p. In what follows, the computed velocities are denoted as u_c.

When performing dynamic simulations, the temporal resolution of MRI measurement is not sufficient. Due to the noisy MRI velocities, strict interpolation schemes enforcing precise agreement with the observed data are not appropriate to generate denser sampling and we rely on an approximation approach by defining a function $s : [0, T] \times (\Gamma_i \cup \Gamma_p) \to \mathbb{R}^3$ (2.5), whose components are spline regression model functions used to prescribe the observed velocity components,

$\tilde{\boldsymbol{u}}^{\star}$, on $\Gamma_i \cup \Gamma_p$. The defined model functions are cubic splines of class C^2 with uniformly distributed nodes. To obtain the model coefficients, the penalized regression spline method (2.7) was applied to minimize the sum of squares fitting error and (weighted by λ) the parameter irregularity. This was used as the interpolation function for the BCs on the inlet and partial layer (2.5). For each space position in $\Gamma_i \cup \Gamma_p$, the interpolation in time reads

$$\forall t \in [0, T], \quad s(t) = \arg\min_{\mathbf{a}} \left(\sum_k |\tilde{\boldsymbol{u}}^{\star}(t^k) - \mathbf{a}(t^k)|^2 + \lambda \int |\mathbf{a}''(\tau)|^2 d\tau \right) \quad (2.7)$$

3   Experimental Setup

In-vitro experiments were performed on a 3-D print of a rigid replica realistically mimicking the geometry of the human aortic root, ascending aorta, the arch without its branches and descending aorta (see Fig. 2a). A centrifugal pump (of 3.9 bar maximum pressure) was connected to the aorta and an open circuit was created by connecting the inlet and outlet tubes to a reservoir. The flow rates were controlled through a ball bearing valve. Linear phase correction were applied to compensate for the background phase induced by Eddy-current. The scans were performed with a 3T Philips scanner using a 6-element cardiac coil.

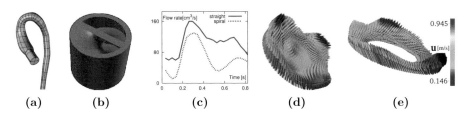

(a)   (b)   (c)   (d)   (e)

Fig. 2. (a): Rigid phantom, (b): 3-D printed screw to create the spiral motion, (c): Flow rates $[cm^3/s]$ for straight and spiral cases, (d and e): Spiral flow pattern visualized at inlet of full and partial domain at peak systole.

Measurements were taken with straight and spiral motion patterns. In order to generate the spiral motion as shown in Fig. 2d and 2e, a small 3-D printed device was additionally placed at the inlet, forcing the incoming fluid to develop a helical flow (see Fig. 2b). The acquisition parameters for straight flow were TR/TE: 5.63/3.25 ms, flip angle: 10°, VENC: 150 cm/s, FOV: $[160 \times 260 \times 50]$ mm^3, acquired voxel size: $[1.25 \times 1.25 \times 1.25]$ mm^3, temporal resolution: 28.0 ms. The parameters for spiral flow were TR/TE: 4.87/2.99 ms, flip angle: 10°, VENC: 100 cm/s, FOV: $[160 \times 320 \times 50]$ mm^3, acquired voxel size: $[2 \times 2.08 \times 2]$ mm^3, temporal resolution: 34.16 ms. As a working fluid, a mixture of H_2O and carboxymethyl cellulose (CMC) was used to increase the viscosity of water. To ensure laminar flow, the viscosity of the mixture was increased to the range of blood viscosity in the aorta. Fig. 2c shows the acquired flow rates in cm^3/s.

4   Preprocessing

Reconstructed MR images provide anatomical and three-directional flow data. The aortic geometry was segmented using snake evolution method in ITK-SNAP (www.itksnap.org) and smoothed using the VMTK framework (www.vmtk.org). In addition, a high resolution surface description was available from the model's 3-D print. This was rigidly registered to each segmentation using the ITK point-set to point-set registration method (www.itk.org). A hexahedral mesh was generated within the high resolution surface using OpenFOAM's snappyHexMesh and transfered to each segmentation using the registration result.

A general outlier detection scheme [1] initially applied to particle image velocimetry data, was implemented to detect spurious velocity vectors of the MRI. The method is based on normalization of the usual median test respecting the local fluctuations of the velocity field. The applicability of the normalized median test has been verified by Westerweel and Scarano [1] for a large variety of flow conditions with Reynolds numbers ranging from 10^{-1} to 10^{7}.

The detected outliers have to be replaced by some values such as from linear interpolation. However, thereby the divergence-free property of the flow field most probably gets lost. We therefore apply Helmholtz-Hodge decomposition [11]. The space of square integrable functions can be decomposed into divergence-free, curl-free and gradient of harmonic components as in (4.1) and (4.2). Let $\bar{u}_{\mathrm{MRI}}$ be the projection of already denoised MRI flow data on Ω. The orthogonal space splitting states $\bar{u}_{\mathrm{MRI}} = \tilde{u} + u_{\wedge} + u^{\star}$. Hence, the divergence free component can be extracted from $\tilde{u}^{\star} = \tilde{u} + u^{\star} = \bar{u}_{\mathrm{MRI}} - u_{\wedge}$, which reads as $\mathscr{P}_{\perp}$ (4.3).

The data were first linearly interpolated onto the computational domain and the decomposition was applied thereafter for each available heart phase. The applied Helmholtz-Hodge decomposition recovers the divergence-free property of the flow field to a great extent (Fig. 3). In [9], the feasibility of the decomposition was validated for a steady state. This is extended to a dynamic case under pulsatile flow conditions to enable robust comparisons between CFD and MRI.

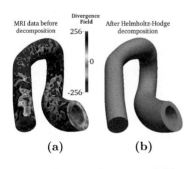

(a)   (b)

Fig. 3. Systolic divergence fields.

$$\left(L^{2}\left(\Omega\right)\right)^{3} = \mathrm{H}_{\mathrm{div},0}\left(\Omega\right) \oplus \mathrm{H}_{\mathrm{curl},0}\left(\Omega\right) \oplus \mathrm{H}_{\mathrm{har}}\left(\Omega\right) \quad (4.1)$$

$$\mathrm{H}_{\mathrm{div},0}\left(\Omega\right) = \left\{\tilde{u} \in (L^{2}(\Omega))^{3} : \; u \cdot n|_{\partial\Omega} = 0, \right.$$
$$\left. \nabla \cdot \tilde{u} \in L^{2}(\Omega), \nabla \cdot \tilde{u} = 0\right\}$$
$$\mathrm{H}_{\mathrm{curl},0}\left(\Omega\right) = \left\{u_{\wedge} = \nabla q : \; q \in H_{0}^{1}(\Omega)\right\} \quad (4.2)$$
$$\mathrm{H}_{\mathrm{har}}\left(\Omega\right) = \left\{u^{\star} = \nabla h : \; h \in H^{1}(\Omega), \; \Delta h = 0\right\}$$

$$\mathscr{P}_{\perp} : \; find \; \tilde{u}^{\star} = \bar{u}_{\mathrm{MRI}} - \nabla q, \; such \; that :$$
$$\Delta q = \nabla \cdot \bar{u}_{\mathrm{MRI}} \; in \; \Omega \quad (4.3)$$
$$q = 0 \; on \; \Gamma_{w} \quad and \quad \nabla q \cdot n = 0 \; on \; \partial\Omega \backslash \Gamma_{w}$$

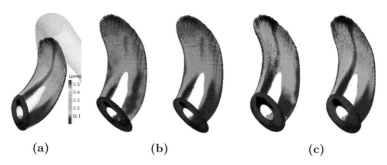

Fig. 4. Illustration of (a): cross-sectional partial domain, (b/c): mid/peak systole for measured (b/c left) and computed (b/c right) velocities.

5   Results

We tested the ability of the partial domain approach to reproduce MRI measurements in the selected domain similarly well as the traditional CFD method on the full domain of the aortic lumen. For this, we performed simulations with both methods and compared them with the MRI data acquired under straight flow conditions. Flow patterns were first qualitatively compared by visual inspection. Fig. 4 illustrates mid and peak systole on a cross-sectional slice of the data with straight flow generated by partial domain simulation. The left most Fig. 4a shows the position of a slice cut at the aortic root for further investigation. The orientation of the slice was chosen to cover both the partial domain and the flow domain immediately thereafter. In Fig. 4b and 4c, flow patterns of measured velocities are illustrated on the left side and the computed velocities on the right side of each sub-figure with respect to peak (Fig. 4c) and mid systole (Fig. 4b), respectively. It can be seen that the pattern is reasonably similar between the left and right plots of each sub-figure.

In order to confirm these qualitative observations, the simulation results of the velocities, $\boldsymbol{u}_c$, have been quantitatively compared to the divergence-free projection of the MRI measurements, $\tilde{\boldsymbol{u}}^\star$. The comparisons consist of root mean square error (nRMSE) normalized against the maximum velocity of the measurements (5.1). Furthermore, we evaluate the flow direction error (FDE) and the relative velocity magnitude error (rVME) defined in (5.2). The FDE delivers a dimensionless value between 0 (same direction) and 2 (opposite directions). These error measurements are less accurate near the wall boundaries in comparison to the middle of the lumen due to segmentation and registration errors. In addition, the phantom material delivers almost no relevant signal (i.e. mainly noise) at and near the boundaries, but noise. Respecting these uncertainties, the errors were also evaluated on a contracted domain within the lumen at a distance d (in mm) away from the aortic surface. We will refer to these errors as nRMSE$_d$, FDE$_d$ and rVME$_d$, respectively. In addition, defining $\boldsymbol{x} \in \Omega$, we introduce the characteristic function $\chi_d(\boldsymbol{x})$, which is equal to 1 if the position $\boldsymbol{x}$ is more than

d apart from the nearest surface point, and 0 otherwise. Furthermore, we define $\Omega_d = \{\boldsymbol{x} \in \Omega : \chi_d(\boldsymbol{x}) = 1\}$, V_d its volume and T is the time of one cardiac cycle.

$$\text{nRMSE}_d = \left(\frac{100}{\max\limits_{t,\Omega_d}|\tilde{\boldsymbol{u}}^\star|}\right)\sqrt{\frac{1}{V_d \cdot T}\int_t\int_{\Omega_d}|\tilde{\boldsymbol{u}}^\star - \boldsymbol{u}_c|^2} \qquad (5.1)$$

$$\text{FDE}_d(t) = \sqrt{\int_{\Omega_d}\left(1 - \frac{\tilde{\boldsymbol{u}}^\star \cdot \boldsymbol{u}_c}{|\tilde{\boldsymbol{u}}^\star||\boldsymbol{u}_c|}\right)^2 \frac{1}{V_d}} \quad \text{rVME}_d(t) = \sqrt{\int_{\Omega_d}\frac{|\tilde{\boldsymbol{u}}^\star - \boldsymbol{u}_c|^2}{|\tilde{\boldsymbol{u}}^\star|^2 V_d}} \qquad (5.2)$$

Table 1. Dimensionless flow direction errors (FDE_d) and relative velocity magnitude errors (rVME_d) for full domain (Full) and partial domain (Part) cases measured at peak systole and early diastole phase within the whole ($d = 0$ mm) and contracted ($d = 2$ mm) volume (Ω_d).

Straight flow		Systole		Diastole		Spiral flow		Systole		Diastole	
		FDE_d	rVME_d	FDE_d	rVME_d			FDE_d	rVME_d	FDE_d	rVME_d
Full	$d = 0$	0.27	0.48	0.28	0.70	Full	$d = 0$	0.12	0.47	0.17	0.55
Part	$d = 0$	0.26	0.45	0.27	0.68	Part	$d = 0$	0.12	0.47	0.18	0.60
Full	$d = 2$	0.19	0.35	0.24	0.48	Full	$d = 2$	0.14	0.45	0.06	0.38
Part	$d = 2$	0.18	0.33	0.21	0.49	Part	$d = 2$	0.08	0.41	0.07	0.41

We evaluated the errors for the entire lumen ($d = 0$ mm) and for the contracted domain by $d = 2$ mm. The evaluations were performed on the peak systole and end diastole over both the partial and the full domain. Furthermore, to assess the performance over the pulsation for one cardiac cycle, we evaluated the time integrated errors nRMSE_d for $d = 0$ and $d = 2$ mm. All simulations were performed using ≈ 95.000 cell volumes. To perform a consistency check and mesh analysis, the straight flow with partial domain case was also simulated with a much finer mesh, using ≈ 600.000 cell volumes.

For straight flow, the results presented on Table 1 (left) show very similar deviations between measured and calculated flow for most measures. The time integrated nRMSE_d errors were for $d = 0$, 13.62% and 15.60%, and for $d = 2$, 12.73% and 13.19% for full and partial domains, respectively. Furthermore, the partial domain case with the finer mesh resulted in $\text{nRMSE}_0 = 14.82\%$ and $\text{nRMSE}_2 = 12.92\%$. This suggests that partial domain simulations can well replace full domain calculation which cannot be performed under turbulent flow conditions. Note that, it could be more appropriate to consider the errors for $d = 2$, as MRI flow measurements are unreliable near to the boundary. In order to investigate the dependency of this observation on the complexity of the flow field, we performed the same comparison using the spiral flow measurements. The results for FDE and rVME are listed in Table 1 (right). In addition, nRMSE_2 were 16.34% for full domain and 18.83% for partial domain, respectively.

6   Discussion and Conclusion

A novel approach based on partial domains has been proposed for vascular flow simulations. The velocity measurements were projected onto the computational domain by linear interpolation and Helmholtz-Hodge decomposition was applied to recover the divergence-free property of the flow field. The simulation results were compared against the decomposed field both qualitatively and quantitatively. The work is still in an early stage and we have presented preliminary results. The centrifugal pump cannot capture the backflow, hence does not fully reflect the pulsating nature of blood flow. In-vitro MRI experiments under straight and spiral motion patterns with pulsatile flow showed the feasibility of the application. The partial domain approach reveals a great potential to investigate hemodynamics related parameters near the wall regions of tubular structures.

References

1. Westerweel, J., Scarano, F.: Universal outlier detection for PIV data. Exp. Fluids 39, 1096–1100 (2005)
2. Markl, M., Frydrychowicz, A., Kozerke, S., Hope, M., Wieben, O.: 4D flow MRI. Magn. Reson. Im. 36, 1015–1036 (2012)
3. Stankovic, Z., Allen, B.D., Garcia, J., Jarvis, K.B., Markl, M.: 4D flow imaging with MRI. Cardio. Diag. and Thera. 4(2), 173–192 (2014)
4. Katritsis, D., Kaiktsis, L., Chaniotis, A., Pantos, J., Efstathopoulos, E.P., Marmarelis, V.: Wall shear stress: theoretical considerations and methods of measurement. Prog. Cardiovasc. Dis. 49(5), 307–329 (2007)
5. Leuprecht, A., Kozerke, S., Boesiger, P., Perktold, K.: Blood flow in the human ascending aorta: a combined MRI and CFD study. J. of Eng. Maths. 47(3-4), 387–404 (2003)
6. Morbiducci, U., Ponzini, R., Gallo, D., Bignardi, C., Rizzo, G.: Inflow boundary conditions for image-based computational hemodynamics: Impact of idealized versus measured velocity profiles in the human aorta. J. of Biomech. 46(1), 102–109 (2013)
7. Gupta, S., Boomsma, K., Poulikakos, D., Boutsianis, E.: Boundary Conditions by Schwarz-Christoffel Mapping in Anatomically Accurate Hemodynamics. Ann. of Biomed. Eng. 36(12), 2068–2084 (2008)
8. Steinman, D.A., Milner, J.S., Norley, C.J., Lownie, S.P., Holdsworth, D.W.: Image-Based Computational Simulation of Flow Dynamics in a Giant Intracranial Aneurysm. American J. of Neurorad. 24, 559–566 (2003)
9. Koltukluoglu, T.S., Hirsch, S., Binter, C., Kozerke, S., Székely, G., Laadhari, A.: A Robust Comparison Approach of Velocity Data Between MRI and CFD Based on Divergence-Free Space Projection. In: Intern. Symp. on Biomed. Imag. (2015)
10. Stein, P.D., Sabbah, H.N.: Turbulent Blood Flow in the Ascending Aorta of Humans with Normal and Diseased Aortic Valves. Cir. Res. 39, 58–65 (1976)
11. Denaro, F.M.: On the application of the Helmholtz-Hodge decomposition in projection methods for incompressible flows with general boundary conditions. Int. J. Numer. Meth. Fluids 46, 43–69 (2003)

Discussion and Conclusion

Reconstruction, Image Formation, Advanced Acquisition – Computational Imaging

Flexible Reconstruction and Correction of Unpredictable Motion from Stacks of 2D Images

Bernhard Kainz[1,2], Amir Alansary[1], Christina Malamateniou[2], Kevin
Keraudren[1], Mary Rutherford[2], Joseph V. Hajnal[2], and Daniel Rueckert[1]

Department of Computing, Imperial College London, UK
{b.kainz,kevin.keraudren10,d.rueckert}@imperial.ac.uk
King's College London, Division of Imaging Sciences, London, UK
{christina.malamateniou,mary.rutherford,jo.hajnal}@kcl.ac.uk

Abstract. We present a method to correct motion in fetal in-utero scan
sequences. The proposed approach avoids previously necessary manual
segmentation of a region of interest. We solve the problem of non-rigid
motion by splitting motion corrupted slices into overlapping patches of
finite size. In these patches the assumption of rigid motion approximately holds and they can thus be used to perform a slice-to-volume-
based (SVR) reconstruction during which their consistency with the
other patches is learned. The learned information is used to reject patches
that are not conform with the motion corrected reconstruction in their
local areas. We evaluate rectangular and evenly distributed patches for
the reconstruction as well as patches that have been derived from superpixels. Both approaches achieve on 29 subjects aged between 22–37 weeks
a sufficient reconstruction quality and facilitate following 3D segmentation of fetal organs and the placenta.

1 Introduction

Evaluation of fetal organs and the placenta is an important diagnostic tool during
prenatal screening and is considered to be an indicator for fetal health after birth.
Fetal Magnetic Resonance Imaging (MRI) allows to acquire high resolution slices
from the fetus at a large field of view and with good tissue contrast [9]. However,
the fetus is not sedated during these scans and may move freely inside the uterus.
Because of a scan time of up to 500 ms per slice, motion artefacts are likely to
corrupt volumetric scans. Therefore, several (usually 3–12) orthogonal stacks of
slices are acquired and reconstructed using approaches based on slice-to-volume
registration (SVR) to obtain an artefact free, high resolution volume of a fetal
target region [8,5]. So far, this process has been applied only to small regions and
organs with rigid body characteristic such as the fetal brain. Usually, these areas
have to be identified by manual labor intensive segmentation methods. Such
approaches cannot be applied to the whole fetal body and uterus because of the
assumption of rigid motion in the 2D to 3D registration step of SVR methods.

© Springer International Publishing Switzerland 2015
N. Navab et al. (Eds.): MICCAI 2015, Part II, LNCS 9350, pp. 555–562, 2015.
DOI: 10.1007/978-3-319-24571-3_66

Different areas in each slice that are likely to move in different directions will break this assumption. Because an extension of 2D-3D registration to non-rigid deformations is not well-constrained, current SVR approaches will fail for non-rigid deformations and movements.

Contribution: We solve the motion compensation problem for large field of views in stacks of 2D slices. We split the input into small overlapping areas and find these, which contain rigid components. This allows to iteratively learn their consistency compared to a global reconstruction volume and to exclude corrupted data automatically. This approach paves the way to fully automatically reconstruct whole collections of motion corrupted stacks without the need for manually segmented input. The method also finds rigidly connected areas automatically, which can be used for further refinement or as segmentation prior.

Related Work: Fetal MRI is increasingly used as a complementary diagnostic tool to ultrasound sonography. Currently, the brain [8], thorax [6], and the appearance of the whole fetus [10] are qualitatively examined using MRI in the clinical practice. Fetal motion and its unpredictable nature make the acquisition of 3D MR sequences very challenging. Fast MR sequences such as single shot fast spin echo (ssFSE) [9] are often used in order to freeze motion within a single 2D image. Using several overlapping stacks of 2D images provides coverage of a 3D volume of a target region of interest. However, the resulting stacks are usually corrupted by relative motion between individual slices. Often six to twelve stacks need to be acquired to sufficiently oversample a 3D volume. Segmentation and localization of selected organs can be automated, however, the available approaches provide either a very rough segmentation of the central slices of a stack [7] or require less motion corrupted stacks [4]. Furthermore, they are only applicable to a specificity trained region, *c.g.*, the fetal brain.

2   Method

The proposed method is based on the fact that certain regions of a scanned anatomy are rigid and can be reconstructed with SVR super-resolution algorithms. These methods usually use manually defined rigid regions of the 2D input images (slices) and register them to an iteratively improving global 3D reconstruction volume. Robust statistics can be used to identify mis-registered or heavily corrupted data [8,11]. Data consistency is reached by oversampling a region of interest with different scan orientations. We propose to reduce the granularity of the input data by using 2D data *patches* of arbitrary shape instead of whole slices for SVR reconstruction. That way, multiple, large motion

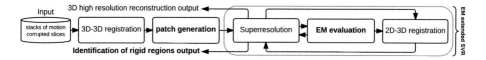

Fig. 1. An overview over our approach. Bold parts are extensions to SVR.

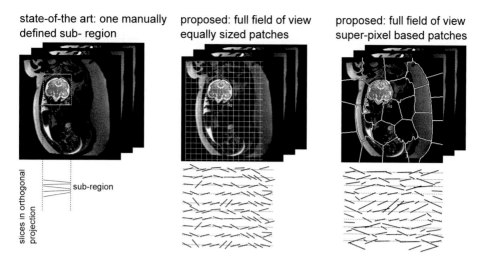

Fig. 2. Comparison of the proposed reconstruction methods to the state-of-the-art.

corrupted field of views can be reconstructed and regions with rigid motion can be found automatically. Fig. 1 gives a schematic overview over our approach and Fig. 2 shows a high level overviews over the current state-of-the-art manual segmentation-based reconstruction paradigm compared to the here presented fully automatic, full field of view reconstruction method.

The input data can be represented as stacks of 2D images consisting of $Y = \{y_s | s \in S\}$, where y_s is a 2D patch indexed by the location s and S is the set of all locations in all p stacks, $S = \{s_1, s_2, ...s_M\}$. y_s can have arbitrary (2D) shape. In this work we explore using overlapping square patches as a general application of our novel reconstruction method and Simple Linear Iterative Clustering (SLIC) super-pixels [1] as a method to reduce the required data redundancy.

SVR: We can reconstruct a high resolution image X from a number of motion corrupted y_s using 2D-3D registration-based super-resolution [8,5]. After initial 3D-3D alignment a gradually improving approximation of X (super-resolution with the measured point spread function of the used MRI sequence) is used to initialize and perform 2D-3D registration and robust statistics. To provide enough structural information for rigid registration of y_s to X we dilate each y_s by γ pixels using a flat structuring element b with a fixed (26 in our case) pixels neighbourhood, hence $\bar{y}_s = y_s \oplus b$.

Patch Generation: The shape of y_s can be square with similar edge sizes in the simplest naïve case. These patches can be defined by their edge length a and stride ω. While this definition is likely to be generally applicable to any kind of oversampled motion corrupted data, it does not assume any knowledge about the data and a and ω are likely to depend on for example the gestational age. Ideally, each y_s corresponds to a subregion of the volume in which the motion can be characterized as rigid. A good trade-off between the size of the patch region and the likelihood of rigid motion has to be found. The larger the chosen patch regions are the less likely they will cover rigidly moving areas. An alternative to naïve shape definitions of y_s is to use correlation between each pixel and its neighbors. Such correlations can be found by popular unsupervised image segmentation techniques like *super-pixels*. Super-pixels clusters the image into areas of pixels with local correlations. Correlated regions may define rigidly connected areas, which can support the image reconstruction step with less but more useful data blocks. In the literature, there are different techniques for generating super-pixels. We aim for clinical applicability of our method. Therefore, we selected a super-pixel algorithm, which is fast to compute, i.e., we use Simple Linear Iterative Clustering (SLIC) [1]. SLIC allows to segment 2D image slices into compact and uniform super-pixels as shown in Fig. 2. This approach is also computationally more efficient for image reconstruction because larger rigid areas require less redundant image registration and super-resolution effort, independent from data parameters like gestational age. To determine the number of super-pixels N_{sp} for each 2D slice, we use the rule of thumb proposed by [3], which is based on the total number of pixels n. To handle the high variability of the size and shape of our data, we have weighted this generation rule with a constant factor k, where $k \in \mathbb{R}_{>0}$ and is chosen depending on the resolution of the input data and thus $N_{sp} \approx k \cdot \sqrt{(n/2)}$.

EM Evaluation: We aim to use only voxels from $\bar{y}_s$ that can be well registered and that have a minimal error e when compared to the originally scanned data. To achieve this we propose to classify $\bar{y}_s$ and the included pixels into an inlier and an outlier class using an expectation maximization (EM) framework. Inspired by [2,8], we use a zero-mean Gaussian distribution $G_\sigma(e)$ with variance σ^2 for the inliers and a uniform distribution with constant density $m = \frac{1}{max(e)-min(e)}$ for the outliers. This allows us to use redundant information, i.e., overlapping $\bar{y}_s$, to find partly matching patches and to depreciate or fully reject erroneous voxels of each $\bar{y}_s$. For these regions we try to maximize the log-likelihood for each patch $y_s|logP(Y,\Phi) = \sum logP(e|\sigma,c)$ to be part of an area that undergoes rigid motion. Φ contains the current estimate of the reconstructed volume X, the variance σ^2 of the errors e, and the proportion of correctly matched voxels c. The posterior probability for a pixel $\in \bar{y}_s$ being identified as inlier is $p = \frac{G_\sigma(e)c}{G_\sigma(e)c+m(1-c)}$. We perform the updates of c and σ^2 similar to [8]. Using $\bar{p} = \sqrt{(\sum_{\bar{y}_s} p^2)/N}$ (with N the number of pixels in $\bar{y}_s$) we can also define an inlier and outlier probability for each patch $\bar{y}_s$ and stop processing this patch if it gets classified as outlier.

Identification of Rigid Regions: Keeping track of the probability p of each pixel of every $\bar{y}_s$ allows to identify areas that best fit the rigid 2D-3D registration constraint of SVR methods. Integrating p and $\bar{p}$ into a separate probability volume P using the same slice to volume integration scheme as used by SVR can be used to identify candidate regions, which contain only rigid motion components. This can be useful to apply the classic SVR reconstruction approach at a higher level of detail only in these regions. As shown by [7], tight region of interest masks can lead to a higher reconstruction quality for rigid regions like the fetal brain. In practice we can identify such rigid regions by blurring P using a 3D Gaussian filter with σ related to the size of the desired regions followed by blob detection. These regions can subsequently be reconstructed and motion corrected in the high-resolution volume and used for automatic classification, *e.g.*, in organ classes with machine learning. Fig. 5(g) shows cross section views through P, which was generated using super-pixels at $k = 0.2$.

3   Evaluation and Results

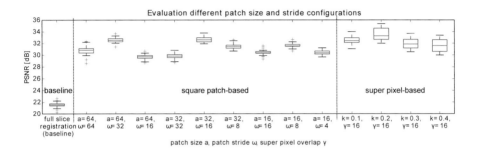

Fig. 3. PSNR comparison in the brain region of 29 subjects between using the slices of the input stacks directly for full field of view SVR reconstruction (baseline, most left whisker-box) to different regular patch sizes a with varying stride ω. The last four whisker-box plots are using super pixels with varying k and an overlap $\gamma = 16$ pixels, which yielded good results during our experiments. A PSNR above 30 dB shows that all the proposed configurations produce a result, which is very similar to a reconstruction when using a tight manually defined mask. Small square patches with $a = 32$, $\omega = 16$ and super pixels with $k = 0.2$, $\gamma = 16$ produced the best results during this experiment.

We evaluate our method with experiments using 29 data sets from fetuses with gestational ages between 22–37 weeks. To the best of our knowledge our method

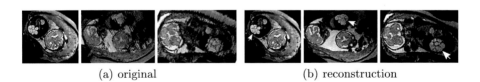

      (a) original   (b) reconstruction

Fig. 4. Three viewing planes through the originally scanned (a) and the reconstruction (b) of a motion corrupted scan from moving twins with a gestational age of 28 weeks using super-pixels $k = 0.2$ $\gamma = 16$. For this dataset we used a mask of the uterus so save unnecessary computation time in areas containing maternal tissue. The white arrow points at a unilateral multicystic kidney of one of the twins.

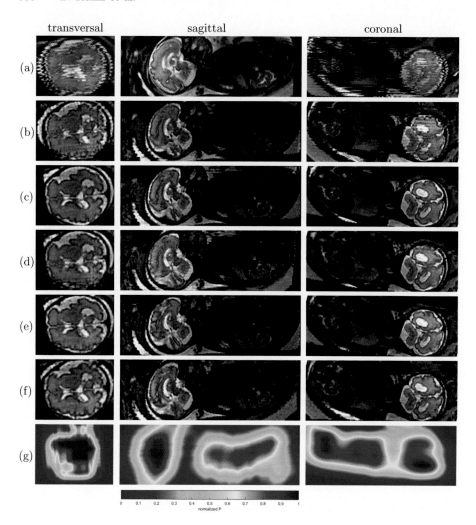

Fig. 5. Visual comparison between the input data (a) and different configurations for full fetal body reconstruction of a motion corrupted 3T MRI dataset with gestational age of 33 weeks. The categorization into best and worst has been made by an expert. (b): reconstruction with full slices and [8]; (c): best: $s = 32 \times 16, \omega = 16$; (d): worst $s = 64 \times 64, \omega = 64$; (e): best: super-pixels $k = 0.2\ \gamma = 16$, (f): worst: $k = 0.05$ super-pixels/slice $\gamma = 16$. (g) indicates which regions move as a rigid body as a function of P ($\sigma = 15$ with super-pixels $k = 0.2$, $\gamma = 16$) for subsequent automatic identification of rigid regions.

provides the first approach to reconstruct other areas than the brain or the lung, hence there is no ground truth for the full fetal body to compare with. However, we can compare the reconstruction quality with a well researched organ: the fetal brain. Our hypothesis is that our method provides similar reconstruction and motion correction quality for the brain as it would be the case if a tight mask [7] for a region of interest would have been used for SVR. We expect the quality of our results to be close to the results from the state-of-the-art SVR approach [5] for rigid regions. Fig. 3 shows peak signal-to-noise ratio (PSNR) comparisons with a defined region in the fetal brain for different patch sizes (a) and super-pixel sizes (b) with different strides and overlaps compared to a full field of view reconstruction using the slices directly without masking or splitting into patches (baseline). Fig. 5 shows an expert quality assessment of the results from different image parcellations applied to a full fetal body 3T ssFSE dataset.

Our method allows for the first time the reconstruction and motion correction of scans of the whole uterus with more than one fetus. Up to now only selected regions could be reconstructed and malformations in multiple births as shown in the kidney of one twin in Fig. 4 were difficult to examine.

Runtime: Super-pixels can be generated for all slices of motion corrupted stacks within a few seconds ($\sim$ 800 2D images/examination). Our approach becomes slower the more patches/super-pixels and the more overlap is used (approx. quadratically). We use a parallelized and hardware accelerated SVR reconstruction method based on [5]. A full field of view reconstruction of 8 input stacks at $288 \times 288 \times 100$ voxels takes up to $1 - 2$ hours using a small patch size (*e.g.*, $a = 32$, $\omega = 16$) on a multi GPU System (Intel Xeon E5-2630 2.60GHz system with 16 GB RAM, an Nvidia Tesla K40 and a Geforce 780). Using large ($k = 0.1$) overlapping super-pixels reduces this time to approximately $45min$ for a full field-of-view volume, while maintaining a comparable result to the best configuration of overlapping square patches.

4   Discussion and Conclusion

We have presented a method to fully automatically reconstruct the full overlapping field of view of multiple motion corrupted stacks of 2D slices. This method is generally applicable to motion corrupted scan protocols and especially useful for fetal MRI. We discuss how data patches can be used to tackle the problem of locally rigid body movements between different body parts. The presented method can be used to provide a segmentation prior for rigid and stable regions like the fetal brain and the thorax and provides a motion corrected overview over the whole uterus in 3D including multiple births and the placenta. For certain configurations our method might produce a slightly less accurate reconstruction of specific body parts as it would be the case when using tight masks of these regions. However, this can be solved by using standard slice-based SVR reconstruction as a subsequent step, applied only to the automatically detected rigid areas or an automatically derived mask. In fact our method provides an excellent starting point to apply state-of-the-art but motion sensitive 3D volume analysis and segmentation methods directly to the motion corrected result. We introduce the use of super-pixels as an alternative to naïve overlapping square patches. While the parameter configuration for naïve patches is likely to be data dependent (*e.g.*, gestational age), super-pixels provide a framework, which is invariant towards such variations in the data. In future work we will investigate potential improvements of the super-resolution step in SVR methods by using consistent patches for dictionary learning methods to provide a sparse representation of the desired high-resolution volume.

Acknowledgements. We used MITK [12]. This work was supported by Wellcome Trust and EPSRC IEH award [102431] for the iFIND project.

References

1. Achanta, R., Shaji, A., Smith, K., Lucchi, A., Fua, P., Susstrunk, S.: SLIC superpixels compared to state-of-the-art superpixel methods. IEEE Trans. Pattern Analysis and Machine Intelligence 34(11), 2274–2282 (2012)
2. Gholipour, A., Estroff, J.A., Warfield, S.K.: Robust super-resolution volume reconstruction from slice acquisitions: application to fetal brain MRI. IEEE Trans. Med. Imaging 29(10), 1739–1758 (2010)
3. Hair, J.F., Black, W.C., Babin, B.J., Anderson, R.E., Tatham, R.L.: Multivariate data analysis, vol. 6. Pearson Prentice Hall, Upper Saddle River (2006)
4. Kainz, B., Keraudren, K., Kyriakopoulou, V., Rutherford, M., Hajnal, J.V., Rueckert, D.: Fast Fully Automatic Brain Detection in Foetal MRI Using Dense Rotation Invariant Image Descriptors. In: IEEE ISBI 2014, pp. 1230–1233 (2014)
5. Kainz, B., Steinberger, M., Wein, W., Murgasova, M., Malamateniou, C., Keraudren, K., Torsney-Weir, T.K., Aljabar, P., Rutherford, M., Hajnal, J., Rueckert, D.: Fast Volume Reconstruction from Motion Corrupted Stacks of 2D Slices. IEEE Trans. Med. Imaging 34(9), 1901 1913 (2015)
6. Kainz, B., Malamateniou, C., Murgasova, M., Keraudren, K., Rutherford, M., Hajnal, J.V., Rueckert, D.: Motion Corrected 3D Reconstruction of the Fetal Thorax from Prenatal MRI. In: Golland, P., Hata, N., Barillot, C., Hornegger, J., Howe, R. (eds.) MICCAI 2014, Part II. LNCS, vol. 8674, pp. 284–291. Springer, Heidelberg (2014)
7. Keraudren, K., Murgasova, M., Kyriakopoulou, V., Malamateniou, C., Rutherford, M., Kainz, B., Hajnal, J., Rueckert, D.: Automated Fetal Brain Segmentation from 2D MRI Slices for Motion Correction. NeuroImage 101, 633–643 (2014)
8. Kuklisova-Murgasova, M., Quaghebeur, G., Rutherford, M.A., Hajnal, J.V., Schnabel, J.A.: Reconstruction of Fetal Brain MRI with Intensity Matching and Complete Outlier Removal. Medical Image Analysis 16(8), 1550–1560 (2012)
9. Levine, D.: Fetal Magnetic Resonance Imaging. J. Matern. Fetal Neonatal Med. 15(2), 85–94 (2004)
10. Prayer, D., Brugger, P., Prayer, L.: Fetal MRI: techniques and protocols. Pediatric Radiology 34(9), 685–693 (2004)
11. Rousseau, F., Glenn, O.A., Iordanova, B., Rodriguez-Carranza, C., Vigneron, D.B., Barkovich, J.A., Studholme, C.: Registration-Based Approach for Reconstruction of High-Resolution In Utero Fetal MR Brain Images. Academic Radiology 13(9), 1072–1081 (2006)
12. Wolf, I., Vetter, M., Wegner, I., Böttger, T., Nolden, M., Schöbinger, M., Hastenteufel, M., Kunert, T., Meinze, H.P.: The medical imaging interaction toolkit. Medical Image Analysis 9(6), 594–604 (2005)

Efficient Preconditioning in Joint Total Variation Regularized Parallel MRI Reconstruction[*]

Zheng Xu[1], Yeqing Li[1], Leon Axel[2], and Junzhou Huang[1,**]

[1] Department of Computer Science and Engineering,
University of Texas at Arlington, Arlington TX 76019, USA
[2] Department of Radiology, New York University, New York, NY 10016, USA
jzhuang@uta.edu

Abstract. Parallel magnetic resonance imaging (pMRI) is a useful technique to aid clinical diagnosis. In this paper, we develop an accelerated algorithm for joint total variation (JTV) regularized calibrationless Parallel MR image reconstruction. The algorithm minimizes a linear combination of least squares data fitting term and the joint total variation regularization. This model has been demonstrated as a very powerful tool for parallel MRI reconstruction. The proposed algorithm is based on the iteratively reweighted least squares (IRLS) framework, which converges exponentially fast. It is further accelerated by preconditioned conjugate gradient method with a well-designed preconditioner. Numerous experiments demonstrate the superior performance of the proposed algorithm for parallel MRI reconstruction in terms of both accuracy and efficiency.

1 Introduction

Parallel MR imaging is a powerful method that uses multiple receiver coils for reducing scanning time in MRI[5,6]. Based on the way in utilizing the sensitivity information and local kernel in k-space, these methods are classified broadly into two main types. Reconstruction techniques such as SENSE[11] and CSSENSE[8] expect accurate estimation of reception profiles from each coil element to optimally reconstruct undersampled MR image. However, it is often very difficult to accurately and robustly measure the sensitivities and even small errors can result in inconsistencies that lead to visible artifacts in the image. These disadvantages therefore motivate the other type of methods, termed auto-calibrating methods, e.g. GRAPPA[4] and SPIRiT[9], that derive sensitivity information from auto-calibration signals (ACSs) and thus avoid side effects brought by the difficult and inaccurate sensitivity map estimation. However, it is often limiting or totally infeasible to acquire sufficient ACSs. For example, for non-Cartesian imaging, ACS acquisition requires much longer time and can probably lead to artifacts due to off-resonance. To overcome these shortcomings, several calibrationless methods have been proposed recently, e.g. CaLMMRI[10], FISTA_JTV[2] and SAKE[15].

---

[*] This work was partially supported by U.S. NSF IIS-1423056, CMMI-1434401, CNS-1405985.
[**] Corresponding author.

© Springer International Publishing Switzerland 2015
N. Navab et al. (Eds.): MICCAI 2015, Part II, LNCS 9350, pp. 563–570, 2015.
DOI: 10.1007/978-3-319-24571-3_67

Among these methods, joint total variation (JTV) model has been demonstrated as a powerful tool for calibrationless parallel MR image reconstruction. The JTV model is designed based on the observation of the gradient sparsity of each coil image and the cross-channel similarity of parallel MR images. Previous attempt to solve this model is shown in [2] which is based on FISTA_JTV algorithms. The numerical experiments exhibit its effectiveness and efficiency on the parallel MR images with real measurements. However, real world parallel MR images are often sampled in complex measurements. For complex parallel MR images, the FISTA_JTV algorithm usually fails to solve the model efficiently as it requires more inner loop iterations to converge.

Here, we propose a novel optimization scheme to solve the joint total variation model more efficiently based on the iteratively reweighted least squares (IRLS) framework. It preserves the fast convergence speed of traditional IRLS which converges exponentially fast. Since it requires solving a linear inverse subproblem in each IRLS step, we propose a new pseudo-diagonal preconditioner to significantly accelerate this process with preconditioned conjugate gradient method. Extensive experiment results show that it impressively outperforms previous state-of-art methods for the MR image reconstruction in terms of both reconstruction accuracy and computational complexity.

2   Joint Total Variation Regularized Model

Based on the assumption that the gradients of aliased images from all the coils are jointly sparse, the formulation of joint total variation (JTV) model is designed as follows[2]:

$$\min_{x} \frac{1}{2}\|\mathcal{R}\mathcal{F}x - b\|^2 + \lambda\|[\nabla_h x, \nabla_v x]\|_{2,1}. \tag{1}$$

where $x \in \mathbb{C}^{m \times n \times c}$, is the c-channel parallel MR image with each coil size $m \times n$. $\mathcal{R}$ is the subsampling operator in frequency domain, and $\mathcal{F}$ is the Fourier transform operator. λ is the non-negative tunning parameter balancing the data fitting and JTV regularization. The JTV regularization term $\|[\nabla_h x, \nabla_v x]\|_{2,1} = \sum_{i=1}^{m} \sum_{j=1}^{n} \sqrt{\sum_{k=1}^{c} (\nabla_h x_{i,j,k})^2 + (\nabla_v x_{i,j,k})^2}$ and ∇_h and ∇_v are the horizontal and vertical discrete gradient operators (i.e. $\nabla_h x_{i,j,k} = x_{i,j+1,k} - x_{i,j,k}$, $\nabla_v x_{i,j,k} = x_{i+1,j,k} - x_{i,j,k}$). The JTV regularization sums up the horizontal and vertical discrete gradients across all data channels. Therefore, minimizing the JTV regularization can lead to the joint gradient sparse solution for pMRI reconstruction.

Due to the non-smoothness of JTV regularization, it's hard to optimize the JTV objective function efficiently. Although FISTA_JTV[2] has been proposed as an accelerated algorithm and experimentally proven as a fast method for parallel MR images with real number measurements, it remains challenging to efficiently reconstruct parallel MR images in complex measurements. This situation therefore motivates us to develop a faster algorithm, especially for complex measurements, to solve JTV model in the next section.

3 Algorithm

3.1 Iteratively Reweighted Least Squares Framework

In this section, we first briefly review the iteratively reweighted least squares (IRLS) method[1,3] and show how to fit JTV model into the IRLS framework. The key idea of the IRLS method is to approximate the ℓ_1 regularization by a weighted ℓ_2 regularization, making the loss function strongly convex. The formulation is then able to be optimized in a linear convergence rate as shown in Theorem 1.

Theorem 1. *(Theorem 6.1 in [3]) Let $\{x^t\}$ be the sequence generated by IRLS method, x^* be the $\ell_1-minimizer$ with $\mu \in (0,1)$, thus*

$$\|x^t - x^*\|_1 \le \mu^t \|x^0 - x^*\|_1. \tag{2}$$

Using the techniques introduced in [7], we have the weighted ℓ_2 form for the JTV model (1).

$$\min_x \frac{1}{2}\|\mathcal{R}\mathcal{F}x - b\|^2 + \frac{\lambda}{2}\langle \nabla_h x, W^t \nabla_h x\rangle + \frac{\lambda}{2}\langle \nabla_v x, W^t \nabla_v x\rangle. \tag{3}$$

where $\langle \nabla_h x, W^t \nabla_h x\rangle \; = \; \sum_{i=1}^{m}\sum_{j=1}^{n}\sum_{k=1}^{c} W_{i,j,k}^t (\nabla_h x_{i,j,k})^2,$ and   simi-

larly $\langle \nabla_v x, W^t \nabla_v x\rangle \; = \; \sum_{i=1}^{m}\sum_{j=1}^{n}\sum_{k=1}^{c} W_{i,j,k}^t (\nabla_v x_{i,j,k})^2.$ Here $W_{i,j,k}^t \; =$

$(\sqrt{\sum_{p=1}^{c} (\nabla_h x_{i,j,p}^t)^2 + (\nabla_v x_{i,j,p}^t)^2} + \varepsilon)^{-1}$ for $k = 1, 2, \ldots, c$ and ε is a real infinitesimal added to avoid $W_{i,j,k}^t$ to be infinite.

By solving the Euler-Lagrange equation of (3), we have the least squares subproblem in each IRLS iteration

$$(\mathcal{F}^H \mathcal{R}^H \mathcal{R} \mathcal{F} + \lambda \langle \nabla_h, W^t \nabla_h\rangle + \lambda \langle \nabla_v, W^t \nabla_v\rangle)x = \mathcal{F}^H \mathcal{R}^H b. \tag{4}$$

where the superscript H denotes the conjugate transpose of a linear bounded operator. However, it is not feasible to calculate exact matrix inverse since it requires $\mathcal{O}(pq^2)$ time for a $p \times q$ matrix. Another option is to use the classical iterative methods, e.g. Jacobian, Gauss-Seidel iteration whose convergence are not guaranteed. Therefore, it is challenging to design an efficient algorithm with clear theoretical convergence justification to solve the subproblem (4).

3.2 Preconditioned Conjugate Gradient Descent

In the sequel, we study the preconditioned conjugate gradient (PCG) method aiming at solving subproblem (4) efficiently. We first show, in Theorem 2, the conjugate gradient(CG) algorithm is able to solve the least squares problem in a linear convergence rate.

Theorem 2. *(Section 9.2 in [14]) Let $\{x^t\}$ be the sequence generated by conjugate gradient iteration, x^* be the optimal solution for $b = Ax$. Let κ be the condition number of A, $\|x\|_A = \langle x, Ax \rangle$ be the energy norm, we have*

$$\|x^t - x^*\|_A \leq 2 \left(\frac{\sqrt{\kappa} - 1}{\sqrt{\kappa} + 1} \right)^t \|x^0 - x^*\|_A. \tag{5}$$

The practical convergence speed of CG highly depends on the condition number κ of A. When κ is relatively large, the coefficient of convergence $\frac{\sqrt{\kappa}-1}{\sqrt{\kappa}+1}$ approaches 1, leading to the arbitrarily slow convergence of CG. However, in practices, the A is usually with high condition number. It thus motivates the preconditioning techniques which is typically related to reducing condition number of A by designing a transformation P. The design of preconditioner is problem-dependent and the preconditioner not only needs to be as close as possible to the original system matrix A but also be able to be inverted efficiently.

For least squares subproblem (4), we design a novel preconditioner to accelerate the CG method. Observing $\mathcal{F}^H \mathcal{R}^H \mathcal{R} \mathcal{F}$ is diagonal dominant, we can discard the non-diagonal elements in $\mathcal{F}^H \mathcal{R}^H \mathcal{R} \mathcal{F}$ without bringing in large error. In this way, we can design the following preconditioner for solving subproblem (4)

$$P = \overline{\mathcal{F}^H \mathcal{R}^H \mathcal{R} \mathcal{F}} I + \lambda \langle \nabla_h, W^t \nabla_h \rangle + \lambda \langle \nabla_v, W^t \nabla_v \rangle. \tag{6}$$

where $\overline{\mathcal{F}^H \mathcal{R}^H \mathcal{R} \mathcal{F}}$ denotes the mean of diagonal elements of $\mathcal{F}^H \mathcal{R}^H \mathcal{R} \mathcal{F}$ and I is the identity matrix. The $\overline{\mathcal{F}^H \mathcal{R}^H \mathcal{R} \mathcal{F}} I$ is bounded and the parameter λ is usually small (e.g. 10^{-6}) hence successfully suppressing the condition number of the preconditioner P. Moreover, this preconditioner is observed as a penta-diagonal matrix, whose inverse can be evaluated in linear time by [12]. Therefore, the proposed preconditioner is able to solve problem (4) more accurately, while, in the meantime, it does not increase time complexity.

The proposed algorithm is summarized in Algorithm 1. We denoted this algorithm as *PRIM* which is short for PReconditioned Iterative reweighted Method for parallel MRI reconstruction. Although the proposed algorithm has inner loop, we observe that usually ten PCG iterations are sufficient to obtain a solution very close to the optimal one for the parallel MRI reconstruction. This is because both the inner and outer loops have linear convergence rates. The theoretically fast convergence constitutes a key feature of the proposed method.

Another key feature of our method is the cost of each iteration is only $\mathcal{O}(cmn \log(mn))$. The step of updating $W_{i,j,k}^t$ and P^t requires $\mathcal{O}(cmn)$ time. Updating S^t requires $\mathcal{O}(cmn \log(mn))$ time since in each step it requires to evaluate Fast Fourier Transformation. The inverse of P^t can be calculated in $\mathcal{O}(cmn)$ time as shown in [12]. As a result, the time complexity of each iteration in PRIM is $\mathcal{O}(cmn \log(mn))$.

With these two key features, the PRIM efficiently solves the compressive sensing parallel MR image reconstruction model regularized by joint total variation. The experiment results in the next section demonstrate its superior performance compared with all previous state-of-art methods for pMRI reconstruction.

Algorithm 1. PRIM

Input: $\mathcal{R}$, b, x^0, λ, $t = 0$, ε

while not meet the stopping criterion **do**

$$W_{i,j,k}^t := 1/(\sqrt{\sum_{p=1}^{c}(\nabla_h x_{i,j,p}^t)^2 + (\nabla_v x_{i,j,p}^t)^2 + \varepsilon})$$

$$S^t := \mathcal{F}^H \mathcal{R}^H \mathcal{R} \mathcal{F} + \lambda\langle\nabla_h, W^t\nabla_h\rangle + \lambda\langle\nabla_v, W^t\nabla_v\rangle$$

$$P^t := \overline{\mathcal{F}^H \mathcal{R}^H \mathcal{R} \mathcal{F}} I + \lambda\langle\nabla_h, W^t\nabla_h\rangle + \lambda\langle\nabla_v, W^t\nabla_v\rangle$$

    while not meet the PCG stopping criterion **do**

        Update x^{t+1} by PCG for $S^t x = (\mathcal{R}\mathcal{F})^H b$ with preconditioner P^t

    end while

    $t := t + 1$

end while

---

4   Experiments

4.1   Experiment Setup

The experiments are conducted on three parallel MRI datasets in Figure 1.

3T Knee[13]. The MR image shown in figure 1(a) is a 3D FSE CUBE sequence with proton density weighting scanned on a GE 3T whole body scanner (TE=25ms, TR=1550ms, FOV=160mm, 320×320 matrix). This dataset is open access to public in `http://mridata.org`.

3T Brain[8]. Figure 1(b) shows an image scanned from a GE 3T commercial scanner with an eight-channel head coil using a two-dimensional T1-weighted spin echo protocol (TE = 11ms, TR = 700ms, FOV = 22cm, 256×256 pixels).

Signa-Excite 1.5T Brain[9]. Figure 1(c) shows a T1-weighted image from spoiled gradient echo (SPGR) sequence, scanned on a GE Signa-Excite 1.5-T scanner with an eight-channel receive coil (TE = 8ms, TR=17.6 ms, FOV = 20cm, 200×200 pixels).

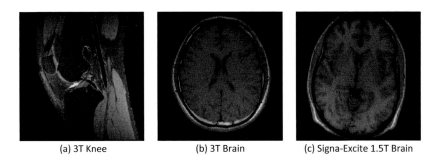

      (a) 3T Knee   (b) 3T Brain   (c) Signa-Excite 1.5T Brain

Fig. 1. Three MR images used in the experiments.

We implemented the proposed method for problem (1) and apply them to MRI k-space data with complex measurements. All experiments are conducted on a PC with Intel i7-4770 @ 3.40 GHz CPU and 16 GB RAM. We compare the proposed method with the state-of-art methods GRAPPA[4], CGSPIRiT[9], and CSSENSE[8]. Moreover, we compare them with SAKE[15] which is another calibrationless method proposed recently. We also compare the proposed method with FISTA_JTV[2] that solves the same JTV model. For fair comparisons, we download the codes from their websites and follow their default parameter settings carefully.

4.2   Numerical Results

Figure 2 shows the reconstruction results on 3T Knee MR image at a reduction factor $R = 4$, together with the ground-truth image. Quantitative comparison results for 3T Knee, 3T Brain and Signa-Excite 1.5T Brain datasets are shown in Table 1, 2 and 3, respectively. Compared to all other methods, the proposed method always preserves most details and suppress most noise (as shown in the zoomed region of interest). It does make sense because the JTV regularization acquires the prior knowledge that the gradients of MR images are typically sparse. The reconstruction results of GRAPPA, CGSPIRiT and SAKE are much more noisy in that their models do not include that assumption. Moreover, the gradient of each image coil(channel) is assumed similar in the JTV model which is the main reason for the better performance than CSSENSE. In this way, the JTV regularization makes the reconstruction result purer and more recognizable compared with other methods.

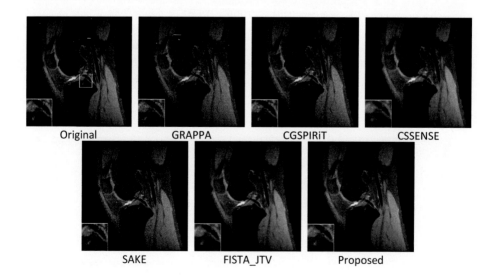

Fig. 2. Visual results of different methods compared with ground-truth. Best viewed in ×2 pdf.

Table 1. Quantitative comparison on 3T Knee dataset.

	GRAPPA	CGSPIRiT	CSSENSE	SAKE	FISTA_JTV	Proposed
RMSE ($\times 10^{-4}$)	11.7595	9.7159	6.9781	9.5650	6.3886	**6.3323**
SNR (db)	9.7149	11.3729	14.2479	11.5089	15.0145	**15.0914**
Time (s)	171.81	9.85	193.21	27.35	115.80	**9.74**

Table 2. Quantitative comparison on 3T Brain dataset.

	GRAPPA	CGSPIRiT	CSSENSE	SAKE	FISTA_JTV	Proposed
RMSE ($\times 10^{-4}$)	4.0159	3.5716	5.7170	3.3266	3.2563	**3.1963**
SNR (db)	21.9516	22.9699	18.8838	23.5871	23.7726	**23.9341**
Time (s)	172.69	9.79	193.40	28.34	113.81	**9.36**

Table 3. Quantitative comparison on Signa-Excite 1.5T Brain dataset.

	GRAPPA	CGSPIRiT	CSSENSE	SAKE	FISTA_JTV	Proposed
RMSE ($\times 10^{-4}$)	6.7155	5.5824	5.5891	4.7867	4.5506	**4.5155**
SNR (db)	17.2415	18.8467	18.8363	20.1823	20.6218	**20.6889**
Time (s)	173.03	9.82	193.47	28.49	116.07	**9.49**

It has also been noticed that our method always consumes least time on each MR image. GRAPPA requires more time for calibration when using random mask. SAKE calculates Singular Value Decomposition (SVD) of the pMRI data tensor in each iteration. The SVD takes $\mathcal{O}(n^3)$ time, resulting in the less efficiency compared with the proposed method. FISTA_JTV requires more inner loop iterations to converge in complex measurements. Overall, the proposed method is able to outperform the other methods in computational performance due to its superior convergence property and lower per-iteration computational cost.

5   Conclusion

We have proposed an novel algorithm PRIM to solve the joint total variation model for parallel MRI reconstruction. It is based on the iteratively reweighted least squares framework and preconditioned conjugate gradient method. Moreover, we have designed a novel preconditioner to strengthen its converge property as it requires to efficiently solve the least squares subproblem. The efficiency of PRIM is theoretically guaranteed and also exhibited in extensive experiments. With the joint gradient sparsity assumption in JTV model, the proposed method is able to provide much more accurate reconstruction result than other state-of-art methods with less time. All these benefits lead us closer to the calibrationless real-time parallel MRI reconstruction than ever before.

References

1. Chen, C., Huang, J., He, L., Li, H.: Preconditioning for accelerated iteratively reweighted least squares in structured sparsity reconstruction. In: CVPR 2014, pp. 2713–2720. IEEE (2014)
2. Chen, C., Li, Y., Huang, J.: Calibrationless parallel MRI with joint total variation regularization. In: Mori, K., Sakuma, I., Sato, Y., Barillot, C., Navab, N. (eds.) MICCAI 2013, Part III. LNCS, vol. 8151, pp. 106–114. Springer, Heidelberg (2013)
3. Daubechies, I., DeVore, R., Fornasier, M., Güntürk, C.S.: Iteratively reweighted least squares minimization for sparse recovery. Comm. on Pure and Applied Math. 63(1), 1–38 (2010)
4. Griswold, M.A., Jakob, P.M., Heidemann, R.M., Nittka, M., Jellus, V., Wang, J., Kiefer, B., Haase, A.: Generalized autocalibrating partially parallel acquisitions (GRAPPA). Magn. Reson. Med. 47(6), 1202–1210 (2002)
5. Huang, J., Zhang, S., Li, H., Metaxas, D.: Composite splitting algorithms for convex optimization. Computer Vision and Image Understanding 115(12), 1610–1622 (2011)
6. Huang, J., Zhang, S., Metaxas, D.: Efficient MR image reconstruction for compressed MR imaging. Medical Image Analysis 15(5), 670–679 (2011)
7. Hunter, D.R., Lange, K.: A tutorial on MM algorithms. The Amer. Stat. 58(1), 30–37 (2004)
8. Liang, D., Liu, B., Wang, J., Ying, L.: Accelerating SENSE using compressed sensing. Magn. Reson. Med. 62(6), 1574–1584 (2009)
9. Lustig, M., Pauly, J.M.: SPIRiT: Iterative self-consistent parallel imaging reconstruction from arbitrary k-space. Magn. Reson. Med. 64(2), 457–471 (2010)
10. Majumdar, A., Ward, R.K.: Calibration-less multi-coil mr image reconstruction. Magn. Reson. Imag. 30(7), 1032–1045 (2012)
11. Pruessmann, K.P., Weiger, M., Scheidegger, M.B., Boesiger, P., et al.: SENSE: sensitivity encoding for fast MRI. Magn. Reson. Med. 42(5), 952–962 (1999)
12. Saad, Y.: Iterative methods for sparse linear systems. Siam (2003)
13. Sawyer, A.M., Lustig, M., Alley, M., Uecker, P., Virtue, P., Lai, P., Vasanawala, S., Healthcare, G.: Creation of fully sampled MR data repository for compressed sensing of the knee (2013)
14. Shewchuk, J.R.: An introduction to the conjugate gradient method without the agonizing pain (1994)
15. Shin, P.J., Larson, P.E., Ohliger, M.A., Elad, M., Pauly, J.M., Vigneron, D.B., Lustig, M.: Calibrationless parallel imaging reconstruction based on structured low-rank matrix completion. Magn. Reson. Med. 72(4), 959–970 (2014)

Accessible Digital Ophthalmoscopy Based on Liquid-Lens Technology

Christos Bergeles, Pierre Berthet-Rayne, Philip McCormac,
Luis C. Garcia-Peraza-Herrera, Kosy Onyenso, Fan Cao,
Khushi Vyas, Melissa Berthelot, and Guang-Zhong Yang

The Hamlyn Centre, Imperial College London, London SW7 2AZ, UK
c.bergeles@imperial.ac.uk

Abstract. Ophthalmoscopes have yet to capitalise on novel low-cost
miniature optomechatronics, which could disrupt ophthalmic monitoring
in rural areas. This paper demonstrates a new design integrating modern components for ophthalmoscopy. Simulations show that the optical
elements can be reduced to just two lenses: an aspheric ophthalmoscopic
lens and a commodity liquid-lens, leading to a compact prototype. Circularly polarised transpupilary illumination, with limited use so far for
ophthalmoscopy, suppresses reflections, while autofocusing preserves image sharpness. Experiments with a human-eye model and cadaver porcine
eyes demonstrate our prototype's clinical value and its potential for accessible imaging when cost is a limiting factor[1].

1 Introduction

Given the extensive worldwide population suffering from a potentially blinding
ophthalmic pathology, innovation on intraocular observation methods is impera-
tive. In rural societies, patients that suffer from detectable and treatable diseases,
such as cataracts or retinopathy of prematurity, would benefit from easily accessible digital ophthalmoscopes. Notably, 80% of blindness is preventable when
detected early [1]. Disruptions in the miniaturisation of lenses, electronics, and
mechanical components, together with ubiquitous computing through micropro-
cessors, should instigate developments in ophthalmoscopy and reshape a field
substantially based on 20th century developments [2].

Retinal fundus imaging is a critical task in ophthalmoscopy, and, thus, the
focus of recent device innovations. Examples of new approaches to fundoscopy
mainly make use of smartphone technologies [3–5]. Initial approaches in 2012 en-
tailed observing the retina using a smartphone's camera and a handheld indirect
ophthalmoscopy lens [3]. Apart from leveraging the smartphone's camera, this
approach did not deviate from the principles of direct observation. The design
was improved in 2014 using a 3D-printed smartphone-attached length-adjustable
"arm" to hold the lens [5]. It was found that this approach was also cumbersome
to use due the requirement for manual mechanical focusing.

---

[1] With partial Fight for Sight, UK, support. Online resources: http://goo.gl/lvYbPp

© Springer International Publishing Switzerland 2015
N. Navab et al. (Eds.): MICCAI 2015, Part II, LNCS 9350, pp. 571–578, 2015.
DOI: 10.1007/978-3-319-24571-3_68

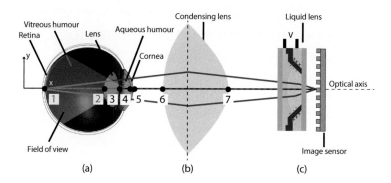

Fig. 1. Indirect ophthalmoscopy entails the use of a condensing lens, (b), held in front of the eye, (a). The image created by the lens is captured either with the clinician's eye, or, in our prototype, with a liquid lens and an image sensor, (c). The optical parameters of surfaces 1-7 are given in Table 1.

A limiting factor of smartphone-based approaches is that they do not account for the expense of the device itself. Thus, the reported costs are misleading and may amount to the cost of a hand-held commercial digital ophthalmoscope. Furthermore, the fact that 90% of blind people live in low-income countries [6] is not considered. Their location should be examined together with the lack of smartphone penetration, *e.g.*, only 37% of population in China, and only 19% in Kenya owns a smartphone [7]. Contrary, truly widespread ophthalmoscopic screening will make use of ubiquitous technology, as "dumb" mobile phones, which represent exceptional penetration (*e.g.*, 82% in Kenya [7]).

Our motivation is to use new lens technology to bring 21st century retinal imaging to vision care in developing economies, creating a low-cost digital ophthalmoscope that makes no use of a smartphone while minimising the system's optical and mechanical elements. Our device is based on state-of-the-art aspheric lenses and is among the first that uses liquid lenses. Optics simulations, selection of illumination components, and reflection-removal via relatively unexplored, in ophthalmoscopy, circularly polarised light, are described together with the selection of the appropriate autofocusing algorithm. Finally, the performance is evaluated with experiments in a human-eye phantom and porcine eyes.

2   Simulation, Design, and Integration

This section presents simulations, components, and integration of the developed digital ophthalmoscope with autofocusing software.

2.1   Optics

The human eye comprises the optical elements that create images on the curved retinal surface [see Fig. 1(a)]. Indirect digital retinal imaging is typically performed through a series of lenses, starting with a high-magnification lens, termed condensing lens, held in front of the eye [see Fig. 1(b)]. This lens reduces the refractive effect of the eye and creates a retinal image. Subsequently, in conventional ophthalmoscopes, field lenses flatten this image for capture by the image sensor [see Fig. 1(c)]. Each lens increases device cost and size and requires additional light intensity since each lens causes reflections and scattering.

Advanced machining techniques have recently enabled the manufacturing of double aspheric lenses, *i.e.*, precisely manufactured lenses whose surface is described by high-order polynomials:

$$x = \frac{y^2/R}{1 + \sqrt{1 - ((c+1)y^2/(R^2)}} + a_4 y^4 + a_6 y^6 + a_8 y^8 + a_{10} y^{10} \qquad (1)$$

where R is the radius of curvature, c is the conic constant, a_{4-10} are the asphericity coefficients, and the axes x and y are shown in Fig. 1. In theory, this class of lenses removes the optical aberrations of the human eye and create flat images. They are hand-held under direct clinical retinal observation with slit lamps and additional ophthalmoscopy equipment.

Biometric eye models based on human population averages have been created to enable optics' optimisation for ophthalmoscopy. This paper bases its results on Navarro's wide-field eye [8], which is an established biometric model explaining the eye's optical aberrations in a large ($\sim 70°$, measured from the eye's centre) field-of-view [see Fig. 1(a)]. The biometric model and aspheric condensing lens parameters, based on [9], are given in Table 1 for completeness. The double aspheric lenses listed in this paper belong to the family of lenses described in [10], which differ among themselves primarily on the field-of-view and magnification.

Simulations are performed using optical design software (OSLO and Trace Pro) from Lambda Research [see Fig. 2(a)]. Assuming that the system must focus on an intraocular range of distances spanning ± 5 mm around the nominal retinal depth, it is simulated that the images are formed behind the condensing lens at ± 3.5 mm around the focal length. This suggests that a single secondary optical element with a minimum range of focus of 7.0 mm, suffices to capture the retinal images created by this type of aspheric lenses. This leads to compact indirect ophthalmoscopy devices with only two optical elements.

Traditionally, focusing lenses are mechanically actuated. The addition of mechanical components, however, complicates device integration. Liquid-lenses, on the other hand, achieve focusing electrically through electrowetting [11]. The voltage applied on the lens regulates its shape, from concave to convex, and its focal length. The Varioptic Artic 416, retrieved from a Digitus Webcam (DA-708117), satisfies the low-cost criteria, and, with a working distance from 6 cm to infinity, covers the full extent of the simulated retinal image locations. The lens is controlled through our custom electronics, based on the Femtoduino® microcontroller and the Supertex HV892 liquid lens driver for voltage regulation.

The imaging sensor was extracted from Microsoft's LifeStudio® webcam, and was selected due to its reduced cost and high pixel density (720p HD). According to [12], retinal observation systems should have a pixel resolution of 50 per

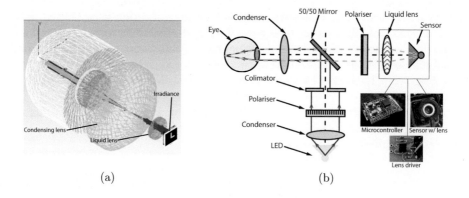

(a)   (b)

Fig. 2. (a) Simulation of optical elements and image sensor irradiance, and (b) Proto-typical optical system schematics.

Table 1. Parameters of the optical system

Surface	Radius	Conic Constant	Thickness	Refractive Index
1	12.00 mm	0.00	16.32 mm	1.336
2	6.00 mm	−1.00	4.00 mm	1.420
3	−10.20 mm	−3.13	3.05 mm	1.337
4	−6.50 mm	0.00	0.55 mm	1.376
5	−7.72 mm	−0.26	3.11 mm	1.000
6	11.65 mm	−9.24	13.00 mm	1.523
7	−9.48 mm	−1.07	∞	

	Asphericity			
	a_4	a_6	a_8	a_{10}
6	4.078×10^{-5}	-1.542×10^{-7}	-2.647×10^{-9}	2.023×10^{-11}

degree. The selected sensor should be used in conjunction with a $\sim 30°$ field-of-view, *e.g.*, with a high magnification condensing lens for observing the macular area, such as the Digital High Mag® from Volk, Inc.. The assembly of the liquid-lens on the camera sensor is shown in Fig. 2(b).

2.2   Illumination

Ophthalmic observation is achieved via transscleral or transpupilary illumina-tion. Diffused illumination through the sclera has been examined in the past by the authors and was found impractical due to scleral specularities and in-sufficient light intensity. Hence, the current prototype uses transpupilary illu-mination. Contrary to conventional Tungsten-lamp-based illumination, this new system uses high-power current-controlled LEDs (Luxon Rebel 4000K LED). Harmful UV-light can be filtered out using a UV-blocking-filter.

Transpupilary illumination suffers from reflections caused by the optical in-terfaces. These reflections are usually avoided with annuli that assign part of the pupil for imaging and the rest for illumination, resulting in a reduced field of view. Alternatively, our prototype uses circularly polarised light whose application in ophthalmoscopy is relatively unexplored [13], and has not been used by any smartphone-based apparatus. Reflection removal is achieved by two perpendicularly crossed polarisers, one placed at the emission LED and one at the imaging sensor. Reflected light retains polarisation, and, hence, is blocked by the second polariser, which permits only the light backscattered from the retina. The reduction of the optical elements minimises light loss due to reflection, and, hence, allows the introduction of the polarisers without a harmful increase in the supplied light energy.

The complete optical schematic of the device is shown in Fig. 2(b). The polarised LED light passes through a condensing lens and a collimator/pinhole, and is reflected by a 45° beam-splitter/mirror (50/50) (beamsplitter plate) towards the ophthalmoscopic condensing lens, which focuses it on the retina. Backscattered light is collimated by the condensing lens, and, through the mirror and the liquid-lens, focuses on the image sensor. Co-axiallity of the components is achieved using a concentric tube approach, where each tube houses an optical element.

2.3   Software

The liquid-lens is driven using Arduino® firmware. The entire system is integrated with software that currently runs on Matlab®; communication is via USB. The software controls video recording, light-intensity control, and autofocusing. Autofocusing is based on adjusting the lens' focus to maximise image information. The user selects the image region to be kept in-focus.

Three common sharpness metrics of increasing complexity were considered: a) the Tenengrad variance, *i.e.* the variance of image gradient, b) the Laplacian variance, and c) the Wavelet variance, *i.e.*, the variance of frequency-enhanced wavelet-transformed images:

$$\delta_{xy,\text{tenengrad}} = \sum_{(i,j)\in\Omega(x,y)} \left(G(i,j) - \overline{G}\right)^2 \tag{2}$$

$$\delta_{xy,\text{laplacian}} = \sum_{(i,j)\in\Omega(x,y)} \left(L(i,j) - \overline{L}\right)^2 \tag{3}$$

$$\delta_{xy,\text{wavelet}} = \sum_{(i,j)\in\Omega(x,y)} \sum_{n\in L,H, m\in L,H} \left[\left(W_{nm}(i,j) - \overline{W_{nm}}\right)^2 \right] \tag{4}$$

where (i,j) span the pixels of the selected region $\Omega(x,y)$, G is the magnitude of the image gradient, $\overline{G}$ the magnitude's average, L is the Laplacian's magnitude, $\overline{L}$ the average, and W_{LH}, W_{HL}, W_{LL}, and W_{HH} correspond to the respective low-and-high image frequency subtends of the wavelet transform (see [14] for details). Maximisation of the focus functions is related to stronger edge information, *i.e.* sharper, images. The computational performance of the sharpness calculations in relation with linear optimal-focus search and bisection search

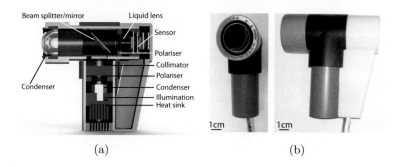

(a)   (b)

Fig. 3. (a) CAD with mechatronics components annotated, and (b) The prototype.

were evaluated. The linear search method exhaustively searches for the best in-focus image throughout the lens' focus range, thus avoiding local minima, while the bisection search method exploits the "bell-shaped" nature of the sharpness function to alternate its search around an estimated optimal focus position. Finally, autofocus is triggered only after loss of focus, *i.e.*, when the calculated focus-score for image region changes by more than a user-specified percentage.

3   Results

Figure 3 shows the actual device and the prototype's CAD with all mechatronics annotated. All housing components are 3D-printed on an Eden 350, with internal components printed in black to minimise light reflection. The prototype is evaluated with experiments in a human-eye phantom and porcine eyes.

3.1   Human Eye Phantom

The human eye phantom from Gwb International, Ltd., is air-filled and has a single lens that mimics the compound effect of the human eye optics. It's hand-painted retina makes it a common platform for ophthalmoscope demonstrations. Reflection removal and autofocusing are evaluated on this phantom.

Figure 4(a)-top demonstrates the extent of reflections without the polarisers. Removal of the reflections via software, as is commonly performed in medical image processing, would only lead to extended image areas with approximated information. The perpendicularly crossed polarisers dramatically reduce the reflections, as shown in Fig. 4(a)-bottom.

Autofocusing using the Tenengrad, Laplacian, and Wavelet variances is evaluated by discretising the range of focus, *i.e.*, the liquid-lens control voltage, into 255 levels, and comparing the selected focus-score maxima. In the representative example of Fig. 4(b), it can be seen that the focus-score functions lead to similar results. Our experiments showed that the Tenengrad variance requires only 4.9 s for a complete focus sweep, compared to 7.4 s for the Laplacian variance and 12.1 s for the Wavelet variance. Hence, the computationally simpler Tenengrad

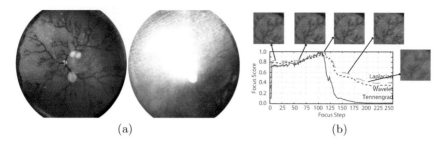

Fig. 4. (a) Reflections on the eye phantom without (left), and with (right), polarisation, and (b) example of focus-point estimation for the three focus-score functions.

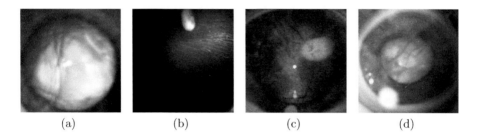

(a)   (b)   (c)   (d)

Fig. 5. Retinal fundus imaging in cadaver porcine eyes. (a) Opaque intraocular lens, (b) retinal haemorrhage, (c), (d) additional retinal images.

focus metric was selected. In addition, the linear search method outperformed the bisection-search method due to the fact that the liquid lens' limited response bandwidth cannot follow the rapid changes in voltage required by the later. Also, the linear sweep avoids local minima. In practice, we sweep the focus range in tuneable steps (every 9 voltage steps, specifically, as decided with preliminary experiments) to achieve faster refocusing; the speed could be further improved by searching in the vicinity of the previous best focus position.

3.2   Ex Vivo Experiments

Porcine eyes are a good model of human eyes in terms of dimension and optical components, so they are routinely used for training. Fresh porcine cadaver eyes were purchased and transported to our lab in ice. During experiments with 20 porcine eyes, the corneas were moisturised to avoid opacification. Since the pupil of the cadaver eyes is relaxed, the intraocular field of view is reduced. Autofocusing is achieved by maximising the Tenengrad measure of a window at the centre of the image.

The ophthalmoscope was used by a clinical student to study the porcine retinas. Figure 5(a) shows an opacified intraocular lens that could indicate cataract. Such examinations are especially useful for rural populations. In Fig. 5(b)-(d), the retina is in focus; extended field of view could be visualised by moving the eye. A pathological case was identified among the porcine samples: Fig. 5(b) shows a haemorrhage resulting in the dark purple colour in the retinal image. Hence, the clinical value of this low-cost device is experimentally supported.

4 Conclusions and Discussion

Routine retinal observations are paramount for disease prevention, and novel optomechatronics support the ophthalmoscope's evolution. Our primary contributions include the integration of a liquid lens and an aspheric lens with cross polarising filters, and autofocusing in a compact device. Its clinical value is supported by *ex vivo* experiments, and its low-cost, $200 excluding the necessary aspheric lens, makes it accessible to developing economies. Ongoing work investigates image improvement and focus estimation on an embedded chip.

References

1. Pascolini, D., Mariotti, S.P.: Global estimates of visual impairment: 2010. British J. Ophthalmology 300538, 1–5 (2011)
2. Keeler, C.R.: A brief history of the ophthalmoscope. Optometry in Practice 4, 137–145 (2003)
3. Bastawrous, A.: Smartphone fundoscopy. Ophthalmology 119(2), 432–433 (2012)
4. Giardini, M.E., Livingstone, I.A.T., Jordan, S., Bolster, N.M., Peto, T., Burton, M., Bastawrous, A.: A smartphone based ophthalmoscope. In: IEEE Int. Conf. Engineering in Medicine and Biology, pp. 2177–2180 (2014)
5. Lin, S.J., Yang, C.M., Yeh, P.T., Ho, T.-C.H.: Smartphone fundoscopy for retinopathy of prematurity. Taiwan J. Ophthalmology 4(2), 82–85 (2014)
6. Bastawrous, A., Hennig, B.D.: The global inverse care law: a distorted map of blindness. British J. Ophthalmology 96, 1357–1358 (2012)
7. Bolster, N.M., Giardini, M.E., Livingstone, I.A.T., Bastawrous, A.: How the smartphone is driving the eye-health imaging resolution. Expert Review on Ophthalmology 9(6), 475–485 (2014)
8. Escudero-Sanz, I., Navarro, R.: Off-axis aberrations of a wide-angle schematic eye model. J. Optical Society of America A 16(8), 1881–1891 (1999)
9. Bergeles, C., Shamaei, K., Abbott, J.J., Nelson, B.J.: Single-camera focus-based localization of intraocular devices. IEEE Trans. Biomedical Engineering 57(8), 2064–2074 (2010)
10. Volk, D.A.: Indirect ophthalmoscopy lens for use with split lamp or other biomicroscope, January 6, 1998. U.S. Patent 5,706,073
11. Kuiper, S., Hendriks, B.H.W.: Variable-focus liquid lens for miniature cameras. Applied Physics Letters 85(7), 1128–1130 (2004)
12. Bernardes, R., Serranho, P., Lobo, C.: Digital ocular fundus imaging: a review. Ophthalmologica 226(4), 161–181 (2011)
13. Tran, K., Mendel, T.A., Holbrook, K.L., Yates, P.A.: Construction of an inexpensive, hand-held fundus camera through modification of a consumer point-and-shoot camera. Investigative Ophthalmology and Visual Science 53(12), 7600–7607 (2012)
14. Yang, G., Nelson, B.J.: Wavelet-based autofocusing and unsupervised segmentation of microscopic images. In: IEEE/RSJ Int. Conf. Intell. Rob. Sys., pp. 2143–2148 (2003)

Estimate, Compensate, Iterate: Joint Motion Estimation and Compensation in 4-D Cardiac C-arm Computed Tomography

Oliver Taubmann[1,2], Günter Lauritsch[3], Andreas Maier[1,2], Rebecca Fahrig[4], and Joachim Hornegger[1,2]

[1] Pattern Recognition Lab., Computer Science Department,
Friedrich-Alexander-University Erlangen-Nuremberg, Germany
[2] Graduate School in Advanced Optical Technologies (SAOT), Erlangen, Germany
[3] Siemens AG, Healthcare, Forchheim, Germany
[4] Radiological Sciences Laboratory, Stanford University, California, USA

Abstract. C-arm computed tomography reconstruction of multiple cardiac phases could provide a highly useful tool to interventional cardiologists in the catheter laboratory. Today, however, for clinically reasonable acquisition protocols the achievable image quality is still severely limited due to undersampling artifacts. We propose an iterative optimization scheme combining image registration, motion compensation and spatio-temporal regularization to improve upon the state-of-the-art w. r. t. image quality and accuracy of motion estimation. Evaluation of clinical cases indicates an improved visual appearance and temporal consistency, evidenced by a strong decrease in temporal variance in uncontrasted regions accompanied by an increased sharpness of the contrasted left ventricular blood pool boundary. In a phantom study, the universal image quality index proposed by Wang et al. is raised from 0.80 to 0.95, with 1.0 corresponding to a perfect match with the ground truth. The results lay a promising foundation for interventional cardiac functional analysis.

1 Introduction

Ventricular wall motion analysis is commonly performed with cardiac magnetic resonance imaging or 3-D echocardiography. However, as these modalities do not readily fit into the workflow of most cardiac interventions, 2-D ventriculography is still frequently used for intraprocedural functional evaluation of cardiac motion. During cardiac resynchronization therapy, volumetric reconstruction of several heart phases, i. e. 4-D imaging, could help physicians find the optimal lead position by providing valuable information regarding the area of latest contraction [2]. Rotational angiography using C-arm devices as they are commonly found in catheter labs in combination with multi-segment retrospective ECG-gating could generate such images [4]. However, for protocols that achieve clinically reasonable acquisition times by performing only a single sweep [1], the gated reconstructions suffer severely from sparse view sampling.

N. Navab et al. (Eds.): MICCAI 2015, Part II, LNCS 9350, pp. 579–586, 2015.
DOI: 10.1007/978-3-319-24571-3_69

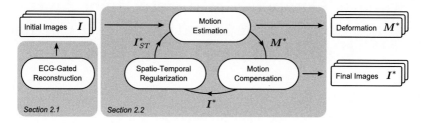

Fig. 1. A schematic overview of our iterative method, notation and paper structure.

In recent literature, several publications have focused on 4-D imaging with C-arm systems. For instance, Mory et al. employ 4-D iterative reconstruction with both spatial and temporal regularization [8]. While this approach can be of use in coping with angular undersampling, the achieved image quality is still severely limited by the small amount of data available for each cardiac phase and the "cartoon-like" appearance of the reconstructed images. Müller et al. attempt to overcome this problem by combining analytical reconstruction with motion compensation [10]. They estimate the motion between all phases of the initial, ECG-gated reconstruction, and then compensate for it in a final reconstruction step using all acquired projection data. However, motion estimation is highly sensitive to the quality of the initial images and artifacts typically propagate into the final images as artificial motion patterns. In this paper, we propose a method to combine the state-of-the-art motion-compensated filtered back-projection reconstruction technique with a novel iterative process incorporating spatio-temporal regularization to reduce artificial motion and further improve both image quality and accuracy of motion estimation.

2   Materials and Methods

Below, we first describe the generation of ECG-gated initial images (section 2.1). They serve as the input to our joint motion estimation and compensation framework presented in section 2.2. An overview of the method is shown in Fig. 1. Afterwards, details regarding our experimental data are provided (section 2.3).

2.1   Initial Image Generation

Initial images for each heart phase are generated using Feldkamp-Davis-Kress (FDK) filtered back-projection reconstruction combined with retrospective ECG-gating using a rectangular window. As only a subset of the projection images is used, we perform the following steps for denoising and reduction of few-view artifacts: **(i)** A two-pass removal of high-density objects such as catheters within the reconstruction field of view (FOV) [9]. **(ii)** A threshold-based masking in the filtered projection images to reduce artifacts caused by cables outside the FOV. **(iii)** An approach by McKinnon and Bates [7] to further reduce undersampling artifacts, in which object-dependent artifact images are estimated and subsequently subtracted from the original images. **(iv)** Denoising with a joint bilateral filter [14] guided by a standard FDK reconstruction from all data.

2.2   Joint Motion Estimation and Compensation

Artifacts in the initial images propagate through motion estimation, leading to inconsistent movement patterns. Motion-compensated images, due to smoothness of the motion model and the no longer incomplete sampling, offer a clearer distinction of structures in the sense that high intensity differences are much more likely to be caused by an actual difference in underlying anatomical properties instead of merely artifacts. This enables us to use more aggressive edge-preserving filtering to eliminate inconsistency in both the spatial and temporal domain while preserving actual motion. In turn, these filtered images allow for a much more robust motion estimation, leading to a motion compensation with fewer inconsistencies. By iteratively filtering, estimating and compensating for motion, we can jointly improve both our images and our motion estimate.

Let $\boldsymbol{I} = \{\boldsymbol{I}^t : t \in \mathcal{N}_{\mathrm{ph}}\}$ denote 3-D images for all cardiac phases t, with $\mathcal{N}_{\mathrm{ph}} = \{1, \ldots, N_{\mathrm{phases}}\}$. Similarly, $\boldsymbol{M} = \{\boldsymbol{M}_{t \to t'} : t, t' \in \mathcal{N}_{\mathrm{ph}}\}$ are deformation operators, where $\boldsymbol{M}_{t \to t'} \boldsymbol{I}^t$ is the image $\boldsymbol{I}^t$ transformed to phase t', i. e. deformed according to the motion between cardiac phases t and t'. $\boldsymbol{M}_{t \to t}$ is defined as the identity transform and not part of the optimization process. The steps of motion estimation, compensation and spatio-temporal regularization described below are performed in an alternating manner.

Motion Estimation is performed by pair-wise 3-D/3-D image registration of all combinations of cardiac phases,

$$\boldsymbol{M}^* = \left\{ \underset{\boldsymbol{M}_{t \to t'}}{\operatorname{argmin}} \left[\mathcal{D} \left(\boldsymbol{I}^{t'}, \boldsymbol{M}_{t \to t'} \boldsymbol{I}^t \right) \right] : t, t' \in \mathcal{N}_{\mathrm{ph}}, \ t \neq t' \right\}, \tag{1}$$

where $\mathcal{D}(\cdot, \cdot)$ is a dissimilarity measure. In our experiments, we use the negative normalized cross correlation and a uniform cubic B-spline motion model [10] with an isotropic control point spacing of 8 mm for the deformation operators $\boldsymbol{M}$. Optimization is performed on a multi-resolution pyramid with 3 levels using a quasi-Newton method, the limited-memory Broyden-Fletcher-Goldfarb-Shanno (L-BFGS) algorithm. 10,000 random image samples per iteration and level are evaluated. For faster convergence, motion estimation is restricted to a manually defined region of interest (ROI) containing the heart and covering roughly $5 - 10\,\%$ of the full volume. Our implementation is based on `elastix`, a toolbox for nonrigid registration of medical images [3]. In the first iteration, $\boldsymbol{I}$ consists of the initial images (cf. section 2.1). In later iterations, we perform registration on the current regularized motion-compensated images, but do not initialize with the previous motion estimate so as not to introduce bias towards a solution potentially converged to an undesirable local minimum.

Motion Compensation amounts to incorporating the current motion estimate in the data fidelity equation of the reconstruction problem for all phases,

$$\boldsymbol{I}^* = \left\{ \boldsymbol{I}^t : \boldsymbol{A}^{t'} \boldsymbol{M}_{t \to t'} \boldsymbol{I}^t = \boldsymbol{P}^{t'}; \ t, t' \in \mathcal{N}_{\mathrm{ph}} \right\}, \tag{2}$$

where $\boldsymbol{A}^{t'}$ is the X-ray projection operator belonging to the measured projection data $\boldsymbol{P}^{t'}$ assigned to phase t' during gating. Thus, for reconstruction of each individual phase t, data belonging to all phases t' are used. The images $\boldsymbol{I}^*$ are found using a variant of FDK-type filtered back-projection which compensates for motion by shifting each voxel according to the given transformation during the back-projection step [11]. This approach is efficient, which is crucial for use in an interventional setting, and at the same time guarantees that we do not lose resolution through repeated interpolation and regularization as we reconstruct anew—directly from the projection images—in each iteration.

Spatio-temporal Filtering is introduced to regularize the optimization. For this purpose, we adopt the common notion of favoring piece-wise constant images and apply spatial and temporal bilateral filters which are straightforward to parameterize and increase sparsity in the gradient domain. They read,

$$\boldsymbol{I}_S^t(\boldsymbol{x}) = \sum_{\boldsymbol{x}' \in N(\boldsymbol{x})} \frac{\boldsymbol{I}^t(\boldsymbol{x}')}{w_S} \cdot \exp\left(-\frac{\|\boldsymbol{x} - \boldsymbol{x}'\|_2^2}{2\sigma_S^2} - \frac{(\boldsymbol{I}^t(\boldsymbol{x}) - \boldsymbol{I}^t(\boldsymbol{x}'))^2}{2\sigma_I^2} \right), \quad (3)$$

$$\boldsymbol{I}_{ST}^t(\boldsymbol{x}) = \sum_{t' \in \mathcal{N}_{\mathrm{ph}}} \frac{\boldsymbol{I}_S^{t'}(\boldsymbol{x})}{w_T} \cdot \exp\left(-\frac{\mathrm{dist}^2(t, t')}{2\sigma_T^2} - \frac{(\boldsymbol{I}^t(\boldsymbol{x}) - \boldsymbol{I}^{t'}(\boldsymbol{x}))^2}{2\sigma_I^2} \right), \quad (4)$$

with σ_S, σ_T and σ_I the Gaussian standard deviations in the spatial, temporal and intensity domain, respectively. $N(\boldsymbol{x})$ is a local neighborhood around $\boldsymbol{x}$, w_S and w_T are normalization factors. $\mathrm{dist}(\cdot, \cdot)$ denotes the distance of two phases in the cardiac cycle, taking periodicity into account. By means of this edge-preserving filtering, we produce cleaner images $\boldsymbol{I}_{ST}^* = \{ \boldsymbol{I}_{ST}^t : t \in \mathcal{N}_{\mathrm{ph}} \}$ with an improved temporal consistency for motion estimation in the next iteration. Note, however, that we stop iterating right after the motion compensation step to avoid an over-smoothed appearance in the final output.

2.3   Experiments

Clinical Data. Three data sets of clinical cases were acquired with an Artis zeego system (Siemens AG, Healthcare, Forchheim, Germany). 381 projection images were captured at approx. 30 Hz with an angular increment of 0.52° during one 14 s long rotation of the C-arm. The isotropic pixel resolution was 0.31 mm/pixel (0.21 in isocenter), the detector size 1240 × 960 pixels. External pacing was applied to ensure a heart rate of 115 bpm. The gating windows cover 10 % of the heart cycle each and are chosen to use all data without overlap, resulting in 10 cardiac phases to be reconstructed for both the initial and motion-compensated images. Undiluted contrast agent was injected in the pulmonary artery at a speed of 7 ml/s (91 ml total). All images were reconstructed on a grid of 256^3 voxels covering a volume of size $(25.6\,\mathrm{cm})^3$.

Phantom Model. For further evaluation, a numerical phantom data set was used [12,5]. 381 projection images of the phantom were simulated using a polychromatic spectrum, discretized in energy bins 2.5 keV wide from 25 keV to 120 keV (peak energy), and a time-current product of 2.5 mAs per X-ray pulse.

For bones and bone marrow, material properties match the mass attenuation coefficients found in the NIST X-ray table[1], while other structures were modeled with the absorption behavior of water for modified densities. For the contrasted left ventricular blood pool, the contrasted blood in the aorta and the myocardium, the densities were set to $2.5\,\mathrm{g/cm}^3$, $2.0\,\mathrm{g/cm}^3$ and $1.5\,\mathrm{g/cm}^3$, respectively. Additionaly, a complete set of projection images for a single cardiac phase (static phantom) was generated for reconstruction of a ground truth image. Other properties of the phantom data set, such as the number of heart beats and the resolution and dimensions of the images, were chosen to reflect the clinical data sets used in this study.

Experimental Setup. Images $I_3^t(x)$ reconstructed with 3 iterations of the proposed method were compared to the the state-of-the-art method by Müller et al. [9], which corresponds to the result $I_1^t(x)$ of the first motion-compensation step. As the preprocessing steps **(ii)** through **(iv)** (cf. section 2.1) have a strong impact on initial image quality, they were also added to their approach to enable a fair comparison with our method. In our experiments, we set $\sigma_S = 5\,\mathrm{mm}$ and $\sigma_T = 60\,\%$ of the cardiac cycle. Although rather large, these spatial and temporal kernel widths proved to work well for all our data sets as we choose σ_I so as to preserve the expected gray value difference between contrasted blood and surrounding tissue. In contrast to typical regularization weights, its value can be intuitively defined on the same scale as the observed intensities, which brings down the common, but often crucially unaddressed problem of proper parameterization to a manageable level.

Evaluation Measures. For quantitative evaluation of the phantom study, we compared the root mean square error (RMSE) as well as the universal image quality index (UQI), a correlation measure proposed by Wang et al. [15], w. r. t. the static ground truth reconstruction. For calculation of the UQI, the volume was divided into regular blocks of size $(16\,\mathrm{mm})^3$ each. Only those fully encompassed by the ROI used for registration (cf. section 2.2) were selected, resulting in a total of 9 blocks. To assess accuracy of motion estimation, we compared the dense motion fields obtained by evaluating the estimated B-spline model on the voxel grid against ground truth motion interpolated from the phantom surface definitions [6] between end-systole and end-diastole. For all data sets, overall visual image quality was scored by 9 experts in medical image processing at our institute. The images were shown in a randomized order to scorers blinded to the employed method. Similar to common approaches for (spatial) signal-to-noise ratio estimation, temporal consistency can also be measured as the temporal variance of intensity values in homogeneous regions consisting of uncontrasted blood and tissue: Ideally, they should appear mostly static over the course of the cardiac cycle as no motion is observed there. At the same time, it is essential to rule out a critical loss of spatial resolution when applying spatio-temporal smoothing. For nonlinear, object-dependent reconstruction methods, standardized modulation transfer function (MTF) evaluations cannot

---

[1] http://physics.nist.gov/PhysRefData/Xcom/html/xcom1.html

Table 1. For all data sets, the observed decrease in temporal variance, $\phi = 1 - \left(\text{var}_t[\boldsymbol{I}_3^t]\right)\left(\text{var}_t[\boldsymbol{I}_1^t]\right)^{-1}$, averaged over homogeneous uncontrasted, i. e. ideally static regions is given. Similarly, ξ_a and ξ_b are the ratios of edge sharpness estimates [13], i. e. descriptors of the relative sharpness increase, in short-axis slices towards the apical and basal ends of the end-diastolic heart, respectively. The visual image quality scores assigned by 9 experts at our institute are given as s_1 for $\boldsymbol{I}_1^t(\boldsymbol{x})$ and s_3 for $\boldsymbol{I}_3^t(\boldsymbol{x})$, ranging from 0 (unacceptable) to 4 (very good).

Data set	$\bar{\phi}$	ξ_a	ξ_b	s_1	s_3
Patient 1	50.1 %	1.22	1.24	2.1 ± 0.60	3.7 ± 0.50
Patient 2	31.5 %	1.02	1.21	1.4 ± 0.73	2.4 ± 0.88
Patient 3	30.8 %	1.03	1.22	1.4 ± 0.53	3.4 ± 0.73
Phantom	87.4 %	1.02	1.05	1.9 ± 0.78	3.7 ± 0.50

be applied, necessitating measurements of edge sharpness instead. Following the approach described in [13] for assessing reduction of motion blur, we measured the sharpness of the contrasted left ventricular blood pool as the anatomical structure of interest. For this purpose, ensembles of line profiles were placed along the edge in short-axis views and then used to robustly estimate its slope.

3   Results and Discussion

For the phantom data set, our method reduced the RMSE over the ROI from 86.3 HU to 73.6 HU (a decrease of 14.7 %), and raised the UQI from 0.80 to 0.95, where 1.0 would correspond to a perfect match. Although, like most, our phantom is piece-wise constant and therefore matches the prior knowledge assumption, rendering it easier to reconstruct with our method, we believe that it is still meaningful to compare the images as they are unregularized filtered backprojections of the same projection data albeit corrected according to different motion estimates. The motion estimation error, computed as the average magnitude of the difference vectors over the ROI, was reduced from 2.08 ± 1.92 mm to 1.52 ± 1.91 mm, a substantial decrease. Note that the numbers are higher than typically expected of target registration errors as we do not limit the evaluation to landmarks for which the motion is known to be observable in the images.

The results of the observer study, listed in Tab. 1, demonstrate a clear preference toward the proposed method as the images are disturbed less by artificial motion patterns. This is also reflected by the fact that our method was able to greatly reduce temporal inconsistency, as seen from the variance measurements in Tab. 1. The same effect is visualized by the difference images in Fig. 2 where we note a reduced amount of noise-like patterns. For visual comparison, animations of reconstructed data sets are available on our website[2]. From the edge sharpness measurements, which are also listed in Tab. 1, we observe a slight overall increase in sharpness. In the phantom, edges already exhibit a high sharpness with the

---

[2] http://www5.cs.fau.de/our-team/taubmann-oliver/supplementary-material

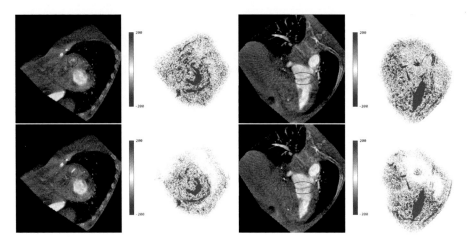

Fig. 2. Short-axis (left) and long-axis (right) views of patient data set 1 in end-diastole reconstructed with both the proposed (bottom) and the state-of-the-art method (top). The color-coded images show the difference between end-diastole and end-systole.

state-of-the-art method, leaving less room for improvement. The lowest values in the clinical data sets occur for the motion-intensive apical regions of patients 2 and 3, which we could confirm visually to have worse contrast than patient 1, thus requiring a more conservatively chosen value of σ_I. This also explains the lower decrease in temporal variance observed in these data sets.

Performance-wise, the motion estimation step constitutes the computational bottleneck of our current implementation. On average, registration of two volumes takes 10-30 s on a machine equipped with a quad-core 2.93 GHz CPU and 12 GB of RAM. Run times of the regularization and reconstruction steps are about 3 s and 85 s per volume, respectively.

4   Conclusion

For advancing accuracy and quality of interventional 4-D cardiac imaging, a scheme for iterative motion estimation and compensation is proposed, enabling the use of stronger regularization. Evaluations on C-arm CT data sets of clinical patients and a numerical heart phantom reveal distinct improvements compared to the state-of-the-art, both in terms of visual quality and accuracy of motion estimation. The results hold promise for efforts toward interventional cardiac functional analysis, which will also be subject of our future work.

Acknowledgments and Disclaimer. The authors gratefully acknowledge funding of the Erlangen Graduate School in Advanced Optical Technologies (SAOT) by the German Research Foundation (DFG) in the framework of the German excellence initiative, and thank Dr. Abt, Centre of Cardiovascular Diseases, Rotenburg a.d. Fulda, for providing the image data. The concepts and information presented in this paper are based on research and are not commercially available.

References

1. De Buck, S., Dauwe, D., Wielandts, J.Y., Claus, P., Janssens, S., Heidbuchel, H., Nuyens, D.: A new approach for prospectively gated cardiac rotational angiography. Proc. SPIE 8668 (2013)
2. Döring, M., Braunschweig, F., Eitel, C., Gaspar, T., Wetzel, U., Nitsche, B., Hindricks, G., Piorkowski, C.: Individually tailored left ventricular lead placement: lessons from multimodality integration between three-dimensional echocardiography and coronary sinus angiogram. Europace 15(5), 718–727 (2013)
3. Klein, S., Staring, M., Murphy, K., Viergever, M., Pluim, J.: elastix: a toolbox for intensity based medical image registration. IEEE Trans. Med. Imag. 29(1), 196–205 (2010)
4. Lauritsch, G., Boese, J., Wigstrom, L., Kemeth, H., Fahrig, R.: Towards cardiac C-arm computed tomography. IEEE Trans. Med. Imag. 25(7), 922–934 (2006)
5. Maier, A., Hofmann, H., Berger, M., Fischer, P., Schwemmer, C., Wu, H., Müller, K., Hornegger, J., Choi, J.H., Riess, C., Keil, A., Fahrig, R.: CONRAD - A software framework for cone-beam imaging in radiology. Med. Phys. 40(11) (2013)
6. Maier, A., Taubmann, O., Wetzl, J., Wasza, J., Forman, C., Fischer, P., Hornegger, J., Fahrig, R.: Fast Interpolation of Dense Motion Fields from Synthetic Phantoms. In: BVM, pp. 168–173 (2014)
7. Mc Kinnon, G.C., Bates, R.: Towards imaging the beating heart usefully with a conventional CT scanner. IEEE Trans. Biomed. Eng. BME 28(2), 123–127 (1981)
8. Mory, C., Auvray, V., Zhang, B., Grass, M., Schäfer, D., Chen, S., Carroll, J., Rit, S., Peyrin, F., Douek, P., Boussel, L.: Cardiac C-arm computed tomography using a 3D + time ROI reconstruction method with spatial and temporal regularization. Med. Phys. 41, 021903 (2014)
9. Müller, K., Lauritsch, G., Schwemmer, C., Maier, A., Taubmann, O., Abt, B., Köhler, H., Nöttling, A., Hornegger, J., Fahrig, R.: Catheter artifact reduction (CAR) in dynamic cardiac chamber imaging with interventional C-arm CT. In: Proc. Intl. Conf. on Image Formation in X-ray CT, pp. 418–421 (2014)
10. Müller, K., Maier, A., Schwemmer, C., Lauritsch, G., Buck, S.D., Wielandts, J.Y., Hornegger, J., Fahrig, R.: Image artefact propagation in motion estimation and reconstruction in interventional cardiac C-arm CT. Phys. Med. Biol. 59(12), 3121–3138 (2014)
11. Schäfer, D., Borgert, J., Rasche, V., Grass, M.: Motion-compensated and gated cone beam filtered back-projection for 3-D rotational X-ray angiography. IEEE Trans. Med. Imag. 25, 898–906 (2006)
12. Segars, W.P., Sturgeon, G., Mendonca, S., Grimes, J., Tsui, B.M.W.: 4D XCAT phantom for multimodality imaging research. Med. Phys. 37, 4902–4915 (2010)
13. Taubmann, O., Wetzl, J., Lauritsch, G., Maier, A., Hornegger, J.: Sharp as a Tack: Measuring and Comparing Edge Sharpness in Motion-Compensated Medical Image Reconstruction. In: BVM, pp. 425–430 (2015)
14. Tomasi, C., Manduchi, R.: Bilateral filtering for gray and color images. In: ICCV, pp. 839–846 (1998)
15. Wang, Z., Bovik, A.: A universal image quality index. IEEE Signal Proc. Let. 9(3), 81–84 (2002)

Robust Prediction of Clinical Deep Brain Stimulation Target Structures via the Estimation of Influential High-Field MR Atlases

Jinyoung Kim[1], Yuval Duchin[2], Hyunsoo Kim[1,3], Jerrold Vitek[4],
Noam Harel[2,5], and Guillermo Sapiro[1,3]

[1] Department of ECE, Duke University, Durham, NC, USA
[2] CMRR, University of Minnesota, Minneapolis, MN, USA
[3] Department of Biomedical Engineering, Duke University, Durham, NC, USA
[4] Department of Neurology, University of Minnesota, Minneapolis, MN, USA
[5] Department of Neurosurgery, University of Minnesota, Minneapolis, MN, USA

Abstract. This work introduces a robust framework for predicting Deep Brain Stimulation (DBS) target structures which are not identifiable on standard clinical MRI. While recent high-field MR imaging allows clear visualization of DBS target structures, such high-fields are not clinically available, and therefore DBS targeting needs to be performed on the standard clinical low contrast data. We first learn via regression models the shape relationships between DBS targets and their potential predictors from high-field (7 Tesla) MR training sets. A bagging procedure is utilized in the regression model, reducing the variability of learned dependencies. Then, given manually or automatically detected predictors on the clinical patient data, the target structure is predicted using the learned high quality information. Moreover, we derive a robust way to properly weight different training subsets, yielding higher accuracy when using an ensemble of predictions. The subthalamic nucleus (STN), the most common DBS target for Parkinson's disease, is used to exemplify within our framework. Experimental validation from Parkinson's patients shows that the proposed approach enables reliable prediction of the STN from the clinical 1.5T MR data.

1 Introduction

Deep brain stimulation (DBS) surgery is commonly used for symptom's treatment in neuro-degenerative diseases such as Parkinson's disease (PD). Precise placement of electrodes within crucial sub-cortical region (e.g., subthalamic nucleus (STN)) leads to successful DBS procedures [1].

Standard DBS targeting approaches today refer to anatomical information based on normalized atlases, particularly based on a single histology sample [1–3]. However, in such indirect methods, the variability in the position and size of the DBS targets needs to be further analyzed in the context of large populations for the reliability [2, 3]. To verify the target location, electrophysiological measurements, such as microelectrode recording (MER), that are lengthy and might result in increased risks for hemorrhage are required during surgery [1–3].

© Springer International Publishing Switzerland 2015
N. Navab et al. (Eds.): MICCAI 2015, Part II, LNCS 9350, pp. 587–594, 2015.
DOI: 10.1007/978-3-319-24571-3_70

Direct visualization and localization of the targets on the *individual* patient are needed for reliable, safe, and time-efficient DBS targeting. With advances in high-field MR (e.g., 7 Tesla (7T)), the superior contrast and high resolution imaging allow to directly identify and visualize the DBS targets, reducing the need for MER and other lengthy intra-operative burdensome steps [1, 3–6]. However, such high-fields are limited in clinical use, and thus the targets need to be localized on standard clinical low-field MR data. Unfortunately, clear visualization of DBS targets is not feasible with such standard clinical MRI protocols.

The aim of this work is to predict the location and shape of the DBS targets that are not normally identifiable on clinical 1.5T MRI. Recent studies have introduced regression approaches to estimate limited shape information within regions of interest from given predictors in the data [7–10]. In our scenario, it is hard to even manually localize DBS targets on the clinical low-field MRI, and thus it is still challenging to build high quality training data for such regression models from just the standard clinical data. In addition, the large variability of learned information from various training subsets might actually increase the uncertainty of the prediction. Furthermore, the influence of such subsets to prediction performance needs to be considered when developing reliable prediction.

In this work we propose a robust prediction framework for reliable DBS targeting on clinical low-field MRI, automatically learning dependencies between targets and predictors from more relevant high-field MR atlases. A key contribution of our work is how to learn shape relationships from high-field MR training sets applicable for DBS targeting on clinical low-field MRI. High quality information on the 7T MR training data is then transferred for DBS targeting onto the 1.5T MRI from a query patient. We apply bagging [11] in a regression model to predict location and shape of anatomical targets, reducing the variability (uncertainty) of learned relationships and obtaining confidence regions with high value for the DBS procedure. The training subsets producing the most accurate prediction are estimated via a machine learning approach. The robust prediction model and its application to STN targeting are described in the next section, followed by experiments demonstrating that our proposed framework enables reliable prediction of the STN on clinical 1.5T MRI for Parkinson's patients.

2 Methods

Target structures and their predictors, segmented from high quality 7T MR training sets, are first registered onto the 1.5T MRI pairs of the same subject [12], and then non-linearly registered onto the 1.5T MRI of a different subject [13]. This enables us to correctly extract features of predictors for the 1.5T MR test data from 7T MR training shapes on the common coordinate space.

2.1 Ensemble Prediction

Our approach uses an ensemble of predictions exploiting learned dependencies between targets and predictors from random subsets of 7T MR training sets. We provide now details on the approach.

Pose and Shape Parameterization. Three dimensional (3D) shapes of predictor and target structures for M random subsets of N 7T MR training sets are represented as the coordinates of surface points, $\mathbf{x}_{i,j} \in \mathbb{R}^{n_x \times 3}$ and $\mathbf{y}_{i,j} \in \mathbb{R}^{n_y \times 3}$, respectively, for $i \in \{1, ..., N\}$ and $j \in \{1, ..., M\}$, where n_x and n_y are the number of surface points. To address the correspondence problem across training shapes, we adopt a recent minimum description length based method [14].

The Procrustes analysis [15] is performed on predictors $\mathbf{x}_{i,j}$ and targets $\mathbf{y}_{i,j}$ with respect to the mean of the surfaces, $m_{\mathbf{x}_j} = \frac{1}{N}\sum_{i=1}^{N}\mathbf{x}_{i,j}$ and $m_{\mathbf{y}_j} = \frac{1}{N}\sum_{i=1}^{N}\mathbf{y}_{i,j}$, respectively, across the 7T MR training sets, yielding pose parameter vectors $\gamma_{i,j}^{x}$ and $\gamma_{i,j}^{y}$ that include translations, scaling factors, and entries of a 3D rotation matrix. Poses for a predictor $\mathbf{x}^{(p)} \in \mathbb{R}^{n_x \times 3}$ on the 1.5T MR test data are also parameterized as $\gamma_j^{x^{(p)}}$ with respect to $m_{\mathbf{x}_j}$. Column vectors, $\bar{\mathbf{x}}_{i,j} \in \mathbb{R}^{3n_x}$ and $\bar{\mathbf{y}}_{i,j} \in \mathbb{R}^{3n_y}$ are obtained by concatenating all the coordinates for the surfaces aligned into $m_{\mathbf{x}_j}$ and $m_{\mathbf{y}_j}$, respectively and then modeled in lower dimensional space using kernel PCA in order to increase the predictive potential, considering non-linear relationships between training shapes [16]. Kernel principal components are denoted as $\beta_{i,j}^{x}$ for predictors, $\beta_{i,j}^{y}$ for targets on 7T MR training sets, and $\beta_j^{x^{(p)}}$ for predictors on the 1.5T MR test data.

Bagging Regression. A bagging procedure [11] is applied in the partial least squares regression model [7, 9, 17] to learn shape relationships between targets and predictors, reducing their variability and providing confidence regions for the prediction. Regression coefficients $\mathbf{B}_{PLS,j}^{\beta}$ and $\mathbf{B}_{PLS,j}^{\gamma}$ for the shape parameters and poses, respectively, between targets and its predictors on the 7T MR training sets are obtained by a non-linear iterative partial least squares approach [17]. Given shape parameters $\beta_j^{x^{(p)}}$ and poses $\gamma_j^{x^{(p)}}$ for predictors on the 1.5T MR test data, $\beta_j^{y^{(p)}}$ and $\gamma_j^{y^{(p)}}$ for the target are predicted with the regression coefficients. Pre-image estimation of $\mathbf{y}_{est,j}^{(p)}$ in the original space from $\beta_j^{y^{(p)}}$ is ill-posed since the kernel mapping is not invertible for non-linear functions [16]. We therefore utilize a reconstruction approach using the feature space distance [16].

After iterating the prediction for M random subsets, a final probability map is calculated as an ensemble of binary volumes, reconstructed from $\beta_j^{y^{(p)}}$ and then transformed by $\gamma_j^{y^{(p)}}$: $V_{Pr} = \frac{1}{M}\sum_{j=1}^{M} V\left(\mathbf{y}_j^{(p)}\right)$. This, properly normalized, gives a probability interpretation of the prediction confidence.

2.2 Robust Prediction Model

Properly chosen subsets in the training data, for a particular patient, might contribute to further improvement of the prediction, reducing the bias from the learned information. To estimate the influence of such subsets in the prediction, we learn the dependency between features from random subsets and the prediction accuracy using a machine learning approach. Fig. 1 represents our robust prediction framework.

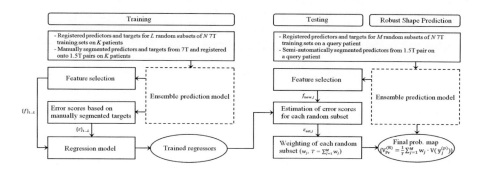

Fig. 1. Robust shape prediction framework.

Estimation of Influential Atlases. During the training, prediction using L random sets of N 7T MR training sets on K patients is performed, and pose parameters (i.e., $\mathbf{B}_{\mathrm{PLS}}^{\gamma}$, $\gamma^{x^{(p)}}$, and $\gamma^{y^{(p)}}$) are selected as features f, since poses for predictors and a predicted target are highly correlated to the prediction accuracy. Each prediction is then evaluated, measuring an error score ε that weighted averages distances from manually segmented targets,

$$\varepsilon = \mu_g(\epsilon_g/\delta_g) + \mu_l(\epsilon_l/\delta_l) + \mu_o(\epsilon_o/\delta_o) + \mu_v(\epsilon_v/\delta_v) + \mu_{\mathrm{DC}}((1-\mathrm{DC})/\delta_{\mathrm{DC}}), \quad (1)$$

where ϵ_g, ϵ_l, ϵ_o, and ϵ_v are errors between each prediction and manual segmentation, respectively, for centers, radii, orientation angles, and volumes. DC is the coefficients $((2\,|V^{(p)} \cap V^{(m)}|) / (|V^{(p)}| + |V^{(m)}|))$, where $V^{(p)}$ and $V^{(m)}$ are predicted and manual volumes, respectively. Also, μ and δ are weights and upper-bounds for corresponding errors. We set $\mu = [0.35\ 0.15\ 0.1\ 0.15\ 0.25]$ and $\delta = [1\mathrm{mm}\ 1\mathrm{mm}\ 30°\ 50\mathrm{mm}^3\ 40\%]$, in this paper, weighting more ϵ_g and DC under acceptable error bounds for DBS targeting ($\varepsilon < 1$).

To address the estimation problem of error scores, we utilize a regression forest model [10], which uses an ensemble of binary trees, learning non-linear mappings between features and error scores. Each tree optimally splits training samples, maximizing information gain among the distribution of error scores, and learned conditionals $p_t(\varepsilon \mid f)$ are stored on leaf nodes. Given a query patient and M random sets $s_{\mathrm{new},j}$ of training sets, each feature $f_{\mathrm{new},j}$ is pushed down on learned trees and stops at leaf nodes, resulting in $p_t(\varepsilon(s_{\mathrm{new},j}) \mid f_{\mathrm{new},j})$. The distributions are averaged over all N_{tree} trees, and finally error scores of each random subset are estimated: $\varepsilon_{\mathrm{est},j} = \arg\max_{\varepsilon_j} \left(\frac{1}{N_{\mathrm{tree}}} \sum_{t=1}^{N_{\mathrm{tree}}} p_t(\varepsilon(s_{\mathrm{new},j}) \mid f_{\mathrm{new},j}) \right)$.

Weighted Ensemble of Prediction. For the M estimated error scores, normalized to $[0\ 1]$, a weighting function is defined as $\mathrm{w}_j = \exp(-(\bar{\varepsilon}_{\mathrm{est},j})^3/\sigma^2)$, where σ is the mean of $\{\bar{\varepsilon}_{\mathrm{est}}\}$. This allows an ensemble of predictions, more weighting learned information from random subsets yielding lower error scores (i.e., more influential atlases for prediction). A final probability map on a query patient is computed by weighted averaging predictions from M random subsets: $V_{\mathrm{Pr}}^{(R)} = \frac{1}{T} \sum_{j=1}^{M} \mathrm{w}_j \cdot V(y_j^{(p)})$, with $T = \sum_{j=1}^{M} \mathrm{w}_j$.

2.3   Application: Prediction of the STN for Clinical Targeting

We apply our proposed framework in DBS targeting problem of the STN which is critical for PD and potentially also for OCD [1, 6]. Predictors in sub-cortical region are introduced by considering the spatial adjacency (high correlation [7]) with the STN and the visibility on the 1.5T MRI. All such structures are easily detected on the 7T MRI [1, 4]. For comparison with the 1.5T MRI, see also [6].

3   Results

7T and 1.5T MR data sets were scanned from 46 patients. The 7T MR structures were manually segmented by anatomical experts, see also [4, 5], and registered onto the corresponding 1.5T MRI pairs, following [12]. We select 10 Parkinson's (PD) patients as 1.5T MR test sets. For each patient, 16 similar patients are chosen, and the corresponding 7T MR structures (registered onto the 1.5T MRIs) are then non-linearly transformed onto the 1.5T MR test data of the query patient using Advanced Normalization Tools [13]. We build training sets with size $N=11$ out of 16 patients and randomly generate $M=10, 50, 100, 150$, and 200 subsets. Predictors are automatically segmented on the 1.5T T_2W MRI of each query patient [5]. We perform forest training with $N_{\text{tree}}=100$, using $L=18000$ random subsets of $N=11$ training sets from $K=9$ PD patients, leaving one out and estimating error scores, given random subsets and predictors on 1 PD patient. Final probability maps are thresholded and then evaluated by calculating errors in (1). Fig. 2 shows average error scores of the prediction results and mean squared error (MSE) of estimated error scores $\{\bar{\varepsilon}_{\text{est}}\}$ from true ones for a different number of random subsets over the 10 PD patients. Average centroid distances and DC values for prediction results from 100 random subsets, as important measurements for DBS targeting, are also presented in Table 1.

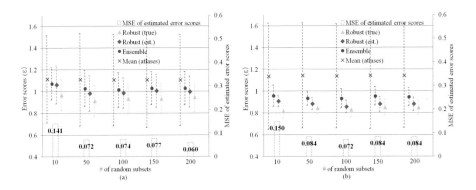

Fig. 2. Average error scores and their variances for 7T MR atlases based mean STN, ensemble prediction, and robust prediction (with estimated error scores and true ones), using a different number of random subsets over the 10 PD patients for (a) left and (b) right STN. Bars indicate MSE of estimated error scores from true ones.

Table 1. Average centroid distances, DC values, and their variances for 7T MR atlases based mean STN, ensemble prediction, and robust prediction using 100 random subsets.

		Mean(atlases)	Ensemble	Robust(est.)	Robust(true)
Left	ϵ_g(mm)	1.69±2.18	1.49±0.73	1.41±0.63	1.29±0.6
	DC(%)	54.7±5.4	60.4±2.1	60.9±2.2	62.4±2
Right	ϵ_g(mm)	1.76±2.61	1.34±0.51	1.16±0.38	1.1±0.4
	DC(%)	52.8±5.5	63.2±1.5	64.2±1.5	65.9±1.1

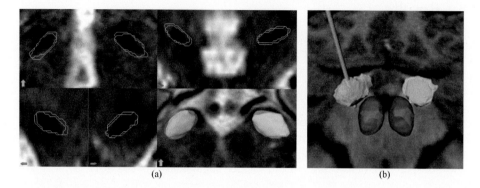

(a)   (b)

Fig. 3. (a) Robust prediction with estimated error scores (green) using 100 random subsets on the 1.5T T_2W MRI from a specific PD patient, and the manually segmented STN (yellow). Contours on the axial plane (top left), the coronal plane (top right), and the sagittal plane (bottom left) are shown, respectively, followed by their 3D surfaces (bottom right). Arrows indicate anterior direction. (b) Post-operative placement of electrodes on the DBS motor sub-region within the predicted STN (green), along with the manually segmented STN (yellow) and the red nucleus (red) provided for validation and ease of 3D orienteering.

Overall prediction results on the 1.5T MR datasets are much closer to the manually segmented STN than the 7T MR atlases based mean STN (probability maps of binary volumes from m_{y_j}), showing the prediction power of our proposed framework. Particularly, learned shape relationships are more effective to the prediction of the right STN, yielding lower error scores (the left STN have large variability over patients). Moreover, predictions are improved with the large number of random sets, showing the bagging effect (see differences in error scores between 10 and over 50 subsets, especially, for the left STN in Fig. 2).

We also observe that the proposed robust prediction with estimated error scores produces more accurate results than ensemble prediction (prediction results with true error scores are also presented for comparison). Particularly, for the number of subsets over 50, robust predictions are further improved, and centroid errors of the predicted right STN with 100 subsets are lowered over 10% (Table 1). This illustrates that random subsets with lower error scores, meaning more influential atlases for prediction, contribute to increasing the accuracy. Additionally, the smaller the number of random subsets, the higher the MSE between estimated error scores and true ones. This might also explain why the robust prediction is more effective with large enough number of subsets.

Low DC (<70%) might be attributed to thresholding an ensemble of predictions. However, note that we provide the probability interpretation of confident target regions rather than the whole shape. Additionally, although our proposed robust prediction shows improvement in error scores, centroid distance, and DC, for its practical use, it is required to validate if the prediction results are clinically acceptable. For that purpose, we qualitatively investigated if small sub-regions (posterior-lateral) of the predictions are completely inside the DBS target sub-region (e.g., motor territory) of true STN and observed that 95% of the predictions (19 out of 20 – both sides of 10 patients) hit the target regions. Fig. 3 shows that our proposed robust prediction provides confident targeting regions on the 1.5T MRI from a PD patient, with clinically feasible measurements (ε=0.48 and 0.58, ϵ_g=0.27mm and 0.76mm, and DC=76.8% and 78.2% for left and right STN, respectively). The DBS lead into the motor region of the STN is accurately placed on sub-regions within our prediction (Fig. 3(b)).

4   Conclusion

We presented a shape prediction framework that enables direct targeting for Deep Brain Stimulation (DBS) surgery based on standard clinical MR images. This is obtained by ensemble learning spatial relationships between DBS targets and their predictors using highly detailed information from 7T MR imaging. We proposed a robust way to improve the prediction, estimating the contribution of different training subsets. Given each subset on a patient, the influence to the prediction is estimated based on error scores and weighted to produce the final accurate and robust prediction.

Experimental results validated that our approach can fully predict the STN on the clinical 1.5T MRI from PD patients, where it is not possible to directly identify it. Ensemble prediction results were much closer to the ground truth manually segmented STN from the 7T MRI than atlases based mean STN, showing the predictive potential and further improved with large number of training subsets, reducing the variability of the learned information. The proposed robust prediction showed more accurate results, considering the contribution of random subsets to the prediction accuracy that leads to bias reduction from atlases. Moreover, small posterior-lateral regions of the predictions provided clinically acceptable localization of the patient-specific DBS lead within true STN.

Accurate estimation of error scores as a measure for the influence to prediction produces more reliable prediction, and thus relevant features need to be further investigated. Additionally, improving quality of predictors on the 1.5T MRI might considerably increase the prediction accuracy. Our ongoing efforts include the study of additional potential predictors and applications to other DBS targets (e.g., internal globus pallidus and ventralis intermedius). Ultimately, to reduce the need for MER in practice, it also remains challenging to minimize registration errors within our prediction framework and validate the manually segmented STN from 7T MRI using the MER mapping to address brain shift.

References

1. Abosch, A., Yacoub, E., Ugurbil, K., Harel, N.: An assessment of current brain targets for deep brain stimulation surgery with susceptibility weighted imaging at 7 tesla. Neurosurgery 67(6), 1745–1756 (2010)
2. Daniluk, S., Davies, K.G., Ellias, S.A., Novak, P., Nazzaro, J.M.: Asssessment of the variability in the anatomical position and size of the subthalamic nucleus among patients with advanced Parkinsons disease using magnetic resonance imaging. Acta Neurochirurgica 152(2), 201–210 (2010)
3. Xiao, Y., Jannin, P., D'Albis, T., Guizard, N., Haegelen, C., Lalys, F., Vérin, M., Collins, D.L.: Investigation of Morphometric Variability of Subthalamic Nucleus, Red Nucleus, and Substantia Nigra in Advanced Parkinsons Disease Patients Using Automatic Segmentation and PCA-Based Analysis. Human Brain Mapping 35(9), 4330–4344 (2014)
4. Lenglet, C., Abosch, A., Yacoub, E., De Martino, F., Sapiro, G., Harel, N.: Comprehensive in vivo mapping of the human basal ganglia and thalamic connectome in individuals using 7T MRI. PLoS One 7, e29153 (2012)
5. Kim, J., Lenglet, C., Duchin, Y., Sapiro, G., Harel, N.: Semiautomatic segmentation of brain subcortical structures from high-field MRI. IEEE J. Biomed. Health Inform. 18(5), 1678–1695 (2014)
6. Cho, Z., Min, H., Oh, S., Han, J., Park, C., Chi, J., Kim, Y., Paek, S.H., Lozano, A.M., Lee, K.H.: Direct visualization of deep brain stimulation targets in Parkinson disease with the use of 7-tesla magnetic resonance imaging. J. Neurosurg. 113(3), 639–647 (2010)
7. Rao, A., Aljabar, P., Rueckert, D.: Hierarchical statistical shape analysis and prediction of sub-cortical brain structures. Med. Image Anal. 12(1), 55–68 (2008)
8. Baka, N., Metz, C., Schaap, M., Lelieveldt, B., Niessen, W., De Bruijne, M.: Comparison of shape regression methods under landmark position uncertainty. In: Fichtinger, G., Martel, A., Peters, T. (eds.) MICCAI 2011, Part II. LNCS, vol. 6892, pp. 434–441. Springer, Heidelberg (2011)
9. Blanc, R., Seiler, C., Szekely, G., Nolte, L., Reyes, M.: Statistical model based shape prediction from a combination of direct observations and various surrogates: Application to orthopaedic research. Med. Image Anal. 16(6), 1156–1166 (2012)
10. Criminisi, A., Robertson, D., Konukoglu, E., Shotton, J., Pathak, S., White, S., Siddiqui, K.: Regression forests for efficient anatomy detection and localization in computed tomography scans. Med. Image Anal. 17(8), 1293–1303 (2013)
11. Breiman, L.: Bagging predictors. Machine Learning 24(2), 123–140 (1996)
12. Duchin, Y., Abosch, A., Yacoub, E., Sapiro, G., Harel, N.: Feasibility of using ultra-high field (7T) MRI for clinical surgical targeting. PLoS One 7, e37328 (2012)
13. Avants, B.B., Tustison, N.J., Song, G., Cook, P.A., Klein, A., Gee, J.C.: A reproducible evaluation of ANTs similarity metric performance in brain image registration. Neuroimage 54(3), 2033–2044 (2011)
14. Heimann, T., Wolf, I., Williams, T., Meinzer, H.: 3d active shape models using gradient descent optimization of description length. In: Christensen, G.E., Sonka, M. (eds.) IPMI 2005. LNCS, vol. 3565, pp. 566–577. Springer, Heidelberg (2005)
15. Cootes, T.F., Taylor, C.J., Cooper, D.H., Graham, J.: Active shape models – Their training and application. Comput. Vis. Image Understand 61(1), 38–59 (1995)
16. Rathi, Y., Dambreville, S., Tannenbaum, A.: Statistical shape analysis using kernel PCA. In: SPIE-IS&T Electronic Imaging (2010)
17. Abdi, H.: Partial least squares regression and projection on latent structure regression (PLS Regression). Wiley Interdiscip. Rev. Comp. Stat. 2(1), 97–106 (2010)

RF Ultrasound Distribution-Based Confidence Maps

Tassilo Klein and William M. Wells III

Brigham and Women's Hospital, Harvard Medical School, Boston, USA

Abstract. Ultrasound is becoming an ever increasingly important modality in medical care. However, underlying physical acquisition principles are prone to image artifacts and result in overall quality variation. Therefore processing medical ultrasound data remains a challenging task. We propose a novel distribution-based measure of assessing the confidence in the signal, which emphasizes uncertainty in attenuated as well as shadow regions. In contrast to the similar recently proposed method that relies on image intensities, the new approach makes use of the enveloped-detected radio-frequency data, facilitating the use of Nakagami speckle statistics. Employing J-divergence as distance measure for the random-walk based algorithm, provides a natural measure of similarity, yielding a more reliable estimate of confidence. For evaluation of the model's performance, tests are conducted on the application of shadow detection. Additionally, computed maps are presented for different organs such as neck, liver and prostate, showcasing the properties of the model. The probabilistic approach is shown to have beneficial features for image processing tasks.

Keywords: Envelope-Detected RF, Ultrasound, Confidence, Nakagami.

1 Introduction

Ultrasound (US) image processing is still commonly performed in the B-mode domain. However, proprietary filtering and non-linear compression to obtain B-mode from raw data distort the signal and effectively reduce the information content in the data in a non-linear fashion, which reduces its suitability for statistical modeling. A more natural way is to deal with the US characteristics in a statistical framework using unprocessed, radio frequency (RF) data. As US imaging is largely driven by patterns referred to as speckle noise, literature suggests a multitude of different models that accommodate the different noise scenarios, e.g. the Rician, generalized K, homodyned K, Rayleigh and Nakagami distribution. Shankar [13] showed that the envelope detected RF signal follows the Nakagami distribution [10]. This distribution has been shown to be a very general model for a multitude of speckle scenarios, often making it the model of choice as it is in this paper.

We propose a novel method for estimating confidence maps [7] in envelope detected RF US images, which emphasizes uncertainty in attenuated as well as

© Springer International Publishing Switzerland 2015
N. Navab et al. (Eds.): MICCAI 2015, Part II, LNCS 9350, pp. 595–602, 2015.
DOI: 10.1007/978-3-319-24571-3_71

shadow regions. Confidence maps have shown to be useful for a number of applications such as registration, segmentation and shadow detection [7,14]. However, in contrast to the previously proposed method [7] that relies on B-mode image intensities, the novel approach makes use of the envelope detected RF data, facilitating the use of Nakagami speckle statistics. The main novelty lies in the use of a probabilistic distance measure that is used within the random walks framework originally introduced for segmentation by Grady [5]. The proposed approach employs J-divergence (JDIV) as the distance measure, which provides a more natural measure of similarity in US imagery, yielding a more reliable confidence measure. The use of JDIV for RF US processing was first proposed by Klein et al. [8] in the context of multi-view reconstruction.

To show-case the advanced performance of the probabilistic confidence maps we show application on different kinds of data as well evaluate performance for the detection of acoustic shadows in a machine learning approach. Shadowing is an US specific artifact caused by an abrupt change in acoustic impedance. A large difference causes strong reflection and limited transmission of sound beyond resulting in a shadow. Although considered an artifact, it is useful for detecting gallstones, calcification, and bone structures [6]. However, for many applications shadows pose a problem, which includes registration and 3D reconstruction. In particular, multi-view 3D reconstruction of US in the presence of shadow artifacts requires processing in order to yield useful results, e.g. avoiding mixing shadow and non shadow information [7]. Consequently, it is important to accurately and reliably detect these artifacts for both diagnostic and image processing applications [6]. Karamalis et al. [7] propose the use of confidence maps for shadow detection based on thresholding. Sheet et al. [14] use confidence maps together with machine learning to detect necrosis in IVUS imagery. In Penney et. al. [11] each US scanline is sampled and marked as shadow upon reaching an empirical threshold. In [9] breast lesions are discriminated from posterior acoustic shadowing in a machine learning approach by previously extracting multi-scale texture features from a training data set. In Hellier et al. [6] possible shadow starting points are detected along each scanline and tested for shadowing by evaluating local patch statistics.

Most of the previously proposed approaches assume that acoustic shadow features a low SNR. However, the US image area after interfaces, like bone-tissue and lung-liver interface, contains a broad range of signal amplitudes and noise (see Fig. 3) because of reverberation, mirroring, and backscattered echo. These effects complicate shadow detection and necessitate specialized approaches. We demonstrate that statistical confidence maps embedded in a machine learning framework allow for a more robust shadow detection.

2   Method

The proposed approach is based on a modification of the ultrasound confidence maps proposed by Karamalis et al. [7]. In contrast to the previous approach we do not use intensity gradients for the graph underlying the random walks algorithm.

Rather we employ a statistical measure, J-divergence, using the distributional change as measure. In the following section we at first provide the confidence map preliminaries before presenting the details on the novel approach.

2.1 Confidence Maps

The confidence/uncertainty estimation problem originally presented in [7] is modeled as a random walk under ultrasound specific constraints. For this purpose the US image is represented as a weighted connected graph, similar as described in the work of Grady [5], where each node corresponds to an image pixel/sample. The weights of the graph Laplacian are given as:

$$w_{ij} = \begin{cases} w_{ij}^H = \exp(-\beta((c_i - c_j)^2 + \gamma)) & \text{if } i,j \text{ adjacent and } e_{ij} \in E_H \\ w_{ij}^D = \exp(-\beta((c_i - c_j)^2 + \sqrt{2} \cdot \gamma)) & \text{if } i,j \text{ adjacent and } e_{ij} \in E_D \\ w_{ij}^V = \exp(-\beta((c_i - c_j)^2)) & \text{if } i,j \text{ adjacent and } e_{ij} \in E_V \\ 0 & \text{otherwise} \end{cases}$$
(1)

where e_{ij} is an edge connecting node i and j, E_H, E_D, E_V are edges along horizontal, diagonal, and vertical graph directions respectively, $E_H \ominus E_D \ominus E_V = E$, $\beta = 90$ is a algorithmic constant (similar to [5]), $c_i = |r_i| \exp(-\alpha x_i)$, α is the attenuation coefficient, r_i is the (intensity/RF) signal, and x_i is the normalized closest distance from node v_i to the virtual transducer elements, which are located in the pixels next to the transducer and function as random walker sources. The random walks solution [5,7] to the graph Laplacian with the previously defined weights yields the desired confidence estimate, which becomes more apparent when analyzing the weights individually and seems more intuitive when discussed in terms of potential theory (as described in [5]). The proportionality of reflected and transmitted acoustic energy is represented by the gradient term $c_i - c_j$, which effectively reduces the potential along possible circuit paths with increasing magnitude. In [7] the depth dependent attenuation of the model is integrated into the c_i function. The beam-width is modeled with the γ term, which effectively results in an accumulative increase in circuit resistance with increasing horizontal/diagonal distance to the originating scanline.

2.2 Probabilistic Graph Distance

In contrast to the originally proposed work Karamalis et al. [7], we do not employ intensity difference as edge weight in the graph as specified by the gradient term $c_i - c_j$ in Eq. 1. Rather we make use of the statistical information within the post-beamformed ultrasound data. The distribution of the envelope of the RF signal I, resulting from backscattered tissue echo, has been shown to be modeled by the Nakagami distribution [13]. Instead of the Nakagami distribution, the gamma distribution g may be used, since squaring a Nakagami distributed random variable yields one that is gamma distributed [10]. For the following we assume the squared envelope-detected RF to follow the Gamma distribution

$$I^2 \sim g(x|\mu,\nu) = \frac{(\nu/\mu)^\nu}{\Gamma(\nu)} x^{(\nu-1)} \exp\left(-\frac{\nu}{\mu}x\right), \tag{2}$$

with μ,ν the shape and scale parameters respectively. As a first step the Gamma distribution parameters are estimated from I^2 by means of a sliding window MLE approach, yielding Gamma image $I_\Gamma \in \mathcal{R}^2$. In order to obtain smooth and denoised maps we employ a variant of Total-Variation (TV) smoothing for vectorial data. The basic concept of TV regularization for image denoising was originally proposed by Rudin, Osher and Fatemi with their ROF model [12], which is an an edge-preserving noise-removal method endowed with a L^2 data fidelity term [3]. Given that $I_\Gamma \in \mathcal{R}^2$ and the inherent shape and scale coupling, we use Vectorial Rudin-Osher-Fatemi (VROF) [2] for joint smoothing of shape and scale. Specifically, this implies the minimization of

$$\inf_{\mathbf{u}} \sup_{|\mathbf{p}|\leq 1} \left\{ \langle \mathbf{u}, \nabla \cdot \mathbf{p}\rangle + \|I_\Gamma - \mathbf{u}\|^2 \right\}, \tag{3}$$

with the dual definition of total variation of function $\mathbf{u} : \mathrm{R}^2 \to \mathrm{R}$, given by

$$\int_{\mathrm{R}^2} |D\mathbf{u}| := \sup_{|\mathbf{p}|\leq 1} \left\{ \int_{\mathrm{R}^2} \langle \mathbf{u}, \nabla \cdot \mathbf{p}\rangle dx \right\} \tag{4}$$

where the dual variable $\mathbf{p} \in C_c^1(\mathrm{R}^2, \mathrm{R}^{2\times 2})$ is a smooth function with compact support. It should be noted that first term of Eq. 3 corresponds to total variation and the last term is L^2 data fidelity. Employing L^2 data fidelity serves as an approximation of a distance measure on the Gamma manifold, which in turn facilitates efficient estimation. The resulting convex regularization problem allows for fast solving by using Chambolle's algorithm [4,2]. In the following we will denote the VROF smoothed image I_Γ as I_Γ^*.

Given the smoothed shape and scale Gamma MLE estimates I_Γ^*, we compute the JDIV, i.e. the sum of two non-symmetric Kullback-Leibler (KL) distances with switched arguments. JDIV for two Gamma distribution $a,b \in g(x|\mu,\nu)$ is given by

$$D_{JDIV}(a,b) \int \log\frac{a(x)}{b(x)} \left(a(x) - b(x)\right) dx = (\mu_a - 1)\,\psi(\mu_a) - \log\nu_a - \mu_a$$
$$- \log\frac{\Gamma(\mu_a)}{\Gamma(\mu_b)} + \mu_b \log\nu_b - (\mu_b - 1)\left(\psi(\mu_a) + \log\nu_a\right) + \frac{\nu_a\mu_a}{\nu_b},$$

where $\psi(.)$ denotes the digamma function.

Next, we replace the gradient gradient term $c_i - c_j$ with JDIV between to Gamma distributions. Solving a family of linear equations based on the graph Laplacian yields the statistics-based confidence maps, which implies for each pixel (graph node) the probability for the random walker to arrive there. It should be noted that compared to the approach of Karamalis et al. [7], we do not explicitly integrate attenuation. Change due to attenuation is intrinsically

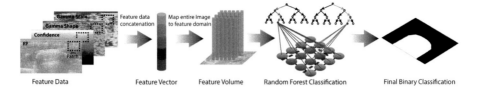

Fig. 1. Shadow detection pipeline (from left to right): 1) Computation of feature such as confidence maps and Gamma image 2) Patchwise feature concatenation 3) Classification using Random Forest

encoded in a change of distribution pattern. This independence w.r.t. to attenuation compensation such as provided by US machines (time gain compensation) suggests increased robustness compared to intensity-based approaches.

2.3 Shadow Classification

For shadow classification we employ Random Forests [1]. Assuming a two class model $C = \{c_0 = \text{shadow}, c_1 = \text{no shadow}\}$ the posterior probability in terms of classification is defined by

$$p(C|\theta) = \frac{1}{T} \sum_{t=1}^{T} p_t(C|\theta), \tag{5}$$

assuming a forest consisting of T trees and $\theta \in \mathcal{R}^n$ the feature-vector space. Consequently, the classifier **H** is obtained as the mode of the posterior

$$H(\theta) = \underset{k}{\text{argmax}}\ p(C = c_k|\theta) \tag{6}$$

The feature space consists of a combination of various patch statistics (e.g. mean, variance etc.), which are extracted separately from RF data, confidence maps, and gamma maps. Individual features are then concatenated yielding a feature vector. See Fig 1 for an illustration for the shadow detection pipeline.

3 Experiments

3.1 Shadow Detection

For testing the performance of the shadow detection in RF ultrasound, numerous data sequences of the Humerus were acquired from five volunteers using an Ultrasonix MDP machine in combination with a linear transducer L14-5/38 GPS. Each data set was recorded with depth 4 cm and 5 MHz, yielding RF images of resolution 1304×256 pixels and 150 frames. For validation, manual segmentation of the shadow regions was performed in each frame for each data set by an US expert. Image sequences for segmentation were selected to

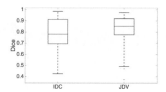

	IDC	JDV
Median	0.78	0.85
Mean	0.79	0.83
STD	0.12	0.11

Fig. 2. Shadow detection results: Left box-plot, Right: corresponding table of results

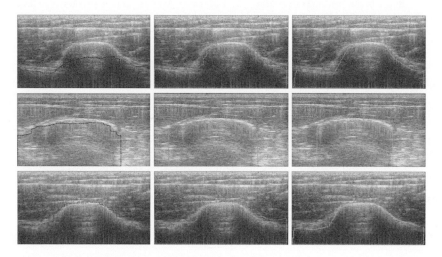

Fig. 3. Shadow prediction for different frames and approaches. From left to right: IDC, JDV and manual ground truth segmentation.

contain various mirroring/reverberation artifact scenarios ranging from low to high. For comparing the information content and the robustness of the confidence maps, two different confidence maps were used as feature vectors. The other feature components, such as Gamma image, remained identical for all approaches. Patch size for feature estimation was set to 5×5. The random forest consisted of 50 trees. Compared were intensity distance (IDC) confidence map [7] ($\alpha = 2.0, \beta = 90.0, \gamma = 0.1$) and the proposed approach based on J-divergence (JDV) ($\beta = 90.0, \gamma = 0.1$) with a patch size of 4×25 for Gamma MLE. For performance estimation 10-fold cross validation was conducted. Figure 2 shows the results for the dice coefficients on shadow classification. The difference between dice coefficients is statistically significant. The Mann-Whitney U-test yields p-values $5.5 \cdot 10^{-5}$. The corresponding t-test on logit transformed dice coefficient yields p-values $3.0 \cdot 10^{-34}$, respectively. In terms of computational complexity obtained on an average state of the art machine using MATLAB, estimation of a single patch requires around $8.0 \cdot 10^{-4}$ sec and $2 - 10$ sec. for an entire image. VROF smoothing takes around $0.5 - 1.5$ sec. for the entire image.

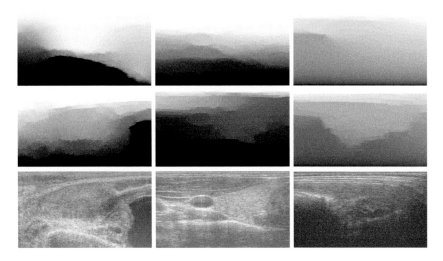

Fig. 4. Maps for different approaches and organs. From left to right: prostate, neck and liver. From top to bottom: IDC, JDV and the ultrasound image, which was used to compute the map.

3.2 Estimation for Different Organs

In order to assess the performance, confidence maps were computed for different kinds of organs. Cross-sections of organs include prostate, liver and neck. The corresponding data shows a variety of image scenarios including low to strong intensity gradients as well as tissue patterns changes. The parameters used for estimating the maps were equal in all approaches: $\alpha = 2.0$, $\beta = 90.0, \gamma = 0.05$. For Gamma MLE, a patch size of of 4×25 was chosen, to match the anisotropy of the underlying RF image.

4 Result and Conclusion

We presented a novel technique for confidence map estimation employing statistical measure as edge weight for the underlying graph. It has shown to outperform intensity approaches for application such as shadow detection, even in regions containing severe reverberation and mirroring artifacts. Evaluation on US image series of the Humerus demonstrates good results that are consistent with manual segmentation, with a comparably lower mean, median and variance in dice coefficient using the proposed approach. Examples on different characteristic organ cross-sections demonstrate the robustness of the proposed approach. Within the novel approach, confidence consistency and coherence is not based directly on brightness changes and is therefore more robust and general. Compared to intensity-based methods, no large brightness gradient is necessary to preserve consistency, e.g. organs that do not have a strongly pronounced outline or tissue parts have a characteristic tissue pattern are captured nicely. This can be seen in Fig. 4 at muscle tissue next to carotid artery, liver boundary or prostate gland. For future work different statistical distances and models will be investigated. Specifically, metrics close to the true geodesic distance on the Gamma manifold are of interest. Additionally, extension to 3D as well as real-time capability will be investigated.

Acknowledgments. This work was supported in part by the DFG (KL 2724/2) and the NIH (P41EB015898, R01CA111288).

References

1. Breiman, L.: Random forests. Machine Learning 45(1), 5–32 (2001)
2. Bresson, X., Chan, T.F.: Fast dual minimization of the vectorial total variation norm and applications to color image processing. Inverse Problems and Imaging 2(4), 455–484 (2008)
3. Burger, M., Osher, S.: A guide to the TV zoo. In: Level Set and PDE Based Reconstruction Methods in Imaging. LNCS, vol. 2090, pp. 1–70. Springer, Heidelberg (2013)
4. Chambolle, A.: An algorithm for total variation minimization and applications. Journal of Mathematical Imaging and Vision 20(1-2), 89–97 (2004)
5. Grady, L.: Random walks for image segmentation. IEEE Trans. Pattern Anal. Mach. Intell 28(11), 1768–1783 (2006)
6. Hellier, P., Coupé, P., Morandi, X., Collins, D.: An automatic geometrical and statistical method to detect acoustic shadows in intraoperative ultrasound brain images. Medical Image Analysis 14(2), 195–204 (2010)
7. Karamalis, A., Wein, W., Klein, T., Navab, N.: Ultrasound confidence maps using random walks. Med. Image Anal. 16(6), 1101–1112 (2012)
8. Klein, T., Hansson, M., Navab, N.: Modeling of multi-view 3d freehand radio frequency ultrasound. In: Ayache, N., Delingette, H., Golland, P., Mori, K. (eds.) MICCAI 2012, Part I. LNCS, vol. 7510, pp. 422–429. Springer, Heidelberg (2012)
9. Madabhushi, A., Yang, P., Rosen, M., Weinstein, S.: Distinguishing lesions from posterior acoustic shadowing in breast ultrasound via non-linear dimensionality reduction. In: EMBS, pp. 3070–3073 (2006)
10. Nakagami, N.: The m-distribution, a general formula for intensity distribution of rapid fadings. In: Hoffman, W.G. (ed.) Statistical Methods in Radio Wave Propagation. Pergamon, Oxford (1960)
11. Penney, G., Blackall, J., Hamady, M., Sabharwal, T., Adam, A., Hawkes, D.: Registration of freehand 3D ultrasound and magnetic resonance liver images. Med. Image Anal. 8(1), 81–91 (2004)
12. Rudin, L.I., Osher, S.J., Fatemi, E.: Nonlinear total variation based noise removal algorithms. Physica D: Nonlinear Phenomena 60, 259–268 (1992)
13. Shankar, P.M.: A general statistical model for ultrasonic scattering from tissues. IEEE Trans. Ultrason Ferroelectr Freq. Control 47(3), 339–343 (2000)
14. Sheet, D., Karamalis, A., Eslami, A., Noël, P., Virmani, R., Nakano, M., Chatterjee, J., Ray, A.K., Laine, A.F., Carlier, S.G., Navab, N., Katouzian, A.: Hunting for necrosis in the shadows of intravascular ultrasound. Comput. Med. Imag. Grap. 38(2), 104–112 (2014)

Prospective Prediction of Thin-Cap Fibroatheromas from Baseline Virtual Histology Intravascular Ultrasound Data

Ling Zhang[1], Andreas Wahle[1] Zhi Chen[1], John Lopez[2], Tomas Kovarnik[3], and Milan Sonka[1]

[1] Iowa Institute for Biomedical Imaging and Department of Electrical and Computer Engineering, University of Iowa, Iowa City IA, USA
[2] Department of Medicine, Cardiology, Loyola University, Maywood, IL, USA
[3] 2nd Department of Internal Medicine of General University Hospital in Prague and Charles University, Prague, Czech Republic
ling-zhang@uiowa.edu

Abstract. Thin-cap fibroatheroma (TCFA) is particularly prone to rupture, which may result in myocardial infarction and death. Virtual histology intravascular ultrasound (VH-IVUS) provides quantitative information about plaque composition and enables TCFA identification. However, prospective prediction of future development of TCFA has not been previously possible. The aim of our study was to determine whether subsequent development of TCFA can be predicted from baseline VH-IVUS data. Corresponding VH-IVUS images of baseline and follow-up examinations were identified by a highly automated approach to register IVUS pullback pairs from 24 patients (2,331 image pairs). Next, 20 location-specific VH-based and IVUS-based features including plaque phenotype and morphology, and 15 systemic patient-specific features were extracted and ranked using a support vector machine recursive feature elimination (SVM RFE) technique. SVM was applied to assess the prediction power of different feature sets, by adding the first n-ranked features to the classification procedure (leave-one-patient-out cross validation) iteratively until all features were considered. The experimental results showed that the prospective prediction of TCFA achieves a sensitivity of 72.6% and a specificity of 73.3%, when an optimal set of the five best selected features is used. The results indicate the feasibility of prospective prediction of TCFA formation based on baseline VH-IVUS data.

1 Motivation

Thrombotic coronary occlusion after rupture of a thin fibrous cap covering a lipid-rich necrotic core (NC) [thin-cap fibroatheroma (TCFA)] is the most common cause of myocardial infarction and death [11]. Virtual histology intravascular ultrasound (VH-IVUS) provides quantitative information about plaque composition and enables TCFA identification. The VH-IVUS-derived TCFA is strongly and independently predictive of major adverse cardiac events [3]. However, it is still a daunting challenge to predict whether, and if so, where any TCFA will occur in the future. Pioneer studies have found significant correlations between IVUS-derived morphological features and TCFA treatment outcome (healed or remaining) [7], and between plaque phenotype and increasing

© Springer International Publishing Switzerland 2015
N. Navab et al. (Eds.): MICCAI 2015, Part II, LNCS 9350, pp. 603–610, 2015.
DOI: 10.1007/978-3-319-24571-3_72

necrotic core (NC) area [4], respectively. However, these correlations do not necessarily imply the ability to successfully predict subsequent development of TCFA.

In order to learn how to prospectively predict TCFA, frame-to-frame registration of baseline and follow-up VH-IVUS pullback data is of paramount importance. Most previous studies examined plaque progression in entire lesions or over long vessel segments [3, 7, 11], in part because accurate frame-to-frame registration of IVUS pullbacks at two time points is challenging [1, 13, 15]. Using longer coronary segments fails to reflect the focal nature of clinical events and leads to over-averaging of focal plaque morphology/composition indices [4]. Recently, we proposed an automated approach for frame-to-frame registration of baseline and follow-up IVUS pullback pair based on 3D graph-based optimization [15]. The registration reported there was robust to the changes of vessel morphology due to automatically higher-weighted perivascular tissue similarity. Pilot validation on four patients showed that the registration accuracy outperformed the distance-normalization-based approach [13]. Our registration method thus enables focal studies of development of coronary plaque phenotypes (e.g., TCFA).

Machine learning techniques (e.g., support vector machines, SVM [2, 5]) provide an effective way to learn complex relationships from empirical data and to facilitate decision making [14]. Specifically, machine learning approaches have been applied to help physicians predict disease outcome and patient survival, such as breast cancer and prostate cancer [9]. Therefore, we hypothesize that machine learning approaches applied to serial studies of registered VH-IVUS data from patients with CAD will allow predicting subsequent development of TCFA.

Our goal is to train a predictive classifier to identify locations on the coronary artery that are likely to demonstrate TCFA development in the future based solely on baseline VH-IVUS data. Fig. 1 shows an overview of classifier training and its use for TCFA prediction. Baseline and one-year-follow-up in vivo IVUS pullback data are initially segmented and registered. The location-specific (frame-level) features and systemic information (biomarkers) at baseline are selected to form an optimal feature subset. The predictive classifier is trained considering corresponding follow-up plaque phenotype (TCFA or non-TCFA) as a to-be-learned response. Consequently, all locations (frame-level) in coronary vessels imaged at baseline will be classified as destined to developing or not-developing TCFA at follow-up. To the best of our knowledge, this is the first work tackling computer-aided prediction of location-specific TCFA development in vivo.

2   TCFA Prediction from Baseline VH-IVUS Data

2.1   Segmentation and Registration of Baseline and Follow-up IVUS Pullbacks

For each frame of each IVUS pullback, lumen and external elastic lamina (EEL) surfaces are automatically segmented using a fully three-dimensional graph-search approach [8] and further reviewed and algorithmically refined by expert cardiologist using an operator-guided computer-aided interface [12]. EEL and lumen surfaces/contours serve as the input for off-line VH computation using Volcano's research software, which

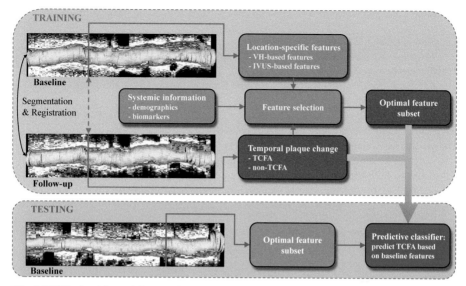

Fig. 1. TCFA classifier training and its use for TCFA prediction. Lumen shown in orange, plaques color-coded by VH composed of four types: dense calcium [DC] (white), necrotic core [NC] (red), fibrofatty [FF] (light green), and fibrotic tissue [FT] (dark green).

is functionally identical to that available on the Volcano IVUS console (Volcano Corp., Rancho Cordoba, CA). Registration of each image frame in corresponding baseline and follow-up IVUS pullback data is performed by a novel IVUS pullback pair registration approach based on 3D graph-based optimization [15]. An example of the computer segmentation and registration result is shown in the upper left panel of Fig. 1.

2.2   Feature Extraction

In this study, two categories of features are extracted for TCFA prediction including location-specific features (VH-based and IVUS-based) and systemic information, as shown in Table 1. Many of these features are those generally accepted as reflecting local vascular disease severity or plaque progression [3, 4, 7, 11], others were designed by us to specifically describe TCFA morphology and axial context (e.g., F2, F11-F13).

VH-Based Features (F1–F13). Using quantitative assessment of VH tissue types, phenotypes of all frames were automatically classified into 6 categories (no lesion [NL], pathological intimal thickening [PIT], fibrous plaque [FP], fibrocalcific plaque [FcP], thick-cap fibroatheroma [ThCFA], and TCFA) according to the definitions of American Heart Association's Committee on Vascular Lesions [10]. The scores for each phenotype were assigned values of 0–5, as shown in Fig. 2. Note that confluent NC $> 10\%$ and NC abutting the lumen $> 30°$ thresholds were used to define the TCFA category as in [11]. We further extracted the contextual plaque phenotype by computing the average plaque phenotype score of the adjacent distal and proximal frames. Such a strategy not

Table 1. Location-specific VH-based and IVUS-based features, systemic information.

Location-specific VH features
F1: Phenotype, F2: Phenotype context, F3: DC CSA, F4: NC CSA, F5: FF CSA, F6: FT CSA, F7: DC percentage (%), F8: NC percentage (%), F9: FF percentage (%), F10: FT percentage (%), F11: Max. confluent NC (%), F12: Ang. NC-abutting-lumen, F13: # NC-abutting-lumen
Location-specific IVUS features
F14: lumen CSA, F15: EEL CSA, F16: plaque CSA, F17: plaque burden, F18: mean plaque thickness, F19: std. plaque thickness, F20: eccentricity
Patient-specific systemic information (biomarkers)
F21: weight, F22: family history, F23: smoking history, F24: current smoker, F25: hypertension, F26: diabetes, F27: hyperlipidemia, F28: previous MI, F29: beta blockers, F30: acinhibitors, F31: statins, F32: bl-choltotal, F33: bl-cholldl, F34: bl-cholhdl, F35: bl-tag

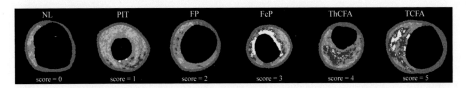

Fig. 2. Plaque phenotype classification. All plaque phenotypes other than "TCFA" were categorized as "non-TCFA" at follow-up.

only limits the impact of noise (inaccurate frame-to-frame registration) but also incorporates surrounding-lesion information. Furthermore, the cross-sectional areas (CSAs) and percentages of each plaque component (DC/NC/FF/FT) were extracted. Considering that NC is likely the most important component of TCFA plaque, three NC-related features were introduced: percentage of the maximal confluent NC region, angle and size of NC-region abutting the vessel lumen.

IVUS-Based Features (F14–F20). Graylevel-IVUS-based measurements of CSAs of lumen, EEL, plaque (defined as EEL area minus lumen area), and plaque burden (defined as the ratio of plaque area to EEL area) were obtained for all frame locations. The mean and standard deviation of plaque thickness (defined as the distance between lumen and EEL borders at 360 circumferential wedges centered at the lumen centroid) were also calculated. Eccentricity (defined as the ratio of minimal to maximal plaque thickness) was measured to quantify the asymmetric distribution of plaque.

2.3   Feature Selection and Predictive Classifier Validation

Robust feature selection cannot be always cleanly separated from classifier design. The SVM [2, 5] methods based on recursive feature elimination (RFE) [6], which is an application of RFE using the weight magnitude as ranking criterion, is a very effective technique for discovering/ranking informative features. In this study, we adopt the SVM RFE method for feature ranking using a leave-one-patient-out cross-validation procedure. Because of the heavy imbalance in the class labels in our study, under-sampling

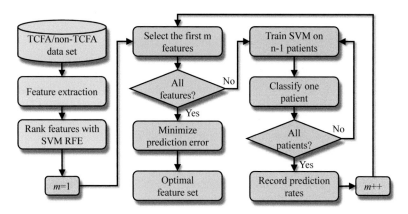

Fig. 3. Flowchart describing feature selection and predictive model validation.

of the non-TCFA class was performed to increase the sensitivity of the prediction to the TCFA class. Note that the percentages of under-sampling for each phenotype in the non-TCFA class were the same.

After ranking the feature set, in which the top-ranked features have strong relations with the TCFA/non-TCFA classifications, the features were normalized to the range of [0 1] and the first m features were iteratively added one by one to the prediction procedure until all features were considered. In each iteration, leave-one-patient-out cross-validation was performed where one patient (whose frames were subsequently used for testing) was left out from each SVM predictor, which was trained on n-1 patients (with said under-sampling of the non-TCFA class). The prediction rates including sensitivity and specificity were calculated and recorded after testing all n patients. Finally, the feature set that minimized the prediction error was selected as the optimal feature set, and the final TCFA prediction rates were obtained. The feature selection and predictive model validation procedure is shown in Fig. 3.

3   Experiments and Results

3.1   Patient Data

The patient data in this study consisted of 29 serial (baseline and one-year follow-up) IVUS images from patients with stable coronary artery disease during lipid-lowering therapy enrolled in the PREDICT study at the Charles University Hospital, Prague (ClinicalTrials.gov identifier: NCT01773512). IVUS imaging was performed in the standard fashion using the IVUS phased-array probe (Eagle Eye 20 MHz 2.9F monorail, Volcano Corporation, Rancho Cordova, California), IVUS console with Gold standard software, and motorized pullback at 0.5 mm/s (research pullback device, model R-100, Volcano Corporation). The Volcano IVUS imaging system provided EKG-gated IVUS image sequences with 8,622 gated frames in total (72 to 235 frames per pullback), 0.27 to 0.67 mm distances between adjacent frames depending on the heart rate, and 500 × 500 pixels per image frame.

3.2   Evaluation of IVUS Pullback Registration

To evaluate the performance of the registration, 262 frame pairs with well-identifiable landmarks (baseline ↔ follow-up) were determined by Expert 1. Two other experts (Experts 2 and 3) were provided the 262 landmarks in baseline and were asked to find corresponding follow-up frames to determine inter-observer variability of manual registration. Distances (numbers of gated frames) between the expert-identified follow-up frames and the computer-registered frames were used as the registration performance measure. For our location-specific prediction task, high registration accuracy of image pairs used in the classifier training is necessary. Therefore, only patients with a mean registration error of <2 frames were used to train the predictive classifier.

Table 2 quantitatively compares inter-observer variability with the registration errors of our method. Our 3D-graph-based method achieved registration results with mean distance errors ranging from 1.36 to 1.48 frames. There were no significant differences between our method and experts in the registration performance as judged by the Wilcoxon signed-ranks test (p=NS); 24 out of 29 patients were successfully registered with mean error <2 frames. Note that the one-time error of 23 frames was due to data acquisition "jump". The affected patient was excluded.

Table 2. Distance error (in frames) of registration for inter-observer variability and our method.

Inter-observer	Mean + std. error	Max error	Our method	Mean + std. error	Max error
Exp. 1 vs. Exp. 2	1.41 ± 2.72	23	Auto vs. Exp. 1	1.45 ± 2.22	18
Exp. 1 vs. Exp. 3	1.30 ± 1.95	12	Auto vs. Exp. 2	1.48 ± 2.31	17
Exp. 2 vs. Exp. 3	1.41 ± 2.77	23	Auto vs. Exp. 3	1.36 ± 2.03	18

3.3   Evaluation of TCFA Prediction

At baseline, IVUS pullbacks from 24 patients exhibited 425 TCFAs and 1,906 non-TCFAs. During the time until follow-up, 325 (76.5%) TCFAs transitioned to another (less advanced, non-TCFA) form of plaque and 131 (6.9%) non-TCFAs became TCFAs. To establish a benchmark for comparisons, let us assume a naive strategy for prediction that would assume that all baseline TCFAs and non-TCFAs remain unchanged at follow-up. Under such a hypothetical scenario, a relatively low sensitivity of 43.3% and a specificity of 84.5% would result for TCFA prediction.

At follow-up, 231 TCFAs and 2,100 non-TCFAs were included in our registered VH-IVUS data. To alleviate the severely of data distribution imbalance between the two classes, 1/6 under-sampling was performed for the non-TCFA class to obtain a total of 349 non-TCFA samples for feature ranking. Other percentages of under-sampling were also tested in a preliminary experiment, with 1/6 producing the most reasonable prediction rates.

Fig. 4 illustrates the classification performance results for the evaluated feature set ranked by the SVM RFE technique. Reasonable prediction rates were obtained when employing 1–9 features, exhibiting a fair sensitivity and specificity (both higher than 65% in all these cases). The prediction performance diminished notably as the number

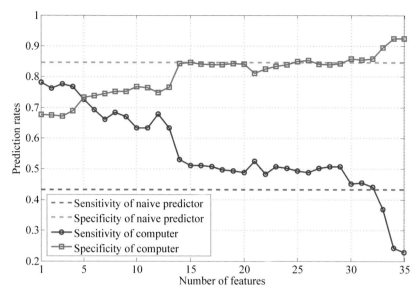

Fig. 4. Estimation of TCFA prediction rates as the number of ranked features.

of features increased beyond 13. The best performance with sensitivity of 72.6% and specificity of 73.3% was achieved when using the five highest-ranked features. This best-performing feature set consisted of: contextual plaque phenotype (F2), fibrotic tissue CSA (F6), hyperlipidemia (F27), standard deviation of plaque thickness (F19), and eccentricity (F20). It is worth mention that the first ranked feature (F2) was specifically designed for this study, which indicates TCFA-prediction value of information context reflecting disease severity in adjacent frames at baseline. Clearly, comparison with the naive prediction scenario outline above shows a notable improvement.

4   Conclusion

We have reported the first computer-aided prediction method to identify locations on the coronary artery that are likely to develop TCFA in the future that exhibits both promising sensitivity and specificity. Our prediction system is highly automated with the expert-guidance-based segmentation refinement being the only interactive step. Frame-to-frame correspondences between baseline and follow-up VH-IVUS pullbacks were determined using a 3D graph-based registration algorithm. The accuracy of segmentation and registration was statistically identical to experts. VH-IVUS derived features combined with systemic patient-specific biomarkers contained information relevant for prospective prediction of TCFA. One of our newly designed features – the contextual plaque phenotype – exhibited leading performance in the prediction task.

The major limitation of this research is that the VH-IVUS imaging alone might be insufficient for detecting TCFA, because of its limited image resolution unable to directly visualize thin fibrous caps. However, this limitation does not detract from the significance of the present results. Our work has clearly demonstrated that VH-IVUS derived indices of plaque morphology, combined with patient-specific biomarkers, are indeed capable of predicting plaque changes that have been shown to lead to major adverse cardiac events [3, 11]. Future work will incorporate 3-frame-based definition to identify 3-frame-TCFA lesions. We anticipate that our efforts will help stratify and identify those patients who have a high probability of developing multiple at-risk lesions so that they can be treated more aggressively with preventive measures.

Acknowledgment. Support of Volcano Corp. providing access to a research version of the IVUS-VH software is gratefully acknowledged. This research was supported - in part - by the NIH grants R01 EB004640 and R01 HL063373.

References

1. Alberti, M., Balocco, S., Carrillo, X., Mauri, J., Radeva, P.: Automatic non-rigid temporal alignment of IVUS sequences. In: Ayache, N., Delingette, H., Golland, P., Mori, K. (eds.) MICCAI 2012, Part I. LNCS, vol. 7510, pp. 642–650. Springer, Heidelberg (2012)
2. Chang, C.C., Lin, C.J.: Libsvm: a library for support vector machines. TIST 2(3), 27 (2011)
3. Cheng, J.M., Garcia-Garcia, H.M., de Boer, S.P., et al.: In vivo detection of high-risk coronary plaques by radiofrequency intravascular ultrasound and cardiovascular outcome: results of the ATHEROREMO-IVUS study. European Heart Journal 35(10), 639–647 (2014)
4. Corban, M.T., Eshtehardi, P., Suo, J., et al.: Combination of plaque burden, wall shear stress, and plaque phenotype has incremental value for prediction of coronary atherosclerotic plaque progression and vulnerability. Atherosclerosis 232(2), 271–276 (2014)
5. Cortes, C., Vapnik, V.: Support-vector networks. Machine Learning 20(3), 273–297 (1995)
6. Guyon, I., Weston, J., Barnhill, S., Vapnik, V.: Gene selection for cancer classification using support vector machines. Machine Learning 46(1-3), 389–422 (2002)
7. Kubo, T., Maehara, A., Mintz, G.S., et al.: The dynamic nature of coronary artery lesion morphology assessed by serial virtual histology intravascular ultrasound tissue characterization. Journal of the American College of Cardiology 55(15), 1590–1597 (2010)
8. Li, K., Wu, X., Chen, D.Z., Sonka, M.: Optimal surface segmentation in volumetric images - a graph-theoretic approach. TPAMI 28(1), 119–134 (2006)
9. Madabhushi, A., Agner, S., Basavanhally, A., Doyle, S., Lee, G.: Computer-aided prognosis: predicting patient and disease outcome via quantitative fusion of multi-scale, multi-modal data. CMIG 35(7), 506–514 (2011)
10. Stary, H.C.: Natural history and histological classification of atherosclerotic lesions an update. Arteriosclerosis, Thrombosis, and Vascular Biology 20(5), 1177–1178 (2000)
11. Stone, G.W., Maehara, A., Lansky, A.J., et al.: A prospective natural-history study of coronary atherosclerosis. New England Journal of Medicine 364(3), 226–235 (2011)
12. Sun, S., Sonka, M., Beichel, R.R.: Graph-based IVUS segmentation with efficient computer-aided refinement. TMI 32(8), 1536–1549 (2013)
13. Timmins, L., Suever, J., Eshtehardi, P., McDaniel, M., Oshinski, J., Samady, H., Giddens, D.: Framework to co-register longitudinal virtual histology-intravascular ultrasound data in the circumferential direction. TMI 32(11), 1989–1996 (2013)
14. Wang, S., Summers, R.M.: Machine learning and radiology. MedIA 16(5), 933–951 (2012)
15. Zhang, L., Wahle, A., Chen, Z., Zhang, L., Downe, R.W., Kovarnik, T., Sonka, M.: Joint registration of location and orientation of intravascular ultrasound pullbacks using a 3D graph based method. In: SPIE Medical Imaging, pp. 94131I–94131I (2015)

Cooperative Robotic Gamma Imaging: Enhancing US-guided Needle Biopsy*

Marco Esposito[1], Benjamin Busam[1,3], Christoph Hennersperger[1],
Julia Rackerseder[1], An Lu[1], Nassir Navab[1,2], and Benjamin Frisch[1]

[1] Computer Aided Medical Procedures (CAMP) Technische Universität München,
Germany
[2] Computer Aided Medical Procedures Johns Hopkins University, US
[3] FRAMOS GmbH, Taufkirchen, Germany

Abstract. Sentinel lymph node (sLN) biopsy mostly requires an invasive surgical intervention to remove sLNs under radioguidance. We present an alternative method where live ultrasound is combined with live robotic gamma imaging to provide real-time anatomical and nuclear guidance of punch biopsies. The robotic arm holding a gamma camera is equipped with a system for inside-out tracking to directly retrieve the relative position of the US transducer with respect to itself. Based on this, the system cooperatively positions the gamma camera parallel to the US imaging plane selected by the physician for real-time multi-modal visualization. We validate the feasibility of this approach with a dedicated gelatine/agar biopsy phantom and show that lymph nodes separated by at least 10 mm can be distinguished.

1   Introduction

The concept of multi-modal imaging is well established in the domain of nuclear medicine, where SPECT/CT, PET/CT, and PET/MR all combine functional with anatomical information. As such, the combination of these modalities is mostly limited to whole-body systems, with notable exceptions being the ClearPEM-Sonic [1] and endoTOFPET-US [2] projects for organ-specific PET and ultrasound (US) imaging. A procedure likely to benefit from a combination of functional and anatomical data is the sentinel lymph node (sLN) biopsy for breast cancer patients, where a radiotracer or colored dye is injected close to the cancer and its spread through the lymphatic system is monitored to identify the first series of nodes that are biopsied for histological assessment. The presence of cancer cells is a key element in staging the disease.

Classic radio-guided surgery uses a 1D gamma probe or a 2D gamma camera to identify radioactive-positive lymph nodes in open surgery [3]. Since these techniques provide functional information only, open surgery is required for the

---

* This work was partially funded by the the Bayerische Forschungsstiftung (project Ro-BildOR). We would like to thank the Department of Nuclear Medicine at Klinikum Rechts der Isar for their kind support with the experiments.

N. Navab et al. (Eds.): MICCAI 2015, Part II, LNCS 9350, pp. 611–618, 2015.
DOI: 10.1007/978-3-319-24571-3_73

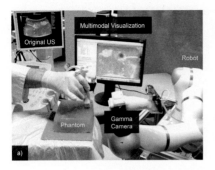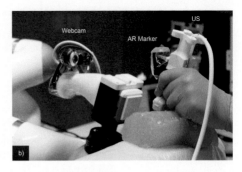

Fig. 1. a) View of the full setup and b) close-up of the multimodal image acquisition.

removal of sLNs. The possibility of punch biopsy under multi-modal guidance was recently introduced by combining freehand SPECT with 3D compounded ultrasound [4] and extended to thyroid imaging [5]. The current approach, whilst allowing for a combination of nuclear and anatomical information, suffers from having to conduct two subsequent acquisitions. This not only extends the procedure, but further does not provide any correction of anatomical deformations during the US scan or a real-time update of the information in the case of a displacement of the tissues of interest. Finally, they rely on external tracking systems, hampered either by the limited accuracy of electromagnetic tracking or the requirement for a line of sight between the tracked devices and an external optical tracking system respectively.

In this work we suggest a novel approach where the sLN punch biopsy can be performed by a single physician under the assistance of a cooperative robotic arm holding the gamma camera. The arm is equipped with a camera system for inside-out tracking, based on the detection of a 2D-marker as suggested by [6]. Using this tracking approach, the robotic arm cooperatively follows the US transducer during the intervention, where the gamma camera is positioned in a way to provide real-time 2D/2D gamma information and ultrasound images to guide the biopsy needle. While the idea of collaborative robotics has been introduced in the medical environment for telemanipulated systems [7] or laparoscopic camera placement [8], this paper introduces the combination of a light-weight robotic arm with camera-in-hand visual servoing in the context of a combination of functional and anatomical information.

2   Materials and Methods

2.1   Setup

The key element of our setup, as shown in Fig. 1, is a LBR 4+ (KUKA, Germany) light-weight robotic arm. A custom-designed 3D-printed mount attached to the tip of the robot arm is used in order to support both a CrystalCam (Crystal Photonics, Germany) gamma camera as well as a QuickCam Pro 9000 (Logitech, Switzerland) wide angle video camera. Ultrasound imaging is provided by an UltraSonix RP US system (Ultrasonix, MA, USA) with a curvilinear probe (model C5/60). The camera detects the position and orientation of a 2D ArUco marker [6] which is rigidly attached to the ultrasound transducer. We further use an infrared optical tracking system (Polaris Vicra, Northern Digital Inc., Ontario, Canada) during the calibration procedure. A standard punch biopsy needle (HistoCore 250 mm, BIP GmbH, Germany) was used in the experiments.

The system consists of two major software components. The first one is a collection of concurrent processes dedicated to tracking and robot control, while the main purpose of the second is visualization. The only communication between them regards the position of the gamma camera with respect to the US probe, expressed as a 6DoF transform, which is necessary in order to correctly merge the images received from both devices.

2.2 Tracking and Robot Control

Our setup is based on the ROS framework [9], and in particular we leveraged the TF library[1] to maintain a global knowledge of the current position of the individual objects of interest in space. Most notably, this includes the robot, the gamma camera and the US probe.

We make use of a wide-angle camera as tracking device in order to retrieve the relative position of the US probe with respect to the gamma camera, and in turn to the robotic arm. This is achieved through the tracking of an AR marker attached to the probe, which provides the transform $^{webcam}_{marker}T$. As the main interest lies in the pose of the tip of the gamma camera with respect to the tip of the US probe, two more transforms are necessary to constitute the calibration of the system: i) a transform from the AR marker to the tip of the US probe defined as a reference frame in the middle of the scanning surface, with the x axis pointing along the probe and z pointing out of the scanning plane, and ii) a transform from the camera to the tip of the gamma camera defined as the center of the sensor, with x pointing to the gamma camera handle and z pointing inside the sensor. This convention minimizes the rotational component between the two tip reference frames.

Calibration. The system requires a one-time calibration in order to find the relative position of the components (robot hand-gamma camera-webcam, AR marker-tip of US probe).

The transformation between the RGB data and gamma camera tip is composed of two individual calibrations with respect to the robot end effector, c.f. Fig. 2a

$$^{webcam}_{gamma}T = {}^{webcam}_{ee}T \; ^{ee}_{gamma}T, \tag{1}$$

where $gamma$ is the gamma tip, ee is the robot end effector and $webcam$ is the camera reference frame. The transformation $^{webcam}_{ee}T$ is found with a procedure based on the Tsai-Lenz algorithm [10] in the eye-on-hand variant, with the

---

[1] http://wiki.ros.org/tf

implementation provided by the ViSP library [11]. In this regard, the robot is moved to several poses such that the camera can observe the AR marker and the ArUco [6] tracking library can estimate the transform from the camera to the marker for each position. The resulting series of corresponding transforms are used as input for the calibration algorithm in order to compute the transform between the camera and the robotic arm end effector.

Next, we retrieve the transform $^{ee}_{gamma}T$ using a NDI tracking device and a dedicated instrument that replaces the gamma camera collimator. The transformation between the tracking system and the basis of the robot is found with the eye-on-base variant of the aforementioned Tsai-Lenz algorithm, which requires a marker attached to the robot end effector. Then, the transformation between the calibration tool and the end effector is computed as

$$^{ee}_{gamma}T = {}^{ee}_{tool}T = {}^{ee}_{base}T \; {}^{base}_{NDI}T \; {}^{NDI}_{tool}T, \tag{2}$$

where $base$ is the robot base, NDI the NDI tracking device, and $tool$ the calibration tool reference frame which by definition coincides with the $gamma$ reference frame that is the objective of the calibration procedure.

Finally, the calibration of the US tip, $i.e.$ the transform $^{marker}_{us}T$ from the AR marker to the desired reference frame is retrieved through an analogous procedure. After calibrating the NDI to the robot, an NDI pointer tool is positioned on the tip of the probe. The final transform is then computed from the following transform chain:

$$^{marker}_{us}T = {}^{marker}_{pointer}T = {}^{marker}_{webcam}T \; {}^{webcam}_{ee}T \; {}^{ee}_{base}T \; {}^{base}_{NDI}T \; {}^{NDI}_{pointer}T \tag{3}$$

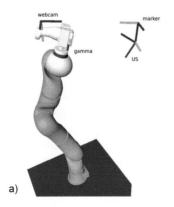
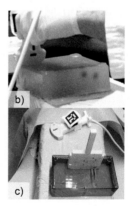

Fig. 2. a) Overview of the reference frames. b) and c) respectively show the gelatine/agar and the plastic sphere phantom.

2.3   Cooperative Path Planning

A static transform is added to the scene in order to represent the desired position of the gamma camera tip with respect to the ultrasound tip. To do so, the gamma frame is placed at a distance of 10 cm and 2 cm in the z and x directions, in order to align the top of the gamma camera and US images and keep a comfortable distance to the patient. The planning software consists of a control loop that runs in a dedicated process, which brings the gamma camera tip in position (0,0,0) with respect to the target reference frame in order to obtain the desired motion:

> **while** *not shutdown* **do**
> > wait for tracking data;
> > compute trajectory;
> > **if** *success* **then**
> > > execute trajectory;
> > > sleep 0.1 seconds;
> >
> > **end**
>
> **end**

Algorithm 1. Robot control loop

Thereby, the sleeping step has a normalization effect and avoids robot vibration and controller overload. The robot movement happens at considerably slow speed (240 mm/s) for various reasons, first of all safety. Furthermore, a slow speed prevents the robot from overshooting the movement in one direction, which would cause the marker to exit the camera image and the tracking to get interrupted. Moreover, a slower movement is also reassuring for both the user and operator. As a safety measure, movement is interrupted when tracking is lost; furthermore, complete trajectory planning is performed at every iteration in order to avoid problems at singular positions or joint limits.

2.4   Image Visualization

The visualization is implemented as a pipeline for the CAMPVis framework [12]. This includes modules to connect to the gamma camera, an OpenIGTLink client receiving images from the US device, and a client for the transformation between the two images, respectively. The US acquisition module provides a live streaming of the US rays, while the gamma camera transmits single events being only visible by integrating them in time for each pixel individually. Hence, the intensity at a given pixel is represented as the number of events that have been observed in the last period of time and is thresholded in order to exclude single random events. In order to resemble the probabilistic nature of the gamma information, pixel information is blurred before visualization using a Gaussian window and alpha blending. For live fusion of US and gamma information, the latter is projected into the US plane along the normal represented by the gamma tip z axis. Thereby, the translation and the varying spatial resolutions are taken into account in order to create a geometrically correct image, resulting in a labeled US image, where radiation is blended in red.

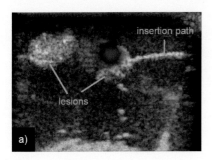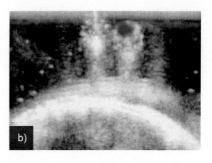

Fig. 3. Multimodal nuclear and US visualization of a) two lesions in the gelatine/Agar phantom and b) two spheres in the accuracy phantom.

3   Experimental Validation

Biopsy Phantom. We evaluate the suitability of the proposed system under two aspects. A first experiment shows the qualitative benefit of the system for a physician performing a sentinel lymph node biospy, provided that it is possible to correctly identify radioactive lymph nodes with this technique. To do so, we use gelatine and agar phantoms for multimodal SPECT (Fig. 2b), CT and US imaging that can be biopsied, following the procedure proposed by [13]. The lymph nodes are mimicked by a mix of 12 weight percent (wt%) of gelatine and 8 wt% of agar, while the surrounding tissue is made of 4 wt% and 1.5 wt% of Agar. 1 MBq of ^{99m}Tc is added to some of the lymph nodes and both, hot and cold nodes are inserted at an average depth of 2 cm into the tissue mimicking material and visually distinguished by blue and red food coloring.

The procedure starts by guiding the gamma camera towards the phantom. In this sense, a medical expert holds the ultrasound transducer into the field of view of the camera mounted on the robot. The ArUco marker is then recognized and the gamma camera follows the US. In the following, a scan for lymph nodes is performed, where the fusion of SPECT and ultrasound helps the examiner to localize the two radioactive nodes within the phantom. If a radioactive-positive target is found, a biopsy is performed under US guidance.

Fig. 3a shows a typical visualization of the combined nuclear and US information for two adjacent nodes. The radioactive-positive lesion is clearly identified. The insertion path of the biopsy needle is also clearly visible. A biopsy study was conducted on 4 lesions, two of which were radioactively labelled. The biopsies confirmed that all lesions were correctly identified in the multi-modal images.

Accuracy. A second experiment evaluates the minimum distance between two nodules, one of which being radioactive-positive, to be distinguished from the other. As shown in Fig. 2c, two plastic spheres with a diameter of 9 mm are filled with 0.5 MBq of ^{99m}Tc each and mounted rigidly on two bars on an evaluation board, where it is possible to change the distance between their centers in steps of 10 mm. The board is set up in a box of water such that the spheres are positioned 3 cm away from the edge of the box and the spheres are covered by

2 cm of water. The ultrasound probe is immersed into the water in order to scan the spheres. The augmented images are visually evaluated to estimate the minimal distance allowing for a clear identification of the radioactive-positive sphere. Fig. 3b shows the multimodal image acquired with the hot and cold spheres adjacent to each other, at a distance of 10 mm between their centers. The hot sphere can be clearly identified.

Marker Tracking Accuracy. As a side experiment we evaluated the precision of the marker tracking application. A marker was fixed to a surface and kept in the field of view of the camera while moving the robot arm. We compared the motion as detected from the marker tracker and the robot controller, and the standard deviation between the two resulted to be 1.7 mm. We deemed the accuracy as appropriate to the needs of the particular clinical application.

4   Discussion

The first part of the experimental validation shows that our approach allows for a clear identification of radioactive-positive nodules, as they can be successfully differentiated from cold nodules in a dedicated multi-modal phantom. The outcome of the biopsy, where every nodule was correctly targeted, confirms that this system can be used to guide a punch biopsy needle. The second experiment shows that even closely located nodules can be distinguished. The system proved to be stable to allow for a full scan of the region of interest to detect and identify nodules and to perform the biopsy during intervention. The robotic arm followed the ultrasound device at a stable distance, providing for an intuitive handling and constant image quality.

On the contrary of [5] and [4], the presented solution provides real-time simultaneous multi-modal nuclear and US imaging, without requiring for consecutive imaging and the need to correct for deformations due to the US acquisition. The use of the camera-in-hand inside-out tracking voids the necessity for an external optical tracking system, relieving the operator from having to pay attention to not obstructing the line of sight. Moreover, the workflow is extremely similar to a standard US-guided punch biopsy, which is familiar to many physicians. On the other side, however, our system does not provide 3D volumetric imaging, consequently requiring the physician to take acquisitions from different directions to be able to distinguish nodes that would be hidden in one particular 2D view. Although using a lightweight robot might seem like an exaggeration at this stage of the development, our system opens the way to further developments on the path of collaborative robotics in the medical environment. In particular, the inclusion of an external RGBD monitoring would provide for live collision avoidance while voice control of the robot would facilitate additional interaction with the robot. Finally, a clinical study will be required in order to evaluate the full feasibility and potential of such an approach.

5   Conclusion

This paper presents the first prototype for cooperative robotic gamma imaging to enhance US-guided needle biopsy and offers a real-time imaging solution that could contribute to reducing the number of open sentinel lymph node resections. It introduces the use of camera-in-hand visual servoing for multi-modal medical image acquisition and opens the way for further developments in this domain.

References

1. Frisch, B.: Development of ClearPEM-Sonic: A multimodal positron emission mammograph and ultrasound scanner. In: 2011 IEEE Nuclear Science Symposium and Medical Imaging Conference (NSS/MIC), pp. 2267–2272 (October 2011)
2. Zvolsky, M.: the EndoTOFPET-US Collaboration: EndoTOFPET-US a miniaturised calorimeter for endoscopic time-of-flight positron emission tomography. Journal of Physics: Conference Series 587(1), 012068 (2015)
3. Vidal-Sicart, S., Valdes Olmos, R.: Sentinel node mapping for breast cancer: Current situation. Journal of Oncology (2012)
4. Okur, A., Hennersperger, C., Runyan, B., Gardiazabal, J., Keicher, M., Paepke, S., Wendler, T., Navab, N.: fhSPECT-US guided needle biopsy of sentinel lymph nodes in the axilla: Is it feasible? In: Golland, P., Hata, N., Barillot, C., Hornegger, J., Howe, R. (eds.) MICCAI 2014, Part I. LNCS, vol. 8673, pp. 577–584. Springer, Heidelberg (2014)
5. Freesmeyer, M., Opfermann, T., Winkens, T.: Hybrid integration of real-time us and freehand spect: Proof of concept in patients with thyroid diseases. Radiology 271(3), 856–861 (2014); PMID: 24475866
6. Garrido-Jurado, S., Munoz-Salinas, R., Madrid-Cuevas, F.J., Marin-Jimenez, M.J.: Automatic generation and detection of highly reliable fiducial markers under occlusion. Pattern Recognition 47(6), 2280–2292 (2014)
7. Padoy, N., Hager, G.: Human-machine collaborative surgery using learned models. In: 2011 IEEE International Conference on Robotics and Automation (ICRA), pp. 5285–5292 (May 2011)
8. Rivas-Blanco, I., Estebanez, B., Cuevas-Rodriguez, M., Bauzano, E., Munoz, V.: Towards a cognitive camera robotic assistant. In: 5th IEEE International Conference on Biomedical Robotics and Biomechatronics, pp. 739–744 (August 2014)
9. Quigley, M., Conley, K., Gerkey, B., Faust, J., Foote, T., Leibs, J., Wheeler, R., Ng, A.Y.: ROS: an open-source robot operating system. In: ICRA Workshop on Open Source Software, vol. 3, p. 5 (2009)
10. Tsai, R., Lenz, R.: A new technique for fully autonomous and efficient 3D robotics hand/eye calibration. IEEE Transactions on Robotics and Automation 5(3), 345–358 (1989)
11. Marchand, É., Spindler, F., Chaumette, F.: ViSP for visual servoing: a generic software platform with a wide class of robot control skills. IEEE Robotics & Automation Magazine 12(4), 40–52 (2005)
12. Schulte zu Berge, C., Grunau, A., Mahmud, H., Navab, N.: CAMPVis – A Game Engine-inspired Research Framework for Medical Imaging and Visualization. Technical report, Technische Universität München (2014)
13. Dang, J., Frisch, B., Lasaygues, P., Zhang, D., Tavernier, S., Felix, N., Lecoq, P., Auffray, E., Varela, J., Mensah, S., Wan, M.: Development of an anthropomorphic breast phantom for combined PET, b-mode ultrasound and elastographic imaging. IEEE Transactions on Nuclear Science 58(3), 660–667 (2011)

Bayesian Tomographic Reconstruction Using Riemannian MCMC

Stefano Pedemonte[1,2], Ciprian Catana[1], and Koen Van Leemput[1,2,3]

[1] Athinoula A. Martinos Center for Biomedical Imaging, MGH/Harvard, MA, USA
[2] Department of Computer Science and Department of Neuroscience and Biomedical
Engineering, Aalto University, Aalto, Finland
[3] Department of Applied Mathematics and Computer Science,
Technical University of Denmark, Lyngby, Denmark

Abstract. This paper describes the use of Monte Carlo sampling for tomographic image reconstruction. We describe an efficient sampling strategy, based on the Riemannian Manifold Markov Chain Monte Carlo algorithm, that exploits the peculiar structure of tomographic data, enabling efficient sampling of the high-dimensional probability densities that arise in tomographic imaging. Experiments with positron emission tomography (PET) show that the method enables the quantification of the uncertainty associated with tomographic acquisitions and allows the use of arbitrary risk functions in the reconstruction process.

1 Introduction

A tomographic imaging device produces an indirect measurement of a spatially-dependent quantity. In the case of positron emission tomography, the interaction of photons with the array of detection crystals provides information about the rate of nuclear decay. In the early days, the tomographic reconstruction problem was addressed with a mathematical formulation arising in the context of integral geometry: the Radon transform. Such idealized formulation provides an exact inversion formula under the assumptions of noiseless measurements and infinitesimally small detection elements. Starting with Shepp and Vardi [1], the formulation of the reconstruction problem in the probabilistic framework has enabled the development of algorithms that account for the uncertainty associated to the measurements and employ accurate models of the characteristics of the imaging devices. While in the context of tomographic imaging the research community has focused on the development of algorithms to compute a *best guess* of the unknown parameters, under the *maximum likelihood* (ML) and *maximum a posteriori* (MAP) point estimation criteria, in the context of low-level vision, starting with Geman and Geman [2], there has been a growing interest in the fully Bayesian approach to probabilistic reasoning, based on Markov Chain Monte Carlo (MCMC) sampling. In contrast to point-estimation criteria, which aim to maximize a density function, the fully Bayesian approach aims to characterize the entire posterior probability density induced by the imaging experiment. This enables the quantification of the uncertainty, as reported

© Springer International Publishing Switzerland 2015
N. Navab et al. (Eds.): MICCAI 2015, Part II, LNCS 9350, pp. 619–626, 2015.
DOI: 10.1007/978-3-319-24571-3_74

in recent applications in low-level vision, including image restoration [3], super-resolution [4], optical-flow [5], *etc.* and in numerous applications in the field of spatial statistics.

The computational complexity of the fully Bayesian approach via sampling techniques has hindered its application in high-dimensional problems that present strong non-local interdependence of the parameters, such as occurs in tomographic imaging due to the integral measurements along lines-of-response (LORs). Recently, Girolami and Calderhead [7] have presented a new class of MCMC algorithms, based on concepts of differential geometry, that exploit the natural structure of probability density functions, achieving significantly improved computational efficiency in high-dimensional problems with strongly correlated parameters. Such formulation is an extension of Hamiltonian Monte Carlo (HMC), a sampling technique based on data-augmentation that was first introduced by Duane *et al.* [8].

In this paper we describe a sampling algorithm for tomographic imaging based on the formulation of Girolami and Calderhead [7]. We describe a strategy that exploits the natural geometry of the probability density function and the spatial structure of tomographic data to enable sampling from the high-dimensional probability densities that arise in tomographic imaging. In the experiments we highlight how the algorithm enables the quantification of uncertainty and enables the use of risk functions in the reconstruction other than the one that leads to MAP estimation.

2   Efficient Sampling of Tomographic Imaging Data

This section first introduces the imaging model for PET and gives an overview of state-of-the-art Hamiltonian Monte Carlo; then it introduces the details of the computational strategy that enables efficient sampling of tomographic data.

2.1   Imaging Model and Overall Sampling Procedure

PET imaging operates in the photon-limited regime. Discretizing the problem on an image lattice, with discrete locations indexed by v, and letting d index the LORs; the probability density associated to the number of counts $\boldsymbol{y} = [y_1, \ldots, y_d, \ldots, y_D]^T$, conditional to the rates of emission $\boldsymbol{x} = [x_1, \ldots, x_v, \ldots, x_N]^T$, is a product of Poisson functions (see e.g. [1]):

$$p(\boldsymbol{y}|\boldsymbol{x}) = \prod_{d=1}^{D} \frac{e^{-[\boldsymbol{Ax}]_d} [\boldsymbol{Ax}]_d^{y_d}}{y_d!}, \tag{1}$$

where each element of the system matrix $\boldsymbol{A} = \{a_{dv}\}$ expresses the probability that a pair of photons emitted from location v is detected in LOR d. Given a prior probability density $p(\boldsymbol{x})$, MAP estimation consists in finding the value of $\boldsymbol{x}$ that maximizes the posterior probability density $p(\boldsymbol{x}|\boldsymbol{y}) \propto p(\boldsymbol{y}|\boldsymbol{x})p(\boldsymbol{x})$. Numerous algorithms have been reported for the maximization of the posterior, the most notables being the MLEM algorithm for non-informative uniform priors, first described by Shepp and Vardi [1], and the one-step-late MAP-EM algorithm for arbitrary log-differentiable priors, introduced by Green [6]. Rather than computing the maximizer, the aim of the algorithm described in the following is to characterize the full posterior density by MCMC sampling.

The samples are generated using a Markov Chain with equilibrium $p(\boldsymbol{x}|\boldsymbol{y})$, obtained with the Metropolis-Hastings (MH) method. A new candidate is generated according to a proposal distribution $q(\boldsymbol{x}^*|\boldsymbol{x}^s)$ and accepted/rejected according to the MH criterion. Letting s index the samples:

$$\boldsymbol{x}^* \sim q(\boldsymbol{x}^*|\boldsymbol{x}^s) \tag{2}$$

$$u \sim \mathrm{unif}(0,1) \tag{3}$$

$$\alpha = \min\left[1, \frac{p(\boldsymbol{x}^*|\boldsymbol{y})q(\boldsymbol{x}^s|\boldsymbol{x}^*)}{p(\boldsymbol{x}^s|\boldsymbol{y})q(\boldsymbol{x}^*|\boldsymbol{x}^s)}\right] \tag{4}$$

$$\boldsymbol{x}^{s+1} := \begin{cases} \boldsymbol{x}^* & \text{if } u < \alpha \\ \boldsymbol{x}^s & \text{if } u \geq \alpha \end{cases} \tag{5}$$

Under the MH criterion, if the proposal $q(\boldsymbol{x}^*|\boldsymbol{x}^s)$ is *reversible* (see e.g. [9]), the sequence is guaranteed to be distributed, at equilibrium, according to the probability density $p(\boldsymbol{x}|\boldsymbol{y})$. A usual choice is to let the proposal $q(\boldsymbol{x}^*|\boldsymbol{x}^s)$ be a Gaussian distribution centered in $\boldsymbol{x}^s$, so that points closer to $\boldsymbol{x}^s$ are more likely to be visited next. Such choice makes the sequence of samples a random-walk, producing high acceptance rate, but slow exploration of the space of the solutions. In order to scale to high-dimensions, it is necessary to make large steps in the proposal of the MH algorithm, while maintaining the probability of acceptance α high. Duane *et al.* [8] introduced a proposal based on data-augmentation that, unlike random walk, uses the derivatives of the posterior density to allow for large steps with high probability of acceptance. The technique consists in introducing a variable $\boldsymbol{z}$ of the same dimensionality of $\boldsymbol{x}$, independent from $\boldsymbol{x}$ and normally distributed with covariance $\boldsymbol{M}$ (denominated *mass-matrix*): $\log p(\boldsymbol{x}, \boldsymbol{z}|\boldsymbol{y}) = \log p(\boldsymbol{x}|\boldsymbol{y}) - \frac{1}{2}\log\{(2\pi)^N|\boldsymbol{M}|\} - \frac{1}{2}\boldsymbol{z}^T\boldsymbol{M}^{-1}\boldsymbol{z}$; the new candidate is computed by drawing a random sample of $\boldsymbol{z}$ and moving along the iso-curve of the joint probability density of $\boldsymbol{x}$ and $\boldsymbol{z}$, described by the Hamiltonian equations with fictitious time t:

$$\boldsymbol{z}^* \sim \mathcal{N}(\boldsymbol{z}; 0, \boldsymbol{M}) \tag{6}$$

$$\begin{bmatrix} \frac{dx_i}{dt} = -\frac{\partial \log p(\boldsymbol{x},\boldsymbol{z}|\boldsymbol{y})}{\partial z_i} = [\boldsymbol{M}^{-1}\boldsymbol{z}]_i \\ \frac{dz_i}{dt} = \frac{\partial \log p(\boldsymbol{x},\boldsymbol{z}|\boldsymbol{y})}{\partial x_i} = [\nabla_{\boldsymbol{x}}\log p(\boldsymbol{x}|\boldsymbol{y})]_i \end{bmatrix} \tag{7}$$

This procedure generates samples from $p(\boldsymbol{x}, \boldsymbol{z}|\boldsymbol{y})$. The samples from the marginal density $p(\boldsymbol{x}|\boldsymbol{y})$ are obtained simply by discarding the samples of $\boldsymbol{z}$. To discretize the Hamiltonian dynamics, we employ the Stormer-Verlet leapfrog integrator, employed by Duane and others. With N_K integration steps ($k = 1, \ldots, N_K$):

$$\begin{bmatrix} \boldsymbol{x}^{*k+1} = \boldsymbol{x}^{*k} + \epsilon\,\boldsymbol{M}^{-1}\left[\boldsymbol{z}^{*k} + \frac{\epsilon}{2}\nabla_{\boldsymbol{x}}\log p(\boldsymbol{x}^{*k}|\boldsymbol{y})\right] \\ \boldsymbol{z}^{*k+1} = \boldsymbol{z}^{*k} + \frac{\epsilon}{2}\nabla_{\boldsymbol{x}}\log p(\boldsymbol{x}^{*k}|\boldsymbol{y}) + \frac{\epsilon}{2}\nabla_{\boldsymbol{x}}\log p(\boldsymbol{x}^{*k+1}|\boldsymbol{y}) \end{bmatrix} \tag{8}$$

The Stormer-Verlet integrator is perfectly time-reversible (see Neal [9] and Giro-lami [7]), therefore guaranteeing reversibility of the overal proposal function for any positive definite mass matrix $\boldsymbol{M}$. The choice of the mass-matrix and of the integration step, addressed next, is critical for the performance of the sampler, especially when the problem exhibits strong correlations [7].

2.2   Efficient Sampling of Tomographic Data

While HMC is well established across multiple domains of computational science, its application to tomographic imaging is challenging. First, the rate of emission $\boldsymbol{x}$ is non-negative. We propose to impose non-negativity by simulating an elastic boundary [9]:

$$\left.\begin{aligned} x_i^{*k+1} &:= -x_i^{*k+1} \\ z_i^{*k+1} &:= -z_i^{*k+1} \end{aligned}\right\} \text{ if } x_i^{*k+1} < 0 \tag{9}$$

Second, the variables are strongly correlated, leading to high rates of rejection for naive implementation of the HMC algorithm. As pointed out in the recent for-mulation of Girolami and Calderhead [7], the Fisher Information Matrix (FIM) of the likelihood term, defined, for the PET imaging model, as:

$$\boldsymbol{H_x}: \ h_{ij} = -\frac{\partial^2}{\partial x_i \partial x_j} \log p(\boldsymbol{x}|\boldsymbol{y}) = \sum_{d=1}^{D} \frac{a_{di} a_{dj} \, y_d}{\left(\sum_{v=1}^{N} u_{dv} \boldsymbol{x}_v\right)^2}, \tag{10}$$

constitutes a piece-wise constant approximation of the metric tensor of the Rie-mann structure of the parameter space. The choice $\boldsymbol{M} = \boldsymbol{H_x}^{-1}$ yields effective transitions that respect and exploit the geometry of the manifold, with the ef-fect of increasing the performance of the sampler and making the choice of the integration step ϵ non-critical.

In tomographic imaging, the FIM is too large to be evaluated numerically and stored. However the spatial organization of the parameters allows for approxi-mations. Assuming periodic boundary conditions, the FIM (10) is well approx-imated by a block-circulant matrix with circulant blocks (BCCB), an approxi-mation commonly utilized, in various ways, in imaging applications [10]. By the Fourier diagonalisation properties of BCCB matrices:

$$\boldsymbol{H_x}^{\mathrm{BCCB}} = \boldsymbol{F}^\dagger \boldsymbol{\Lambda} \boldsymbol{F} \tag{11}$$

$$\boldsymbol{\Lambda} = \mathrm{diag}(\sqrt{N} \boldsymbol{F} \boldsymbol{h}_1), \tag{12}$$

where $\boldsymbol{F}$ is the Discrete Fourier Transform matrix, $\boldsymbol{F}^\dagger$ its complex conjugate, and $\boldsymbol{h}_1$ the first column of the FIM. Following (12), the BCCB approximation reduces the matrix-vector multiplication in (8) to a convolution. Furthermore, sampling the hidden variable $\boldsymbol{z}^*$ becomes trivial using the method of the affine transformation:

$$\boldsymbol{v} \sim \mathcal{N}(0, I) \tag{13}$$

$$\boldsymbol{z} = \boldsymbol{F}^\dagger \boldsymbol{\Lambda}^{-\frac{1}{2}} \boldsymbol{v} \tag{14}$$

The sample of z^* is obtained by generating a vector of independent normal variates and computing an inverse Fourier transformation (14).

A further approximation is introduced by computing the BCCB FIM just once, for x equal to the MAP estimate (the ML estimate in case of uninformative prior).

2.3 Summary of the Algorithm

In summary, the algorithm consists in first constructing an estimate of the BCCB FIM, obtained by performing an initial reconstruction with the MAP-EM algorithm [6] and by computing the first column of the Hessian matrix and its Fourier transform; then, at each iteration, the new candidate is obtained by sampling the hidden variable z^{*0} and integrating the Hamiltonian dynamics with elastic boundary; the resulting candidate is accepted or rejected according to the MH criterion for the joint density. Samples of z are discarded:

Fisher Information
$$\begin{bmatrix} x^{MAP} = \arg\min_x - \log p(x|y) \\ h_1^{BCCB} : \quad h_{1j}^{BCCB} = \sum_{d=1}^{D} \frac{a_{d1} a_{dj} y_d}{\left(\sum_{i=1}^{N} a_{di} x_i^{MAP} \right)^2} \\ \Lambda = \mathrm{diag} \left(\sqrt{N} F h_1^{BCCB} \right) \end{bmatrix} \tag{15}$$

New candidate
$$\begin{bmatrix} \text{for } s = 1 : N_S \\ v \sim \mathcal{N}(0, I) \\ z^{*0} = F^\dagger \Lambda^{-\frac{1}{2}}(v) \\ x^{*0} = x^{s-1} \end{bmatrix} \tag{16}$$

Hamiltonian dynamics
$$\begin{bmatrix} \text{for } k = 0 : N_K \\ w = z^{*k} + \frac{\epsilon}{2} \nabla_x \log p(x^{*k}|y) \\ x^{*k+1} = x^{*k} + \epsilon \, F^\dagger \Lambda F w \\ z^{*k+1} = w + \frac{\epsilon}{2} \nabla_x \log p(x^{*k+1}|y) \\ \left. \begin{array}{l} x_i^{*k+1} := -x_i^{*k+1} \\ z_i^{*k+1} := -z_i^{*k+1} \end{array} \right\} \text{ if } x_i^{*k+1} < 0 \end{bmatrix} \tag{17}$$

Accept / reject
$$\begin{bmatrix} u \sim \mathrm{unif}(0,1) \\ \alpha = \min \left[1, \frac{p(x^*|y)}{p(x^s|y)} e^{-\frac{1}{2}(z^*)^T F^\dagger \Lambda F z^* + \frac{1}{2}(z^{*0})^T F^\dagger \Lambda F z^{*0}} \right] \\ x^{s+1} := \begin{cases} x^* & \text{if } u < \alpha \\ x^s & \text{if } u \geq \alpha \end{cases} \end{bmatrix} \tag{18}$$

With the BCCB approximation, the calculation of the gradient $\nabla_x \log p(x|y) = \nabla_x \log p(x) + A^T \left(\frac{y}{Ax} - \bar{1} \right)$ constitutes the most computationally expensive step, entailing a projection (i.e. the simulation of the light propagation process) and a back-projection. In the experiments that follow, in order to speed up the computations, we utilize a GPU-accelerated ray-tracer, achieving a rate of 50 gradient evaluations per sec with a 64^3 image lattice, using a GPU NVidia Tesla K20.

3   Experiments

The following experiments were performed to investigate the use of MCMC for tomographic image formation. A healthy volunteer was administered 170 MBq of FDG and scanned for 60 min with a Siemens Biograph mMR scanner. The list-mode data was binned (discarding intra-ring coincidences, to reduce the complexity) into three sinograms of duration 20 min, 40 min and 60 min since the start of the acquisition. For each sinogram, an initial reconstruction on a image lattice of 64^3 4 mm isotropic voxels was obtained by running the standard MLEM algorithm until approximate convergence. The first column of the Hessian matrix was computed, for each of the three measurements, using the initial reconstruction. A total of $N_S = 5000$ samples was drawn for each of the three measurements using the uninformative prior (the number of samples was selected empirically to obtain smooth marginals - Fig. 3). The number of integration steps was set to $N_K = 10$ and the integration step size was set empirically to $\epsilon = 0.08$ to obtain acceptance rate near 0.5 – see in Fig. 1-(I). Fig. 1-(II-IV) provides a visualization of the BCCB approximation for the 40 min experiment.

3.1   Uncertainty Quantification

The samples of the posterior density can be used to quantify and visualize the uncertainty associated to the tomographic measurement. Fig. 2(III) displays the sample variance for the 40 min acquisition and Fig. 3 reports the histograms of the samples relative to the three voxels A,B,C, indicated in Fig. 2(I), for the three acquisition times. Providing uncertainty images such as 2(III) alongside the reconstructions themselves is of direct potential clinical use in e.g., tumor imaging to improve diagnosis/detection and interpretation of clinical images. The plots in Fig. 3 demonstrate that the method allows one to capture the increase of information obtained by increasing the scanning time – something that conventional reconstruction algorithms based on point estimation cannot provide. With (much) more powerful computers, this may ultimately provide application-specific real-time feedback on when to stop scanning.

3.2   Decision Theoretic Criteria for Image Reconstruction

Decision theory allows us to obtain estimates that are optimal according to certain risk criteria. In the decision theoretic framework, estimates are obtained by minimizing the expected risk:

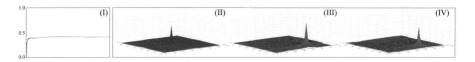

Fig. 1. 20 min scan: (I) Acceptance rate; (II) Column of the FIM matrix, central voxel; (III) Column of the FIM matrix, peripheral voxel; (IV) Column of the BCCB FIM matrix, peripheral voxel.

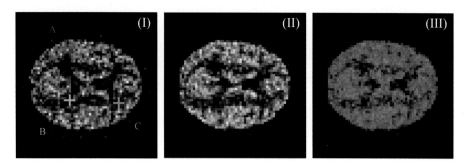

Fig. 2. 40 *min* scan: (I) MAP estimate - MLEM; (II) MMSE estimate (sample mean); (III) Sample variance of each voxel's marginal posterior distribution. A,B,C see Fig.3.

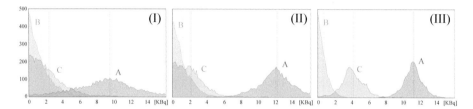

Fig. 3. Histograms of the posterior samples for voxels A,B,C in Fig. 2. (I) 20 *min* scan; (II) 40 *min* scan; (III) 60 *min* scan. Dotted lines indicate the MLE estimates and dashed lines the MMSE estimates (i.e., the sample means). Note the reduction in reconstruction uncertainty with longer acquisition time.

$$\hat{\boldsymbol{x}} = \arg\min_{\tilde{\boldsymbol{x}}} \int L(\tilde{\boldsymbol{x}} - \boldsymbol{x}) \, p(\boldsymbol{x}|\boldsymbol{y}) \, \mathrm{d}\boldsymbol{x}, \qquad (19)$$

where $L(\tilde{\boldsymbol{x}} - \boldsymbol{x})$ represents the loss associated to choosing $\tilde{\boldsymbol{x}}$ when the true underlying value is $\boldsymbol{x}$. The MAP estimation criterion corresponds to the particular choice of the loss function that assigns the same penalty whenever the estimate is not the true underlying variable and none otherwise: $L(\tilde{\boldsymbol{x}} - \boldsymbol{x}) = 1 - \delta_{\tilde{\boldsymbol{x}}\boldsymbol{x}}$, where δ is the Kronecker Delta function. In this case, the minimum risk solution simplifies to $\hat{\boldsymbol{x}} = \arg\max_{\tilde{\boldsymbol{x}}} p(\tilde{\boldsymbol{x}}|\boldsymbol{y})$. In general, however, the integral (19) is intractable. The posterior sampling approach via MCMC enables us to approximate the integral in equation (19) as a finite sum over the samples, allowing the definition of arbitrary risk criteria.

As an example we can perform image reconstruction by computing the Bayesian minimum mean squared error estimate (MMSE), which assigns cost in proportion to the distance of an estimate from the true value, in the sense of the $L2$-norm: $\hat{\boldsymbol{x}} = \arg\min_{\tilde{\boldsymbol{x}}} \int \|\tilde{\boldsymbol{x}} - \boldsymbol{x}\|^2 p(\boldsymbol{x}|\boldsymbol{y}) \, \mathrm{d}\boldsymbol{x} = \int \boldsymbol{x} \, p(\boldsymbol{x}|\boldsymbol{y}) \, \mathrm{d}\boldsymbol{x} \approx \frac{1}{N_S} \sum_{s=1}^{N_S} \boldsymbol{x}^s$. MMSE is equal to the mean of the posterior distribution and approximated by the sample mean. Fig. 2 displays the central transverse slice of (I) the MAP estimate (with non-informative prior) obtained with the MLEM algorithm iterated until approximate convergence and of (II) the MMSE estimate obtained by averaging the samples. The vertical lines in Fig.3 indicate the MMSE and MAP estimates for voxels A,B and C, indicating how the two differ quantitatively. Note that sampling allows for more general reconstruction loss functions than the two reported in Fig. 2, e.g., functions that in tumor detection penalize false negatives more heavily than false positives. Exploring this further is left for future work.

4   Conclusion

In this paper, we have introduced an algorithm for the posterior sampling of the unknown parameters in tomographic imaging. The algorithm enables a number of new possibilities. These include the quantification of the uncertainty of tomographic measurements and the possibility to define arbitrary risk criteria at a very low level of the image formation process. We have described the algorithm in detail and explored its use with simple experiments in PET. Future work will evaluate the comparison of MAP estimation and reconstruction under the MMSE criterion, will explore other risk criteria, and will consider the Bayesian variational framework in search of solutions with increased computational efficiency.

Acknowledgements.   This research was supported by the NIH NCRR (P41-RR14075), the NIH NIBIB (R01EB013565), TEKES (ComBrain), the Lundbeck Foundation (R141-2013-13117), NVIDIA Corporation.

References

1. Shepp, L.A., Vardi, Y.: Maximum Likelihood Reconstruction for Emission Tomography. IEEE TMI 1(2), 113–122 (1982)
2. Geman, S., Geman, D.: Stochastic relaxation, Gibbs distributions, and the Bayesian restoration of images. IEEE TPAMI 6(6), 721–741 (1984)
3. Roth, S., Black, M.J.: Fields of experts. IJCV 82(2), 205–229 (2009)
4. Tappen, M.F., Russell, B.C., Freeman, W.T.: Exploiting the sparse derivative prior for super-resolution and image demosaicing. In: Int. Workshop SCTV (2003)
5. Li, Y., Huttenlocher, D.P.: Learning for optical flow using stochastic optimization. In: Forsyth, D., Torr, P., Zisserman, A. (eds.) ECCV 2008, Part II. LNCS, vol. 5303, pp. 379–391. Springer, Heidelberg (2008)
6. Green, P.J.: Bayesian reconstructions from emission tomography data using a modified EM algorithm. IEEE TMI 9(1), 84–93 (1990)
7. Girolami, M., Calderhead, B.: Riemann Manifold Langevin and Hamiltonian Monte Carlo Methods. J. of the Royal Stat. Soc. 73(2), 123–214 (2014)
8. Duane, S., et al.: Hybrid Monte Carlo. Physics Letters B 195(2), 216–222 (1987)
9. Neal, R.M.: Probabilistic Inference Using Markov Chain Monte Carlo Methods. Technical Report CRG-TR-93-1, University of Toronto (1993)
10. Fischer, B., Modersitzki, J.: Fast inversion of matrices arising in image processing. Numerical Algorithms 22(1), 1–11 (2000)

A Landmark-Based Approach
for Robust Estimation of Exposure Index Values
in Digital Radiography

Paolo Irrera[1,2], Isabelle Bloch[1], and Maurice Delplanque[2]

[1] Institut Mines Telecom, Telecom ParisTech, CNRS LTCI, Paris, France
[2] EOS Imaging, Paris, France

Abstract. The exposure index (EI) gives a feedback to radiographers
on the image quality in digital radiography, but its estimation on clinical images raises many challenges. In this paper we provide a critical
overview of state of the art methods that address this problem and we
show that more robust results can be obtained by detecting anatomical
structures. This new approach implicitly manages the presence of multiple structures in the field-of-view. Moreover, we propose a landmark-
based method that, by exploiting redundancy of local estimates, is more
robust to potential detection errors.

Keywords: Exposure index, anatomical structures detection, local estimates, full-body X-ray imaging.

1 Introduction

The exposure index (EI) is a standardized image quality measure for 2D digital
radiography (DR) [1] that expresses the amount of signal level reaching the
detector and is proportional to the squared signal to noise ratio [2]. Therefore, it
can be used to define the *as low as reasonably achievable* (ALARA) amount of
dose for an exam according to the associated medical purpose. While the physical
meaning of the EI has been extensively justified, how to correctly define it on
clinical images has been less addressed. Only the attenuated X-rays relevant for
the diagnosis need to be taken into account, which in practice requires to define
a region of interest (ROI). In this paper, we show that, by detecting anatomical
structures of interest, the estimated EI values are more consistent compared
with those obtained with methods suggested in the literature [3]. Moreover, we
propose to compute multiple local EI estimates associated with landmarks that
belong to a given structure of interest. The regional EI is then computed as a
weighted mean of the local estimates. This paper also addresses the problem
due to the presence of different anatomical structures in the field-of-view. In
this case, the method should be capable of computing an EI value for each
structure to quantify image quality according to the most relevant anatomical
region for the diagnosis. Our experiments are performed on images acquired with
EOS system, that is dedicated to the full-body analysis of the musculoskeletal

© Springer International Publishing Switzerland 2015
N. Navab et al. (Eds.): MICCAI 2015, Part II, LNCS 9350, pp. 627–634, 2015.
DOI: 10.1007/978-3-319-24571-3_75

apparatus [4]. However, the discussion and the method proposed in this paper can be generalized to other DR systems.

The paper is organized as follows. Section 2 overviews the theoretical background. Section 3 introduces the proposed approaches. Section 4 presents the results. Finally, Section 5 summarizes the contributions and perspectives.

2   Exposure Index Algorithm

2.1   Overview

The EI is computed from the raw image $\mathbf{q}$ that is processed to correct imperfections of the detector and geometric distortions. Other image processing steps such as noise reduction and contrast enhancement must be avoided because they significantly influence the image quality. Then, a subset Ψ of the whole pixel space Ω is defined to associate the EI with X-rays that are attenuated by meaningful structures according to the medical purpose of the undergoing exam. In the literature, this step is called ROI selection and, in this paper, we quantify its importance and propose alternative solutions. From the distribution of the gray levels of the pixels $x_t \in \Psi$, a value of interest (VOI) v is extracted. Since v has to represent the central tendency of the distribution, it is equal to the median of $\mathbf{q}(x_t)$, $x_t \in \Psi$ [3]. Finally, the EI value is computed as follows:

$$EI = c_0 g(v) \tag{1}$$

where c_0^{-1} is a constant fixed at 0.01 μGy according to the norm [1] and $g(.)$ is a calibration function. The value returned by $g(v)$ is the Kerma in the air at the receptor and is expressed in μGy. The function $g(.)$ depends on the X-ray system and must be defined in the X-ray standard beam geometry and calibration conditions specified in the norm [1]. Since the final goal is to assess the quality with respect to ideal ALARA dose conditions, a deviation index (DI) is associated with the EI. The optimal exposure is represented by a target EI value (EI_t), and the DI value is formally defined as follows:

$$DI = 10 \log_{10} \left(\frac{EI}{EI_t} \right) \tag{2}$$

where $DI < 0$ and $DI > 0$ indicate under- and overexposure, respectively.

2.2   State of the Art Methods of Region of Interest Definition

The algorithms for the selection of the ROI suggested in the norm [1] require to initially separate the background, i.e. where X-rays are not attenuated, from the anatomical region. This can be simply achieved by applying to the image $\mathbf{q}$ a threshold defined according to the properties of the system. Therefore, once a subset of anatomical pixel $\Phi \subset \Omega$ is identified, the following methods can be used to define the ROI $\Psi \subset \Phi$.

Histogram Threshold. Two thresholds $\bar{\tau} = [\tau_l; \tau_h]$ are applied to the gray levels histogram of $\mathbf{u}(x_t)$ where $x_t \in \Phi$. These thresholds are defined as function of two percentile values of the histogram, that, in our experiments, are 1% and 24% for τ_l and τ_h, respectively. The percentile values are defined according to prior assumptions on the link between intensity values and related physical meaning: the leftmost part of the histogram is associated with strong absorption that is intuitively higher in bone tissues, which are the information of interest. Nevertheless, changes in patient morphotypes, acquisition conditions, presence of metallic objects and so on, influence the gray level distribution and, hence, this way of defining the ROI Ψ_τ may not be consistent across different exams.

Center of the Image. The ROI can be placed at the center of the image by assuming that the most significant information is centered. The ROI is then, for example, a square or a circle that covers at least 20% of Φ [1]. In our experiments, we use a square Ψ_s that covers 50% of Φ. Potential problems may occur if the anatomical information of interest is dislocated with respect to the central axis inferred from the indicated collimation limits, e.g. spine in bending exams.

3 Estimation of the Exposure Index from Local Measures Associated with Landmarks

3.1 Anatomical Structures Detection

In order to overcome the mentioned drawbacks of state of the art methods, we propose to detect structures of interest in the full-body image. The minimal area bounding boxes that surround the structures of interest are used as ROIs for computing EI values. The detection of such bounding boxes has been widely addressed in the recent literature on medical applications (see [5] and references therein). When 2D images are processed, the bounding box is an oriented rectangle that depends on five parameters: the coordinates of the upper left corner, the width, the height and the orientation. In this paper we do not aim at defining a detection algorithm on full-body X-rays images, but rather at evaluating the application of such techniques to the definition of consistent EI values and, hence, we use the ideal bounding boxes. Nevertheless, in Section 4.2 we study how localization errors influence the EI estimates.

3.2 Proposed Landmark-Based Approach

We suggest to associate with an anatomical ROI a cluster of points l_j within the structure and, then, get the EI from measures computed in local patches P_j centered at these points. In detail, we propose to estimate a local EI measure from the distribution of intensity levels associated with pixels $x_t \in P$. We use circular patches of radius equal to 128 pixels. The circle has to be large enough to avoid the measure to be excessively affected by noise and, at the same time, small enough to guarantee the gray level distribution to be approximately mono-modal.

In this way, the central tendency of a distribution will be a more representative descriptor of the actual amount of signal and, then, of the EI value in a region. Formally, given a set of landmarks $l_j \in \mathcal{L}_r$, where $\mathcal{L}_r$ is the cluster associated with the ROI $\mathcal{A}_r$, the corresponding VOIs $v(l_j)$ and, then, the local EI values $e(l_j)$ are computed (Equation 1). The EI value at the ROI $\mathcal{A}_r$ is then estimated by using the following weighted sum of local EI values:

$$EI_r = \frac{\sum\limits_{l_j \in \mathcal{L}_r} \omega(l_j) e(l_j)}{\sum\limits_{l_j \in \mathcal{L}_r} \omega(l_j)} \tag{3}$$

where the weights $\omega(l_j)$ assess the accuracy of the measure provided by the landmarks $l_j \in \mathcal{L}_r$ by giving higher importance to $e(l_j)$ values that are computed from homogeneous gray level distributions because the corresponding VOI, computed as the median, is a good descriptor of the signal level. Formally, we use the entropy of the intensity levels inside the circular patches P_j centered at the landmarks $l_j \in \mathcal{L}_r$ to compute $\omega(l_j)$ and the weights are defined as follows:

$$\omega(l_j) = \exp\left(\frac{-H(l_j)}{\alpha_H}\right) \tag{4}$$

where $H(l_j)$ is the entropy computed at the patch P_j centered at the landmark l_j and α_H is a constant smoothing parameter set to 2 in our tests. The definition of the landmark positions is out of the scope of this paper, but the effect of detection errors on the measure is quantified in Section 4.2.

4   Results

The methods presented in Section 3 are evaluated on EOS full-body images. We will make reference to the histogram-based, to the centered square-based, to the bounding box-based and landmark-based methods with the abbreviations $hROI$, $sROI$, $bbDet$ and $lDet$, respectively. On each full-body image, eight regions of interest are studied: head ($\mathcal{A}_1$), thoracic spine ($\mathcal{A}_2$), lungs ($\mathcal{A}_3$), lumbar spine ($\mathcal{A}_4$), pelvis ($\mathcal{A}_5$), femur ($\mathcal{A}_6$), knee ($\mathcal{A}_7$) and tibia ($\mathcal{A}_8$). Figure 1a shows an example of manually defined ROIs and the relative EI values are assumed to represent the ground truth. In order to evaluate $hROI$ and $sROI$, the full-body images are divided into sub-windows where only one anatomical structure of interest is present because, if the whole anatomical pixel space was taken into account, the estimation errors would clearly be very high. The ideal bounding boxes correspond to the minimal area oriented rectangles that surround these regions, whereas Figure 1b shows an example of manually annotated landmarks. The methods are evaluated according to the DI between the manual and automatic EI values and the standard deviation of DI values ($\sigma(DI)$) over patients in a database associated with each region $\mathcal{A}_i$. Similarly to Equation 2, a DI value from the ground truth is computed as follows:

$$DI = 10 \log_{10}\left(\frac{EI}{EI_{gt}}\right) \tag{5}$$

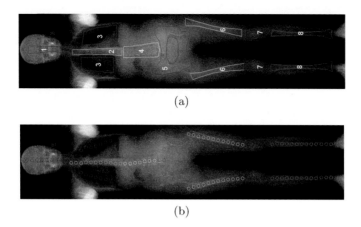

(a)

(b)

Fig. 1. In order to define ground truth EI values, the ROI relative to $\mathcal{A}_i$, $i = 1, \ldots, 8$ are manually defined (a). The structures can also be associated with clusters of points (b). The images in the Figures (a) and (b) are not the raw images $\mathbf{q}$ but the post-processed ones for which the grayscale look-up-table is inverted.

where EI_{gt} is the ground truth value associated with a given anatomical ROI. The ideal result is a DI equal to zero, but a margin of error is accepted and different degrees of errors are, thus, considered: $|DI| \in [0, 0.25)$, $|DI| \in [0.25, 0.5)$, $|DI| \in [0.5, 0.75)$, $|DI| \in [0.75, 1)$ and $|DI| \in [1, +\inf)$ mean, respectively, negligible, low, medium, high and extreme errors. The measure $\sigma(DI)$ quantifies if a given method provides a stable measure over different exams. The methods have been qualitatively compared on a database composed of 82 full-body images by including patients of different ages, and pathological or normal. In the following sections we provide a quantitative evaluation from manually segmented structures on a subset of 6 images that well represents the variability of the data. The parameters specified in Sections 2 and 3 do not change among the tested cases.

4.1   Comparison of the Methods

Figures 2a and 2b show the root mean-squared-error (RMSE), where the errors are the DI values, and the $\sigma(DI)$ associated with each anatomical structure $\mathcal{A}_i$, respectively. The graphs in Figures 2a and 2b do not present $\mathcal{A}_3$ because the thresholds $\bar{\tau}$ chosen for the method $hROI$ are not adapted to the lungs. In other experiments we have focused on the region $\mathcal{A}_3$ and, hence, adapted the parameters. The analysis from the associated results is comparable to the one relative to the region $\mathcal{A}_2$ that is described in the following comparison.

The method $hROI$ provides acceptable results only in regions $\mathcal{A}_4$, $\mathcal{A}_5$ and $\mathcal{A}_7$ as in these areas the signal is quite homogeneous ($\mathcal{A}_{4-5}$) or the highest absorption well matches the anatomical structure ($\mathcal{A}_7$). However, $hROI$ fails in providing a good exposure indicator in the other regions and, in particular, high errors occur in regions $\mathcal{A}_2$ and $\mathcal{A}_6$. This happens because the ROI associated with $\mathcal{A}_2$ contains the thoracic spine and the soft tissues in the upper part of

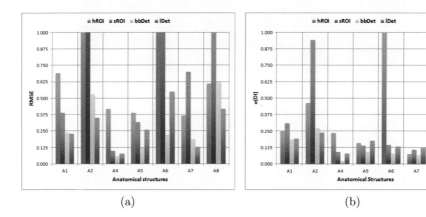

Fig. 2. Comparison of the methods in terms of: (a) RMSE, (b) $\sigma(DI)$. The graphs show values in the range $[0, 1]$.

the lumbar region, while the upper part of the thoracic spine is not included. A similar effect occurs in $\mathcal{A}_6$ where the lower part of the pelvis is retained in place of the femurs. Note that the $\sigma(DI)$ values are also high in these regions and, hence, proves that this method does not give consistent EI estimates. By changing $\bar{\tau}$ settings, the results do not improve.

The results with method $sROI$ are good in $\mathcal{A}_1$ and $\mathcal{A}_5$ and even negligible errors are observed in $\mathcal{A}_4$. In other regions the RMSEs are higher as the anatomical structures are misplaced with respect to the central axis ($\mathcal{A}_{6-8}$) or tissues of different densities are included in the ROI Ψ_s ($\mathcal{A}_2$). Nevertheless, the $\sigma(DI)$ values associated with $\mathcal{A}_{6-8}$ are very low, which means that the estimated EI values are consistent. This is however not the case in region $\mathcal{A}_2$ and, hence, $sROI$ is sub-optimal. Moreover, we expect that the performances of this method would decrease in presence of deformed structures (e.g. idiopathic scoliosis) or if the patient is not correctly placed before the acquisition.

The methods $bbDet$ and $lDet$ work very well in all the regions[1]. In detail, $bbDet$ presents RMSE values higher than 0.50 only in regions $\mathcal{A}_2$ and $\mathcal{A}_8$. In the thoracic spine, the rectangles take into account some of the surrounding pulmonary tissues, which increases the EI value. In region $\mathcal{A}_8$, the signal is not very homogeneous, and, hence, the imperfect correspondence between the rectangle and the tibia entails a slight increase of EI value. The method $lDet$ allows reducing the DI values associated with $\mathcal{A}_2$ because by using landmarks the bending of the spine is better respected, whereas in $\mathcal{A}_6$ RMSE slightly increases because some soft tissues on the side of the femur are considered in the local measures. However, the $\sigma(DI)$ values obtained with both $bbDet$ and $lDet$ are very low, which proves that in order to obtain consistent EI measures the ROI definition in the EI algorithm should be replaced by anatomical structure detection.

---

[1] This is also true for the lungs where the RMSE are equal to 0.22 and 0.13 and $\sigma(DI)$ equal to 0.10 and 0.11 for, respectively, $bbDet$ and $lDet$.

Table 1. Misplacement in mm at which the error on the EI values become negligible (< 0.25) with bounding boxes, 100%, 50% and 25% misplaced landmarks for each $\mathcal{A}_i$. The higher the value the more robust the method is.

	$\mathcal{A}_1$	$\mathcal{A}_2$	$\mathcal{A}_3$	$\mathcal{A}_4$	$\mathcal{A}_5$	$\mathcal{A}_6$	$\mathcal{A}_7$	$\mathcal{A}_8$
bbDet	10	< 5	< 5	30	15	5	5	30
lDet-100%	30	10	10	30	30	15	15	10
lDet-50%	30	20	15	30	30	30	30	20
lDet-25%	30	30	20	30	30	30	30	30

Moreover, the presence of multiple structures in the field-of-view is implicitly controlled and localization methods can be efficiently implemented [5].

4.2   Robustness to Misplacement Errors

So far only ideal bounding boxes and landmarks have been considered and it remains to quantify the impact of misplaced bounding boxes or landmarks on the estimation of EI values. Therefore, we measure how the EI values change according to simulated localization errors of 5, 10, 15, 20, 25 and 30 mm. For each simulation, the bounding boxes or the landmarks are misplaced with respect to their ground truth positions. The errors for bounding boxes could be induced by mistaken estimation of the position, orientation and size parameters. At first, only errors on the position are taken into account, but changes in orientation or size could probably cause wrong estimation of the EI values as well. As for the landmarks, we evaluate how the performances decrease as the positions of all or part of the landmarks are incorrectly estimated. For each degree of error in distance, 100 simulations are executed and the mean EI values are computed. Then, the DI values are computed with respect to the ideal EI measures, i.e. those obtained from not displaced landmarks or bounding boxes.

The $|DI|$ clearly increases at higher displacement in mm and Table 1 reports at which distance the errors on EI measure become negligible, i.e. $|DI| < 0.25$, according to the method and region $\mathcal{A}_i$. In general, the approach based on landmark detection is more robust than the bounding box one. This is due to the redundancy that is introduced in the proposed landmark-based method: if the whole region is misplaced, the central tendency of the gray level distribution will be biased as well, whereas measures from local patches only partially count in the final estimation. As a consequence, if part of the landmarks is correctly located, the EI estimates will be exact within a wide range of spatial error. Quantitatively, all the EI values are correctly estimated if, for example, at least 75% (50%) of landmarks are correctly located within 20 (15) mm, whereas to obtain the same results with bbDet the spatial error has to be inferior to 5 mm. Given these results, we consider unnecessary to simulate errors on the orientation or the size of the bounding boxes that probably would lead to similar conclusions. Finally, Table 1 also highlights that the errors significantly change according to the regions $\mathcal{A}_i$, which is coherent with the analysis conducted in Section 4.1.

The EI values are good in regions $\mathcal{A}_{4-5}$ regardless the detection method and the error degree and, therefore, it will be easy to provide correct measures in these areas. On the other hand, in the chest $\mathcal{A}_{2-3}$ the estimation is more complex given the proximity of structures at low and high density (i.e. the lungs and the thoracic spine) and, hence, the proposed landmark-based method is even more interesting.

5 Conclusion

In this paper, we have studied the state of the art methods that are used to estimate EI values from clinical images and then concluded that they may introduce severe errors and are not consistent, especially the histogram-based one. Then, we have shown that more robust and reproducible EI measures can be obtained by relying on anatomical structure detection. Besides, this allows managing the presence of different anatomical structures in the field-of-view, while being efficient. Moreover, we have proposed a landmark-based approach that, by exploiting redundancy of local estimates, is more robust to detection errors than the bounding box-based method. In future works we will present how to automatically detect the landmark clusters. This can be achieved by combining global and local information. A global model encodes the sizes of anatomical structures and the relative landmark positions. The search space is then sequentially narrowed by increasing both efficiency and robustness of the algorithm. The local analysis exploits the positions of salient points associated with peaks of absorption at the detector. The adaptation of the patch shapes to the anatomical structures to which the landmarks are associated is a further perspective.

Acknowledgments. Work in part supported by an ANRT grant (2012/0202).

References

1. IEC 62494-1: Medical electrical equipement - Exposure index of digital X-ray imaging systems - Part 1: Definitions and requirements for general radiography. International Electrotechnical Commission Norm (2008)
2. Seibert, A., Shelton, D.K., Moore, E.H.: The standardized exposure index for digital radiography: an opportunity for optimization of radiation dose to the pediatric population. Pediatric Radiology 41, 573–581 (2011)
3. Shepard, S.J., Wang, J., Flynn, M., Gingold, E., Goldman, L., Krugh, K., Leong, D.L., Mah, E., Ogden, K., Peck, D., Samei, E., Wang, J., Willis, C.E.: An exposure indicator for digital radiography: AAPM Task Group 116 (Executive Summary). Medical Physics 36, 2898–2914 (2009)
4. Illés, S., Somoskeöy, S.: The EOS imaging system and its uses in daily orthopaedic practice. International Orthopaedics 36, 1325–1331 (2012)
5. Zhou, S.K.: Discriminative anatomy detection: classification vs regression. Pattern Recognition Letters 43, 25–38 (2014)

Accelerated Dynamic MRI Reconstruction with Total Variation and Nuclear Norm Regularization[*]

Jiawen Yao[1], Zheng Xu[1], Xiaolei Huang[2], and Junzhou Huang[1,**]

[1] Department of Computer Science and Engineering,
University of Texas at Arlington, Arlington TX 76019, USA
[2] Computer Science and Engineering Department, Lehigh University,
Bethlehem, PA 18015, USA
jzhuang@uta.edu

Abstract. In this paper, we propose a novel compressive sensing model for dynamic MR reconstruction. With total variation (TV) and nuclear norm (NN) regularization, our method can utilize both spatial and temporal redundancy in dynamic MR images. Due to the non-smoothness and non-separability of TV and NN terms, it is difficult to optimize the primal problem. To address this issue, we propose a fast algorithm by solving a primal-dual form of the original problem. The ergodic convergence rate of the proposed method is $\mathcal{O}(1/N)$ for N iterations. In comparison with six state-of-the-art methods, extensive experiments on single-coil and multi-coil dynamic MR data demonstrate the superior performance of the proposed method in terms of both reconstruction accuracy and time complexity.

1 Introduction

Dynamic magnetic resonance imaging (dMRI) is an important medical imaging technique that has been widely used for multiple clinical applications. To reduce scanning time, partial k-space data are typically required for reconstruction instead of full sampling. However, when k-space is under sampled, the Nyquist criterion is violated and the inverse Fourier transform will exhibit aliasing artifacts. Fortunately, dynamic MR sequences often provide both redundant spatial and temporal information, which makes the use of Compressive Sensing (CS) theory repeatedly successful [6,14,13].

There are two kinds of prior knowledge about dynamic MR images which can be used by CS methods. First, a dynamic MR sequence has the piece-wise smooth property in the spatial domain. In traditional CS-MRI reconstructions, the piece-wise smooth property of MR images plays a very important role. With the sparsity-induced regularization such as Wavelets [13] or Total Variation [9,8], it is possible to reconstruct high quality MR images using far fewer measurements.

---

[*] This work was partially supported by U.S. NSF IIS-1423056, CMMI-1434401, CNS-1405985.

[**] Corresponding author.

N. Navab et al. (Eds.): MICCAI 2015, Part II, LNCS 9350, pp. 635–642, 2015.
DOI: 10.1007/978-3-319-24571-3_76

Second, dynamic MR images actually are temporally correlated due to very slow changes of the same organ(s) through the whole image sequence. Such high correlation in the temporal domain becomes another piece of important prior knowledge for guiding dynamic MRI reconstruction.

In recent years, researchers have proposed two types of dMRI reconstructions based on temporal information of dynamic MR images. The first type of methods applies a sparsity constraint in the temporal domain, e.g. Dictionary Learning with Temporal Gradients (DLTG) [2] and Dynamic Total Variation (DTV) [5]. Instead of using sparsity in the temporal domain, another type of methods exploits the low-rank property of matrices. Based on rank minimization, low-rank plus sparse decomposition methods are proposed for dMRI reconstruction [16,18]. Because these methods collect the data from all frames in the reconstruction, they can exploit the redundancies of the whole dataset and reconstruct more accurate results. However, drawbacks are their sensitivity to noise. They may fail in recovering clean images when the acquired data are contaminated with noise because the sparse prior cannot exploit the local spatial consistency or piece-wise smoothness of dynamic MR images.

In this paper, by exploiting redundancies in both the temporal and spatial domains, we propose a Total Variation and Nuclear Norm Regularization (TVNNR) model for dMRI reconstruction. In our TVNNR, nuclear norm (NN) exploits the low-rank property of dynamic MR images while total variation encourages each MR frame's intensities to be locally consistent which can enforce the piece-wise smoothness constraint and make reconstruction more robust to noise. The intuition of combining TV and NN terms is simple, but the joint TV/NN minimization problem is actually difficult to solve because of the non-separability and non-smoothness of the two terms. A fast algorithm (FTVNNR) is then proposed to efficiently solve this problem. It can obtain a $\mathcal{O}(1/N)$ convergence rate for N iterations. Extensive experiments on dynamic MR data demonstrate its superior performance over all previous methods in terms of both reconstruction accuracy and computational complexity.

2   Model

Here we assume $x_1, ..., x_T$ as one dynamic MR sequence to be reconstructed. At time t, $x_t \in \mathbb{C}^{m \times n}$ is one dynamic MR frame, the physical model for the undersampled k-space measurement of x_t can be formulated as

$$b_t = R_t(Fx_t + n), \tag{1}$$

where b_t is the measurement vector which may contain noise (n represents noise in k-space); R_t denotes the undersampling mask to acquire only a subset of k-space and F performs a 2D Discrete Fourier Transform (DFT).

With prior knowledge in the temporal and spatial domains, it is possible to reconstruct x_t with fewer k-space measurements b_t. Based on a batch scheme, the proposed TVNNR model for dMRI reconstruction is defined as follows

$$\min_X \frac{1}{2}||RFX - B||_F^2 + \lambda_1||X||_{TV} + \lambda_2||X||_*, \tag{2}$$

where $X \in \mathbb{R}^{mn \times t}$ denotes the whole dynamic MR images. $||X||_*$ is the nuclear norm—the sum of singular values of the matrix X. $||X||_{TV}$ denotes the anisotropic total variation of the matrix X. It is defined as $\sum_{t=1}^{T} \sum_{ij} (|\nabla_1 x_{i,j,t}| + |\nabla_2 x_{i,j,t}|)$ where ∇_1 and ∇_2 denote the forward finite difference operators on the first and second coordinates, respectively. If we define $\nabla = [\nabla_1, \nabla_2]$, $||X||_{TV}$ can be simplified as $||\nabla X||_1$. $B = [b_1, b_2, ..., b_T]^T$ represents the collection of all the measurements.

Although the problem (2) is the single coil case, it has the potential to process multi-coil parallel MRI data. When the coil sensitivities are available, it can be combined with SENSE in the k-t SPARSE-SENSE framework [17] by multiplying coil sensitivities E after the undersampled Fourier transform, which means the least square term in (2) will be $||RFEX - B||_F^2$.

3   Algorithm

Due to the non-smoothness and non-separability of both the TV and NN functions, it is very difficult to efficiently solve the primal problem (2). Instead of directly solving the primal problem, it is suggested in [3,4] that TV regularization can be solved by its dual form. By using the Legendre-Fenchel transformation of total variation (see Ref. [1], Example. 3. 26, p. 93), we can have the primal-dual form of the primal problem (2) as

$$\min_X \max_Y \frac{1}{2} ||RFX - B||_F^2 + \lambda_2 ||X||_* + \lambda_1 \langle \nabla X, Y \rangle - I_{B_\infty}(Y), \qquad (3)$$

where Y is the dual variable and $I_{B_\infty}(Y)$ is the indicator function of the ℓ_∞ unit norm ball

$$I_{B_\infty}(Y) = \begin{cases} 0 & ||Y||_\infty \le 1, \\ +\infty & \text{otherwise.} \end{cases} \qquad (4)$$

The min-max problem (3) can be solved by a splitting scheme [7] as

$$X^{n+1} = \arg\min_X \frac{1}{2} ||X - X^n||_F^2 + \frac{t_1}{2} ||RFX - B||_F^2 + t_1 \lambda_1 \langle \nabla X, Y^n \rangle + t_1 \lambda_2 ||X||_* \qquad (5)$$

$$Y^{n+1} = \arg\min_Y \frac{1}{2} ||Y - Y^n||_F^2 + I_{B_\infty}(Y) - t_2 \lambda_1 \langle \nabla(2X^{n+1} - X^n), Y \rangle, \qquad (6)$$

where X^n, Y^n are the primal and dual variables in the n-th iteration, respectively. t_1, t_2 are the corresponding iteration step sizes.

First, for the X **subproblem** (5), it can be reduced to a de-noising problem by [4] as

$$X^{n+1} = \arg\min_X \frac{1}{2} ||X - \bar{X}^n||_F^2 + \lambda ||X||_*, \qquad (7)$$

where

$$\bar{X}^n = X^n - \frac{t_1}{1 + t_1 L} \mathcal{A}^T (\mathcal{A} X^n - B) - \frac{t_1 \lambda_1}{1 + t_1 L} \nabla^T Y^n, \quad \lambda = \frac{t_1 \lambda_2}{1 + t_1 L}.$$

Here $\mathcal{A} = RF$ and $L = \lambda_{max}(\mathcal{A}^T \mathcal{A})$. ∇^T is the adjoint operator of ∇. Suppose that $\bar{X}^n = U diag(\sigma(\bar{X}^n)) V^H$ is any singular value decomposition of $\bar{X}^n$. Then the solution of (7) can be obtained by the matrix shrinkage operator [15] as $X^{n+1} = S_\lambda(\bar{X}^n) = U diag(\bar{\sigma}_\lambda(\bar{X}^n)) V^H$ where $\bar{\sigma}_\lambda(\bar{X}^n) = max(\sigma(\bar{X}^n) - \lambda, 0)$

Then we consider the Y **subproblem** in (6)

$$Y^{n+1} = \arg\min_Y \frac{1}{2}\|Y - Y^n\|_F^2 + I_{B_\infty}(Y) - t_2\lambda_1\langle\nabla(2X^{n+1} - X^n), Y\rangle, \quad (8)$$

After simplification, it becomes

$$Y^{n+1} = \arg\min_Y \frac{1}{2}\|Y - \bar{Y}^n\|_F^2 + I_{B_\infty}(Y), \quad (9)$$

where

$$\bar{Y}^n = Y^n + t_2\lambda_1\nabla(2X^{n+1} - X^n).$$

The solution of (9) can be obtained by the Euclidean projection of $\bar{Y}^n$ onto a ℓ_∞ unit ball, which could be evaluated by

$$Y^{n+1} = sgn(\bar{Y}^n) \cdot \min(|\bar{Y}^n|, 1), \quad (10)$$

where $sgn(x)$ is the sign function; it outputs 1 if $x > 0$, -1 if $x < 0$ and zero otherwise. All the operations in (10) are element-wise.

Now, the X, Y subproblems have been solved and we summarize the proposed FTVNNR in Algorithm 1. A key feature of the FTVNNR is its fast convergence performance. It can be proved that the ergodic convergence rate of FTVNNR is $\mathcal{O}(1/N)$ for N iteration [4].

Algorithm 1. FTVNNR

---

input: $\mathcal{A} = RF$, B, λ_1, λ_2
initialization: $X_0, Y_0, t_1, t_2, \lambda = t_1\lambda_2/(1 + t_1 L)$
while not converged **do**
  1) Compute: $\bar{X}^n = X^n - \frac{t_1}{1+t_1 L}\mathcal{A}^T(\mathcal{A}X^n - B) - \frac{t_1\lambda_1}{1+t_1 L}\nabla^T Y^n$ in (7)
  2) Evaluate Matrix Shrinkage Operator: $X^{n+1} = S_\lambda(\bar{X}^n)$
  3) Compute: $\bar{Y}^n = Y^n + t_2\lambda_1\nabla(2X^{n+1} - X^n)$ in (9)
  4) Project $\bar{Y}^n$ onto ℓ^∞ unit ball: $Y^{n+1} = sgn(\bar{Y}^n) \cdot \min(|\bar{Y}^n|, 1)$ (element-wise)
end while

---

4 Experiments

4.1 Reconstruction Accuracy

We first evaluate our method on two noisy dynamic MR sequences. To simulate such noisy dynamic MR images, we use the in-vivo breath-hold cardiac perfusion ($128 \times 128 \times 40$) and cine data ($256 \times 256 \times 24$) from [16] and then add Gaussian white noise with standard derivation $\sigma = 0.05$ in the k-space data followed by the equation (1). We apply the most practical Cartesian mask with 25% sampling ratio as the undersampling mask in our experiments. For quantitative evaluation, Peak Signal-to-Noise Ratio (PSNR) is adopted as the metric. All experiments are conducted using MATLAB 2013b on a desktop with 3.4GHz Intel core i7 4770 3.4GHz CPU and 16.0 GB RAM.

We compare our method with four state-of-the-art methods, the undersampled (k,t)-Space via Low-rank plus sparse prior (ktRPCA) [18], dictionary learning based method DLTG [2], the dynamic Total Variation (DTV) [5] and k-t SLR [12]. The source codes for these methods are downloaded from each author's website and we use their default parameter settings for all experiments. For the proposed method, we set $\lambda_1 = 0.001$ and $\lambda_2 = 3$ for both sequences.

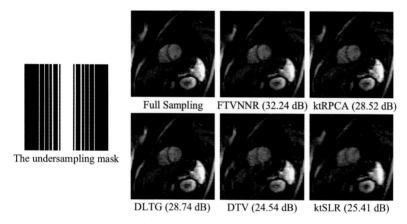

Fig. 1. Results of the 21st frame of the perfusion sequence at sampling ratio 1/4.

Fig. 1 shows the 21st reconstructed frame of the perfusion data. Clearly visible artifacts can be observed on the images by DTV and k-t SLR. Such results show that both methods are very sensitive to noise. Although it is reported that DTV gives very good performances [5], the method requires the reconstruction on the first frame to be very accurate, therefore it may not recover good results when there is no specific high sampling ratio for the first frame. Comparing the rest of the two approaches, DLTG reconstructs better results than ktRPCA. However, when looking at the time cost in Table. 1, one can see that DLTG requires nearly 2-3 hours for processing. Moreover, images obtained by both methods are still not very clear. Compared with the other four methods, the proposed FTVNNR can achieve the best reconstruction and cost the least amount of processing time.

Quantitative results of a whole sequence on two dynamic MR data are shown in Fig. 2. From the figure, one can clearly see that the proposed FTVNNR achieves the highest mean PSNR.

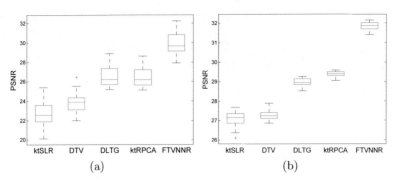

| | ktSLR | DTV | DLTG | ktRPCA | FTVNNR |

(a)   (b)

Fig. 2. Bxplot of PSNR results for (a) Perfusion data and (b) for Cine data. The proposed FTVNNR method outperforms all other methods being compared.

Table 1. The time cost of different methods

Time (Seconds)	Proposed	ktRPCA	DTV	k-t SLR	DLTG
Perfusion ($128 \times 128 \times 40$)	38	527	55	252	6614
Cine ($256 \times 256 \times 24$)	92	1282	121	609	11462

4.2   Multi-coil Parallel Imaging

To further evaluate performances, we use two multi-coil pMRI data from [16]; the number of coils is 12 and the coil sensitivities were known. The perfusion and cine data were acquired by Cartesian masks with 12.5% and 25% sampling ratio for all frames, respectively. We compare the proposed method with three state-of-the-art parallel MRI approaches including low-rank plus sparse reconstruction (L+S) [16], dynamic Total Variation (DTV) [5] and k-t SPARSE-SENSE [17].

The running time of all methods on the Perfusion and Cine data can be found in Table. 2. One can see that the proposed method has the fastest reconstruction speed compared to others, due to its fewer iterations and faster convergence.

Table 2. The time cost of different methods. "ktSS" is k-t SPARSE-SENSE

Time (Seconds)	Proposed	L+S	ktSS	DTV
Perfusion ($128 \times 128 \times 40$)	44.3	66.5	155.9	112.8
Cine ($256 \times 256 \times 24$)	56.5	78.9	115.5	291.9

Reconstruction results on the Cine data are shown in Fig. 3. All methods were able to reconstruct high quality images. However, when looking at details and temporal cross sections in Fig. 4, it can be observed that FTVNNR presents less noisy and lower residual aliasing artifacts on the cardiac surface. This is because the FTVNNR can utilize the local consistency in the spatial domain while the temporal FFT used in k-t SPARSE-SENSE and sparse prior in L+S can not exploit the spatial sparsity.

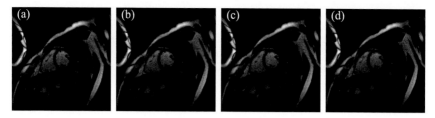

Fig. 3. Results of the 22nd frame of the Cine data. (a) DTV; (b) k-t SPARSE-SENSE; (c) L+S; (d) The proposed FTVNNR.

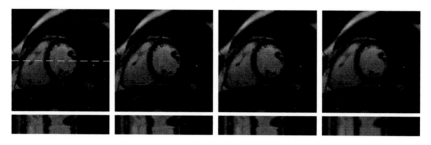

Fig. 4. Zoomed in areas of interest. The bottom are temporal cross sections by the yellow dashed line. From left to right are methods: (a) DTV; (b) k-t SPARSE-SENSE; (c) L+S; (d) The proposed FTVNNR.

5   Conclusion

We have proposed an efficient algorithm for dynamic MRI. The contributions of our work are as follows. First, the proposed FTVNNR achieves the best reconstruction performance when compared to four other state-of-the art methods. Second, it can obtain an $\mathcal{O}(1/N)$ convergence rate and experiments demonstrate that it is faster than other dMRI methods. These properties make the proposed method more powerful than conventional dMRI methods in terms of both accuracy and time efficiency. Moreover, the proposed method can be easily extended to parallel MRI. The parallel version of FTVNNR can also share good properties like fast convergence. Numerous experiments were conducted to show its better performance. In our future work, we will introduce existing online learning techniques [10,11] to further speed up the proposed FTVNNR and explore other applications in medical imaging.

References

1. Boyd, S., Vandenberghe, L.: Convex Optimization. Cambridge University Press, Cambridge (2004)
2. Caballero, J., Price, A.N., Rueckert, D., Hajnal, J.: Dictionary learning and time sparsity for dynamic MR data reconstruction. IEEE Transactions on Medical Imaging 33(4), 979–994 (2014)

3. Chambolle, A.: An algorithm for total variation minimization and applications. Journal of Mathematical Imaging and Vision 20(1-2), 89–97 (2004)
4. Chambolle, A., Pock, T.: On the ergodic convergence rates of a first-order primal-dual algorithm. Technical report, Optimization online preprint No. 4532 (2014)
5. Chen, C., Li, Y., Axel, L., Huang, J.: Real time dynamic MRI with dynamic total variation. In: Golland, P., Hata, N., Barillot, C., Hornegger, J., Howe, R. (eds.) MICCAI 2014, Part I. LNCS, vol. 8673, pp. 138–145. Springer, Heidelberg (2014)
6. Gamper, U., Boesiger, P., Kozerke, S.: Compressed sensing in dynamic MRI. Magnetic Resonance in Medicine 59(2), 365–373 (2008)
7. He, B., Yuan, X.: Convergence analysis of primal-dual algorithms for a saddle-point problem: From contraction perspective. SIAM Journal on Imaging Sciences 5(1), 119–149 (2012)
8. Huang, J., Zhang, S., Li, H., Metaxas, D.: Composite splitting algorithms for convex optimization. Computer Vision and Image Understanding 115(12), 1610–1622 (2011)
9. Huang, J., Zhang, S., Metaxas, D.: Efficient MR image reconstruction for compressed MR imaging. Medical Image Analysis 15(5), 670–679 (2011)
10. Li, Y., Chen, C., Huang, X., Huang, J.: Instrument tracking via online learning in retinal microsurgery. In: Golland, P., Hata, N., Barillot, C., Hornegger, J., Howe, R. (eds.) MICCAI 2014, Part I. LNCS, vol. 8673, pp. 464–471. Springer, Heidelberg (2014)
11. Li, Y., Chen, C., Liu, W., Huang, J.: Sub-selective quantization for large-scale image search. In: Proc. AAAI Conference on Artificial Intelligence (AAAI), pp. 2803–2809 (2014)
12. Lingala, S.G., Hu, Y., DiBella, E., Jacob, M.: Accelerated dynamic MRI exploiting sparsity and low-rank structure: k-t SLR. IEEE Transactions on Medical Imaging 30(5), 1042–1054 (2011)
13. Lustig, M., Donoho, D., Pauly, J.M.: Sparse MRI: The application of compressed sensing for rapid MR imaging. Magnetic Resonance in Medicine 58(6), 1182–1195 (2007)
14. Lustig, M., Santos, J.M., Donoho, D.L., Pauly, J.M.: k-t SPARSE: High frame rate dynamic MRI exploiting spatio-temporal sparsity. In: Proceedings of the Annual Meeting of ISMRM, p. 2420 (2006)
15. Ma, S., Goldfarb, D., Chen, L.: Fixed point and bregman iterative methods for matrix rank minimization. Mathematical Programming 128(1-2), 321–353 (2011)
16. Otazo, R., Cands, E., Sodickson, D.K.: Low-rank plus sparse matrix decomposition for accelerated dynamic MRI with separation of background and dynamic components. Magnetic Resonance in Medicine 73(3), 1125–1136 (2015)
17. Otazo, R., Kim, D., Axel, L., Sodickson, D.K.: Combination of compressed sensing and parallel imaging for highly accelerated first-pass cardiac perfusion MRI. Magnetic Resonance in Medicine 64(3), 767–776 (2010)
18. Trémoulhéac, B., Dikaios, N., Atkinson, D., Arridge, S.: Dynamic MR image reconstruction-separation from under-sampled (k,t)-space via low-rank plus sparse prior. IEEE Transactions on Medical Imaging 33(8), 1689–1701 (2014)

Robust PET Motion Correction
Using Non-local Spatio-temporal Priors

S. Thiruvenkadam[1], K.S. Shriram[1], R. Manjeshwar[2],
and S.D. Wollenweber[3]

[1] GE Global Research, Bangalore, India
[2] GE Global Research, Niskayuna, USA
[3] GE Healthcare, Waukesha, USA

Abstract. Respiratory motion presents significant challenges for PET/
CT acquisitions, potentially leading to inaccurate SUV quantitation. Non
Rigid Registration [NRR] of gated PET images is quite challenging due to
large motion, intrinsic noise, and the need to preserve definitive features
like tumors. In this work, we use non-local spatio-temporal constraints
within group-wise NRR to get a stable framework which can work with
few number of PET gates, and handle the above challenges of PET data.
Additionally, we propose metrics for measuring alignment and artifacts
introduced by NRR which is rarely addressed. Our results are quantitatively compared to related works, on 20 clinical PET cases.

1 Introduction

Patient respiratory motion is a key challenge for PET/CT imaging, which could
lead to blurring of clinically definitive features such as tumors. Such blurring in
turn affects detectability of tumors, accuracy of SUV values, and could lead to
sub-optimal radiation therapy planning. Motion compensation can be done by
factoring in CT/MR derived motion fields within PET reconstruction [1] or using
joint frameworks for motion/attenuation correction [2]. An alternative approach
is to reconstruct, non-rigidly register and then average [RRA] to get a higher SNR
PET image [3, 4]. Although the more sophisticated approaches where motion
compensation is treated within reconstruction such as [1, 2] are theoretically
preferable, the RRA method is simpler from a computational perspective. In
this work, we address PET motion correction within the RRA framework.

Fundamentally, this is the problem of non-rigidly aligning multiple 3D images.
The 'reference' based approach as in [3,4] would be to pick one of the images as
reference and non-rigidly register the other images to it. Alternatively, one could
use *groupwise* NRR. Unlike pairwise formulations, group wise motion correction
is 'reference free' and is not biased by the choice of the reference image. In
gated PET data, reconstruction artifacts e.g. due to PET-CT phase mismatch
or incorrect gating may occur in some of the gates. Thus, pronounced differences
in registration results occur with a different choice of the reference image.

Groupwise NRR [5–8] is used for aligning large populations of data without
the problem of reference bias. Simply put, group-wise registration iteratively

© Springer International Publishing Switzerland 2015
N. Navab et al. (Eds.): MICCAI 2015, Part II, LNCS 9350, pp. 643–650, 2015.
DOI: 10.1007/978-3-319-24571-3_77

estimates the 'reference image' and the transforms to map the images to the reference domain. The issue however is, the bare groupwise NRR formulation is unstable and additional constraints are essential for stability especially for NRR of small populations. Current works have enhanced groupwise NRR using spatial constraints on the deformation [5,6], temporal constraints [9] and feature based metrics [8]. Additionally, NRR of gated PET images is quite challenging due to large motion, intrisic noise, and the need to preserve small features like tumors. Large motion impacts structures such as small tumors leading to collapse, splits etc. resulting in quantitation inaccuracies. Thus, group-wise NRR in addition to handling the stabilty issue, has to robustly handle above data challenges.

Many of the previous groupwise NRR efforts have been in Atlas building where these efforts typically work with large populations and there is no correlation of motion expected across the population. The main challenge these works have tried to address is multiple modes of variation in the population. However, the problem here is different, gated PET data has frequently as few as 4 to 6 gates. Thus, standard groupwise NRR formulations are unstable since, even locally, there might be multiple solution pairs for the jointly estimated reference image and transforms. Also, in 4D data having respiratory/cardiac motion, there is strong correlation of motion across frames and across faraway regions. For example, the effects of respiration can be seen as low as the pelvic region. The above motion correlation, if modeled, could be effective in tackling the instability issue of groupwise NRR, and the large motion/noise challenges of PET data. Although not completely representative, non-local penalties on the motion fields come close in modeling such correlations between faraway regions. Non-local regularization ([10], [11]) of the motion fields is shown to give increased robustness to large motion, noise, and small structures compared to local approaches.

In this work, we propose non-local spatio-temporal constraints within groupwise NRR to get a stable 4D framework which can also handle above challenges of PET data. The non-local penalties differentiates our work from above prior groupwise NRR works, and is key in robust prediction of definitive PET features under large motion. The reasoning is that at a location where a small structure exhibits large motion, a non-local neighbour such as lung/cardiac interface where it is easier to capture the motion, can help in predicting the structure's motion. We also carefully address the important aspect of NRR validation using lesion profile based metrics. These metrics measure two aspects of NRR quality, namely, alignment and artifacts. Alignment is a common attribute that is measured in Registration works. Here, we additionally propose measures for artifacts introduced by NRR which is rarely addressed. We compare our results to level set NRR which is part of ITK (Vemuri et al. [12], used for PET motion correction [4]) and a Groupwise NRR algorithm similar to [6].

2 Methods

We assume a monomodal scenario since large intensity changes are not expected in gated PET data. Intensity/contrast changes that could occur e.g. due to gating induced count variations, can be handled using preprocess normalization steps. Given N PET gates $\{I_k\}_{k=1}^N$ defined on Ω, we seek a reference image μ and deformation fields $\{u_k\}_{k=1}^N$, $\mathbf{u} = [u_1, u_2, ..., u_N]$, which minimizes:

$$E[\mu, \mathbf{u}] = \sum_{k=1}^N \int_\Omega |I_k(. + u_k) - \mu|^2 dx + \lambda \int_\Omega |\nabla u_k|^2 dx \qquad (1)$$

The above objective function [**GW**] is the basic formulation of groupwise NRR, posed on smooth motion fields and measures pixel level variance of the PET images. [**GW**] can be minimized by iteratively updating $\mu = \frac{1}{N} \sum_{k=1}^N I_k(. + u_k)$ and motion fields $\mathbf{u}$. It is however seen that the above formulation is illposed since there might be, even locally, several solutions of $\mu, \mathbf{u}$ with the same energy E. One way to address this instability is to use a penalty that seeks, $\sum_{k=1}^N \int_\Omega u_k dx = 0$ as in [6], which is called the 'zero deformation' penalty. We refer to the Groupwise NRR framework with the zero deformation penalty as [**GW-zD**].

As highlighted in the introduction, we augment Eq. 1 with non-local spatio-temporal penalties to give a stable framework, able to handle the data challenges of PET modality. Specifically, we look at proposed energy [**GW-NL**]:

$$E_{nl}[\mu, \mathbf{u}] = \sum_{k=1}^N \int_\Omega |I_k(. + u_k) - \mu|^2 dx + \lambda_s \int_\Omega \int_\Omega w(x,y)|u_k(x) - u_k(y)|^2 dx dy$$

$$+ \lambda_t \int_\Omega \int_\Omega \hat{w}(x,y)|v_k(x) - v_k(y)|^2 dx dy \qquad (2)$$

The first regularization term is a *spatial* penalty, on the motion fields $\mathbf{u}$, which captures correlations in the motion field between 'non-local' regions. The second regularization is a *temporal* penalty term which captures the non-local spatial correlations of velocity $v_k = u_{k+1} - u_k$. The above term captures temporal trend of motion across non-local pixels which would help NRR in the case of noise, large motion, low contrast etc.. Also, the temporal penalty is less restrictive on the motion fields than the spatial penalty since only spatial variations in velocity are penalized. λ_s, λ_t are scalars that balance the terms. $w(x,y), \hat{w}(x,y)$ are weight functions that are used to set the active pixels y that are correlated with the current pixel x. For simplicity, we have used a $L2$ metric for the regularization term and a straight forward Gaussian choice for the weight functions $w(x,y) = G_\sigma(|x - y|), \hat{w}(x,y) = G_{\hat{\sigma}}(|x - y|)$. To minimize Eq. 2, we use time descent given by the EL and discretized using semi-implicit finite differences, in a multi-resolution framework. For gaussian weights $w, \hat{w}$, the descent equation involves just convolutions which is fast to compute. Also, the descent equation contains linear terms which can be posed in simple implict schemes for fast convergence.

In Fig 1, we show experiments on two synthetic examples which have a combination of noise, large motion and presence of small structures as in PET data. The top row in both examples shows 4 images we want to register. The bottom row shows the resulting mean using [**GW**], [**GW-zD**], and proposed [**GW-NL**].

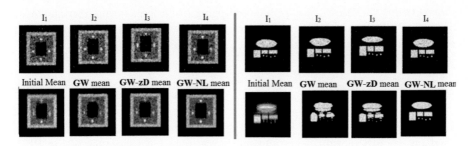

Fig. 1. Robustness comparison of [**GW**], [**GW-zD**], [**GW-NL**] in the presence of large motion, noise and small structures. Resulting mean images are shown at the bottom row with [**GW-NL**] giving the best results.

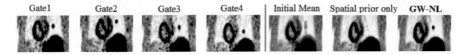

Fig. 2. Role of Temporal term in [**GW-NL**]: Better recovery of motion than just using the spatial penalty term.

It is clear from the illustrations that [**GW-NL**] is able to preserve integrity of small structures and handle the challenges of large motion/noise. Fig. 2 highlights the need for the temporal penalty term in [**GW-NL**]. With just the spatial penalty term, i.e. $\lambda_t = 0$ in Eq. 2, we see in a case of extreme motion, the lesion has collapsed.

3   Experiments

We present results on 20 datasets which were acquired using a GE Discovery 600 PET-CT system. These data were phase matched with acquired cine CT and reconstructed to form gated PET images (typically 4 to 6 gates). Comparisons of proposed approach [**GW-NL**] is performed with pair-wise NRR [**PW**] available in ITK (Vemuri et al. [12], used for PET motion correction [4]). Next, we compare against Groupwise NRR with zero-deformation penalty (as in [6]) [**GW-zD**]. For [**GW-zD**], we have used the formulation, Eq 1, augmented with the zero-deformation penalty, and minimized using steepest descent.

3.1   Illustrative Examples on Two PET Cases

In Fig. 3, we look at qualitative comparisons on 2 gated PET cases, each with 4 gates. For the first PET data example, the data is shown gate-wise (top row), the mean of the gates is shown in the last column. This case exhibits a few challenges. The right lung lesion exhibits large motion (relative to lesion size). The other challenge is contrast variations which are seen in Gate 4. Also, features in the

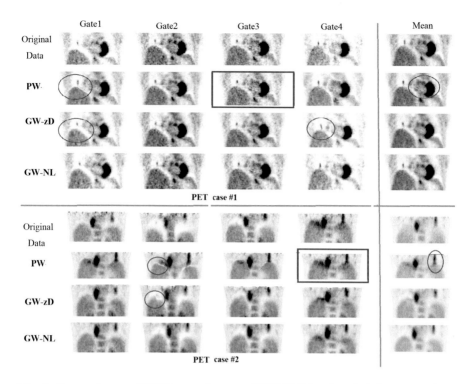

Fig. 3. Comparison on 2 PET example cases: [**GW-NL**] has handled the motion/data challenges better than [**PW**], [**GW-zD**]. Artifacts are highlighted by the red circle. The reference gate for [**PW**] is highlighted by the blue rectangle.

cardiac region are not consistently visible in all the gates. The second to fourth rows shows results (registered gates and resultant mean) using [**PW**], [**GW-zD**], and [**GW-NL**] respectively. The [**PW**] approach suffers from registration artifacts in Gates 1 and 4. The effect of bias to reference for [**PW**] is clearly seen in the 2nd gate where distinct features in the cardiac region have collapsed since the reference image (the 3rd gate) does not have it. In the second PET data illustration in Fig. 3, [**PW**] shows similar artifacts due to large motion in the 2nd gate. The issue of bias to reference is also seen here, where in, the lesion on the top of left lung looks more like the reference image (gate 4 in this case). [**GW-zD**] has done reasonably well with minor artifacts due to large motion (highlighted by the red circles). For both examples, as seen in Fig. 3, the proposed approach [**GW-NL**] has handled the challenges highlighted above and shows clean results in the registered gates and the resultant mean image.

A note on timing comparison between the methods. For a gated PET dataset (126x128x47x6), [**PW**] took 90 sec, [**GW-zD**] took 65 sec, and [**GW-NL**] took 80 sec, for convergence. The timing for [**GW-NL**] is quite remarkable considering the noticable improvement in results. Note that, [**PW**], [**GW-zD**], and [**GW-NL**] are all implemented in C++, using standard libraries from ITK.

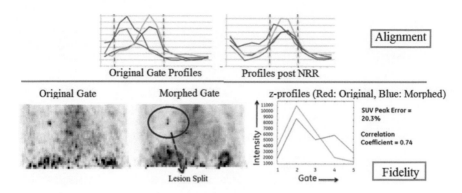

Fig. 4. Top row: Alignment metric measures spread in extrema locations of gate profiles (curves shown in the plot). Bottom row: Fidelity metrics (SUV peak, profile correlation) used to measure closeness of lesion profile before and after NRR, to catch artifacts. E.g. The lesion split results in a z-profile (blue curve) with 2 peaks and is captured by the reduced correlation value with the gate profile (red curve)

3.2   Quantitative Validation

Here, we use validation based on lesions which are key clinical features in PET data. For this purpose, lesion location was manually annotated on the RRA (average of motion corrected gates) and on each of the original gates of 20 clinical datasets.

Most of validation of NRR is around measuring alignment and very few works (e.g. NIREP, [13]) address artifacts introduced by NRR. Measuring the fidelity/artifacts of registration is very challenging and use of general purpose metrics such as Jacobian of the deformation field might not completely be representative of NRR quality in noisy data as in PET. For gated PET NRR, as discussed in the previous subsection, we want to look at 3 types of artifacts (e.g. see results of [**PW**] in Fig 3), namely, a) stretch type artifacts due to large motion, b) splits, collapse of lesions, and c) bias in results introduced due to artifacts in some gates (we term this as *NRR bias*). While it is difficult to measure the above artifacts in general cases, it is relatively straightforward to do it for lesions. Since lesions remain close to rigid under physiological motion, it is fair to expect lesions to preserve their intensity and shape, post NRR. Thus, to measure both alignment and artifacts(fidelity), we introduce metrics linked to the *z-profiles* of lesions. Since the motion in PET gates is mostly due to respiration, the z-profile (a 1D profile of intensity values in z direction passing through the lesion centroid) characterizes the lesion motion.

The *alignment* of the gates post NRR can be deduced by capturing the spatial spread (using standard deviation) of high intensity values in the z-profiles across all gates (Fig 4, Top row). The better the alignment, the tighter the spread of high intensity values in the ensemble. To capture *fidelity* (Fig 4, Bottom row), we first compute percentage difference between the z-profile peaks of gates

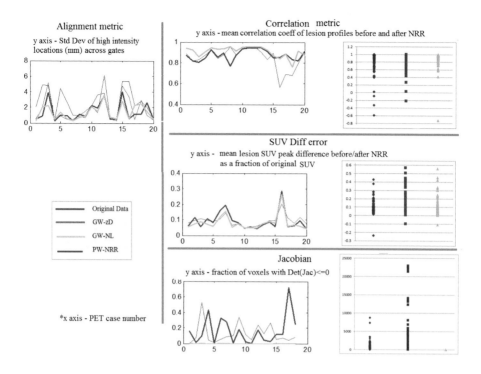

Fig. 5. Quantitative comparison on 20 PET Datasets with ≈120 gates in total. Note on metric values: Alignment: lower better, Correlation: higher better, SUV error: lower better, Jacobian: lower better. Left column: Mean across gates for alignment values for 20 cases, Middle column: Mean across gates for fidelity metric values for 20 cases. Last Column: scatter plot of the fidelity metric values across all gates from all cases. The plots show similar alignment, and better fidelity values for [**GW-NL**].

before and after NRR (*SUV peak* error). The SUV peak error indicates whether intensity values in the original gates have been flattened by NRR. Next, we compute *correlation of z-profiles* of individual gates before and after NRR. The correlation coefficient would be high if there is not much of a deviation in the shape of the z-profile post NRR. The above metric can capture issues of lesion splits/collapse and NRR bias to outlier gates. Lastly, to capture artifacts in general at any location, we use *Jacobian* of motion fields to capture crossovers and stretch artifacts (i.e. where Det(Jac) ≤ 0).

The quantitative results on 20 PET cases are shown in Fig 5. The data had a good mix of cases with varying lesion motion and noise. A few cases showed motion almost twice the lesion size, in addition to deviation in SUV values as much as 40 % of the mean SUV value across gates. From the alignment plot (Low value indicates good alignment), we see that [**GW-zD**](Magenta), [**GW-NL**](cyan) show better alignment than [**PW**](Red). In the fidelity (correlation, SUV, Jacobian) plots, the first column has the mean metric values across gates, for each PET case. The last column shows scatter plots of metric values for all gates across the 20 PET cases. The correlation plots (High value indicates good fidelity of lesion shape) show least lesion artifacts for [**GW-NL**]. The SUV peak difference (measures change in SUV, post NRR) is comparable for [**PW**], [**GW-NL**], and slightly higher for [**GW-zD**]. Finally, the Jacobian plot (showing number of voxels with $\text{Det}(\text{Jac}) \leq 0$), indicative of amount of crossovers and tears is close to zero for [**GW-NL**], overwhelmingly lesser compared to [**PW**], [**GW-zD**]. To summarize, [**GW-NL**] is seen to be comparable in alignment to the other 2 methods, but has resulted in reduced NRR artifacts.

4   Conclusion

Robust NRR for gated PET is key to accurate quantitation. Here, we have captured non-local correlations in motion within the group-wise NRR framework. This has clearly resulted in stability of solutions, robustness to large motion, noise and small structure challenges of PET data. Our results are quantitatively compared with related works using lesion based validation metrics, on 20 cases.

References

1. Manjeshwar, R.M., Xiaodong, T., et al.: Motion compensated image reconstruction of respiratory gated pet/ct. In: ISBI (2006)
2. Blume, M., Martinez-Moller, et al.: Joint reconstruction of image and motion in gated positron emission tomography. TMI, 1892–1906 (2010)
3. Dawood, M., Buther, F., Schafers, X.J., Respiratory, K.: motion correction in 3d pet data with advanced optical flow algorithms. In: TMI (2008)
4. Wollenweber, S.D., et al.: Eval. of the accuracy and robustness of a motion correction algorithm for pet using a novel phantom approach. In: TNS (2012)
5. Joshi, S., Davis, B., Jomier, M., Gerig, G.: Unbiased diffeomorphic atlas construction for computational. NeuroImage (2004)
6. Bhatia, K.K., Hajnal, J.V., Puri, B.K., Edwards, A.D., Rueckert, D.: Consistent groupwise non-rigid registration for atlas construction. In: ISBI (2004)
7. Wu, G., Jia, H., Wang, Q.: Sharpmean groupwise registration guided by sharp mean image and treebased registration. NeuroImage (2011)
8. Wang, Q., Wu, G., Yap, P.-T., Shen, D.: Attribute vector guided groupwise registration. NeuroImage (2010)
9. Metz, C.T., Klein, S., et al.: Nonrigid registration of dynamic medical imaging data using ndt bsplines. In: MIA (2010)
10. Werlberger: Motion estimation with non-local total variation regularization. CVPR 13, 234–778 (2010)
11. Thiruvenkadam: Dense multi-modal registration with structural integrity using non-local gradients. In: VISAPP (2013)
12. Vemuri, B.C., Ye, J., et al.: Image registration via level-set motion, applications to atlas-based segmentation. In: MMBIA (2003)
13. Christensen, G.E., Geng, X., Kuhl, J.G., Bruss, J., Grabowski, T.J., Pirwani, I.A., Vannier, M.W., Allen, J.S., Damasio, H.: Introduction to the Non-Rigid Image Registration Evaluation Project (NIREP). In: Pluim, J.P.W., Likar, B., Gerritsen, F.A. (eds.) WBIR 2006. LNCS, vol. 4057, pp. 128–135. Springer, Heidelberg (2006)

Subject-specific Models for the Analysis of Pathological FDG PET Data

Ninon Burgos[1], M. Jorge Cardoso[1,2], Alex F. Mendelson[1],
Jonathan M. Schott[2], David Atkinson[3], Simon R. Arridge[4],
Brian F. Hutton[5,6], and Sébastien Ourselin[1,2]

[1] Translational Imaging Group, CMIC, University College London, London, UK
[2] Dementia Research Centre, University College London, London, UK
[3] Centre for Medical Imaging, University College London, London, UK
[4] Centre for Medical Image Computing, University College London, London, UK
[5] Institute of Nuclear Medicine, University College London, London, UK
[6] Centre for Medical Radiation Physics, University of Wollongong, NSW, Australia

Abstract. Abnormalities in cerebral glucose metabolism detectable on fluorodeoxyglucose positron emission tomography (FDG PET) can be assessed on a regional or voxel-wise basis. In regional analysis, the average relative uptake over a region of interest is compared with the average relative uptake obtained for normal controls. Prior knowledge is required to determine the regions where abnormal uptake is expected, which can limit its usability. On the other hand, voxel-wise analysis consists of comparing the metabolic activity of the patient to the normal controls voxel-by-voxel, usually in a groupwise space. Voxel-based techniques are limited by the inter-subject morphological and metabolic variability in the normal population, which can limit their sensitivity.

In this paper, we combine the advantages of both regional and voxel-wise approaches through the use of subject-specific PET models for glucose metabolism. By accounting for inter-subject morphological differences, the proposed method aims to remove confounding variation and increase the sensitivity of group-wise approaches. The method was applied to a dataset of 22 individuals: 17 presenting four distinct neurodegenerative syndromes, and 5 controls. The proposed method more accurately distinguishes subgroups in this set, and improves the delineation of disease-specific metabolic patterns.

1   Introduction

In current clinical practice, fluorodeoxyglucose positron emission tomography (FDG PET) is commonly used to diagnose dementias. FDG uptake reflects glucose consumption, which is reduced by synaptic dysfunction and neuronal degeneration [1]. Different neurodegenerative diseases affect different areas of the brain, and localising abnormalities is essential for differential diagnosis [2–4].

Cerebral glucose metabolism as measured by FDG PET can be quantitatively evaluated either regionally or on a voxel-by-voxel basis. In regional analysis, the regional standardised uptake value ratio, defined as the average uptake in a

N. Navab et al. (Eds.): MICCAI 2015, Part II, LNCS 9350, pp. 651–658, 2015.
DOI: 10.1007/978-3-319-24571-3_78

region of interest (ROI) relative to a reference region (commonly the pons or cerebellar grey matter), is compared with the regional SUVR expected in a normal control population. This analysis usually requires prior knowledge regarding the selection of relevant discriminant regions, limiting its use [5]. In voxel-wise analysis, a subject's PET image is usually aligned to a standardised group space to compare the metabolic activity of the spatially normalised scan on a voxel-by-voxel basis to a distribution obtained from normal control scans, e.g. to produce a Z-score [6]. Exploratory in nature, voxel-wise techniques require less prior information than regional SUVR analysis, but their sensitivity is limited by inter-subject variability in non-pathological tracer uptake, making pathological effects harder to detect [5]. Furthermore, there is theoretical uncertainty regarding how to appropriately resample PET data to the group space, how to match the PET point spread function with the group-wise model under linear and non-linear transformations, and how to map the PET data to the group space in a biologically plausible manner.

In this paper, we combine the advantages of both regional and voxel-wise approaches by analysing PET data in the original subject space (as in regional SUVR approaches) while still providing voxel-by-voxel statistics (as in group-wise approaches). This is achieved through a subject-specific PET model based on the propagation of morphologically-matched PET scans. The local morphological matching reduces both the bias and variance of the healthy patient-specific model, increasing sensitivity.

2   Method

In the following, 4 approaches analysing FDG PET images are explored: a regional analysis based on SUVR (section 2.3), a voxel-wise analysis in a group space (section 2.4), a voxel-wise analysis in the subject's space (section 2.5) and the proposed subject-specific analysis (section 2.6).

2.1   Data

Twenty-two sets of ^{18}F-FDG PET and T1-weighted MRI brain images were used to evaluate the proposed methodology, here denoted validation dataset. Of these subjects, 5 were diagnosed with posterior cortical atrophy (PCA), 5 with semantic dementia (SD), 4 with progressive non-fluent aphasia (PNFA), 3 with logopenic progressive aphasia (LPA) and 5 were healthy controls. The T1-weighted magnetisation-prepared rapid gradient-echo (3.0 T; TE/TR/TI, 2.9 ms/2200 ms/900 ms; voxel size $1.1 \times 1.1 \times 1.1$ mm^3) scans were acquired on a 3T Siemens Magnetom Trio scanner (Siemens Healthcare, Erlangen, Germany). PET images (voxel size $1.95 \times 1.95 \times 3.27$ mm^3) were acquired on a GE Discovery ST PET/CT scanner (GE Healthcare systems, Waukesha, WI) for 20 minutes, 30 minutes after injection of 185 MBq ^{18}F-FDG. The local ethics committee approved the study and all subjects gave written, informed consent.

To create fully independent healthy population statistics and to demonstrate the applicability of the proposed patient-specific modelling strategy to multi-site data, a dataset of 29 healthy controls with T1-weighted MRI and ^{18}F-FDG PET were selected from the ADNI2 database[1]. From here on, this dataset is referred to as the control dataset.

2.2 Data Preprocessing

T1 images from the validation dataset were corrected for intensity non-uniformity following a nonparametric intensity non-uniformity normalisation method [7]. The T1 images from both the validation and control datasets were then parcellated into 143 different regions using a multi-atlas propagation and fusion algorithm implemented in NiftySeg [8]. PET images were intensity normalised using the mean uptake of the pons [9].

2.3 Regional Analysis

Regional analysis consisted of computing the average standardised uptake in a region of interest to produce a regional SUVR (rSUVR) for each subject independently. This value is then compared with those obtained for normal controls (NC) by its expression as a Z-score, i.e.

$$Z_{\text{rSUVR}} = \frac{\text{rSUVR} - \mu^{\text{NC}}_{\text{rSUVR}}}{\sigma^{\text{NC}}_{\text{rSUVR}}} \, , \qquad (1)$$

where $\mu^{\text{NC}}_{\text{rSUVR}}$ and $\sigma^{\text{NC}}_{\text{rSUVR}}$ are the mean and standard deviation of the 29 control subjects' rSUVRs.

2.4 Voxel-by-Voxel Analysis in the Group Space

For the voxel-by-voxel group-wise analysis, all image pairs from the control and the validation datasets were mapped to a common space defined through iterative group-wise non-rigid registration of the T1 data [10]. PET images were brought to the group space by composing the rigid transformations between paired PET and T1 images and the non-rigid transformation between the native T1 images and the group space. After resampling, PET images were smoothed with a Gaussian filter with 5 mm FWHM.

The 22 PET images of the validation dataset were compared with the 29 of the control dataset by expressing the value at each voxel x as a Z-score

$$Z_{\text{group-wise}}(x) = \frac{I_G(x) - \mu^{\text{NC}}_G(x)}{\sigma^{\text{NC}}_G(x)} \, , \qquad (2)$$

where I_G corresponds to the subject's PET in the group space, and μ^{NC}_G and σ^{NC}_G are the mean and standard deviation of the 29 subjects of the control dataset in the group space.

---

[1] Imaging data were provided by the Alzheimer's disease neuroimaging initiative (http://adni.loni.ucla.edu/).

2.5 Voxel-Wise Analysis in the Subject's Space

Analysing the subject's PET image in its native space requires the control dataset to be transported to the target subject space. To do so, each of the 29 MRI images of the control dataset was deformed to the target image using an affine followed by a non-rigid registration [11]. The PET images of the control dataset, pre-aligned to the MRI images, were then mapped using the same transformation to the subject MRI image. The Z-score between the subject's PET and the entire control dataset aligned to the subject is defined as

$$Z_{\text{native}}(x) = \frac{I(x) - \mu^{\text{NC}}(x)}{\sigma^{\text{NC}}(x)} \quad , \tag{3}$$

where I corresponds to the subject's PET image, and μ^{NC} and σ^{NC} are the arithmetic mean and standard deviation of the 29 ADNI2 controls mapped into the native subject space, respectively.

2.6 Proposed Voxel-Wise Subject-Specific Analysis

This paper proposes a novel analysis framework that consists of creating a subject-specific healthy PET template. As in the previous approach (section 2.5), the control dataset is transported into the target subject space. A local image similarity measure, here the local normalised cross-correlation (LNCC), is then used to estimate the morphological similarity between the subject's MRI and the set of registered MRIs from the control dataset. To generate the subject-specific PET Z-score parameters, namely the patient-specific healthy-population mean and standard deviation, the set of registered PETs is locally selected and fused using a voxel-wise weighting scheme. As in [12], for all of the N control dataset MRIs propagated to the target subject's MRI, the LNCC at each voxel is ranked across all images. This ranking, denoted $r_n(x)$ (with x indexing the voxel and n indexing the propagated MRI) is converted to a weight by applying an exponential decay function $w_n(x) = e^{-\beta r_n(x)}$, with $\beta = 0.5$. Here, $w_n(x)$ represents the weight or contribution of subject n at voxel x to the patient specific model. For each of the N subjects in the control dataset, let the nth mapped PET image be denoted by J_n. The subject-specific Z-score model parameters (I_μ, I_σ) are obtained by a spatially varying weighted average

$$I_\mu(x) = \frac{\sum_{n=1}^{N} w_n(x) \cdot J_n(x)}{\sum_{n=1}^{N} w_n(x)} \tag{4}$$

$$I_\sigma(x) = \sqrt{\frac{N_w}{N_w - 1} \frac{\sum_{n=1}^{N} w_n(x) \cdot (J_n(x) - I_\mu(x))^2}{\sum_{n=1}^{N} w_n(x)}} \tag{5}$$

where N_w is the number of non-zero weights. Finally, the subject-specific Z-score is defined as

$$Z_{\text{subject-specific}}(x) = \frac{I(x) - I_\mu(x)}{I_\sigma(x)} \quad . \tag{6}$$

3   Validation and Results

The ^{18}F-FDG PET images of the 22 subjects from the validation dataset were examined using the regional, group-wise, native and proposed subject-specific analyses. Comparisons were restricted to 8 clinically relevant regions (Figure 1, top) for the sake of brevity. These regions were selected to represent the areas where abnormal uptake, compared with controls, is expected for the four pathologies represented in our dataset:

 - a frontal region, comprising the inferior frontal gyrus, precentral gyrus and anterior insula, was defined as relevant for PNFA subjects [2,3];
 - the anterior temporal region, comprising the hippocampus, amygdala and temporal pole, was defined as relevant for SD [3];
 - the tempoparietal region, comprising the inferior parietal lobule, posterior middle and superior temporal gyri, was defined as relevant for LPA [3];
 - finally, the occipital region, comprising the inferior, middle and superior occipital gyri, was defined as relevant for PCA [4].

Each hemisphere was analysed separately to account for left/right asymmetry.

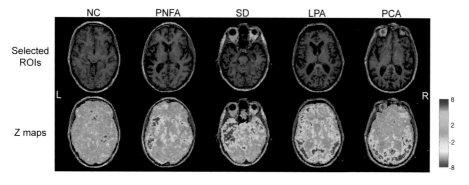

Fig. 1. T1 images overlaid with the selected ROIs (top) and the patient-specific Z-scores (bottom) for a representative subject of each condition.

3.1   Subject-Specific Z-Maps

As a first evaluation of the proposed method, we visually assessed the subject-specific Z-scores. Z-maps obtained for a representative subject of each condition are displayed in Figure 1 (bottom). A highly negative Z-score (red) indicates a reduced FDG uptake in the subject relative to the controls. Note that the Z-scores coincide with the regions where uptake abnormalities are expected for each pathology, and that the left/right asymmetries observed for the PNFA, SD, LPA and PCA subjects match the clinical syndromes: PNFA, SD and LPA subjects are expected to have greater left hypometabolism [3] while a greater right hypometabolism can be observed on subjects with PCA [4].

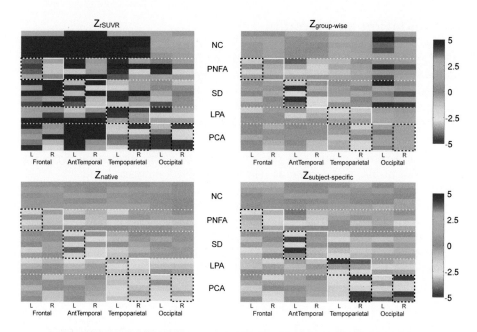

Fig. 2. Displayed above are the average Z-scores obtained for the rSUVR, group-wise, native and subject-specific methods in each ROI. The white boxes correspond to the regions where abnormal uptake is expected for each of the four pathologies while the black boxes indicate the predominant side when asymmetry is expected.

3.2 Z-Score Comparison in Predefined Regions-of-Interest

The Z-scores obtained from the rSUVR, and average regional Z-scores obtained using the group-wise, native and proposed subject-specific methods in each ROI are displayed in Figure 2. We first note that, using the native and subject-specific methods, the controls have approximately zero Z-scores in all regions, while high Z-scores are observed in the occipital region with the group-wise method. We also note that, when using the proposed method, highly negative Z-scores are observed for each pathology in regions where a reduced uptake is expected when compared with healthy controls. Moreover, the left/right observed asymmetries match the clinical syndromes. These highly relevant Z-score results were stable for all the subjects in each pathological group. The same significance and stability was not observed in the native or group-wise methods.

A Wilcoxon-Mann-Whitney test was used to assess whether the different analysis methods were able to differentiate controls and subjects with pathology. Results showed that the Z_{rSUVR}, Z_{native} and the proposed $Z_{subject-specific}$ scores could distinguish controls from each of the pathologies at a 5% significance level. With the $Z_{group-wise}$ score, only controls and PCA subjects were significantly different. These results suggest an improvement in sensitivity with the Z_{rSUVR}, Z_{native} and $Z_{subject-specific}$ scores when compared with the $Z_{group-wise}$ score.

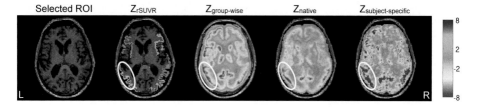

Fig. 3. Z-maps obtained with the different analysis methods for a subject with LPA. The white ellipses indicate the predominant side where abnormal uptake is expected.

Z-maps obtained for a representative LPA subject with the different analysis methods are displayed in Figure 3. We observe higher negative Z-scores in the relevant ROIs with the subject-specific approach than with the other methods.

4   Discussion and Conclusion

In this paper, we analyse ^{18}F-FDG PET data in the original subject space by providing voxel-wise statistics of normality/abnormality. The subject PET image is compared using a Z-score to a subject-specific PET model obtained through the propagation of morphologically-matched PET scans from a control dataset.

We first observed that, when analysing the PET images in the native subject space, the normal controls have low Z-scores in all regions, which was not always the case with the other methods (Figure 2). We note that the Z-scores obtained with the proposed method coincide with the regions where uptake abnormalities are expected for each of the pathologies studied and respect the left/right asymmetry (Figures 1 & 2). Finally, it appears that these highly negative Z-score results are stable across all subjects in each pathological group, which is not the case with the other methods (Figure 2).

The group-wise analysis seems strongly affected by uncertainties in the group-wise registration, driven by subjects with a large amount of atrophy (i.e. subjects with PCA), and the large variations in the normal population. Analysing the PET data in the native space avoids registering and resampling the subject PET into the group space. Furthermore, in the subject-specific method, only the most morphologically similar controls per target are selected to build the model, which reduces the variance of the normal population used for comparison in the Z-score, thus increasing the sensitivity. The low Z-scores systematically observed for the healthy subjects suggest that the subject-specific analysis is less prone to false positives. Finally, in contrast with rSUVR-based methods, the proposed analysis is not restricted to predefined regions.

While our method offers greater sensitivity, this is not its only purpose. It is our hope that, by disentangling the measurement of atrophy and metabolic decline, our method may provide a greater understanding of neurodegenerative diseases. Future work will involve validating the method on a larger dataset to provide more quantitative results.

Acknowledgements. This work was supported by an IMPACT studentship funded by Siemens and the UCL FES. Funding was received from the EPSRC (EP/H046410/1, EP/J020990/1, EP/K005278), the MRC (MR/J01107X/1), the EU-FP7 project VPH-DARE@IT (FP7-ICT-2011-9-601055), Alzheimer's Research UK, the Brain Research Trust, and the NIHR Biomedical Research Unit (Dementia). This work was also supported by funding from AVID Radiopharmaceuticals (a wholly owned subsidiary of Eli Lilly) and by researchers at the NIHR UCLH Biomedical Research Centre (including the High Impact Initiative).

References

1. Herholz, K.: PET studies in dementia. Annals of Nuclear Medicine 17(2) (2003)
2. Nestor, P.J., Graham, N.L., Fryer, T.D., Williams, G.B., Patterson, K., Hodges, J.R.: Progressive non-fluent aphasia is associated with hypometabolism centred on the left anterior insula. Brain 126(11), 2406–2418 (2003)
3. Rabinovici, G.D., Jagust, W.J., Furst, A.J., Ogar, J.M., Racine, C.A., Mormino, E.C., O'Neil, J.P., Lal, R.A., Dronkers, N.F., Miller, B.L., Gorno-Tempini, M.L.: Ab Amyloid and Glucose Metabolism in Three Variants of Primary Progressive Aphasia. Annals of Neurology 64(4), 388–401 (2008), doi:10.1002/ana.21451
4. Crutch, S.J., Lehmann, M., Schott, J.M., Rabinovici, G.D., Rossor, M.N., Fox, N.C.: Posterior cortical atrophy. The Lancet Neurology 11(2), 170 (2012)
5. Signorini, M., Paulesu, E., Friston, K., Perani, D., Colleluori, A., Lucignani, G., Grassi, F., Bettinardi, V., Frackowiak, R.S.J., Fazio, F.: Rapid Assessment of Regional Cerebral Metabolic Abnormalities in Single Subjects with Quantitative and Nonquantitative [^{18}F]FDG PET: A Clinical Validation of Statistical Parametric Mapping. Neuroimage 9(1), 63–80 (1999)
6. Drzezga, A., Grimmer, T., Riemenschneider, M., Lautenschlager, N., Siebner, H., Alexopoulus, P., Minoshima, S., Schwaiger, M., Kurz, A.: Prediction of Individual Clinical Outcome in MCI by Means of Genetic Assessment and ^{18}F-FDG PET. Journal of Nuclear Medicine 46(10), 1625–1632 (2005)
7. Sled, J.G., Zijdenbos, A.P., Evans, A.C.: A nonparametric method for automatic correction of intensity nonuniformity in MRI data.. IEEE Transactions on Medical Imaging 17(1), 87–97 (1998)
8. Cardoso, M., Wolz, R., Modat, M., Fox, N.C., Rueckert, D., Ourselin, S.: Geodesic Information Flows. In: Ayache, N., Delingette, H., Golland, P., Mori, K. (eds.) MICCAI 2012, Part II. LNCS, vol. 7511, pp. 262–270. Springer, Heidelberg (2012)
9. Minoshima, S., Frey, K.A., Foster, N.L., Kuhl, D.E.: Preserved Pontine Glucose Metabolism in Alzheimer Disease A Reference Region for Functional Brain Image (PET) Analysis. Journal of Computer Assisted Tomography 19(4), 541–547 (1995)
10. Rohlfing, T., Brandt, R., Maurer, Jr., C.R., Menzel, R.: Bee brains, B-splines and computational democracy: generating an average shape atlas. In: Proc. IEEE Workshop Mathematical Methods in Biomedical Image Analysis, pp. 187–194 (2001)
11. Modat, M., Ridgway, G.R., Taylor, Z.A., Lehmann, M., Barnes, J., Hawkes, D.J., Fox, N.C., Ourselin, S.: Fast free-form deformation using graphics processing units. Computer Methods and Programs in Biomedicine 98(3), 278–284 (2010)
12. Burgos, N., Cardoso, M.J., Thielemans, K., Modat, M., Pedemonte, S., Dickson, J., Barnes, A., Ahmed, R., Mahoney, C.J., Schott, J.M., Duncan, J.S., Atkinson, D., Arridge, S.R., Hutton, B.F., Ourselin, S.: Attenuation Correction Synthesis for Hybrid PET-MR Scanners: Application to Brain Studies. IEEE Transactions on Medical Imaging 33(12), 2332–2341 (2014)

Hierarchical Reconstruction of 7T-like Images from 3T MRI Using Multi-level CCA and Group Sparsity

Khosro Bahrami[1], Feng Shi[1], Xiaopeng Zong[1], Hae Won Shin[2], Hongyu An[1], and Dinggang Shen[1]

[1] Department of Radiology and BRIC, University of North Carolina at Chapel Hill, NC
[2] Department of Neurology, University of North Carolina at Chapel Hill, NC

Abstract. Advancements in 7T MR imaging bring higher spatial resolution and clearer tissue contrast, in comparison to the conventional 3T and 1.5T MR scanners. However, 7T MRI scanners are less accessible at the current stage due to higher costs. Through analyzing the appearances of 7T images, we could improve both the resolution and quality of 3T images by properly mapping them to 7T-like images; thus, promoting more accurate post-processing tasks, such as segmentation. To achieve this method based on an unique dataset acquired both 3T and 7T images from same subjects, we propose novel multi-level Canonical Correlation Analysis (CCA) method and group sparsity as a hierarchical framework to reconstruct 7T-like MRI from 3T MRI. First, the input 3T MR image is partitioned into a set of overlapping patches. For each patch, the local coupled 3T and 7T dictionaries are constructed by extracting the patches from a neighboring region from all aligned 3T and 7T images in the training set. In the training phase, we have both 3T and 7T MR images scanned from each training subject. Then, these two patch sets are mapped to the same space using multi-level CCA. Next, each input 3T MRI patch is sparsely represented by the 3T dictionary and then the obtained sparse coefficients are utilized to reconstruct the 7T patch with the corresponding 7T dictionary. Group sparsity is further utilized to maintain the consistency between neighboring patches. Such reconstruction is performed hierarchically with adaptive patch size. The experiments were performed on 10 subjects who had both 3T and 7T MR images. Experimental results demonstrate that our proposed method is capable of recovering rich structural details and outperforms other methods, including the sparse representation method and CCA method.

1 Introduction

Magnetic Resonance Imaging (MRI) is a noninvasive method of observing the human body without the use of surgery, harmful dyes or x-rays, making this approach widely used in medical imaging, as using MRIs can help to detect problems at early stages. High resolution MRI is always desirable in research and

N. Navab et al. (Eds.): MICCAI 2015, Part II, LNCS 9350, pp. 659–666, 2015.
DOI: 10.1007/978-3-319-24571-3_79

clinical practice, since it has smaller voxel size, which provides greater structural details. In contrast, low-resolution MRI is affected by partial volume effect, in which a voxel captures signals from multiple tissue types, resulting in fuzzy tissue boundaries. The introduction of ultra-high-field MR (7 Tesla (7T)) scanners have allowed for high resolution MRI scanning. In theory, the signal-to-noise ratio (SNR) should be almost linearly related to the magnetic field. For instance, the SNR of 7T should be 2.3 times of the SNR of 3T. Therefore, 7T MRI should provide images with higher resolution. In this regard, it has been shown that 7T MRI is more effective in the diagnosis of multiple sclerosis, cerebrovascular diseases, brain tumors, and degenerative diseases than 3T and 1.5T MRI [1].

In Fig. 1, we show the axial views of 3T and 7T MR images acquired from the same subject, as well as a close-up view of the bottom-left part of the images. Compared to 3T, the 7T MRI shows much higher tissue contrast between the white matter and gray matter and clearer boundaries between cerebrospinal fluid (CSF) and gray matter. However, due to the low availability and higher prices for 7T scanners, accessibility to high-resolution 7T MRI is limited. For instance, there are approximately more than 20000 3T scanners in the world while there are only around 40 7T scanners [2]. Therefore, it is significant to predict 7T-like MR images from 3T MR images to help increase both the resolution and quality of these input 3T images. This motivates us to propose a method to reconstruct images of 7T from 3T MRI.

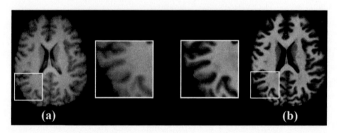

Fig. 1. Axial views of (a) 3T MRI and (b) 7T MRI of the same subject, along with the zoomed regions. Better anatomical details could be observed in 7T MRI.

In the reconstruction of high-resolution (HR) from low-resolution (LR) images, most resolution enhancement methods can be categorized into motion-based and example-based. The motion-based methods use multiple observations [3,4], while example-based methods use the dictionaries of paired high and low resolution patches in a sparse representation framework [5,6]. Such methods have also been employed for resolution enhancement of MRI [7,8]. In this work, we follow the example-based methods based on sparse representation through incorporating the dictionary of 3T (LR) and 7T (HR) MR images. In such methods, it is assumed that the LR and HR images have similar distributions and high correlation. However, in general, such assumption may not be satisfied completely. To overcome this weakness, in human face super-resolution work [9], LR and HR images are mapped into canonical correlation analysis (CCA) space to increase the correlation of LR and HR images. However, the mapping with CCA only improves the correlation between all data pairs in 3T and 7T dictionaries, without considering the structure of input 3T patch in reconstructing 7T patch.

In this paper, we propose an extension of CCA called multi-level CCA to further improve the correlation of 3T and 7T dictionaries with respect to the input 3T patch. Our main contributions include: 1) We propose a novel common space called multi-level CCA space to increase the correlation of 3T and 7T dictionaries; 2) We incorporate the group sparsity in the multi-level CCA space to share the sparsity among the neighboring 3T patches for reliable and accurate 7T MRI reconstruction; 3) We propose a hierarchical patch-based reconstruction to reconstruct the overall structure of 7T MRI at the early stage and then the details at the final stage. To the best of our knowledge, this is the first work that has been proposed for the reconstruction of 7T MRI from 3T MRI. The rest of this paper is organized as follows. In Section 2, we introduce our proposed method. In Section 3, experimental results are provided. In Section 4, the conclusion of our paper is stated.

2   Proposed Method

Overview: In this paper, we propose a hierarchical framework for the reconstruction of 7T MRI from 3T MRI based on group sparsity in multi-level CCA space, as shown in Fig. 2. First, the input 3T MRI is partitioned into overlapping patches. For each patch, the 3T and 7T local dictionaries are constructed from all subjects in the training set, each with both 3T and 7T MRI scans. Then, each 3T MRI patch is sparsely represented by the 3T local dictionary, while the obtained sparse coefficients are utilized to reconstruct the 7T patch with the corresponding 7T dictionary in multi-level CCA space. To do so, the similarity of sparse representation from nearby patches in the input 3T image is also enforced using group sparsity. Such reconstruction is achieved through adaptive patch size, by hierarchically reducing the patch size in multi-step iterations. The following sections provide detailed steps of our proposed method.

Local Dictionary Building: In this step, the goal is to build local 3T and 7T dictionaries for each patch of the input 3T MRI. The local 3T dictionary is used to sparsely represent the 3T patch in the input 3T MRI, while the local 7T dictionary is used for reconstruction of the corresponding 7T patch based on the estimated sparse coefficients.

Let $\mathbf{y}$ be a column vector representing a 3T patch of size $m \times m \times m$ extracted from the input 3T MR image $\mathbf{Y}$. We build the local 3T dictionary $\mathbf{D}_{3T}$ and 7T dictionary $\mathbf{D}_{7T}$ for $\mathbf{y}$ from the patches with the same location and immediate neighboring locations in all N pairs of aligned 3T and 7T training MR images from N training subjects. To build the local dictionaries, we define P to be a neighborhood search window size, in which the patches are extracted from each training (3T or 7T) image from N pairs of aligned images.

Multi-level CCA Representation: Followed by the generation of local dictionaries $\mathbf{D}_{3T}$ and $\mathbf{D}_{7T}$, in this step the objective is to reconstruct the 7T patch

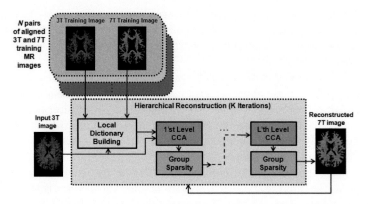

Fig. 2. Proposed framework for reconstruction of 7T MRI from 3T MRI.

$\mathbf{x}$ from the 3T input patch $\mathbf{y}$ using $\mathbf{D}_{3T}$ and $\mathbf{D}_{7T}$. In the example-based methods [5], $\mathbf{y}$ can be sparsely represented with respect to $\mathbf{D}_{3T}$ via

$$\hat{\boldsymbol{\alpha}} = \arg \min ||\mathbf{y} - \mathbf{D}_{3T}\boldsymbol{\alpha}||_2^2 + \lambda_1||\boldsymbol{\alpha}||_1 \tag{1}$$

where $\boldsymbol{\alpha}$ is the column vector of the sparse coefficients. Then, the estimated coefficients $\boldsymbol{\alpha}$ can be utilized to reconstruct the 7T patch $\mathbf{x}$ using $\mathbf{D}_{7T}$, as follows

$$\mathbf{x} = \mathbf{D}_{7T}\hat{\boldsymbol{\alpha}} \tag{2}$$

However, the sparse representation in the spatial domain assumes that there is a high correlation between the paired 3T and 7T image patches, which may not be completely satisfying in practice. Instead, we use the sparse representation in the CCA space. Generally, CCA is used to find the basis vectors for two sets of variables such that the correlation between the projections of these two sets of variables is maximized [9]. Here, for the two dictionaries $\mathbf{D}_{3T}$ and $\mathbf{D}_{7T}$, we incorporate CCA to obtain two basis vectors $\mathbf{b}_{3T}$ and $\mathbf{b}_{7T}$ such that the correlation of $\mathbf{D}_{3T}$ and $\mathbf{D}_{7T}$ in CCA space (i.e., between $\mathbf{b}_{3T}\mathbf{D}_{3T}$ and $\mathbf{b}_{7T}\mathbf{D}_{7T}$) is maximized. Then, the 3T patch $\mathbf{y}$ is also projected into CCA subspace using the base vector $\mathbf{b}_{3T}$. In the CCA subspace, we sparsely represent $\mathbf{y}$ with respect to $\mathbf{D}_{3T}$ by modifying Eq.(1) as

$$\hat{\boldsymbol{\alpha}} = \arg \min ||\mathbf{b}_{3T}\mathbf{y} - \mathbf{b}_{3T}\mathbf{D}_{3T}\boldsymbol{\alpha}||_2^2 + \lambda_1||\boldsymbol{\alpha}||_1 \tag{3}$$

Although CCA improves the correlation between all pairs of patches in 3T and 7T dictionaries, it does not consider the structure of the input 3T patch in reconstructing 7T patch. To address this limitation, we propose an extension of CCA, called multi-level CCA, as shown in Fig. 3, to further improve the correlation based on the input 3T patch.

In Fig. 3, suppose the red filled circles and green unfilled circles correspond to the elements of 3T and 7T local dictionaries in image space. In the first level, after CCA projection, the input 3T patch is sparsely represented using 3T dictionary in CCA space using Eq.(3). In such representation, the non-zero sparse

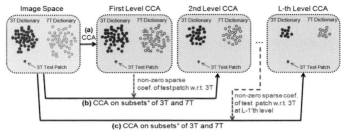

Fig. 3. The multi-level CCA. (a) CCA, (b) 2nd level CCA, and (c) L-th level CCA.

coefficients show the most important part of the 3T dictionary in representation of the input 3T patch. In the 2nd level, instead of using the whole 3T and 7T dictionaries, a subset of 3T dictionary, with elements corresponding to the non-zero coefficients, is transformed from the image space into the CCA space together with the corresponding subset of 7T dictionary (Fig. 3(b)). Then, the input 3T patch is sparsely represented using this subset of 3T dictionary in CCA space using Eq.(3). With this data-driven dictionary refinement, the prediction using the learned reconstruction coefficients is more effective in the next level of representation. This process can be done in L levels to further improve the sparse representation of the input 3T patch. At each level, followed by the sparsely representation of $\mathbf{y}$ with respect to D_{3T} using Eq.(3), the non-zero sparse coefficients, which indicate the most important patches of 3T and 7T dictionaries to be mapped from image space to the CCA space in the next level.

Group Sparse Regularization: In the multi-level CCA space, instead of sparse representation of a single 3T patch, we incorporate the group sparsity using neighboring 3T patches in order to share the same sparsity to make the local structure consistent for the reconstructed patches. We refer the current input 3T patch and its G immediately neighboring patches as a group. Besides solving the sparse representation for the current patch, we simultaneously solve the sparse representation for G neighboring patches, to construct the sparse coefficients for the entire group. We reformulate the Eq.(3) to have multi-level CCA using group sparsity as below

$$\hat{\mathbf{A}} = \arg\min \sum_{i=1}^{G+1} ||\mathbf{b}_{3T,i}\mathbf{y}_i - \mathbf{b}_{3T,i}\mathbf{D}_{3T,i}\boldsymbol{\alpha}_i||_2^2 + \lambda_1||\mathbf{A}||_{2,1} \qquad (4)$$

where $\mathbf{A} = [\boldsymbol{\alpha}_1, ... \boldsymbol{\alpha}_{G+1}]$ is a matrix where each column includes the sparse coefficients of a patch in the group, and $\mathbf{D}_{3T,i}$, $\mathbf{y}_i$, and $\boldsymbol{\alpha}_i$ denote the local 3T dictionary, 3T input patch, and sparse coefficient vector of the i-th patch in the group, respectively. The first term is the multi-task least square minimizer for all $G+1$ neighboring patches. The second term is the regularization term, which is a combination of L_1 and L_2 norms. The L_2 norm is imposed to each row of

A to make the neighboring patches have similar sparsity, while the L_1 norm is imposed to the all rows of **A** to ensure the sparsity.

Hierarchical Reconstruction: Using our proposed method based on group sparsity in multi-level CCA space, each patch of 7T image can be reconstructed from 3T patch. However, in the reconstruction of 7T patches, choosing the appropriate size of patches is very important. If we choose small patch sizes, the patches can capture the details, but the final reconstructed 7T image can be very noisy. In contrast, by choosing large patch sizes, the patches can capture the whole structure, but the result can be blurry. To overcame this problem, we propose an adaptive patch size. Starting from a large patch size, we hierarchically decrease the patch size in multi-iterations. In such case, in the first iteration the whole structure is estimated by reconstructing the initial 7T image, while in the next iterations by decreasing the patch size the image details are gradually recovered by hierarchical reconstruction of 7T image, as explained bellow.

- **First Iteration: Reconstruction of Initial 7T Image.** First, Eq.(4) is incorporated to represent each input 3T patch **y** using the local dictionary $\mathbf{D}_{3T}$ to estimate sparse coefficients. Using the estimated sparse coefficients, the corresponding 7T patch **x** is estimated. Then, the whole 7T image is reconstructed by taking the average of all reconstructed 7T patches if they are overlapped.
- **The 2nd ... K-th iterations: Hierarchical reconstruction of 7T image.** Using the reconstructed 7T image in the first iteration, in the 2nd to K-th iterations, we propose Eq.(5) by adding a regularization term to Eq.(4) as

$$\hat{\mathbf{A}}^k = \arg\min \sum_{i=1}^{G+1} ||\mathbf{b}_{3T,i}^k \mathbf{y}_i^k - \mathbf{b}_{3T,i}^k \mathbf{D}_{3T,i}^k \boldsymbol{\alpha}_i^k||_2^2 + \lambda_1 ||\mathbf{A}^k||_{2,1}$$

$$+ \lambda_2 \sum_{i=1}^{G+1} ||\mathbf{b}_{7T,i}^k \mathbf{x}_i^{k-1} - \mathbf{b}_{7T,i}^k \mathbf{D}_{7T,i}^k \boldsymbol{\alpha}_i^k||_2^2 \tag{5}$$

where $k = \{2, ..., K\}$ denotes the iteration number and $\mathbf{x}_i^{k-1}$ is a patch from the reconstructed 7T image from the previous iteration $k-1$. The first and second terms are as explained for Eq.(4), and the last term is the penalty term, which is proposed to ensure that there is consistency between iterations.

After estimating 7T-like patches in the CCA space, we use the inverse of base vector $\mathbf{b}_{7T}$ to transform the 7T-like patches to the image space.

3   Experimental Results

We evaluated the performance of our proposed method with the related works including the sparse representation in image space [5] and the sparse representation in CCA space [9].

Data and Preprocessing: We recruited 10 volunteers (4M/6F) for this study with ages between 30 ± 8 years. Of these 10 volunteers, 5 subjects were healthy and 5 subjects were patient with epilepsy. They were scanned using both a 3T Siemens Trio scanner and a 7T Siemens scanner. For each subject, the 3T and 7T images were rigidly aligned together, followed by a skull stripping to remove the non-brain tissues. The resolutions of 3T and 7T images are $1 \times 1 \times 1 \ mm^3$ and $0.65 \times 0.65 \times 0.65 \ mm^3$, respectively.

Experiment Settings: To evaluate our proposed method, a leave-one-out cross-validation strategy is adopted by considering one image for testing and the rest of the images for training. We consider 2 levels CCA ($L = 2$). For the group sparsity, we consider 6 neighborhoods ($G = 6$) for each input 3T patch. We set $\lambda_1 = 0.1$ and $\lambda_2 = 0.01$. For the hierarchical reconstruction, we use 3 iterations ($K = 3$) where the patch size ($m \times m \times m$) is adaptively changed from $9 \times 9 \times 9, 5 \times 5 \times 5$ to $3 \times 3 \times 3$. Similarly, neighborhood size P for dictionary is set to $13 \times 13 \times 13$, $7 \times 7 \times 7$ and $5 \times 5 \times 5$, respectively. To select these parameters, we evaluated our proposed method for different parameter values in cross validation. In all iterations, we consider the overlap of 1 voxel between the adjacent patches.

Visual Inspection: Fig. 4 compares the reconstructed 7T-like MRI based on different methods. Top row shows the axial views of the reconstructed 7T-like images for a subject by different methods, and the bottom row shows the close-up views of the bottom-left part of the reconstructed 7T-like images. Compared to the previous methods, the reconstructed 7T-like image by our proposed method is closer to the 7T ground truth on the right of Fig. 4. Also, it contains much more details while the other two results lack clarity.

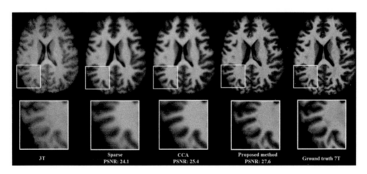

Fig. 4. Visual comparison of the reconstructed 7T-like images based on sparse representation [5], CCA based sparse representation [9] and our proposed method.

Quantitative Evaluation: We evaluate our proposed method by comparing the reconstructed 7T-like image with the ground truth 7T image of the same subject. We adopt two measures, peak-signal-to-noise ratio (PSNR) and root mean square error (RMSE). Higher PSNR and lower RMSE indicate that the reconstructed images are much closer to the ground truth 7T image. Table 1 compares the reconstruction results of each subject by different methods. Also, the last row shows the averages of PSNR and RMSE for all 10 subjects. Compared to the previous methods, our proposed method has a much higher PSNR and a much lower RMSE for all 10 subjects.

Table 1. Performance comparison of three methods in terms of PSNR and RMSE.

(a) PSNR

Method	Sparse [5]	CCA [9]	Proposed
Subject 1	22.6	24.2	**26.1**
Subject 2	24.8	26.4	**27.7**
Subject 3	23.3	24.3	**26.3**
Subject 4	24.8	25.7	**27.3**
Subject 5	25.6	26.4	**28.1**
Subject 6	25.2	26.2	**27.9**
Subject 7	25.6	27.1	**29.0**
Subject 8	24.9	26.2	**28.0**
Subject 9	22.4	23.4	**24.9**
Subject 10	24.1	26.0	**29.1**
Average	24.3	25.5	**27.4**

(b) RMSE

Method	Sparse [5]	CCA [9]	Proposed
Subject 1	17.0	15.1	**12.0**
Subject 2	14.5	12.2	**10.5**
Subject 3	17.3	15.5	**12.3**
Subject 4	14.5	13.1	**11.0**
Subject 5	13.4	12.2	**10.1**
Subject 6	13.9	12.4	**10.2**
Subject 7	13.3	11.2	**9.0**
Subject 8	14.5	12.5	**10.1**
Subject 9	19.2	17.7	**14.5**
Subject 10	15.7	12.7	**8.9**
Average	15.3	13.4	**10.8**

4   Conclusion and Discussion

In this work, we proposed a hierarchical framework for reconstruction of 7T-like MR image from 3T MR image based on group sparsity in multi-level Canonical Correlation Analysis (CCA) space. The experiments performed on 10 subjects using 3T and 7T MR images demonstrate that our proposed method is capable of recovering more structural details and outperforms previous methods such as sparse representation in image space and CCA space. In future works, we will perform more experiments to further evaluate the influence of the proposed 7T-like reconstruction on subsequent image processing such as brain tissue segmentation.

References

1. Kolka, A.G., Hendriksea, J., Zwanenburg, J.J.M., Vissera, F., Luijtena, P.R.: Clinical applications of 7T MRI in the brain. Eur. Jour. of Radiology 82, 708–718 (2013)
2. DOTmed Daily News (2012). http://www.dotmed.com/news/story/17820
3. Tian, J., Ma, K.: A survey on super-resolution imaging. Signal Image Video Process. 5(3), 329–342 (2011)
4. Farsiu, S., Robinson, M.D., Elad, M., Milanfar, P.: Fast and robust multiframe super resolution. IEEE Trans. Image Process. 13(10), 1327–1344 (2004)
5. Yang, J., Wright, J., Huang, T.S., Ma, Y.: Image super-resolution via sparse representation. IEEE Trans. Image Process. 19(11), 2861–2873 (2010)
6. Freeman, W.T., Jones, T.R., Pasztor, E.C.: Example-based superresolution. IEEE Comput. Graphics Appl. 22(2), 56–65 (2002)
7. Shilling, R.Z., Robbie, T.Q., Bailloeul, T., Mewes, K., Mersereau, R.M., Brummer, M.E.: A super-resolution framework for 3-D high-resolution and high-contrast imaging using 2-D multislice MRI. IEEE Trans. Med. Imaging 28(5), 633–644 (2009)
8. Rueda, A., Malpica, N., Romero, E.: Single-image super-resolution of brain MR images using overcomplete dictionaries. Med. Image Anal. 17, 113–132 (2013)
9. Huang, H., He, H., Fan, X., Zhang, J.: Super-resolution of human face image using canonical correlation analysis. Pattern Recognition 43, 2532–2543 (2010)

Robust Spectral Denoising for Water-Fat Separation in Magnetic Resonance Imaging

Felix Lugauer[1], Dominik Nickel[2], Jens Wetzl[1], Stephan A.R. Kannengiesser[2], Andreas Maier[1], and Joachim Hornegger[1]

[1] Pattern Recognition Lab, Friedrich-Alexander-Universität Erlangen-Nürnberg, Erlangen, Germany
[2] MR Applications Predevelopment, Siemens Healthcare, Erlangen, Germany

Abstract. Fat quantification based on the multi-echo Dixon method is gaining importance in clinical practice as it can match the accuracy of spectroscopy but provides high spatial resolution. Accurate quantification protocols, though, are limited to low SNR and suffer from a high noise bias. As the clinically relevant water and fat components are estimated by fitting a non-linear signal model to the data, the uncertainty is further amplified. In this work, we first establish the low-rank property and its locality assumptions for water-fat MRI and, consequently, propose a model-consistent but adaptive spectral denoising. A robust noise estimation in combination with a risk-minimizing threshold adds to a fully-automatic method. We demonstrate its capabilities on abdominal fat quantification data from in-vivo experiments. The denoising reduces the fit error on average by 37 % and the uncertainty of the fat fraction by 58 % in comparison to the original data while being edge-preserving.

Keywords: Robust Denoising, Water-Fat MRI, Locally Low-Rank.

1 Introduction

Tissue fat concentration is an established indicator for various disorders like hepatic steatosis or fatty liver disease. Even though liver biopsy is invasive and risk-involving, it is still widely used in clinical practice [1].

Recently, validated biomarkers, foremost the proton density fat fraction (PDFF), could be obtained non-invasively by MR spectroscopy (MRS) and MRI [2]. While the latter enables a larger coverage, it can only quantify the tissue fat concentration accurately when confounding effects like T_1 bias, R_2^* relaxation and magnet imperfections are sufficiently mitigated [3]. As a consequence, clinical fat quantification protocols based on MRI are limited in resolution and flip angle as to reduce T_1-bias and noise bias [4]. Also, a larger series of contrast images (e.g. 6 echos) must be acquired to enable the estimation of iron as well and to reduce the remaining confounding factors [5]. As this signal is used to determine the clinically relevant biomarkers by a non-linear voxel-wise fit, further noise amplification arises. Suppressing this noise—depending on breath-hold, resolution and flip angle parameters—by exploiting the shared information in the data series is desirable. However, typical priors promoting similarities of intensity or

© Springer International Publishing Switzerland 2015
N. Navab et al. (Eds.): MICCAI 2015, Part II, LNCS 9350, pp. 667–674, 2015.
DOI: 10.1007/978-3-319-24571-3_80

gradient data cannot be enforced directly due to strong variations in contrast. Yet, in multi-contrast imaging there is a spectral sparsity when the number of modeled components is less than the acquired contrast images. Previously, this sparsity motivated the use of singular value filtering [6] for multi-echo denoising, assuming a low-rank (LR) signal. Advances in matrix completion [7] leveraged LR regularization based on the nuclear norm for various applications. [8] showed the benefit of local over global LR priors for dynamic MRI. Recently, extending the unbiased risk estimator for singular value thresholding (SVT) enables risk-minimizing denoising for a given noise estimate [9]. We adopt these concepts, and first show that the LR property of multi-contrast images is well-justified for local correlations of the signal, lending itself ideally for local processing. Then, the noise level of the signal is robustly estimated from local estimates which feeds an adaptive block-wise SVT. Our proposed method is validated both qualitatively and quantitatively using in-vivo experiments.

2 Water-Fat Imaging

Water-fat separation and quantification is based on the known difference of spectral properties between hydrogen nuclei bound in water and fat. An exact determination requires multiple echos for estimating and correcting the phase evolution $\boldsymbol{\Phi} \in \mathbb{C}^{N \times E}$ incorporating R_2^* relaxation, field inhomogeneities, gradient delays and eddy currents. The relation between the spectral components of water and fat and the e-th echo image $\boldsymbol{w}, \boldsymbol{f}, \boldsymbol{x}_e \in \mathbb{C}^N$ at time t_e is modeled as,

$$\boldsymbol{x}_e(j) = (\boldsymbol{w}(j) + c_{t_e}\boldsymbol{f}(j))\,e^{i\boldsymbol{\Phi}(j,e)}, \; j = 1 \ldots N, \; e = 1 \ldots E, \tag{1}$$

for the j-th out of N voxels and E contrast images. A pre-calibrated multi-peak fat spectrum is given by $c_{t_e} \in \mathbb{C}$ while the phase effects are modeled with $e^{i\boldsymbol{\Phi}(j,e)}$.

Biomarker Estimation. The clinically relevant signals of water, fat and R_2^*—an indicator for increased iron deposits—are determined voxel-wise by a non-linear fit of either the complex- or absolute-valued contrast images [10]. Then, the fat fraction (PDFF), an important biomarker, is simply $\boldsymbol{f}(j)/(\boldsymbol{w}(j) + \boldsymbol{f}(j))$.

Low-Rank Property. Signal models based on chemical shift encoding often share the property that they yield series of images which are superpositions of only a limited number of spectral components. For the explicit case of water-fat imaging, the signal variation of a multi-echo series is a combination of water and fat images. Thus, for a series of more than two contrasts there will be a spectral sparsity. To identify this, we rewrite (1) and consider the series of contrasts as

$$\underbrace{\begin{bmatrix} \boldsymbol{x}_1(j) \\ \boldsymbol{x}_2(j) \\ \vdots \\ \boldsymbol{x}_E(j) \end{bmatrix}}_{\boldsymbol{x}(j)} = \underbrace{\begin{bmatrix} e^{i\boldsymbol{\Phi}(j,1)} & 0 & \cdots & 0 \\ 0 & e^{i\boldsymbol{\Phi}(j,2)} & \cdots & 0 \\ \vdots & \vdots & \ddots & \vdots \\ 0 & 0 & \cdots & e^{i\boldsymbol{\Phi}(j,E)} \end{bmatrix}}_{\boldsymbol{D}_\Phi(j)} \cdot \underbrace{\begin{bmatrix} 1 & c_{t_1} \\ 1 & c_{t_2} \\ \vdots & \vdots \\ 1 & c_{t_E} \end{bmatrix}}_{\boldsymbol{A}} \cdot \underbrace{\begin{bmatrix} \boldsymbol{w}(j) \\ \boldsymbol{f}(j) \end{bmatrix}}_{\rho(j)}, \tag{2}$$

with the chemical shift composition $\boldsymbol{A}$ and diagonal matrix $\boldsymbol{D}_\Phi$ combining relaxation and other phase effects while $\boldsymbol{\rho}$ holds the signal of water and fat.

Let $\boldsymbol{X} \in \mathbb{C}^{N \times E}$ denote the signal matrix containing all N voxels and E echos. In order to exploit the spectral sparsity, we correlate small local image regions with N_P elements of all E contrasts in a so called *Casorati* matrix $(N_P \times E)$,

$$\mathcal{B}_P(\boldsymbol{X}) = \begin{bmatrix} (\boldsymbol{D}_\Phi(p_1)\boldsymbol{A}\boldsymbol{\rho}(p_1))^T \\ \vdots \\ (\boldsymbol{D}_\Phi(p_{N_P})\boldsymbol{A}\boldsymbol{\rho}(p_{N_P}))^T \end{bmatrix}, \tag{3}$$

where $\mathcal{B}_P : \mathbb{C}^{N \times E} \to \mathbb{C}^{N_P \times E}$, $(E \ll N_P \ll N)$ denotes the reshape operator and $p_i \in \{1 \ldots N\}$ is the i-th voxel from the set of voxel indices P. Besides being computationally tractable, small image regions are beneficial as we become independent of the phase error map $\boldsymbol{\Phi}$ which is expected to be rather smooth and, thus, can be assumed to be locally constant [2]. Under this assumption, the rank of this matrix is at most 2 and is in general restricted by the number of modeled spectral components: $\mathrm{rank}(\mathcal{B}_P(\boldsymbol{X})) \leq \dim(\boldsymbol{\rho})$. The singular value distribution of sufficiently small image patches confirms this assumption in practice (see Fig. 1).

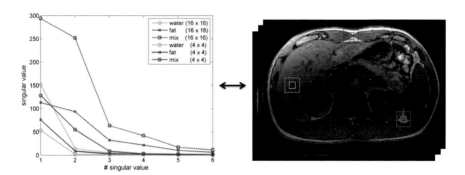

Fig. 1. Low-rank property of multi-echo MRI: Local image patches extracted from all echos yields matrices with low rank for sufficiently small patches. Note the different tissues underlying each patch and their corresponding singular value distribution.

3   Proposed Method

As we have just established, the Casorati formulation for multi-contrast water-fat MRI has a maximum rank of 2 in theory and, thus, lends itself for low-rank denoising. To this end, we find a robust estimate for the noise in the whole image domain and incorporate it into a block-wise low-rank denoising such that the optimal regularization is data-driven. Finally, a weighted averaging of the results from overlapping blocks further improves the robustness of the algorithm. We will refer to this algorithm as Robust Locally Low-Rank (RLLR) denosing.

3.1   Robust Noise Estimation

An accurate noise estimation is vital, as over- or under-estimation can render the subsequent denoising useless, especially in low SNR applications. We assume the acquired data $\hat{\boldsymbol{X}}$ to be affected by complex white noise $\mathcal{W} \overset{\text{iid}}{\sim} \mathcal{N}_{\mathbb{C}}(0, \sigma_\epsilon^2)$ and propose to combine local noise estimates from block-wise processing to a robust estimate. W.l.o.g., the set of blocks Ω tiles the spatial domain in quadratic blocks of length k as to implement a sliding window. Then we define the estimator as

$$\hat{\sigma}_\epsilon = \frac{\text{median}(\sigma_E(\mathcal{B}_P(\hat{\boldsymbol{X}})) \mid P \in \Omega_n)}{\text{median}(\sigma_E(\boldsymbol{M}_i) \mid i = 1 \ldots N_M)}, \tag{4}$$

where $\sigma_E(\cdot)$ denotes the smallest singular value of its argument and $\Omega_n \subseteq \Omega$ is a subset with every n-th block. Assuming that the lowest singular value is dominated by noise for low-rank matrices, we obtain the noise standard deviation by normalizing the median to that of random matrices sampled from the unit normal distribution $\mathcal{N}_{\mathbb{C}}(0, 1)$. For the stability of the median, N_M random matrices are generated. This needs to be computed only once per block configuration.

3.2   Adaptive Block-Wise SVT

We seek to remove the noise $\mathcal{W}$ in the acquired signal $\hat{\boldsymbol{X}}$ to obtain the pure signal $\boldsymbol{X} = \hat{\boldsymbol{X}} - \mathcal{W}$ by processing the image domain in small partitions Ω. For blocks of locally correlated regions, the low rank property can be exploited. Rank optimization, however, is known to be NP-hard; a feasible alternative is needed. Instead of imposing hard constraints, e.g., rank-r approximation which sets all but r singular values to zero, we prefer to minimize the sum of singular values—known as the nuclear norm—for two reasons: 1) it is more robust in the sense that it will not fail when the exact rank property is violated or the modeled spectrum is enlarged and 2) as the tightest convex relaxation of the rank optimization, it can be solved efficiently [7]. Accordingly, the nuclear norm optimization for individual patches P in an unconstrained formulation reads

$$\min \frac{1}{2}\|\mathcal{B}_P(\hat{\boldsymbol{X}}) - \mathcal{B}_P(\boldsymbol{X})\|_F^2 + \lambda\|\mathcal{B}_P(\boldsymbol{X})\|_* , \lambda \geq 0, \tag{5}$$

which is the proximal operator of the nuclear norm $\|\cdot\|_*$, for which the following closed-form solution based on the singular value decomposition exists: $\text{SVT}(\mathcal{B}_P(\hat{\boldsymbol{X}}), \lambda) = \boldsymbol{U}\,\text{diag}((\boldsymbol{\sigma} - \lambda)_+)\boldsymbol{V}^T$; $(t)_+$ is evaluated per component as $\max(t, 0)$, which performs soft-thresholding on the singular values such that values smaller than the threshold become zero while larger ones are drawn towards zero. Then, a denoised signal for the whole image can be obtained by applying SVT to each block and averaging the contribution per voxel [9]. Similarly, we define the weighted and block-adaptive denoising with individual thresholds λ_P,

$$\boldsymbol{X} = \boldsymbol{W} \circ \sum_{P \in \Omega} \mathcal{B}_P^\dagger(r_p^{-1} \text{SVT}(\mathcal{B}_P(\hat{\boldsymbol{X}}), \lambda_P)), \quad \boldsymbol{W} = \sum_{P \in \Omega}(\mathcal{B}_P^\dagger(r_P \boldsymbol{J}_P)) \tag{6}$$

where $\mathcal{B}_P^\dagger$ is the adjoint Casorati transform; W is the normalization matrix due to overlapping as well as weighted patches and J_P is $N_P \times E$ matrix of ones. Sparser, less noisy patches are promoted due to a reciprocal rank-weighting $r_P = \max(1, \|\sigma_P\|_0)$ while an overlap of patches ensures data consistency [11].

The singular value threshold is critical and should be chosen robustly based on the global noise level. A noise-dependent, though fixed threshold might not be adequate for all variations in the data, i.e. the actual singular value distribution, so a block-dependent threshold may be preferred. Consequently, we make use of the SURE formulation derived by Candès et al. that yields the risk involved in SVT with a certain λ solely based on the data and its noise variance [9]. We propose to use adaptive risk-minimizing thresholds $\lambda_P = \mathrm{argmin}_\lambda \, \mathrm{SURE}(\mathcal{B}_P(\hat{X}), \lambda, \hat{\sigma}_\epsilon^2)$ for every image block which can either be found via grid search or approximately as this function is piece-wise smooth.

4   Experiments and Results

We performed various experiments to evaluate the noise reduction of contrast images from water-fat MRI and the effects on the subsequent non-linear estimation of the clinically relevant biomarker PDFF and R_2^*. In addition, we quantified the *fit error*—introduced by the voxel-wise fitting—as further measure:

$$R_{\mathrm{fit}}(j) = \frac{\sum_e \left(\hat{x}_e(j) - x_e(j) \right)^2}{\sum_e \hat{x}_e(j)^2}. \tag{7}$$

Method Parameters. Throughout this study we used quadratic image patches of length $k = 5$, i.e. Casorati matrices of size $25(N_P) \times 6(E)$ as sliding windows with stride $\delta_\mathcal{B} = 1$ for all partitions of the 3-D data. Every 10-th patch was used for noise estimation. Note, the method does not require parameter tuning and is generally applicable as long as sparsity assumptions hold, i.e. $N_P \gg E$. The patch length could be chosen resolution dependent ($\sim 1\,\mathrm{cm}$), but a larger support will increase spatial smoothing while a smaller support lacks statistics and invalidates $N_P \gg E$. On standard hardware (4-core), the C++ prototype implementation runs in under a minute for the data used here.

In-vivo Data. We used data from abdominal MRI examinations of 3 volunteers on a $3\,\mathrm{T}$ MR system (MAGNETOM Skyra, Siemens Healthcare, Erlangen, Germany). A prototype 3-D gradient multi-echo acquisition (VIBE) with PAT acceleration 4 was used in combination with the prototype of a multi-step magnitude fitting technique [10]. Parameters included TR = 16.6 ms, TEs = 1.06, 2.20, 3.69, 6.15, 9.84, 14.76 ms with flip angle = $2°$ and FoV of $420 \times 346 \times 60\,\mathrm{mm}^3$ and matrix $160 \times 132 \times 60$.

Fig. 2 shows an exemplary contrast image of a 6-echo liver examination (row 1). Comparing the original and the denoised image indicates that a constant noise bias was removed while preserving edge sharpness (left to right), which is confirmed by the difference image and by a rise in SNR[1] from 10.3 to 12.6.

---

[1] SNR is averaged over 3 smooth liver ROIs as, $\varnothing(\varnothing(|x|)/\sigma_{(|x|)})$.

The impact of the denoising on the biomarkers and the fit error which are obtained through fitting the echo series to the non-linear signal model are compared in row 2 & 3 of Fig. 2. PDFF, R_2^* and R_{fit} are shown left-to-right. The PDFF using the original data shows highly varying noise, possibly amplified through the fitting and the fraction calculation (SNR=3.1). The noise bias on the R_2^* map is less severe but still prominent (SNR=6.0). The fit error map indicates larger errors in the central FoV, which supports that a low SNR decreases the accuracy of the parameter estimation. The denoising, in consequence, strongly stabilizes the PDFF calculation as the fat concentration in the liver is far more homogeneous

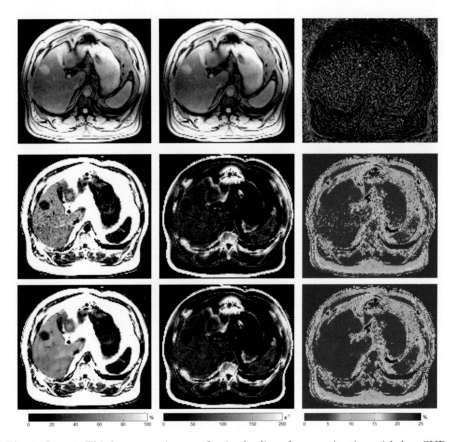

Fig. 2. Row 1: Third contrast image of a 6-echo liver fat examination with low SNR. Original (SNR=10.3), denoised (SNR=12.6) and their difference image (20 × scaled) are shown from left to right. A strong noise bias could be removed while details are enhanced, e.g., blood vessels in the liver.

Row 2 & 3: Impact of the denoising on the biomarker estimation: PDFF, R_2^* and associated fit error (left to right) using original and denoised data (bottom). Noise levels are considerably lower in PDFF (SNR=9.4, before 3.1) and R_2^* (SNR=8.4, before 6.0) maps and fit error is reduced using denoised data.

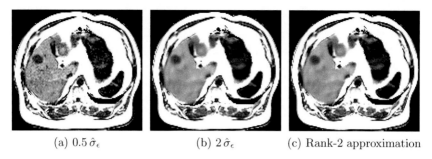

(a) $0.5\,\hat{\sigma}_\epsilon$ (b) $2\,\hat{\sigma}_\epsilon$ (c) Rank-2 approximation

Fig. 3. Noise adaptive technique: automatically obtained noise estimate $\hat{\sigma}_\epsilon$ was altered to demonstrate under-/over regularization for inaccurate estimates (a), (b). A Rank-2 approximation yields blurred edges while our method is edge-preserving (see Fig. 2).

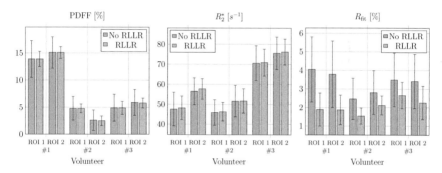

Fig. 4. Mean and standard deviation (SD) of the PDFF, R_2^* and the fit error R_{fit} for two liver ROIs of three volunteers. The SD is reduced consistently for all biomarkers, and the mean of the fit error. On average, the denoising reduced the fit error by 37 % and eliminated uncertainty (SD) of the PDFF by 58 % and that of R_2^* by 24 %.

(SNR=9.4). A milder smoothing is seen for R_2^*, though edges, e.g. blood vessels, are preserved (SNR=8.4). The fit error shows a notable decrease in regions with low signal strength, i.e. the liver and spleen. Fig. 3 demonstrates the sensitivity of the method to the noise level based on the PDFF map. When the automatically obtained noise estimate is altered, or inaccurately estimated, the method either fails to remove noise or blurs over edges. Similarly, a rank-2 approximation overshoots and removes detail. By contrast, our automatic threshold seems both edge-preserving and adaptive.

Fig. 4 shows our quantitative findings as the mean and standard deviation (SD) of the estimated biomarkers and the fit error using the original and the denoised data. For three subjects, average ROI measurements were taken from homogeneous areas of the liver for two slices, belonging to the upper and lower part of the liver. Altogether, the denoising reduced the fit error by 37 % and eliminated uncertainty (SD) of the PDFF by 58 % and that of R_2^* by 24 %.

5 Conclusion

A robust denoising algorithm for contrast-sparse MRI data has been proposed. The inherent low-rank property of locally correlated multi-contrast data is promoted with the nuclear norm in a model-consistent way. The algorithm is also automatic as the noise level is derived from local estimates of the whole image such that a risk-minimizing threshold can be used for a patch-based denoising.

We demonstrated the potential of the method on low SNR fat quantification data. Here, the contrast image series could be greatly improved while an even stronger effect is observed when this data is used for further processing, such as the fat fraction biomarker estimation. This has direct benefits as acquisition protocols with higher spatial resolution and/or lower flip angles become possible.

The integration into existing workflows is straightforward and attractive due to a low runtime and no need for parameter-tuning. Furthermore, the proposed method requires only spectrally sparse data as input and is, thus, widely applicable to instances of dynamic MRI, spectroscopy, and hyperspectral imaging.

References

1. Thampanitchawong, P., Piratvisuth, T.: Liver biopsy: complications and risk factors. World J. of Gastroenterol. 5, 301–304 (1999)
2. Reeder, S.B., Wen, Z., Yu, H., Pineda, A.R., Gold, G.E., Markl, M., Pelc, N.J.: Multicoil dixon chemical species separation with an iterative least-squares estimation method. Magn. Reson. Med. 51(1), 35–45 (2004)
3. Reeder, S.B., Cruite, I., Hamilton, G., Sirlin, C.B.: Quantitative assessment of liver fat with magnetic resonance imaging and spectroscopy. J. of Magn. Reson. Imaging 34(4), 729–749 (2011)
4. Liu, C. Y., McKenzie, C.A., Yu, H., Brittain, J.H., Reeder, S.B.: Fat quantification with ideal gradient echo imaging: correction of bias from t1 and noise. Magn. Reson. Med. 58(2), 354–364 (2007)
5. Sharma, P., Altbach, M., Galons, J.-P., Kalb, B., Martin, D.R.: Measurement of liver fat fraction and iron with mri and mr spectroscopy techniques. Diagn. Interv. Radiol. 20(1), 17–26 (2014)
6. Bydder, M., Du, J.: Noise reduction in multiple-echo data sets using singular value decomposition. Magn. Resonance Imaging 24(7), 849–856 (2006)
7. Cai, J.-F., Candès, E.J., Shen, Z.: A singular value thresholding algorithm for matrix completion. SIAM J. on Optim. 20(4), 1956–1982 (2010)
8. Trzasko, J., Manduca, A., Borisch, A.: Local versus global low-rank promotion in dynamic mri series reconstruction. In: Proc. Int. Symp. Magn. Reson. Med, p. 4371 (2011)
9. Candès, E.J., Sing-Long, C.A., Trzasko, J.D.: Unbiased risk estimates for singular value thresholding and spectral estimators. IEEE Trans. Signal Process. 61(19), 4643–4657 (2013)
10. Zhong, X., Nickel, M.D., Kannengiesser, S.A., Dale, B.M., Kiefer, B., Bashir, M.R.: Liver fat quantification using a multi-step adaptive fitting approach with multi-echo gre imaging. Magn. Reson. Med. 72(5), 1353–1365 (2014)
11. Manjón, J.V., Coupé, P., Buades, A., Collins, D.L., Robles, M.: New methods for mri denoising based on sparseness and self-similarity. Med. Image Analysis 16(1), 18–27 (2012)

Scale Factor Point Spread Function Matching: Beyond Aliasing in Image Resampling

M. Jorge Cardoso, Marc Modat, Tom Vercauteren, and Sebastien Ourselin

Translational Imaging Group, CMIC, University College London, London, UK

Abstract. Imaging devices exploit the Nyquist-Shannon sampling theorem to avoid both aliasing and redundant oversampling by design. Conversely, in medical image resampling, images are considered as continuous functions, are warped by a spatial transformation, and are then sampled on a regular grid. In most cases, the spatial warping changes the frequency characteristics of the continuous function and no special care is taken to ensure that the resampling grid respects the conditions of the sampling theorem. This paper shows that this oversight introduces artefacts, including aliasing, that can lead to important bias in clinical applications. One notable exception to this common practice is when multi-resolution pyramids are constructed, with low-pass "anti-aliasing" filters being applied prior to downsampling. In this work, we illustrate why similar caution is needed when resampling images under general spatial transformations and propose a novel method that is more respectful of the sampling theorem, minimising aliasing and loss of information. We introduce the notion of scale factor point spread function (sfPSF) and employ Gaussian kernels to achieve a computationally tractable resampling scheme that can cope with arbitrary non-linear spatial transformations and grid sizes. Experiments demonstrate significant ($p < 10^{-4}$) technical and clinical implications of the proposed method.

1 Introduction

Image resampling is ubiquitous in medical imaging. Any processing pipeline that requires coordinate mapping, correction for imaging distortions, or simply altering the resolution of an image, needs a representation of the image outside of the digital sampling grid provided by the initial image. The theoretical foundations from the Nyquist-Shannon sampling theorem provide conditions under which perfect continuous reconstruction can be achieved from regularly spaced samples. This theoretical model thus provides a means of interpolating between the discrete samples and underpins the typical resampling procedure used in medical imaging. The Whittaker-Shannon interpolation formula, or sinc interpolation, is optimal for bandlimited signals but the unbounded support of the sinc function calls for approximations. Many interpolating methods, ranging from low order, e.g. piecewise constant and linear interpolation, to high order, e.g. polynomial, piecewise-polynomial (spline) and windowed sinc (Lanczos) methods have thus been developed. Most of these have direct extension to N dimensional data, with different methods being optimal for specific types of signal.

© Springer International Publishing Switzerland 2015
N. Navab et al. (Eds.): MICCAI 2015, Part II, LNCS 9350, pp. 675–683, 2015.
DOI: 10.1007/978-3-319-24571-3_81

Resampling typically relies on one such interpolation method to represent, on a given (discrete) target sampling grid, a continuous image derived from the input source image. In most cases, the (discrete) resampled image is simply assumed to be a faithful representation of the continuous derived image, with no special care taken to ensure the sampling theorem conditions. Within the context of medical imaging, Meijering *et al.* [1] compared multiple resampling kernels, concluding that the quality of the resampling was proportional to the degree of the kernel, with linear, cubic and Lanczos resampling kernels being the best with a 1st, 2nd and 3rd order neighbourhood respectively. This comparison was done with regular grid aligned data under translation, thus respecting the Nyquist criterion. Thus, their conclusions cannot easily be extrapolated to the general resampling case.

Resampling is known to introduce artefacts in medical imaging. One common example arises within the context of image registration [2,3,4] where a source image is typically resampled to the sampling grid of a target image and a similarity function is used to compare the images based on the discrete samples at the target grid location only, thereby discarding the continuous image representation. Pluim *et al.* [2] ameliorated the problem by using partial volume (PV) sampling, Klein *et al.* [3] by random off grid sampling, and more recently Aganj *et al.* [4] by replacing the cost function summation term with an approximate integral. Another main source of artefacts is the fact that aliasing is introduced when resampling an image to lower resolution. While, in multi resolution pyramids [5], aliasing is well addressed by applying a Gaussian filter prior to downsampling, the problem in the general resampling case has surprisingly received little attention in the medical imaging community. Unser *et al.* [6] propose a least-squares spline-based formulation that achieves aliasing-free resampling for affine spatial transformations but to the best of our knowledge no solution has been proposed for general non-linear spatial transformations. Inverse approximation-based resampling has also been proposed. It relies on the inverse of the standard spatial transformation to explicitly transport samples from the source image to the target space and then uses a least-squares grid-based spline reconstruction [7]. While this approach would avoid aliasing problems and can deal with non-linear spatial transformations, it can not easily be adapted to take into account the local anisotropy of the transformations and has the drwback of requiring the inverse transformation which is not always available or easy to compute.

In this paper, we propose to address aliasing artefacts in the general context of resampling with non-linear spatial transformations by associating a scale factor point spread function (sfPSF) to the images and formulating the resampling process as an sfPSF matching problem. In the case of an original image from a known imaging device, the sfPSF is simply the PSF of the device. Our approach models local sfPSF transformations as a result of coordinate mapping, providing a unified and scale-aware way to resample images between grids of arbitrary sizes, under arbitrary spatial transformations.

2   Methods and Methodological Considerations

Nominal Scale Factor Point Spread Function (sfPSF). Observed samples (pixels/voxels) in medical images are not direct Dirac impulse measurements of a biological scene, but are typically samples from the convolution of the unobservable biological scene with an observation kernel, i.e. they have an associated point spread function (PSF). This PSF is commonly a property of the acquisition or reconstruction system. For example, 3D MRI images have approximately Gaussian PSFs due to the low-pass filters in the receiver coils, while CT and PET images have spatially variant PSFs dependent on many parameters including the image reconstruction algorithm.

In this work, we propose to associate a PSF to each image, whether it directly arises from an imaging device or is the result of further transformation or processing, and refer to this as the scale factor PSF (sfPSF) by analogy with the scale factor used in scale space theory [5]. In the case where the image directly arises from an imaging device with known PSF, the sfPSF is simply taken as the closest Gaussian kernel to the PSF of the device. When the actual PSF associated with a given image is unkown, the nominal sfPSF is taken as a Gaussian $\mathcal{G}_\Sigma$, where the covariance matrix Σ is diagonal and the full-width-half-maximum (FWHM) of the Gaussian PSF is classically and without loss of generality matched to the voxel size $D = \{D_x, D_y, D_z\}$: $\Sigma = (2\sqrt{2\ln 2})^{-2} \operatorname{diag}(D_x^2, D_y^2, D_z^2)$. Similarly, when resampling to a target grid not already associated with an image, we associate the same voxel-size matched nominal sfPSF with the grid. The relevance of the sfPSF will become clear in the following section. Intuitively, when an image with an associated sfPSF is smoothed, the resulting smoothed image will be associated with a larger sfPSF. Conversely, when an image is upsampled, the resulting image will be associated with the same sfPSF as the source image if expressed in world (rather than pixel) coordinates.

Compensating for Aliasing When Downsampling. In medical images, frequencies commonly approach the Nyquist limit of their representation (e.g. full k-space sampling in MRI). If one affinely transforms an image onto its own grid with an affine transformation which has a determinant greater than 1, i.e. spatially compressing the samples, or transforms an image into a lower resolution grid, then the Nyquist criterion is not satisfied with typical interpolation. This sub-Nyquist sampling introduces frequency aliasing and loss of information.

In scale-space and pyramidal approaches, when downsampling an image by a factor of $k = 2$, the original image is typically pre-convolved with a Gaussian filter with variance $\sigma_P = 0.7355$. Applying the notion of sfPSF and the notations introduced above, we specify $\mathcal{G}_{\Sigma_S}$ and $\mathcal{G}_{\Sigma_T}$ as the source image and target grid nominal sfPSFs respectively. Following the scale space methodology [5], sfPSF matching consists of finding the best scale-matching PSF $\mathcal{G}_{\Sigma_P}$ that, when combined with the source sfPSF, provides the best approximation of the target sfPSF. If the sfPSFs are Gaussian, then the covariance of $\mathcal{G}_{\Sigma_P}$ can be obtained through simple covariance addition $\Sigma_T = \Sigma_S + \Sigma_P$. In the downsampling example above, without additional knowledge, we have $\mathrm{FWHM}_T = k = 2$

and $\text{FWHM}_S = 1$. We therefore get $\Sigma_P = \Sigma_T - \Sigma_S = (k^2 - 1^2)(2\sqrt{2\log 2})^{-2}\,\text{Id}$ or, in this case, $\sigma_P = 0.7355$. This is equivalent to finding the best Fourier domain filter that limits the bandwidth of the source image frequencies to the representable Nyquist frequencies on the target grid. Similar filtering would be necessary to avoid aliasing when rigidly resampling high resolution images to a lower resolution, e.g. high resolution anatomical MRI and CT images or binary segmentations are transformed to lower resolution MRI (2D FLAIR), metabolic (PET), microstructural (DWI) and functional (fMRI) images. In this work we propose to compensate for the differences in sfPSF when resampling to arbitrary grid sizes under global (affine) or local (non-linear) spatial transformations.

Before presenting our methodological contribution in detail, we illustrate the sfPSF performance in comparison with standard interpolation on a synthetic phantom (Fig. 1) with a low frequency object (square) overlaid on a high-frequency pattern (to highlight aliasing). This phantom is resampled to a grid with 3 times less resolution *per* axis. Note that the proposed sfPSF method appropriately integrates out high frequencies without introducing aliasing.

Pre-Convolution sfPSF Matching. In the restricted affine transformation $\mathcal{A}$ scenario going from the space of T to S, the source image can be pre-convolved with an *anti-aliasing* filter with covariance such that $\Sigma_P^S + \Sigma_S = \mathcal{A} \cdot \Sigma_T \cdot \mathcal{A}^\mathsf{T}$, where we now emphasize that Σ_P^S is defined in the space of S, and then resampled using classical interpolation.

In the general non-linear spatial transformation case, a similar but spatially-variant pre-filtering procedure could be applied by relying on a local affine approximation of the spatial transformation, i.e. using the jacobian matrix. This solution might provide useful results but because the sfPSF matching, or smoothing, is performed before the spatial transformation, and the sfPSF potentially has a large spatial extent, it can be seen as disregarding the non-homogeneous

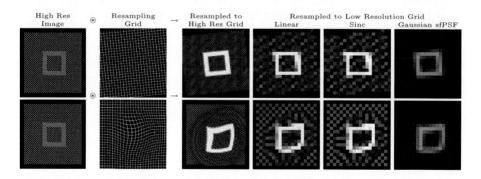

Fig. 1. Left to right: a high resolution (HR) image (63×63 voxels at $1 \times 1mm$ voxel size) with a square on a high frequency pattern; the resampling grid (transformation); the HR image resampled to the original HR grid and to a lower resolution (21×21 voxels at $3 \times 3mm$ voxel size) grid using linear, sinc and a Gaussian sfPSF (proposed) interpolation strategy. Note the aliasing in the linear and sinc examples.

distribution of the samples in target space T. Instead, we propose to model and perform the sfPSF matching in the space of T and thus rely on Σ_P^T.

Target Space sfPSF Matching. Let $\mathcal{F}_{S \leftarrow T}(\mathbf{v})$ be a spatial transformation mapping the location $\mathbf{v} = (v_x, v_y, v_z)$ from the space of T to that of S, given either an affine or non-linear transformation. Let $\mathcal{A}_{S \leftarrow T}(\mathbf{v})$ be the jacobian matrix of $\mathcal{F}$ at $\mathbf{v}$ which provides the best linear approximation of $\mathcal{F}$ at $\mathbf{v}$. Following our previous derivations we have $\Sigma_P^S(\mathbf{v}) + \Sigma_S \approx \mathcal{A}_{S \leftarrow T}(\mathbf{v}) \cdot \Sigma_T \cdot \mathcal{A}_{S \leftarrow T}^{\mathsf{T}}(\mathbf{v})$. Thus, given $\Sigma_P^S(\mathbf{v}) = \mathcal{A}_{S \leftarrow T}(\mathbf{v}) \cdot \Sigma_P^T(\mathbf{v}) \cdot \mathcal{A}_{S \leftarrow T}^{\mathsf{T}}(\mathbf{v})$ we now want $\Sigma_P^T(\mathbf{v}) + \mathcal{A}_{S \leftarrow T}^{-1}(\mathbf{v}) \cdot \Sigma_S \cdot \mathcal{A}_{S \leftarrow T}^{-\mathsf{T}}(\mathbf{v}) \approx \Sigma_T$. In other words, we want to find a *symmetric positive semi-definite* covariance $\Sigma_P^T(\mathbf{v})$ that, when combined with the affinely transformed covariance $\Sigma_S^T(\mathbf{v}) = \mathcal{A}_{S \leftarrow T}^{-1}(\mathbf{v}) \cdot \Sigma_S \cdot \mathcal{A}_{S \leftarrow T}^{-\mathsf{T}}(\mathbf{v})$, best approximates Σ_T. Under the typical assumption that the nominal sfPSF Σ_T is diagonal, this approximation is given by $\tilde{\Sigma}_P^T(\mathbf{v}) = \max(\Sigma_T - \lambda(\mathbf{v}), 0)$ with $\lambda(\mathbf{v})$ being a diagonal scaling matrix containing the components of $\Sigma_S^T(\mathbf{v})$ obtained through polar decomposition and $max(\cdot, \cdot)$ is the element-wise maximum operator between two matrices. It is important to note that under regimes where the Nyquist limit is not violated, e.g. upsampling, rigid transformation between isotropic grids, or non-linear transformations with the Jacobian determinant below 1, then the proposed method leads to a Dirac in the sfPSF matching meaning that our procedure reverts to standard resampling.

Interpolation by Convolution with the sfPSF. Let $I_T(\mathbf{v})$ be the sought resampled intensity in the space of T at location $\mathbf{v}$, and $I_S(\mathbf{v})$ be the intensity of the source image. The interpolated and PSF matched value of I_T at location $(\mathbf{v})$ can be obtained by an *oversampled* discretised convolution

$$I_T(\mathbf{v}) = \frac{1}{Z} \sum_{v_x}^{N_x(\mathbf{v})} \sum_{v_y}^{N_y(\mathbf{v})} \sum_{v_z}^{N_z(\mathbf{v})} I_S(\mathcal{F}_{S \leftarrow T}(\mathbf{v} - v)) \mathcal{G}_{\tilde{\Sigma}_P^T(\mathbf{v})}(v)$$

where $\mathcal{G}_{\tilde{\Sigma}_P^T(\mathbf{v})}(v) = (2\pi)^{-\frac{3}{2}} |\tilde{\Sigma}_P(\mathbf{v})|^{-\frac{1}{2}} e^{-\frac{1}{2} v'(\tilde{\Sigma}_P^T(\mathbf{v}))^{-1} v}$, Z is a normaliser that ensures the (discrete) sum over $\mathcal{G}_{\tilde{\Sigma}_P^T(\mathbf{v})}(v)$ equals 1. $N_x(\mathbf{v})$, $N_y(\mathbf{v})$ and $N_z(\mathbf{v})$ are sampling regions centered at $\mathbf{v}$ in the x, y and z directions respectively. More specifically, $N_x(\mathbf{v})$ are homogeneously spaced samples between -3 and 3 standard deviations, i.e. $N_x(\mathbf{v}) = \{k \sigma_{P_x}(\mathbf{v}) \;\; \forall k \in [-3, 3]\}$, with $\sigma_{P_x}^2(\mathbf{v}) = \tilde{\Sigma}_P^{Txx}(\mathbf{v})$, and equivalently for $N_y(\mathbf{v})$, $N_z(\mathbf{v})$, $\sigma_{P_y}(\mathbf{v})$ and $\sigma_{P_z}(\mathbf{v})$. As S is a discrete image, an appropriate interpolation method, such as linear, cubic or sinc interpolation is used to get the sample values at $\mathcal{F}_{S \leftarrow T}(\mathbf{v} - v)$. Similarly, interpolation is required to compute $\mathcal{F}_{S \leftarrow T}(\mathbf{v} - v)$ if the spatial transformation is represented as a displacement field. Note also that when σ_{P_x} (resp. σ_{P_y} or σ_{P_z}) becomes 0 or very small, care has to be taken to appropriately compute the limit of the Gaussian weight by resorting to an axis aligned Dirac function.

3   Validation and Discussion

Data. 30 healthy control subjects were obtained from the ADNI2 database. All subjects had an associated T1-weighted MRI image, acquired at $1.1 \times 1 \times 1mm$ voxel size, and a ^{18}F-FDG PET image, reconstructed at $3 \times 3 \times 3mm$. For this selected subset of ADNI2, all data (MRI and PET) were acquired on the same scanner with the same scanning parameters, thus removing acquisition confounds. While the effective PSF of PET images can be between 3 and $6mm$ FWHM, in these experiments we will assume a PSF with $3mm$ FWHM.

Frequency Domain Analysis Under Non-linear Transformation. Frequency domain analysis was used to assess whether resampling images under non-linear transformation respects the Nyquist limit and to test whether the proposed method can mitigate any error. The 30 T1 MRIs were zero padded by a factor of 2 in the frequency domain ($0.55 \times 0.5 \times 0.5mm$ voxel size), doubling the representable frequencies. Fig. 2 shows two upsampled images and their frequency magnitude. Note the empty power spectrum outside the Nyquist band (white box). 29 upsampled T1 images were affinely [8] and then non-rigidly [9] registered to the remaining image using standard algorithms. Each upsampled image was resampled to the space of the remaining image using both a three-lobed truncated sinc resampling, and the proposed Gaussian sfPSF method. The Gaussian sfPSF was set to $1.1 \times 1 \times 1mm$ FWHM for both Σ_S and Σ_T. An example of an image resampled using both methods is shown in Fig. 2. Note that, as expected, supra-Nyquist frequencies are created when using sinc interpolation. These frequencies are greatly suppressed when using the proposed method. Analysis of the power spectra of the 29 resampled images showed an average power suppression of 94.4% for frequencies above the Nyquist band when using the Gaussian PSF instead of sinc interpolation. This power suppression results in an equivalent reduction of aliasing at the original resolution.

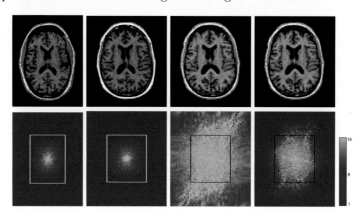

Fig. 2. Left to right: (Top) upsampled source S and target T images followed by S non-linearly resampled to T using sinc and Gaussian sfPSF; (Bottom) their respective frequency domain log magnitude. The white box represents the Nyquist limit before zero-padding. Note the high supra-Nyquist magnitude after sinc resampling.

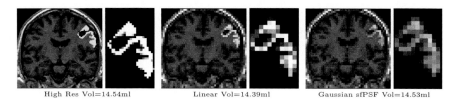

High Res Vol=14.54ml   Linear Vol=14.39ml   Gaussian sfPSF Vol=14.53ml

Fig. 3. Left to right: A segmented region overlaid on a high resolution T1 ($1.1 \times 1 \times 1mm$) image (and zoomed), followed by the same segmentation resampled to the resolution of a PET image ($3 \times 3 \times 3mm$) using linear and the proposed Gaussian sfPSF. The zoomed segmentations are in gray scale between 0 and 1. Given that the cortex is commonly thinner than $3mm$, note the unrealistic large amount of voxels with segmentation probability equal to 1 at PET resolution when using linear resampling.

Volume Preservation and Partial Volume under Rigid Resampling. To demonstrate clinically relevant consequences of aliasing, we tested the effect of resampling within the context of segmentation propagation and partial volume estimation. Specifically, T1 images are segmented into 98 different regions using multi-atlas label propagation and fusion [10] based on the Neuromorphometrics, Inc. labels. The T1 images were then rigidly registered [8] to the PET data, and each one of the segmented regions was resampled to the PET data using both linear interpolation and the Gaussian sfPDF. Linear was chosen here due to the signal-limited $[0, 1]$ nature of probabilities. Example results are shown in Fig. 3.

As all the segmentations are probabilistic, volume was estimated as the sum of all probabilities for all voxels $\mathbf{v}$ times the voxel size $\mathcal{V}$. The volume was estimated in the original T1 space (V_{HR}), and in the PET space after linear (V_{TRI}) and the Gaussian sfPSF (V_{sfPSF}) resampling. Similar volumes were obtained when the probabilistic segmentations were thresholded at 0.5. The relative volume difference RVD= $(V_{sfPSF} - V_{HR})/V_{HR}$ and its absolute value, ARVD = $|RVD|$, were estimated for each of the 30 subjects, 98 cortical regions and 2 resampling methods. The RVD and ARVD were averaged over all subjects for each region, resulting in 98 mean RVD and ARVD values per region, per method. These values are plotted in Fig. 4. A Parzen window mean and STD are also plotted in the

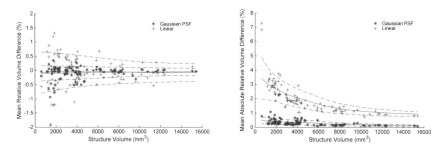

Fig. 4. The mean RVD (Left) and mean ARVD (Right) between a low and high resolution representation of a segmented region averaged over the population. 100 different regions are plotted against the mean volume of the region V_{HR} over the population.

same figure. Both resampling methods are unbiased according to the mean RVD. However, the Gaussian sfPSF method provides significantly lower ($p < 10^{-4}$ - Wilcoxon signed-rank test) errors in terms of mean ARVD for all regions, especially in smaller regions where linear resampling can introduce up to 8% mean absolute volume difference. A 8% mean difference implies even larger local errors, resulting in detrimental effects in partial volume/ compartment modelling, and when estimating biomarkers that rely on structural segmentations.

4   Conclusion

The presented work explores aliasing in medical image resampling and proposes a new interpolation technique that matches the scale factor PSF given arbitrary grid sizes and non-linear transformations. We demonstrate the advantages of using Gaussian sfPSF resampling, both in terms of Nyquist limit and volume preservation, when compared with common resampling techniques. Future work will involve deploying the proposed methodology within image registration algorithms and verifying the impact of the sfPSF in partial volume and compartment modelling. An implementation will be made available at the time of publication.

References

1. Meijering, E.H.W., Niessen, W.J., Pluim, J.P.W., Viergever, M.A.: Quantitative comparison of sinc-approximating kernels for medical image interpolation. In: Taylor, C., Colchester, A. (eds.) MICCAI 1999. LNCS, vol. 1679, pp. 210–217. Springer, Heidelberg (1999)
2. Pluim, J.P., Maintz, J.B.A., Viergever, M.A.: Mutual information matching and interpolation artifacts. In: SPIE Medical Imaging, vol. 3661, pp. 56–65. SPIE Press, May 1999
3. Klein, S., Staring, M., Murphy, K., Viergever, M.A., Pluim, J.P.W.: ElastiX: A toolbox for intensity-based medical image registration. IEEE Trans. Med. Imag. 29(1), 196–205 (2010)
4. Aganj, I., Yeo, B.T.T., Sabuncu, M.R., Fischl, B.: On removing interpolation and resampling artifacts in rigid image registration. IEEE Trans. Image Process. 22(2), 816–827 (2013)
5. Lindeberg, T.: Scale-space for discrete signals. IEEE Trans. Pattern Anal. Mach. Intell. 12(3), 234–254 (1990)
6. Unser, M., Neimark, M., Lee, C.: Affine transformations of images: a least squares formulation. In: Proc. ICIP 1994, vol. 3, pp. 558–561 (1994)
7. Arigovindan, M., Sühling, M., Hunziker, P., Unser, M.: Variational image reconstruction from arbitrarily spaced samples: A fast multiresolution spline solution. IEEE Trans. Image Process. 14(4), 450–460 (2005)
8. Modat, M., Cash, D.M., Daga, P., Winston, G.P., Duncan, J.S., Ourselin, S.: Global image registration using a symmetric block-matching approach. Journal of Medical Imaging 1(2), 024003–024003 (2014)

9. Modat, M., Ridgway, G.R., Taylor, Z.A., Lehmann, M., Barnes, J., Hawkes, D.J., Fox, N.C., Ourselin, S.: Fast free-form deformation using graphics processing units. Computer Methods and Programs in Biomedicine 98(3), 278–284 (2010)
10. Cardoso, M.J., Wolz, R., Modat, M., Fox, N.C., Rueckert, D., Ourselin, S.: Geodesic information flows. In: Ayache, N., Delingette, H., Golland, P., Mori, K. (eds.) MICCAI 2012, Part II. LNCS, vol. 7511, pp. 262–270. Springer, Heidelberg (2012)

Analytic Quantification of Bias and Variance of Coil Sensitivity Profile Estimators for Improved Image Reconstruction in MRI*

Aymeric Stamm, Jolene Singh, Onur Afacan, and Simon K. Warfield

CRL - Boston Children's Hospital, Harvard Medical School, MA, USA
aymeric.stamm@childrens.harvard.edu

Abstract. Magnetic resonance (MR) imaging provides a unique in-vivo capability of visualizing tissue in the human brain non-invasively, which has tremendously improved patient care over the past decades. However, there are still prominent artifacts, such as intensity inhomogeneities due to the use of an array of receiving coils (RC) to measure the MR signal or noise amplification due to accelerated imaging strategies. It is critical to mitigate these artifacts for both visual inspection and quantitative analysis. The cornerstone to address this issue pertains to the knowledge of coil sensitivity profiles (CSP) of the RCs, which describe how the measured complex signal decays with the distance to the RC.

Existing methods for CSP estimation share a number of limitations: (i) they primarily focus on CSP magnitude, while it is known that the solution to the MR image reconstruction problem involves complex CSPs and (ii) they only provide point estimates of the CSPs, which makes the task of optimizing the parameters and acquisition protocol for their estimation difficult. In this paper, we propose a novel statistical framework for estimating complex-valued CSPs. We define a CSP estimator that uses spatial smoothing and additional body coil data for phase normalization. The main contribution is to provide detailed information on the statistical distribution of the CSP estimator, which yields automatic determination of the optimal degree of smoothing for ensuring minimal bias and provides guidelines to the optimal acquisition strategy.

Keywords: coil sensitivity profile, bias, variance, image reconstruction.

1 Introduction

A modern magnetic resonance (MR) scanner collects signal using an array of receiving surface coils (RSC) [5], from which an image reconstruction problem is solved to obtain the highest SNR composite image, which magnitude is of main interest for radiological evaluation. The coil sensitivity profile (CSP) is a spatially varying magnetic field generated by the RSC that characterizes how RSC signal magnitude and phase spatially vary. In most MRI applications, an array

---

* This work was supported in part by NIH Awards RO1 EB013248, RO1 NS079788, RO1 DK100404, RO1 EB019483 and 5R42 MH086984.

N. Navab et al. (Eds.): MICCAI 2015, Part II, LNCS 9350, pp. 684–691, 2015.
DOI: 10.1007/978-3-319-24571-3_82

of RSCs is used because it provides stronger MR signal near the coil location. On the other hand, RSC-measured signal rapidly decays with the distance to the coil and the signal phase is not as spatially homogeneous as with the RBC. Since RSCs are distributed around the coil array, conventional MR imaging suffers from a *shading artifact* that pertains to an important signal loss at the image center, impairing tissue contrast or abnormality detections. Moreover, a number of accelerated MRI acquisition strategies have been devised in the literature to enable the collection of more images in shorter scan times (see [2] for a comprehensive review). They rely on sub-sampling the k-space and resort to inferential procedures for recovering missing data, which represents an additional source of noise, called *g-factor noise*, that is strongly increased by poor CSP estimates.

A number of methods have already been proposed in the literature for addressing this problem (see [10] for a detailed review). With the latest methods emerged the idea of using the RBC measurement to help with the CSP estimation of RSCs. For instance, Siemens online reconstruction offers the possibility to compensate for intensity inhomogeneity via the method proposed in [3], which define the CSP estimator as the ratio of the two low-pass filtered magnitude images measured by the RSC and RBC respectively. In our opinion, these state-of-the art methods present two major limitations. First, they primarily focus on the magnitude of the CSPs, while neglecting phase variations, while it is known that the linear combination of RSC images that yields highest SNR composite image involves complex-valued weights that depend on (i) the real-valued covariance structure of the coil array and (ii) the complex-valued CSPs [9]. Second, they only provide a voxelwise point estimate of the CSPs, while ignoring the distribution of the underlying CSP estimator, which is of critical importance to reason about the choice of the parameters of such estimators or the optimal acquisition strategy to ensure consistent CSP estimates.

The scope of this work is to provide a novel statistical framework for the estimation of complex-valued CSPs. In the same line as [3], the CSP estimator that we aim at studying uses low-pass filtered RSC and RBC images, where the RBC measurement enables phase normalization to mitigate phase-variation artifacts. The important difference with respect to [3]'s estimator resides in the use of complex images rather than their magnitude only and in RBC normalization only affecting the phase of the estimator. The focus is on understanding the statistical distribution of the proposed CSP estimator, for which we derive the analytic expression of bias and variance, which ultimately leads to the automatic determination of the optimal degree of smoothing for ensuring minimal bias. We apply this new approach to the image reconstruction problem. We provide a comparison of the reconstructed image using our CSP estimator, optimized via knowledge of its statistical distribution, and using the approach proposed by [3].

2   Theory

In the rest of the paper, x represents voxel locations. Straight, curved, bold and non-bold symbols designate random variables, fixed values, vectors and scalars, respectively. The upperscripts $\star$, $\top$ and H are the conjugate, transpose and conjugate transpose operators respectively. The symbols $\mathcal{M}$, $\mathcal{P}$, $\mathcal{R}$ and $\mathcal{I}$ denote respectively the magnitude, phase, real and imaginary operators for any complex number. Finally, τ, g and G are respectively the standard deviation, density and distribution functions of the standard Gaussian distribution.

Let $\mathbf{c}(\boldsymbol{x}) = (c_1(\boldsymbol{x}), \ldots, c_L(\boldsymbol{x}))^\top$ be the $\mathbb{C}^L$-valued random variable representing the complex signals measured by an array of L RSCs. Following [9], the linear combination of these signals that yields SNR-maximized signal s($\boldsymbol{x}$) is:

$$s(\boldsymbol{x}) = \frac{\boldsymbol{b}^H(\boldsymbol{x})\Sigma^{-1}\mathbf{c}(\boldsymbol{x})}{\sqrt{\boldsymbol{b}^H(\boldsymbol{x})\Sigma^{-1}\boldsymbol{b}(\boldsymbol{x})}}, \tag{1}$$

where $\boldsymbol{b}(\boldsymbol{x})$ is the $\mathbb{C}^L$-valued vector of CSPs at voxel $\boldsymbol{x}$ and Σ is the $L \times L$ noise covariance structure of the coil array. The above equation can be rewritten more conveniently as s($\boldsymbol{x}$) = $\boldsymbol{\beta}^H(\boldsymbol{x})\Sigma^{-1/2}\mathbf{c}(\boldsymbol{x})$, where:

$$\boldsymbol{\beta}(\boldsymbol{x}) = \frac{\Sigma^{-1/2}\boldsymbol{b}(\boldsymbol{x})}{\sqrt{\boldsymbol{b}^H(\boldsymbol{x})\Sigma^{-1}\boldsymbol{b}(\boldsymbol{x})}}, \tag{2}$$

is the **normalized uncorrelated CSP** vector that we aim at estimating.

2.1 Noise Covariance Estimation

Let $\mathbf{c}(\boldsymbol{x})$ and $c_0(\boldsymbol{x})$ be the $\mathbb{C}^L$-valued and $\mathbb{C}$-valued random variables, representing the complex signals measured by an array of L RSCs and by the RBC respectively at voxel $\boldsymbol{x}$. It is known that the random variable $\mathbf{c}(\boldsymbol{x})$ follows a multivariate complex Gaussian distribution [7]. When the full k-space is sampled, the covariance structure of the coil array can be assumed spatially-invariant [7].

For a voxel $\boldsymbol{x}_B$ in the background of the image, we have $\mathbf{c}(\boldsymbol{x}_B) = 0$. Hence, if N_B denotes the number of background voxels, we can thus think of the complex signals measured in the background as a set of $2N_B$ independent and identically distributed centered Gaussian variables with covariance Σ. The sample covariance estimator on background signals provides an unbiased estimate of Σ:

$$\Sigma = \frac{1}{2N_B - 1}\sum_{\boldsymbol{x}_B}\left[\mathcal{R}\left(\mathbf{c}(\boldsymbol{x}_B)\right)\mathcal{R}\left(\mathbf{c}(\boldsymbol{x}_B)\right)^\top + \mathcal{I}\left(\mathbf{c}(\boldsymbol{x}_B)\right)\mathcal{I}\left(\mathbf{c}(\boldsymbol{x}_B)\right)^\top\right]. \tag{3}$$

Since $N_B \gg 1$ in most MR images ($N_B \approx 2$ millions for a $2 \times 2 \times 2$ mm brain image), this estimator is almost noise-free. We thus assume, from now on, that Σ is completely known and computed via Eq. (3).

2.2 Coil Sensitivity Profile Estimation

The CSP of an RSC is the spatially-referenced map of magnetic field generated per unit current flowing through the RSC. MR physics principles states the following properties of CSPs:

1. The noise-free complex signal $c_k(x)$ measured by the k-th RSC at voxel x is proportional to the CSP $b_k(x)$ at that voxel [9];
2. The CSP $b_k(x)$ at voxel x is inversely proportional to the squared distance between the RSC position and x and, in that respect, is spatially smooth [4].
3. Drifts in the signal phase are introduced due to a number of factors: radiofrequency filtering, noncentered echo, readout compensation gradients and/or static field inhomogeneities and chemical shifts [6].
4. The covariance structure used for decorrelating the CSPs varies in time as pre-amplifiers in the RSCs heat up [7].
5. Motion and physiological noise obviously introduce dramatic distortions.

Properties 1-3 are helpful for designing a sound CSP estimator for Eq. (2) while properties 4-5 provide insights into what type of acquisitions is most suited for CSP estimation. Using properties 1-3, we define the CSP estimator using spatial smoothing and additional RBC data for phase normalization to mitigate phase-variation artifacts. For a proper mathematical definition, let us define:

$$\xi(x) = \sum_{j=1}^{|V|} W\left(\frac{\|x_j - x\|}{\tau}\right) \Sigma^{-1/2} c(x_j), \tag{4}$$

where $W\left(\frac{\|x_j-x\|}{\tau}\right) = \left[\sum_{\ell=1}^{|V|} g\left(\frac{\|x_\ell-x\|}{\tau}\right)\right]^{-1} g\left(\frac{\|x_j-x\|}{\tau}\right)$, with Σ being the noise covariance structure estimator defined in Eq. (3). Likewise, let $\xi_0(x)$ be the same random variable defined from the RBC signals. Our CSP estimator can be formulated in the following terms:

$$\beta(x) = \frac{\xi_0^\star(x)}{\|\xi_0(x)\|} \cdot \frac{\xi(x)}{\|\xi(x)\|}. \tag{5}$$

The k-th component of the CSP estimator proposed in eq. (5) is the product of two complex-valued random variables. It can be expanded as:

$$\beta_k(x) = [R_0(x)R_k(x) + I_0(x)I_k(x)] + j[R_0(x)I_k(x) - I_0(x)R_k(x)], \tag{6}$$

where $R_k(x) := \mathcal{R}(\xi_k(x))/\|\xi(x)\|$ and $I_k(x) := \mathcal{I}(\xi_k(x))/\|\xi(x)\|$, $k \in [\![1, L]\!]$, and $R_0(x)$ and $I_0(x)$ are similarly defined as the real and imaginary parts of the normalized RBC-related variable ξ_0. Hence, determining the bias and variance of $\beta_k(x)$ reduces to determining the bias and variance of $R_k(x)$.

2.3   Distribution of the Squared Norm of the CSP Estimator

The $\mathbb{C}^L$-valued random variable $\xi(x)$ from Eq. (4) is a linear combination of multivariate complex Gaussian variables. Hence, in turn, $\xi(x)$ is a multivariate Gaussian variable with mean and covariance given by:

$$\xi(x) := \sum_{j=1}^{|V|} W\left(\frac{\|x_j - x\|}{\tau}\right) \Sigma^{-\frac{1}{2}} c(x_j) \quad \text{and} \quad \text{Cov}[\xi(x)] := \sigma^2 I_L,$$

with $\sigma^2 := \sum_{j=1}^{|V|} W^2\left(\frac{\|\boldsymbol{x}_j - \boldsymbol{x}\|}{\tau}\right)$. Now, observe that $\mathrm{R}_k^2(\boldsymbol{x}) = \frac{\mathrm{X}}{\mathrm{X+Y}}$, where:

$$\mathrm{X} := \frac{\mathcal{R}\left(\xi_k(\boldsymbol{x})\right)^2}{\sigma^2} \quad \text{and} \quad \mathrm{Y} := \frac{1}{\sigma^2}\left[\mathcal{I}\left(\xi_k(\boldsymbol{x})\right)^2 + \sum_{\substack{\ell=1 \\ \ell \neq k}}^{L}\left(\mathcal{R}\left(\xi_\ell(\boldsymbol{x})\right)^2 + \mathcal{I}\left(\xi_\ell(\boldsymbol{x})\right)^2\right)\right].$$

The real-valued random variables X and Y are independent and both formed of the sum of squared independent Gaussian variables. Hence, they both follow non-central χ^2-distributions, with respective degrees of freedom (DoF) $2\alpha_1 = 1$ and $2\alpha_2 = 2L - 1$ and non-centrality parameters (NcP) λ_1 and λ_2 given by:

$$\lambda_1 = \frac{\mathcal{R}\left(\xi_k(\boldsymbol{x})\right)^2}{\sigma^2} \quad \text{and} \quad \lambda_2 = \frac{1}{\sigma^2}\left[\mathcal{I}\left(\xi_k(\boldsymbol{x})\right)^2 + \sum_{\substack{\ell=1 \\ \ell \neq k}}^{L}\left(\mathcal{R}\left(\xi_\ell(\boldsymbol{x})\right)^2 + \mathcal{I}\left(\xi_\ell(\boldsymbol{x})\right)^2\right)\right].$$

As a result, $\mathrm{R}_k^2(\boldsymbol{x})$ follows a **doubly non-central Beta** (DNcB) distribution [8] with DoFs $\alpha_1 = 1/2$ and $\alpha_2 = L - 1/2$ and NcPs λ_1 and λ_2, respectively.

2.4   Bias and Variance of the CSP Estimator

Let $T = \mathrm{R}_k^2(\boldsymbol{x})$, $\alpha^+ - \alpha_1 + \alpha_2$, $\lambda^+ = \lambda_1 + \lambda_2$ and $\theta_1 = \lambda_1/\lambda^+$. Since T a DNcB random variable, its first two raw moments are given by [8]:

$$\mathbb{E}(T) = \mathbb{E}\left(\frac{\alpha_1 + \theta_1 P}{\alpha^+ + P}\right), \ \mathbb{E}(T^2) = \mathbb{E}\left(\frac{\alpha_1(\alpha_1+1) + (2\alpha_1 + 2 - \theta_1)\theta_1 P + \theta_1^2 P^2}{(\alpha^+ + P)(\alpha^+ + 1 + P)}\right)$$

where P is a Poisson-distributed random variable with parameter $\lambda^+/2$. After some calculations, one can show that the above equations simplify to:

$$\mathbb{E}(T) = \frac{\alpha_1}{\alpha^+ - 1} M\left(1, \alpha^+; -\frac{\lambda^+}{2}\right) + \frac{\theta_1 \lambda^+}{2\alpha^+} M\left(1, \alpha^+ + 1; -\frac{\lambda^+}{2}\right),$$

$$\mathbb{E}(T^2) = \frac{\theta_1^2 \lambda^+}{2\alpha^+} M\left(1, \alpha^+ + 1; -\frac{\lambda^+}{2}\right) + \frac{\alpha_1(\alpha_1+1)}{(\alpha^+ - 1)\alpha^+} M\left(2, \alpha^+ + 1; -\frac{\lambda^+}{2}\right) \quad (7)$$

$$+ \frac{(2(\alpha_1+1) - \theta_1(\alpha^+ + 1))\theta_1 \lambda^+}{2\alpha^+(\alpha^+ + 1)} M\left(2, \alpha^+ + 2; -\frac{\lambda^+}{2}\right),$$

where M denotes Kummer's confluent hypergeometric function [1]. Now, using the Taylor series expansion of the square root around $\mathbb{E}(T)$, we can show that:

$$\mathbb{E}(\mathrm{R}_k(\boldsymbol{x})) \approx [2\mathbb{P}\left(\mathrm{R}_k(\boldsymbol{x}) > 0\right) - 1] \frac{\sqrt{\mathbb{E}(T)}}{8}\left(9 - \frac{\mathbb{E}(T^2)}{\mathbb{E}(T)^2}\right), \quad (8)$$

where the probability of $\mathrm{R}_k(\boldsymbol{x})$ being positive can be analytically derived as:

$$\mathbb{P}\left(\mathrm{R}_k(\boldsymbol{x}) > 0\right) = \mathbb{P}\left(\mathcal{R}\left(\xi_k(\boldsymbol{x})\right) > 0\right) = G\left(\frac{\mathcal{R}\left(\xi_k(\boldsymbol{x})\right)}{\sigma}\right).$$

Equations (7) and (8) provide the first 2 raw moments of $R_k(\boldsymbol{x})$. Similar equations for $I_k(\boldsymbol{x})$, $R_0(\boldsymbol{x})$ and $I_0(\boldsymbol{x})$ can be straightforwardly obtained, which ultimately yields analytic expressions of bias and variance of the magnitude, real and imaginary parts of the CSP estimator $\beta_k(\boldsymbol{x})$ of k-th RSC proposed in Eq. (6).

In particular, the bias of $\beta_k(\boldsymbol{x})$ depends on the smoothing parameter τ and the initial SNRs $\|\Sigma^{-\frac{1}{2}}\boldsymbol{c}(\boldsymbol{x})\|$. Hence, given initial SNRs, the smoothing parameter τ can be optimized in order to guarantee minimally biased CSP estimates.

3 Experiments

3.1 Study of Bias and Variance of Our CSP Estimator

The goal of this simulation is to assess the behavior of the CSP estimator magnitude upon variation of the smoothing parameter τ and the SNR ρ_0 of the RSoS image formed from noise-free complex data. We generated a 33×33 2D image centered in the voxel of interest with SNR ρ_0, attributing decreasing SNRs to the surrounding voxels proportionally to their distance in pixel units to the center voxel. We simulated an array of 32 RSCs uniformly located on the image anti-diagonal, with different uniform phases and magnitude inversely proportional to the distance between the RSC and the voxel of interest. We used a Gaussian kernel of standard deviation τ for smoothing. We assessed evolution of bias and variance of the magnitude of our CSP estimator proposed in Eq. (5) by evaluating numerically the analytic expressions provided in Eqs. (6) to (8). We plotted them against ρ_0 and τ and investigated the optimal smoothing $\tau^\star$ that minimizes the bias of our CSP estimator as a function of initial SNR ρ_0.

3.2 Application to the MR Reconstruction Problem

We applied our CSP estimator for imaging a healthy volunteer at 0.4 mm isotropic. We targeted a T1 MPRAGE image and we imaged the subject with a 3T Siemens Skyra MR scanner. We additionally acquired an independent set of low-resolution (2 mm iso) RSC and RBC images for CSP estimation. The SNR for the RSC images was around 40 dB, which, according to the theory, requires a spatial smoothing of $\tau = 1.5$ mm. Additionally, we also estimated the CSPs using [3]'s method (Siemens prescan normalize). We compare the uncorrected high resolution reconstruction to the ones obtained after intensity inhomogeneity correction (IIC) using both sets of CSP estimates ([3]'s and our optimized one). Quantitatively, we use sharpness measures (image energy M1, gradient magnitude energy M2) to compare the results, for which higher values highlight a better reconstruction.

4 Results

4.1 Study of Bias and Variance of our CSP Estimator

Figure 1a shows the relative bias and the variance of the magnitude of our CSP estimator as a function of the smoothing parameter τ for different SNRs. The first result is that the variance decreases as the amount of smoothing and SNR increase as expected. The two most important messages from Fig. 1a however

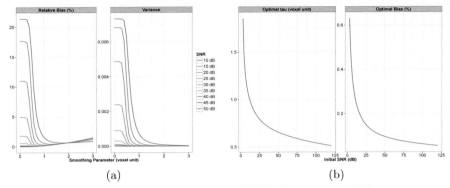

(a)   (b)

Fig. 1. Bias and Variance of Magnitude of CSP Estimator. (a) bias and variance of the magnitude of the CSP estimator as defined in Eq. (5); (b) optimal smoothing parameter as a function of the initial SNR and corresponding value of minimal bias.

are that (i) smoothing does not systematically either introduce bias or reduce bias but there is an optimal degree of smoothness that yields minimal bias, which depends on the SNR. Figure 1b further investigates this phenomenon by plotting the optimal degree of smoothness and corresponding minimal bias against the SNR. If the initial images used for CSP estimation already have high SNR, smoothing will introduce bias in the CSP estimates whereas, if they have low SNR, there is a optimal smoothing that ensures minimally biased CSPs.

4.2   Application to the MR Reconstruction Problem

Figure 2 shows an axial slice of a high resolution brain MPRAGE reconstruction achieved using a SENSE1 reconstruction according to Eq. (1). Image (a)

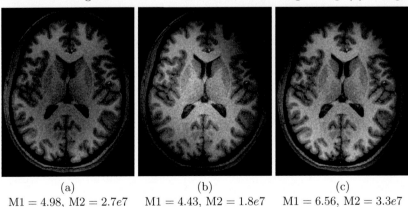

(a)   (b)   (c)
M1 = 4.98, M2 = 2.7e7   M1 = 4.43, M2 = 1.8e7   M1 = 6.56, M2 = 3.3e7

Fig. 2. High Resolution brain MPRAGE reconstruction. Image reconstruction according to Eq. (1) with (a) no IIC, (b) IIC using [3]'s CSPs, (c) IIC using our CSPs.

is obtained with no IIC, which clearly depicts the loss of signal in the center of the image. Image (b) illustrates pre-scan normalization, where we can see an undesirable loss (resp., amplification) of signal in the upper right (resp., middle left) area. Image (c) displays the IIC from our minimally biased CSPs, which is uniform in sensitivity as desired. Sharpness measures M1 and M2 quantitatively confirms the improvement obtained using our CSP estimates.

5 Discussion

In this paper, we generalized the CSP estimator proposed in [3] to infer complex-valued CSP estimates. This estimator uses spatial smoothing and additional body coil data for phase normalization to mitigate phase-variation artifacts.

The main contribution is the derivation of the statistical distribution of our proposed estimator. This allows us to establish that, in order to achieve minimally biased CSP estimates, (i) there is an optimal degree of smoothing that depends on the image SNR and (ii) high SNR in the images used for CSP estimation is highly recommended. In addition, from MR physics considerations, it is even more recommended to acquire low spatial resolution data to keep the acquisition time short and thus avoid the problem of time-varying covariance structures and mitigate motion and physiological noise. To the best of our knowledge, this is the first study that propose a detailed understanding of a CSP estimator. It is shown to resolve intensity inhomogeneities in structural images and to present a significant improvement over the on-line scanner pre-scan normalization, especially for high spatial resolution image reconstructions (in which case, CSPs are still estimated from an independent low-resolution scan).

References

1. Abramowitz, M., Stegun, I.: Handbook of Mathematical Functions: With Formulas, Graphs, and Mathematical Tables. Applied maths, Dover Publications (1964)
2. Blaimer, M., Breuer, F., Mueller, M., Heidemann, R.M., Griswold, M.A., Jakob, P.M.: SMASH, SENSE, PILS, GRAPPA: how to choose the optimal method. Top. Magn. Reson. Imaging 15(4), 223–236 (2004)
3. Brey, W.W., Narayana, P.A.: Correction for intensity falloff in surface coil magnetic resonance imaging. Med. Phys. 15(2), 241–245 (1988)
4. Haacke, E., et al.: Magnetic Resonance Imaging: Physical Principles and Sequence Design, 1st edn. Wiley-Liss (1999)
5. Keil, B., Wald, L.L.: Massively parallel MRI detector arrays. J. Magn. Reson. 229(6), 75–89 (2013)
6. McVeigh, E.R., Bronskill, M.J., Henkelman, R.M.: Phase and sensitivity of receiver coils in magnetic resonance imaging. Med. Phys. 13(6), 806–814 (1986)
7. McVeigh, E., Henkelman, R., Bronskill, M.: Noise and filtration in magnetic resonance imaging. Med. Phys. 12(5), 586 (1985)
8. Ongaro, A., Orsi, C.: On non-central beta distributions. In: Cabras, S., Di Battista, T., Racugno, W. (eds.) 47th SIS Sci. Meet. Ital. Stat. Soc. (2014)
9. Roemer, P., et al.: NMR phased array. Magn. Reson. Med. 16(2), 192–225 (1990)
10. Vovk, U., Pernuš, F., Likar, B.: A review of methods for correction of intensity inhomogeneity in MRI (2007)

Mobile C-arm 3D Reconstruction in the Presence of Uncertain Geometry

Caleb Rottman[1], Lance McBride[2], Arvidas Cheryauka[2],
Ross Whitaker[1], and Sarang Joshi[1]

[1] Scientific Computing and Imaging Institute, University of Utah, Utah, USA
crottman@sci.utah.edu,
[2] GE Healthcare, Salt Lake City, Utah, USA

Abstract. Computed tomography (CT) is a widely used medical technology. Adding 3D imaging to a mobile fluoroscopic C-arm reduces the cost of CT, as a mobile C-arm is much less expensive than a dedicated CT scanner. In this paper we explore the technical challenges to implementing 3D reconstruction on these devices. One of the biggest challenges is the problem of uncertain geometry; mobile C-arms do not have the same geometric consistency that exists in larger dedicated CT scanners. The geometric parameters of an acquisition scan are therefore uncertain, and a naïve reconstruction with these incorrect parameters leads to poor image quality. Our proposed method reconstructs the 3D image using the expectation maximization (EM) framework while jointly estimating the true geometry, thereby improving the feasibility of 3D imaging on mobile C-arms.

Keywords: Cone-beam reconstruction, Expectation maximization, Mobile C-arms.

1 Introduction

Cone-beam CT reconstruction is typically done using large, expensive systems such as dedicated CT scanners and fixed-room C-arms. Mobile C-arms are extremely popular surgical tools due to their affordability and small footprint. Because mobile C-arms are designed to produce high quality 2D images, they have several characteristics that make 3D imaging challenging. Most mobile C-arms are non-isocentric, have limited angular range, and have low-power X-ray acquisition systems. There are currently a few mobile C-arms with 3D imaging in use, however, these C-arms are all isocentric.

Another major limitation of mobile C-arms is their uncertain geometry. For cone-beam reconstruction, we must know the true geometry of the system at each acquisition. This geometry consists of location and orientation in space of the gantry (known as the extrinsic parameters) and the internal alignment of source and detector (known as the intrinsic parameters). Even in fixed room systems, these geometric parameters do not remain constant over the life of the system. Therefore, these systems are often corrected using dedicated calibration

© Springer International Publishing Switzerland 2015
N. Navab et al. (Eds.): MICCAI 2015, Part II, LNCS 9350, pp. 692–699, 2015.
DOI: 10.1007/978-3-319-24571-3_83

phantoms [6]. In mobile C-arms, our uncertain geometry problem is even more challenging: the geometric parameters are not repeatable from scan to scan. Others have proposed image-based calibrations using the Nelder-Mead optimization [3,5].

In this paper, we introduce a novel method for 3D imaging in the presence of uncertain geometry. We derive and implement a full gradient based parameter optimization within the expectation maximization framework. Our method jointly estimates the reconstructed image using an ordered subset expectation maximization and estimates the geometry by performing conjugate gradient updates of the geometric parameters. With this method, we show we are able to improve 3D reconstruction on mobile C-arms.

There are two main applications for our method. First, our method reduces the need for expensive hardware improvements in mobile C-arms to introduce 3D imaging. Since we are estimating the true geometric parameters, the only added cost is computation. Second, our method can be used to retrofit existing mobile C-arms with 3D imaging, even if these C-arms are non-isocentric. This would decrease the cost of and increase the prevalence of 3D imaging, particularly important in developing countries.

2   Mobile Acquisition Setup

We built an experimental system by retrofitting an existing mobile C-arm. We started with a small-footprint GE-OEC 6800 system (see Figure 1(a)) and installed improved acquisition and control components. The clinical applications of the original C-arm device included orthopedic cases performed on human extremities. The original low-watt monoblock was replaced with a pulse-capable high-power source block, and the image intensifier was replaced with a mid-size flat panel detector.

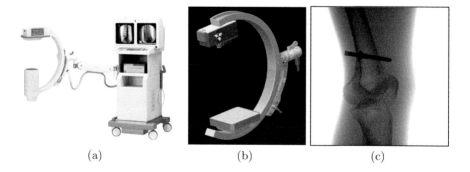

(a)   (b)   (c)

Fig. 1. Left: original C-arm. Center: modified gantry. Right: image from retrofitted system

The orbital range of the imaging gantry was extended to a complete short-scan of approximately 200 degrees with near-centric offset.

Though we have precision tube and detector components, the electro-mechanical characteristics of the new gantry are still considered approximate. For instance, the nominal value of the source-to-detector distance (SID) that corresponds to a weightless model of the gantry is 600 mm. When the gantry is loaded with imaging components, moves along a circular trajectory, and faces gravitational acceleration, the SID becomes a complicated function of several static and dynamic parameters.

The system also utilizes gravitational acceleration vector as measured by a 9DOF MEMS sensor as its initial orientation estimate. By reading the gravity vector from the 3-axis accelerometer during the scan, the system can provide an accurate representation of its orientation prior to reconstruction.

The systematic deviations of the gantry motion can be learned prior to surgical operations and compensated for during a scan of the patient. Within the image reconstruction framework, we intend to re-use some of the repeatable scan chacteristics and refine the non-repeatable portion of the pose during the optimization-based iterative process.

3   Joint Reconstruction and Geometry Estimation

To describe the reconstruction framework, we first define the cone-beam system. The cone-beam system consists of an X-ray source (assumed to be a point) and a 2D X-ray detector (assumed to be flat). Given 2D projection data with corresponding geometric parameters, we estimate the 3D image. The projection data is defined by its *projection coordinates* $(u, v) \in \mathbb{R}^2$ and the reconstructed image $I(\boldsymbol{x})$ is defined by its *world coordinates* $\boldsymbol{x} = (x, y, x) \in \mathbb{R}^3$. To relate these two coordinate systems, we introduce *camera coordinates* $\boldsymbol{x}' = (x', y', z') \in \mathbb{R}^3$. The origin of the camera coordinate system is the X-ray source, and the x' and y' axes point in the same direction as the u and v axes, respectively. The z' axis points directly at the *piercing point*, the unique point (u_0, v_0) on the detector plane that is closest to the source. The distance from the source to the detector is the *source-to-image distance* (or SID) $l \in \mathbb{R}^+$. Together, the SID and piercing point are the *intrinsic parameters* of the system, and they describe the internal characteristics of the C-arm.

The orientation and offset of the projection system relative to world coordinates are described by a 3D rotation $R \in \mathrm{SO}(3)$ and a 3D translation $\boldsymbol{T} \in \mathbb{R}^3$. These together are called the *extrinsic parameters*. With this, we define the relationship between a point $\boldsymbol{p}'$ described by its camera coordinates and the same point $\boldsymbol{p}$:

$$\boldsymbol{p} = R(\boldsymbol{p}' + \boldsymbol{T}). \tag{1}$$

The projection operator defined at a point (u, v) is the line integral of attenuating coefficients from the source to that point. We write this path as $\boldsymbol{p}'(s) = (s(u - u_0), s(v - v_0), sl)$, with $s \in [0, 1]$. Therefore, the projection operator is defined as

$$P\{I(\boldsymbol{x}); \boldsymbol{T}, R, u_0, v_0, l\}(u, v) = \gamma \int_0^1 I(R(\boldsymbol{p}'(s) + \boldsymbol{T})) \, ds. \tag{2}$$

Since we integrate from 0 to 1, we multiply the integral by the real length of the integral path $\gamma = ||p'(1)||$.

3.1 Image Update

Our algorithm alternates between two steps: estimating the image and estimating the geometric parameters. For our image update, we take one iteration using ordered subset expectation maximization (OSEM) [2]. The update is

$$I(\boldsymbol{x}) \mapsto \frac{I(\boldsymbol{x})}{\sum_j P_j^\dagger \{\mathbf{1}\}(\boldsymbol{x}) + \lambda \frac{\partial U(I)}{\partial I(\boldsymbol{x})}} \sum_j P_j^\dagger \left(\frac{f_j^*}{P_j\{I(\boldsymbol{x})\}} \right). \tag{3}$$

In this equation, $\mathbf{1}$ is a 2D image of all ones, $P^\dagger$ is the backprojection operator, f^* is the projection data, and $\frac{\partial U(I)}{\partial I(\boldsymbol{x})}$ is the derivative of a total variation (TV) regularizer. The strength of this regularizer is adjusted by the scalar λ. We use the TV stencil found in [4].

3.2 Geometric Parameter Update

Each projection is paired with current estimates for its extrinsic and intrinsic parameters. We estimate these parameters by using our current estimate of $I(\boldsymbol{x})$ and comparing it to the projection data. We therefore minimize the following energy functional for each projection:

$$E_j = \frac{1}{2} \int_{\Omega_d} ||P_j\{I(\boldsymbol{x})\}(u,v) - f_j^*(u,v)||^2, \tag{4}$$

where Ω_d is the detector. We take the derivative of this functional, which requires that we analytically solve for the gradients of the projection operator with respect to the geometric parameters. We will not derive them here, but these derivatives are:

$$\frac{\partial}{\partial T} P\{I(\boldsymbol{x})\}(u,v) = \gamma R^{\mathrm{T}} \int_0^1 (\nabla I)(R(\boldsymbol{p}'(s) + \boldsymbol{T}))\,ds, \tag{5}$$

$$\frac{\partial}{\partial R} P\{I(\boldsymbol{x})\}(u,v) = \gamma \int_0^1 (\nabla I)(R(p'(s) + \boldsymbol{T})) \times R(p'(s) + \boldsymbol{T})\,ds, \tag{6}$$

$$\frac{\partial}{\partial \boldsymbol{\tau}} P\{I(\boldsymbol{x})\}(u,v) = \frac{-((u,v,0) - \boldsymbol{\tau})}{||(u,v,0) - \boldsymbol{\tau}||^2} P\{I\}(u,v)$$

$$- \gamma(u,v;\boldsymbol{\tau}) R^{\mathrm{T}} \int_0^1 s(\nabla I)(R(\boldsymbol{p}'(s) + \boldsymbol{T}))\,ds. \tag{7}$$

Here we combine the intrinsic parameters in a single variable $\boldsymbol{\tau} = (u_0, v_0, -l)$, and we update R using Rodrigues' rotation formula.

With these gradients, we take one conjugate gradient step to update the parameters, and we alternate between image updates and parameter updates until both are converged.

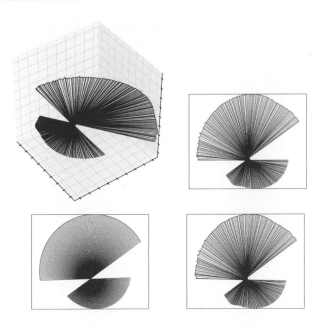

Fig. 2. Acquisition paths. The X-ray source follows the path along the blue curve, and each red line shows the path from the source to the piercing point. Upper left: 3D view of ground truth acquisition path. Upper right: 2D projection of the ground truth acquisition path. Lower left: 2D projection of the nominal path. Lower right: 2D projection of the estimated path.

4   Results

4.1   Ground Truth Image and Geometric Parameters

We evaluate our results in two ways: first by analytically comparing image reconstruction and parameter estimation using ground truth volume and parameters, and second by visually analyzing the reconstructions with real C-arm projection data.

Since we have no ground truth image or ground truth parameters, we create our own simulated dataset given real parameters. We acquired geometric parameters using EM sensors along with high-attenuation markers of a 144 degree limited-angle scan. These results were acquired on a full-size mobile C-arm. This was performed on a non-isocentric C-arm and the gantry was rotated by hand. We used these acquired geometric parameters to create a simulated projection scan of a known CT dataset. We used a skull CT dataset from the University of North Carolina (http://graphics.stanford.edu/data/voldata/) and we simulated 144 projections with Poisson noise. We then created nominal parameters consisting of a 144 degree circular equal-spaced trajectory. We tested our method by comparing three cases: reconstruction with the ground truth parameters, reconstructing with the nominal parameters, and reconstructing given the

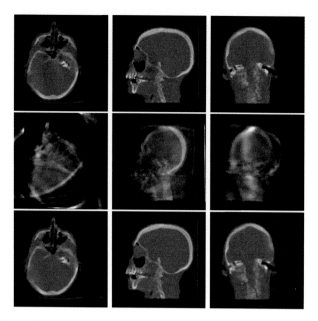

Fig. 3. Top Row: Reconstruction given true geometric parameters. Middle Row: Reconstruction given nominal parameters without parameter estimation. Bottom Row: Reconstruction given nominal parameters with parameter estimation.

nominal parameter while jointly estimating the geometry. These three scans can be seen in Figure 2, and the reconstructions can be seen in Figure 3. The image quality using our joint reconstruction method provides comparable results to reconstruction using the ground truth parameters, whereas the reconstruction without any geometry estimation yields very poor results.

We analytically compared the reconstruction to the ground truth volume. The L^2 error between the reconstructed images and the ground truth image is: 100.1 (given ground truth parameters), 578.0 (given nominal parameters), and 119.2 (given nominal parameters while estimating geometry). We also analytically compared the results to the ground truth parameters. These results are found in Figure 4.

4.2   Real C-Arm Data

We have tested our method on multiple real datasets, and we present results from two of those datasets acquired using the setup described in Section 2.

We reconstructed using 274 projections of a 190 degree scan from a physical knee phantom and a physical skull phantom [1]. We reconstructed these using the given parameters with no estimation and using the given parameters with geometry estimation. The results can be seen in Figure 5. The geometry estimation reduces many of the ghosting artifacts found while reconstructing using the nominal pose.

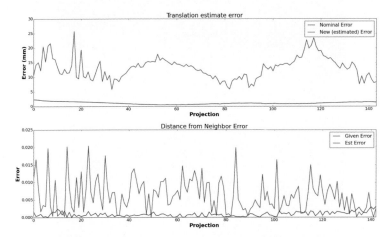

Fig. 4. Nominal parameter error and estimated geometry error for all 144 projections. Each red line is the distance between the nominal parameters and ground truth. Each blue line is the distance between the estimated parameters and ground truth. Top: translation error in $\mathbb{R}^3$. Bottom: neighboring rotation error (geodesic distance).

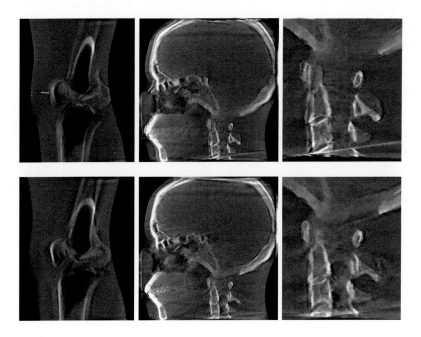

Fig. 5. Top row: reconstruction with nominal parameters of the knee and skull physical phantoms. Bottom row: joint reconstruction and geometry estimation

These algorithms are implemented efficiently on the GPU, and reconstruction with 512^2 projections to a 256^3 volume takes approximately 5 minutes.

5 Conclusion

In this paper, we introduced a novel method for reconstructing a 3D volume given the uncertain geometry of a mobile C-arm. Our method of jointly estimating the geometry and the image produces much improved results over the reconstruction using nominal parameters. In our experiments, we found that optimizing only the extrinsic parameters yields a nearly identical reconstruction as optimizing over all the parameters. Therefore, for efficiency, we only optimize over rotation and translation.

References

1. Cheryauka, A., Breham, S., Christensen, W.: Sequential intrinsic and extrinsic geometry calibration in fluoro CT imaging with a mobile C-arm. In: Proc. SPIE, vol. 6141, pp. 61412H–61412H–8, March 2006
2. Hudson, H.M., Larkin, R.S.: Accelerated Image Reconstruction Using Ordered Subsets of Projection Data. IEEE Transactions on Medical Imaging 13(4), 601–609 (1994)
3. Panetta, D., Belcari, N., Del Guerra, A., Moehrs, S.: An optimization-based method for geometrical calibration in cone-beam CT without dedicated phantoms.. Physics in Medicine and Biology 53(14), 3841–3861 (2008)
4. Panin, V.Y., Zeng, G.L., Gullberg, G.T.: Total Variation Regulated EM Algorithm. IEEE Transactions on Nuclear Science 46(6), 2202–2210 (1999)
5. Wein, W., Ladikos, A., Baumgartner, A.: Self-calibration of geometric and radiometric parameters for cone-beam computed tomography. In: 11th International Meeting on Fully Three-Dimensional Image Reconstruction in Radiology and Nuclear Medicine, vol. (2), pp. 1–4 (2011)
6. Zhang, F., Du, J., Jiang, H., Li, L., Guan, M., Yan, B.: Iterative geometric calibration in circular cone-beam computed tomography. Optik - International Journal for Light and Electron Optics 125(11), 2509–2514 (2014)

Fast Preconditioning for Accelerated Multi-contrast MRI Reconstruction[*]

Ruoyu Li[1], Yeqing Li[1], Ruogu Fang[2], Shaoting Zhang[3], Hao Pan[1,4]
and Junzhou Huang[1,**]

[1] Computer Science and Engineering,
University of Texas at Arlington, Arlington TX 76019, USA
ruoyu.li@mavs.uta.edu, jzhuang@uta.edu
[2] Computing and Information Sciences, Florida International University,
Miami, FL 33199, USA
[3] Computer Science, University of North Carolina at Charlotte,
Charlotte, NC 28223, USA
[4] Information Management, Beijing Institute of Petrochemical Technology,
Beijing, 102617, China

Abstract. Real-time reconstruction in multi-contrast magnetic resonance imaging (MC-MRI) is very challenging due to the slow scanning and reconstruction process. In this study, we propose a novel algorithm to accelerate the MC-MRI reconstruction in the framework of compressed sensing. The problem is formulated as the minimization of the least square data fitting with joint total variation (JTV) regularization term. We first utilized the iterative reweighted least square (IRLS) framework to reformulate the problem. A joint preconditioner is dexterously designed to efficiently compute the inverse of large transform matrix at each iteration. We compared our algorithm with eight cutting-edge compressive sensing MRI algorithms on real MC-MRI dataset. Extensive experiments demonstrate that the proposed algorithm can achieve far better reconstruction performance than all other eight cutting-edge methods.

1 Introduction

The multi-contrast magnetic resonance imaging (MC-MRI) is an important enhancement to MRI technology. The MC-MRI better serves the clinic diagnosis [15], because it generates multiple MR images with different contrast setting for visualizing the same anatomical cross section. However, the primary technical difficulty of real-time MC-MRI is the dramatically increased scanning and processing time for obtaining the examinational results.

The study of compressive sensing (CS) theory [3,7] has shown that, if the transformed data is sparse, an accurate original could be reconstructed from

---

[*] This work was partially supported by U.S. NSF IIS-1423056, CMMI-1434401, CNS-1405985.

[**] Corresponding author.

© Springer International Publishing Switzerland 2015
N. Navab et al. (Eds.): MICCAI 2015, Part II, LNCS 9350, pp. 700–707, 2015.
DOI: 10.1007/978-3-319-24571-3_84

highly under-sampled k-space data, which significantly reduce the amount of required samples and consequently reduce the time cost. Motivated by the aforementioned CS theory, Lustig et al. proposed their pioneering work for compressed sensing MRI [10]. However, the SparseMRI is too slow for real-time MRI. Afterwards, the Operator-splitting [11] and the variable splitting [14] methods were separately proposed to accelerate the MRI reconstruction. Recently, a composite splitting algorithm [9] has been also proposed. However, these single-contrast MRI methods have not addressed the joint reconstruction of MC-MRI. An efficient extension for multiple contrast problem is non-trivial, because of the underlying correlations existing between those contrasts.

There has been some attempts to recover all the contrasts jointly. Among current algorithms, the FCSA-MT [8] delivers best reconstruction accuracy. Given the cross-contrast structural sparsity as prior knowledge, the reconstructed images by FCSA-MT enjoys better accuracy than the individual algorithms and other joint algorithms, e.g. Bayesian CS [2] and SPGL1 [12]. However, the efficiency of FCSA-MT is still impeded by the suboptimal convergence rate of FISTA framework [1]. The IRLS-MIL method [13] solves the regularized least square problem using the matrix inverse lemma. FIRLS [4,5,6] relaxes the sparsity regularization under the IRLS framework and boost the conjugate gradient descent method (CG) by a special preconditioning. However, it is unclear how these IRLS based algorithms can be used to efficiently solve the joint MC-MRI reconstruction with the JTV regularization.

In this paper we propose a novel algorithm for joint reconstruction of MC-MRI. Our method inherits its exponentially convergence property of IRLS framework. Moreover, we dexterously design a joint "pseudo-diagonal" preconditioner $\mathcal{P}$ for efficiently solving the inverse problem in IRLS at each iteration. The proposed algorithm is able to efficiently deliver better fidelity due to the utilization of structural sparsity across contrasts and the more accurate approximation given by $\mathcal{P}$. Extensive experiments have been conducted to compare the proposed algorithm with eight cutting-edge methods for MC-MRI. The experimental results demonstrate that the proposed algorithm can achieve far better performance than all other methods.

2 Algorithm

2.1 Problem Formulation

Joint total variation (JTV) regularization well characterizes the correlated light intensity change in all contrasts. Assuming Gaussian noise, the objective function for joint MC-MRI reconstruction could be formulated as below:

$$\min_{\mathbf{X}} \sum_{s=1}^{T} \|A_s(\mathbf{X}(:,s)) - b_s\|_2^2 + \lambda \|\mathbf{X}\|_{JTV}, \tag{1}$$

where A_s is partial Fourier Transform matrix, $\mathbf{X}$ is the $\mathbb{R}^{N \times T}$ concatenating matrix of all contrasts and b_s is the noisy observation. We have T contrasts, each of which has $N = m \times n$ pixels. The JTV regularizer is $\|[D_1\mathbf{X}, D_2\mathbf{X}]\|_{2,1}$, where D_1 and D_2 are $\mathbb{R}^{N \times N}$ first-order finite difference matrix. Here, the $l_{2,1}$ norm is the summation of the l_2 norm of each row of the matrix concatenated by $[,]$. To avoid repetition, here we only derive the isotropic form of JTV term.

The problem (1) was solved by a FISTA framework [1]. It is not fast enough because at each iteration the solution of problem after the primal-dual relaxation of JTV still takes $1/\mathcal{O}(k^2)$ time to converge, where k is the iteration mark [1]. To further accelerate it, we consider to first approximate the JTV term by IRLS. Applying the Young's inequality and the Majorization Minimization method [4]:

$$Q(\mathbf{X}, W^k) = \sum_{s=1}^{T} \|A_s(\mathbf{X}(:, s)) - b_s\|_2^2 + \frac{\lambda}{2} \left[\sum_{s=1}^{T} \mathbf{X}(:, s)^T \right. \tag{2}$$

$$\left. D_1^T W^k D_1 \mathbf{X}(:, s) + \sum_{s=1}^{T} \mathbf{X}(:, s)^T D_2^T W^k D_2 \mathbf{X}(:, s) + Tr((W^k)^{-1}) \right],$$

where $Tr(\star)$ denotes the trace operator. W^k is the weight matrix at the k-th iteration, and its diagonal elements are:

$$W^k(i) = 1/\sqrt{\sum_{s=1}^{T} G_1^k(i, s)^2 + G_2^k(i, s)^2 + \theta}, \quad i = 1, \ldots, N, \tag{3}$$

where $G_1^k(i, s) = D_1(i, :)X^k(:, s)$ and $G_2^k(i, s) = D_2(i, :)X^k(:, s)$ are the 2-D gradient matrix which are updated along with solution X^k. Small positive constant θ is for avoiding infinite weight. The original non-smooth problem has been approximated by the below smooth problem:

$$\hat{\mathbf{X}}^{k+1} = arg \min_{\mathbf{X}} Q(\mathbf{X}, W^k), \tag{4}$$

the solution of which could converge to the minimizer in exponential rate [4].

Algorithm 1. FMCMRI

Input A_s, b_s, $\mathbf{X}^1$, W^1, D_1, D_2, $Err^1 \Leftarrow$ inf, ϵ, $\lambda \Leftarrow 1e^{-3}$, $k \Leftarrow 1$.
while $Err^k \geq \epsilon$ **do**
   Update W^k by Eq(3);
   Update $\tilde{\mathbf{A}}$ by $\tilde{A}_s = A_s^T A_s + \lambda D_1^T W^k D_1 + \lambda D_2^T W^k D_2$, $s = 1, \ldots, T$;
   Update $\mathcal{P}$ Eq(7);
   while NOT reach the stopping criterion of CG **do**
      Update $\mathbf{X}^k$ through solving Eq(6) by CG;
   end while
   Update $Err^{k+1} = \sum_{s=1}^{T} \|A_s\mathbf{X}^k(:, s) - b_s\|_2^2$, $k \Leftarrow k + 1$;
end while
Output $\mathbf{X}^k$.

2.2   Accelerating IRLS Framework

At each iteration, we need to solve problem (4). After eliminating constant terms and setting the first-order derivative zero, we easily find that the solution could be obtained by solving following linear system:

$$\tilde{\mathbf{A}}\mathbf{X} = \begin{bmatrix} \ddots & & \\ & \tilde{A}_s & \\ & & \ddots \end{bmatrix} \begin{pmatrix} \vdots \\ \mathbf{X}(:,s) \\ \vdots \end{pmatrix} = \tilde{\mathbf{b}}, \quad s = 1,\ldots,T. \tag{5}$$

$\tilde{\mathbf{A}}$ is a block-wise diagonal matrix where $\tilde{A}_s = A_s^T A_s + \lambda D_1^T W^k D_1 + \lambda D_2^T W^k D_2$ and $\tilde{\mathbf{b}}$ consists of $\tilde{b}_s = A_s^T b_s$. While IRLS based algorithms can converge exponentially fast, the final speed is also determined by the time complexity of each iteration. For our scenario where N is large, it is impractical to directly inverse $\tilde{A}$, because the exact inverse of $\tilde{A}$ takes $\mathcal{O}(N^3 T)$ time complexity.

An alternative is the conjugate gradient (CG) descent method. However, the actual convergence rate of CG is largely determined by the condition number of $\tilde{A}_s$, i.e. $k(\tilde{A}_s) = \lambda_{max}/\lambda_{min}$, where λ here is the set of eigenvalues of $\tilde{A}_s$. Unfortunately, in our case, $\tilde{A}_s$ is usually not well-conditioned leading to slow actual convergence. One way to accelerate CG is to precondition on $\tilde{A}_s$ and use CG to solve the below problem for instead:

$$\mathcal{P}^{-1}\tilde{\mathbf{A}}\mathbf{X} = \mathcal{P}^{-1}\mathbf{b}. \tag{6}$$

If $\mathcal{P} = I$, the $\mathcal{P}^{-1}$ is trivial, but the CG is not accelerated. For ideal $\mathcal{P} = \tilde{\mathbf{A}}$, the $\mathcal{P}^{-1}$ will be difficult, but solving (6) becomes fast because every eigenvalue of $\tilde{\mathbf{A}}^{-1}\tilde{\mathbf{A}}$ is one. A good preconditioner should balance the tradeoff. For solving all contrasts jointly, we suggest to use the block-wise diagonal preconditioner:

$$\mathcal{P} = \begin{bmatrix} \ddots & & \\ & P_s & \\ & & \ddots \end{bmatrix}, \quad s = 1,\ldots,T. \tag{7}$$

Penta-diagonal matrix $P_s = \alpha_s I + \lambda D_1^T W^k D_1 + \lambda D_2^T W^k D_2$, where α_s is the mean of diagonal elements of $A_s^T A_s$, and I is an identity matrix of N. This is motivated by the fact that $A_s^T A_s$ is diagonal dominant and the $D_{(1,2)}$ is sparse. The complexity of $\mathcal{P}^{-1}$ could be alleviated by incomplete LU decomposition, $\mathcal{P}_s^{-1} = L^{-1}U^{-1}$. It only takes $\mathcal{O}(NT)$ time to obtain $\mathcal{P}^{-1}$. $P_s^{-1}\tilde{A}_s$ with its eigenvalues more closely clustered makes the convergence of CG faster and accelerates the reconstruction of all contrasts. The preconditioner (7) can also deliver better reconstructed accuracy than other preconditioners, e.g. Jacobi preconditioner, because P_s preserves more non-diagonal information making a more precise approximation of $\tilde{A}_s$.

3 Experiments

3.1 Experimental Setup

Our experiments are conducted on the complex value in-vivo Turbo Spin Echo (TSE) slices images [2]. These 256×256 MR images can cover 24 cm field of view. Besides, we also conducted experiments on SRI24 dataset. White Gaussian noise n_s of standard deviation $\sigma = 0.01$ was added to the measurements b_s, where $b_s = A_s \mathbf{X}(:, s) + n_s$. The regularization weight λ is 1e-3. We computed the SNR and RMSE as the metrics of fidelity and the CPU time for speed comparison. Radial and slice shape sample masks were employed separately. To eliminate the randomness, all experiments were repeated for 100 times before recording. All experiments were executed on PC equipped with Intel i7-4770 CPU.

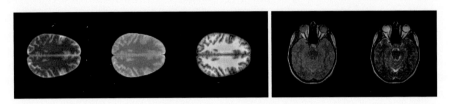

Fig. 1. Original images for experiments. Left: SRI24 three contrast MRI; Right: complex valued in-vivo Turbo Spin Echo (TSE) two contrast MRI.

3.2 Numerical Results

We first conducted experiments to compare the proposed algorithm with the individual algorithms [9,10,11,14], which recover MC-MRI individually. Figure 2(a) shows the comparison results. It is clear to see that our algorithm converged in few seconds, which was resulted from the exponential convergence rate of IRLS framework and the linear time complexity brought by the proposed joint preconditioning.

Moreover, we observe from Figure 2(b) that the slow convergence speed of FCSA-MT [8] was obviously alleviated by the removal of group wavelet sparsity term (FISAT-JTV). This is caused by the massy calculation of wavelet sparsity regularized subproblem in FCSA-MT. Besides, the splitting structure of FCSA-MT algorithm also constrains the speed of the faster subproblem because it can only be updated until the other iterative solution has converged, which takes another $1/\mathcal{O}(k^2)$ time complexity [1]. Fortunately, in this image reconstruction task, the removal of group wavelet sparsity term does not influence too much on the reconstructed accuracy. This evidence, in return, well supports the formulation of our algorithm Eq(1) with only JTV regularization term.

The benefit of our algorithm in accelerating convergence is more clearly presented in Table 1 and Figure 3. We compared the proposed algorithm with the FISTA-JTV, which has the exactly identical formulation as Eq(1). As shown in Figure 3, FISTA-JTV took at least double time to converge under 35% sample ratio, and even more under 25%. Different from the nested primal-dual iterative

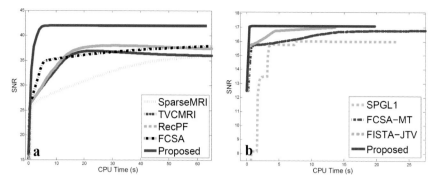

Fig. 2. Performance comparison between the proposed and all existing MC-MRI methods. a: SNR vs Time between the proposed and individual CS-MRI algorithms on SRI24 data; b: SNR vs Time between the proposed and joint CS-MRI algorithms on TSE data. Radial mask with 35% sample ratio was employed.

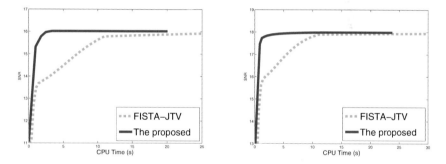

Fig. 3. Convergence time comparison between the proposed and FISTA-JTV under ratio radial mask of 25% (left) and 35% (right) sample ratio on TSE data.

solution, our algorithm inherits both exponentially fast convergence rate from IRLS and the linear time complexity of a well-designed PCG. We also observe in Figure 3 that the speed advantage the proposed method became even more significant when fewer sample data are available. To further verify its potential in reducing the amount of required samples, more comparisons were presented in Table 1. The proposed algorithm has a more robust convergence speed under low sample ratio scenario, e.g. 20%, meanwhile the good SNR is still maintained. For example, the SNR difference between the proposed and SPGL1 increased by 74% when the sample ratio decreased from 30% to 20%.

In Figure 4, we can visually indicate that our algorithm delivered the smallest reconstructed errors. This is because our formulation Eq(1) with JTV better characterized the group gradient sparsity across multiple contrasts. Besides, the exponential convergence rate granted by IRLS guaranteed a more complete convergence to the minimizer after certain number of iterations.

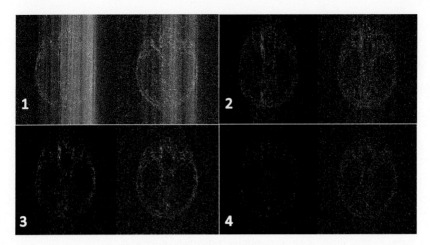

Fig. 4. Reconstructed absolute error comparison for the joint MC-MRI methods. 1) Bayesian CS [2]; 2) SPGL1 [12]; 3) FCSA-MT [8]; 4) the proposed. Best view in × 2 PDF.

Table 1. Additional reconstruction results on TSE data with different type of sample mask under 20% or 30% sample rate. The CPU Time and SNR comparison between Bayesian CS [2], SPGL1 [12], FCSA-MT [8], FISTA-JTV and the proposed algorithm.

Mask	Sample Ratio	Metrics	Bayesian CS	SPGL1	FCSA-MT	FISTA-JTV	The Proposed
Radial	30%	RMSE	0.3068	0.1648	0.1267	0.1255	**0.1248**
		SNR (dB)	11.2806	15.0429	17.0382	17.0770	**17.0962**
		Time (s)	1348.59	56.91	44.73	20.18	**6.62**
	20%	RMSE	0.3712	0.2118	0.1534	0.1541	**0.1521**
		SNR (dB)	9.1084	12.9261	15.5363	15.5223	**15.5427**
		Time (s)	3096.49	89.16	90.09	25.67	**6.72**
Slice	30%	RMSE	0.2913	0.2256	0.2042	0.2052	**0.2030**
		SNR (dB)	10.3723	12.1847	13.0681	13.0414	**13.1571**
		Time (s)	598.51	41.73	58.20	29.01	**5.52**
	20%	RMSE	0.3045	0.2899	0.2283	0.2343	**0.2191**
		SNR (dB)	9.8634	10.3546	12.0297	11.8192	**12.0380**
		Time (s)	2177.41	35.79	51.89	27.52	**9.25**

4   Conclusion

This paper proposes a novel algorithm to accelerate multi-contrast MRI. Our proposed algorithm inherits the exponentially fast convergence from the IRLS and the linear time complexity at each iteration due to the joint pseudo-diagonal preconditioning on CG. These properties make our algorithm more feasible to implement real-time MC-MRI due to the fast reconstruction speed and the reduced sample requirement.

References

1. Beck, A., Teboulle, M.: A fast iterative shrinkage-thresholding algorithm for linear inverse problems. SIAM Journal on Imaging Sciences 2(1), 183–202 (2009)
2. Bilgic, B., Goyal, V., Adalsteinsson, E.: Multi-contrast reconstruction with bayesian compressed sensing. Magnetic Resonance Medicine 66, 1601–1615 (2011)
3. Candès, E.J.: Compressive sampling. In: Proceedings oh the International Congress of Mathematicians, Madrid, August 22-30, invited lectures, pp. 1433–1452 (2006)
4. Chen, C., Huang, J., He, L., Li, H.: Preconditioning for accelerated iteratively reweighted least squares in structured sparsity reconstruction. In: 2014 IEEE Conference on Computer Vision and Pattern Recognition (CVPR), pp. 2713–2720. IEEE (2014)
5. Chen, C., Li, Y., Huang, J.: Calibrationless parallel MRI with joint total variation regularization. In: Mori, K., Sakuma, I., Sato, Y., Barillot, C., Navab, N. (eds.) MICCAI 2013, Part III. LNCS, vol. 8151, pp. 106–114. Springer, Heidelberg (2013)
6. Chen, C., Li, Y., Huang, J.: Forest sparsity for multi-channel compressive sensing. IEEE Transactions on Signal Processing 62(11), 2803–2813 (2014)
7. Huang, J., Zhang, T.: The benefit of group sparsity. Annals of Statistics 38, 1978–2004 (2010)
8. Huang, J., Chen, C., Axel, L.: Fast multi-contrast MRI reconstruction. Magnetic Resonance Imaging 32(10), 1344–1352 (2014)
9. Huang, J., Zhang, S., Metaxas, D.: Efficient MR image reconstruction for compressed MR imaging. In: Jiang, T., Navab, N., Pluim, J.P.W., Viergever, M.A. (eds.) MICCAI 2010, Part I. LNCS, vol. 6361, pp. 135–142. Springer, Heidelberg (2010)
10. Lustig, M., Donoho, D., Pauly, J.: Sparse MRI: The application of compressed sensing for rapid MR imaging. Magnetic Resonance in Medicine 58, 1182–1195 (2007)
11. Ma, S., Yin, W., Zhang, Y., Chakraborty, A.: An efficient algorithm for compressed MR imaging using total variation and wavelets. In: Proceedings of CVPR (2008)
12. Majumdar, A., Ward, R.: Joint reconstruction of multiecho MR images using correlated sparsity. Magnetic Resonance Imaging 29, 899–906 (2011)
13. Ramani, S., Fessler, J.A.: An accelerated iterative reweighted least squares algorithm for compressed sensing mri. In: 2010 IEEE International Symposium on Biomedical Imaging: From Nano to Macro, pp. 257–260. IEEE (2010)
14. Yang, J., Zhang, Y., Yin, W.: A fast alternating direction method for TVL1-L2 signal reconstruction from partial fourier data. IEEE Journal of Selected Topics in Signal Processing, Special Issue on Compressive Sensing 4(2) (2010)
15. Yuan, C., Kerwin, W.S., Yarnykh, V.L., Cai, J., Saam, T., Chu, B., Takaya, N., Ferguson, M.S., Underhill, H., Xu, D., et al.: MRI of atherosclerosis in clinical trials. NMR in Biomedicine 19(6), 636–654 (2006)

Author Index

Printed in the United States
By Bookmasters